Modern Virology

Modern Virology

Editor: Khloe Mackay

AMERICAN
MEDICAL PUBLISHERS
www.americanmedicalpublishers.com

AMERICAN
MEDICAL PUBLISHERS
www.americanmedicalpublishers.com

Cataloging-in-Publication Data

Modern virology / edited by Khloe Mackay.
p. cm.
Includes bibliographical references and index.
ISBN 979-8-88740-276-5
1. Virology. 2. Virus diseases. 3. Viruses. I. Mackay, Khloe.
QR360 .M63 2023
576.64--dc23

American Medical Publishers,
41 Flatbush Avenue,
1st Floor, New York,
NY 11217, USA

ISBN 979-8-88740-276-5 (Hardback)

Contents

Preface

Virology refers to the study of biological viruses. It is a branch of microbiology that aims to detect, structure, classify and study the evolution of viruses. It focuses on detecting the methods of infection and how host cells are exploited for replication of the viruses. Furthermore, it studies the interaction of viruses with the physiology and immunity of the host. Virology also focuses on identifying diseases caused by viruses, isolation techniques and how they can be utilized in the research for developing appropriate therapies. There are various approaches which can be utilized for detecting viruses, including identification of nucleic acids or antigens, and virus particles along with infectivity assays. Various diagnostic tests are utilized in the laboratories for identification of viruses, such as polymerase chain reaction, which is a nucleic acid amplification method. This book contains some path-breaking studies in the field of virology. It presents researches that have transformed this discipline and aided its advancement. This book includes contributions of experts and scientists, which will provide innovative insights into this field.

The researches compiled throughout the book are authentic and of high quality, combining several disciplines and from very diverse regions from around the world. Drawing on the contributions of many researchers from diverse countries, the book's objective is to provide the readers with the latest achievements in the area of research. This book will surely be a source of knowledge to all interested and researching the field.

In the end, I would like to express my deep sense of gratitude to all the authors for meeting the set deadlines in completing and submitting their research chapters. I would also like to thank the publisher for the support offered to us throughout the course of the book. Finally, I extend my sincere thanks to my family for being a constant source of inspiration and encouragement.

Editor

1

Treating Influenza Infection: From Now and into the Future

*Sophia Davidson**

Inflammation Division, The Walter and Eliza Hall Institute of Medical Research, Parkville, VIC, Australia

***Correspondence:**
Sophia Davidson
Davidson.s@wehi.edu.au

Influenza viruses (IVs) are a continual threat to global health. The high mutation rate of the IV genome makes this virus incredibly successful, genetic drift allows for annual epidemics which result in thousands of deaths and millions of hospitalizations. Moreover, the emergence of new strains through genetic shift (e.g., swine-origin influenza A) can cause devastating global outbreaks of infection. Neuraminidase inhibitors (NAIs) are currently used to treat IV infection and act directly on viral proteins to halt IV spread. However, effectivity is limited late in infection and drug resistance can develop. New therapies which target highly conserved features of IV such as antibodies to the stem region of hemagglutinin or the IV RNA polymerase inhibitor: Favipiravir are currently in clinical trials. Compared to NAIs, these treatments have a higher tolerance for resistance and a longer therapeutic window and therefore, may prove more effective. However, clinical and experimental evidence has demonstrated that it is not just viral spread, but also the host inflammatory response and damage to the lung epithelium which dictate the outcome of IV infection. Therapeutic regimens for IV infection should therefore also regulate the host inflammatory response and protect epithelial cells from unnecessary cell death. Anti-inflammatory drugs such as etanercept, statins or cyclooxygenase enzyme 2 inhibitors may temper IV induced inflammation, demonstrating the possibility of repurposing these drugs as single or adjunct therapies for IV infection. IV binds to sialic acid receptors on the host cell surface to initiate infection and productive IV replication is primarily restricted to airway epithelial cells. Accordingly, targeting therapies to the epithelium will directly inhibit IV spread while minimizing off target consequences, such as over activation of immune cells. The neuraminidase mimic Fludase cleaves sialic acid receptors from the epithelium to inhibit IV entry to cells. While type III interferons activate an antiviral gene program in epithelial cells with minimal perturbation to the IV specific immune response. This review discusses the above-mentioned candidate anti-IV therapeutics and others at the preclinical and clinical trial stage.

Keywords: influenza, therapeutics, treatment, antiviral, immunomodulation

INTRODUCTION

Influenza viruses (IVs) are a continual and re-emerging threat to human health. Annual epidemics infect approximately 1 billion individuals, leading to three to five million cases of severe illness and up to half a million fatalities worldwide (1, 2). Influenza A Virus (IAV), Influenza B Virus (IBV) and Influenza C Virus (ICV) are all members of the *Orthomyxoviridae* family. IV genomes are segmented, which allows for reassortment within, but not between, family groups. Although IBV and ICV do cause disease in humans (IBV being responsible for approximately 25% of seasonal influenza infections) IAV strains are responsible for the majority of human infections and are most likely to cause severe disease. IAV are further classified into subtypes based on the antigenic properties of two viral surface glycoproteins, hemagglutinin (HA) and neuraminidase (NA), to date 18 HA (H1–H18) and 10 NA (N1–N10) antigenic subtypes been identified (3, 4). Unlike IBV and ICV, IAV infects a broad range of species including humans, pigs, horses, wild mammals, and birds (5). Due to different preferences for sialic acid moieties direct zoonosis of IAV between birds and humans is rare, however when it does occur, the mortality rate is staggeringly high, approximately 60% for H5N1 and 30% for H7N9 (6). In worrying contrast, transmission of IAV strains from swine to humans is common (7).

In healthy humans, IV infection induces a robust immune memory response, in spite of this the average adult will experience two IV infections per decade throughout their lifetime (8). IVs are able to evade IV-specific host immunity through two mechanisms: antigenic drift and shift. Antigenic drift occurs as IV genomes do not have RNA proofreading enzymes and consequently, point mutations accumulate in the genome through successive replication. This leads to alterations in the appearance of viral antigens and eventual emergence of new IV strains which are unrecognizable to pre-existing host immunity (9). Significantly more dramatic and, within the *Orthomyxoviridae* family, believed to be specific to IAV is antigenic shift. Infection of a single host cell with two or more strains of IAV results in the reassortment of genomic segments. IAV genome segments are packaged into viral particles by the host cell without respect to the original strains, leading to progeny virions which possess new HA and/or HA and NA proteins, such as those of avian or swine origin, but may retain the ability to effectively infect humans. Antigenic shift gives IAV pandemic potential, indeed it is thought that the majority of pandemics of the Twenty-First century have been caused by reassortment events that resulted in avian or swine IAV being able to stably infect humans (10).

The severity of IV induced disease is a function of the interplay between viral virulence and the host immune response. In a mild infection the inflammatory response is controlled and cleared rapidly. However, in highly pathogenic IV infections the host immune response can become excessive. Termed the cytokine storm, severe IV infection in humans is characterized by aberrant cytokine and chemokine responses that associate with infiltration of inflammatory cells, particularly monocytes and neutrophils. This inflammation coincides with destruction of the epithelial layer and consequently, respiratory dysfunction or acute respiratory distress syndrome (ARDS) (11). *Ex vivo* analysis of clinical samples, experimental infection models and clinical trials all indicate that the cytokine storm positively correlates with tissue injury and severe IV induced disease (12–17).

To add to the multifarious nature of IV infection, it can be complicated by secondary bacterial infection. Bacteria which normally colonize the upper respiratory tract such as *Streptococcus pneumoniae* or *Staphylococcus aureus* can cause pneumonia and septicaemia in IV infection (18). It is thought that opportunistic bacteria take advantage of changes in the pulmonary environment wrought by IV infection. Many mechanisms have been proposed to explain this phenomenon, for example IV infection induces a robust type I interferon (IFNαβ) response, which blocks the recruitment of neutrophils, a cell type particularly important for clearance of bacterial infection (19). Furthermore, monocytes and monocyte-derived cells recruited to the lung during IV infection induce the apoptosis of airway epithelial cells via TNF-related apoptosis-inducing ligand (TRAIL), this facilitates bacterial colonization and systemic dissemination by compromising epithelial layer ntegrity (20).

Undeniably, there is a real and present need for effective broad spectrum anti-IV therapies. Given the high mutagenicity of the IV genome vaccine development is fraught with difficulty, current IV vaccines are strain specific and therefore a new immunization is required for each new season (21). Moreover, the rapid emergence of the 2009 H1N1 pandemic strain demonstrated how under prepared we are for a serious IAV pandemic. This review reports current treatments for IV and discusses new therapies at clinical or pre-clinical stage. As IAV has pandemic potential and is most likely to cause severe disease in humans many of the treatments discussed are primarily directed at this virus, however they may be effective against other *Orthomyxoviridae* family members. For clarity, therapies are categorized based on point of action in IV infection, specifically, (1) IV: proteins and genomes, (2) Host immune response: cytokines/chemokines and other inflammatory modulators, and (3) Target cells for IV replication: respiratory epithelium.

DIRECT TARGETING OF IV

Current Treatment

IV surface proteins HA and NA are responsible for virion attachment to and detachment from sialic acid moieties on the host cell surface. HA attaches to cell surface sialic acid receptors to initiate viral entry and promote fusion of viral and cellular membranes, while NA acts as a sialidase, cleaving the α-ketosidic bond linking a terminal neuraminic acid residue to the adjacent oligosaccharide moiety. This enzymatic action of NA releases IV particles from infected cells and thereby allows the spread of IV to naive cells (22). NA sialidase activity also facilitates the movement of IV through the sialic acid-rich mucous of the human respiratory tract (23). NA is essential for productive IV infection and the catalytic sites of NA are conserved across IAV and IBV strains, making this glycoprotein an attractive target for antiviral therapy (24). Accordingly, in the 1990s Neuraminidase inhibitors (NAIs) were developed. NAIs are sialic acid analogs which competitively bind to the active site on NA molecules to inhibit the release of IV progeny from the cell surface (25).

NAIs are the only antivirals currently recommended to treat IV infection, oseltamivir and zanamivir are used worldwide, laninamivir is approved in Japan and peramivir is approved in China, Japan, South Korea, and the United States (26). Oseltamivir (**Table 1**) is most commonly used and has been shown *in vitro* to have activity against human and avian IAV subtypes and IBV strains (27). NAIs have been employed

TABLE 1 | Summary of key treatments discussed.

	Therapy	Stage	Activity	Specificity	Effect on IV replication	Effect on host inflammatory response	Effect on epithelial Cells	Viability
IV	MHAA4549A	Phase II	Antibody to HA stem region, induces cellular cytotoxicity of infected cells	IAV only	Inhibitory	Inhibitory	Not reported	Good
	MEDI8852	Phase II	Antibody to HA stem region, induces cellular cytotoxicity of infected cells	IAV only	Inhibitory	Not reported	Not reported	Good
	VIS-410	Phase II	Antibody to HA stem region, induces cellular cytotoxicity of infected cells	Select IAV strains	Inhibitory	Not reported	Not reported	Good
	JNJ63623872	Phase II	Inhibits IV replication by binding PB2 and preventing 7-methyl GTP docking	IAV only	Inhibitory	Not reported	Not reported	Moderate
	Favipiravir	Approved/phase II	Inhibits generation of viable IV particles by driving mutations in IV genome	None	Inhibitory	Not reported	Not reported	Good
	JJ3297	Preclinical	Inhibits NS1 activity	None	Inhibitory	Stimulatory	Not reported	Unknown
Immune response	Etanercept	Clinically approved for other	TNF receptor decoy, blocks TNFα signaling	None	Inhibitory	Inhibitory	Not reported	Unknown
	IFNαβ	Clinically approved for other	Induces expression of antiviral and inflammatory genes in epithelial cells and immune cells	None	Inhibitory	Stimulatory	Increased cell death	Low
	AAL-R	Preclinical	Inhibits inflammatory cytokine and chemokine secretion and immune cell recruitment by agonism of S1PRs: 1, 3, 4, and 5	None	No effect	Inhibitory	Decreased cell death	Low
	CYM-5442	Preclinical	Inhibits inflammatory cytokine and chemokine secretion and immune cell recruitment by agonism of S1PR1	None	No effect	Inhibitory	Decreased cell death	Moderate
	RP-002	Preclinical	Inhibits inflammatory cytokine and chemokine secretion and immune cell recruitment by agonism of S1PR1	None	No effect	Inhibitory	Decreased cell death	Moderate
	Celecoxib	Clinically approved for other (Phase III for IV)	COX-2 inhibitor, may blunt immunopathology through induction of PGE_2	None	No effect	Inhibitory/no effect	Not reported	Moderate
	Statins	Clinically approved for other	Competitive inhibitors for HMG-CoA reductase, blunts inflammation and viral replication in some settings	None	Inhibitory	Inhibitory	Not reported	Moderate
	Pioglitazone	Clinically approved for other	PPARγ agonist, decreases recruitment of tipDCs	None	No effect	Inhibitory	Not reported	Moderate
Epithelial cells	Fludase	Phase II	Removes IV entry point into epithelial cells by cleaving sialic acid receptors	None	Inhibitory	Not reported	Not reported	Good
	IFNλ	Phase II (other)	Induces expression of antiviral and inflammatory genes primarily in epithelial cells	None	Inhibitory	No effect	Decreased cell death	Good
	Anti-TRAIL	Preclinical	mAb to TRAIL, blocks interaction between TRAIL and its cognate receptors to inhibit extrinsic apoptosis	None	No effect	No effect	Decreased cell death	Unknown
	A-1155463	Preclinical	Bcl-2 family inhibitor, drives apoptosis of IV infected cells	None	Inhibitory	Not reported	Not reported	Unknown

Potential therapeutics for human IV infection are summarized. Treatments are separated based on which aspect of IV infection is targeted. Viability of each therapeutic is rated based on data discussed in this review.

successfully for over decade, however between 2007 and 2009 resistance to oseltamivir in seasonal IAV strains surged from less than 1% to over 90% (28–31). IV strains resistant to NAIs typically contain mutations in the NA which reduce the inhibitor binding ability by altering the shape of the NA catalytic site. Although several resistance conferring mutations have been reported, the most common for IAV is H274Y. In order for oseltamivir to bind correctly, NA must undergo rearrangements to form a binding pocket. Key to these rearrangements, is the amino acid E276 rotating and binding to R224 (32, 33). *In vitro* modeling and X ray crystallography revealed that H274Y inhibits this rotation of the E276 residue thereby preventing pocket formation (32, 34). Such a dramatic uptake of the H274Y mutation at the population level is unlikely to be driven by individual patient use, instead H274Y-mutant IAV strains may have acquired advantageous epidemiologic fitness, allowing for rapid global transmission (35, 36). Fortunately, the 2009 H1N1 IAV pandemic strain did not carry this mutation when it emerged, and as this is the current dominant seasonal strain, the frequency of NAI resistance in circulating IAV strains is now low. However, localized clusters of oseltamivir-resistant IAV have been detected (37), and mutations which confer decreased sensitivity to oseltamivir in IBV strains have also been reported (38). The rapid emergence of oseltamivir-resistance observed between 2008 and 2009 demonstrates that NAI-resistance can develop at no cost to viral fitness and these mutations can easily spread throughout the population.

Aside from concerns regarding resistance, the effectiveness of NAIs is limited when delivered over 48 h after symptom onset. Indeed, multiple systematic reviews have concluded that oseltamivir does not reduce IV related hospitalizations, and that there is little evidence of reduction in complications of IV infection (39–42). Although, another meta-analysis did demonstrate that oseltamivir was effective for prevention of influenza at the individual and household levels (43). Use of oseltamivir and other NAIs has demonstrated the need for development of anti-IV drugs that improve treatment effectiveness, particularly when delivered late in the progression of disease, and have a low propensity for driving the emergence of viral resistance.

Potential IV Targeted Therapies

The IV surface protein HA binds to host cell receptors to initiate infection. This glycoprotein consists of a globular head and a stem region that are folded within six disulfide bonds, plus several N-glycans that produce a homotrimeric complex structure (44). The majority of IV neutralizing antibodies elicited by vaccination or infection bind to the globular head of HA and recognize homologous strains within a given subtype (45). Antibodies to the HA head neutralize virus infectivity by blocking sialic acid receptor binding either directly, by interacting with the receptor binding site at the tip of the molecule, or indirectly, by projecting over the binding site and rendering it inaccessible (46–48). However, N-linked glycosylation sites on the HA globular head are highly variable across different IV subtypes and some IAV strains can further avoid host antibody responses by acquiring additional N-glycan modifications in the HA head region (49, 50). In contrast, N-linked glycosylation sites in the HA stem region are relatively well conserved among IAV strains. Antibodies to IAV HA stem motifs occur naturally and have activity against a broad range of IAV subtypes, however they are immune-subdominant and are only induced in very low titres during natural infection. Mechanistically, anti-stem antibodies control IAV by inducing antibody-dependent cellular cytotoxicity of infected cells (51–53). Given their potential, several monoclonal antibodies targeting the highly conserved stem region of the HA molecule are being evaluated in clinical trials. In particular, MHAA4549A and MEDI8852 have demonstrated high-affinity binding to 16 IAV HA subtypes and VIS410 has confirmed binding to 7 (54–56) (**Table 1**). MHAA4549A, MEDI8852, and VIS410 were all shown to be effective in protecting IV infected hosts by inhibiting pulmonary viral load in preclinical animal models (55–59). VIS410 was found to be safe and well tolerated in a phase 1 study and is now under phase 2 investigation (60). MHAA4549A and MEDI8852 were both reported to control viral shedding in humans in phase 2a clinical trials (58, 59). Furthermore, MHAA4549A was reported to lower patient influenza symptom scores and significantly, levels of inflammatory cytokines in serum and nasopharyngeal samples compared to placebo controls (58).

In a clinical trial setting MHAA4549A and MEDI8852 both performed comparably to oseltamivir, yet neither antibody improved oseltamivir effectiveness when used in combination (clinical trials: NCT02293863 and NCT02603952), indicating that these antibodies do not offer better protection than NAIs. However, compared to oseltamivir, which must be given twice daily (61), HA stem antibodies have superior pharmacokinetics, the half-life of MHAA4549A is approximately 3 weeks in humans (58) and MHAA4549A, MEDI8852 and VIS410 all have demonstrated protection against IV induced disease with only one to two doses (55–59). Furthermore, both MHAA4549A and MEDI8852 have been shown to confer protection beyond 48 h post infection, a point at which oseltamivir has lost effectivity in small animal models (55, 56, 58, 59). Excellent pharmacokinetics and a longer therapeutic window make HA stem antibodies strong candidates for treatment of IV infection.

The IV RNA-dependent RNA-polymerase (RdRp), is responsible for transcription and replication of IV's genome and is highly conserved across different strains. It is a heterotrimeric protein containing three virally encoded subunits: PB1, PB2, and PA. PB1 has polymerase activity, PB2 is involved in cap-binding of host cell pre-mRNAs and PA cleaves capped host pre-mRNAs and initiates transcription (62). Cap-snatching by PB2 essential for RNA transcription, PB2 first binds to the 5′-methyl cap of host pre-mRNA which is then cleaved by PA's endonuclease site to produce a capped primer for IV transcription initiation (62). JNJ63623872 (formerly known as VX-787) (**Table 1**) is a compound that binds to key residues in the PB2 cap binding domain preventing the docking of the natural ligand: 7-methyl GTP. Preclinical *in vivo* and *in vitro* studies have demonstrated that JNJ63623872 has varying degrees of activity against a range of IAV strains, however due to the differences in IAV and IBV PB2 protein JNJ63623872 is ineffective against IBV (63). When directly compared in a mouse model of IAV infection JNJ63623872 was more effective than oseltamivir in controlling IV induced disease severity (64). A placebo-controlled phase IIa study showed JNJ63623872 to be well tolerated and resulted in a 94% reduction in viral shedding and quicker resolution of flu-like symptoms compared to controls (65). However, the dosing regime of JNJ63623872 is similar to oseltamivir and variant strains with reduced susceptibility to JNJ63623872 have been isolated from *in vitro* culture (66), indicating that this therapy in its current form may not supersede NAIs. JNJ63623872 is now in phase II trials alone (NCT02342249) and in combination with oseltamivir (NCT02532283). Interestingly, a phase I trial has been initiated to evaluate the safety and pharmacokinetic interaction of JNJ63623872 with AL-974, a PA inhibitor that is in early-stage development (NCT02888327).

Favipiravir (also known as T705) (**Table 1**) is a ribonucleotide analog (6-fluoro-3-hydroxy-2-pyrazinecarboxamide) that inhibits viral RdRps. However, the mechanism by which this inhibition occurs is not understood, indeed, even the viral proteins targeted by Favipiravir are not yet defined. *In vitro* studies have revealed that serial passage with increasing concentrations of Favipiravir drives guanosine to adenine nucleotide mutations in IV, essentially resulting in the production of non-viable IV particles (67). Several studies in mice have demonstrated Favipiravir administration up to 72 h post infection with seasonal IAV strains such as H1N1 and avian strains: H5N1 and H7N9 result in a dose-dependent reduction lung viral titres and host mortality (68–71). Favipiravir has been shown to be to have potent inhibitory activity against several RNA viruses *in vitro* and appears especially effective for IVs (72). This acute susceptibility of IV may be due to IV's lack of RNA proofreading enzymes. Furthermore, Favipiravir appears to have an exceptionally high barrier for drug resistance, currently only one mutation (V43I in PB1; obtained in virus-infected cell cultures under selection) was found to confer a slight increase in resistance to Favipiravir (73). Favipiravir is highly promising as a broad acting anti-IV therapy and as such, has been approved for select use in Japan and has completed phase III trials in the USA and Europe.

Along with proteins for replication, assembly and infection, IV genomes also code for a protein which can inhibit the host immune response: non-structural protein (NS1). NS1 is a highly conserved multifunctional protein which inhibits host antiviral responses, particularly, induction of types I and III IFNs (IFNαβ and IFNλ). NS1 antagonism of host immunity varies between IV strains; NS1 can prevent IV-mediated activation of key inflammatory transcription factors such as IFN Regulatory Factor 3 (IRF-3) and nuclear factor kappa-light-chain-enhancer of activated B cells (NF-κB) (74–76). NS1 limits host recognition of IV through the pattern recognition receptor (PRR): retinoic acid inducible gene-I (RIG-I) by sequestering dsRNA (which is a RIG-I agonist) and inhibiting RIG-I ubiquitination and therefore activation (77–83). NS1 is key to viral fitness, strains deficient for NS1 induce markedly higher secretion of antiviral IFNs from cells *in vitro* and are non-pathogenic in mouse models of IV infection (84–87). Thus, the NS1 protein is a suitable target for anti-IV therapeutics. JJ3297 (**Table 1**) is a second-generation chemical inhibitor of NS1 function that has been shown in an *in vitro* assay to restore levels of IFNαβ-mRNA to those seen when cells were infected with a NS1 deleted mutant (88). While the exact mechanism of action is not understood, JJ3297 mediated inhibition of NS1 absolutely requires the function of cellular RNase L, indicating that an intact interferon system is essential for function of the compound (88). Further development of JJ3297 has resulted in the generation of another compound: A22 and NS1 inhibitors are now being investigated in *in vivo* models of infection (89). Additionally, SP600125, a C-Jun-N-terminal kinase inhibitor reduces the replication of IV *in vitro* and *in vivo* by indirect inhibition of NS1-mediated functions in the early stages of infection (90) and small molecules such as polyphenol and quinoxaline derivatives have also been proposed to inhibit NS1 (91). More study is required to determine if NS1 inhibitors are suitable for clinical use. However, given the direct correlation between host inflammatory response and IV-induced disease severity, use of NS1 inhibitors, particularly late in infection, should be cautiously evaluated.

STEPPING INTO THE STORM

Limiting IV replication curbs disease severity not only by decreasing number of virions able to propagate the infection, but also by limiting immune stimulation. All cell types will secrete cytokines and chemokines to varying degrees upon recognition of IV pathogen associated molecular patterns. Cytokines and chemokines drive the recruitment and activation of both innate and adaptive immune cells which, while vital for resolution of infection, can also exacerbate disease through tissue damage. Therefore, at later time points in infection when viral load is already limited, it is more important to control the inflammatory response. Use of interventions which target the host response is an excellent strategy to combat severe IV infection. Host directed therapeutics are unlikely to drive the emergence of resistant strains and their effectivity is not strain specific. However, which immune drives are the most appropriate to target remains an open question. Severe IV infection induces many cytokines; IFNαβ, TNFα, IFNγ, C-X-C motif chemokine (CXCL) 10 (CXCL10), CXCL9, C-C motif ligand (CCL) 2 (CCL2), CCL4, CCL5 and interleukin (IL)−6 (IL-6), IL-2, IL-8, and IL-10 have all be observed to be upregulated during severe IV infection in humans (14, 15, 17, 92, 93). Yet studies in animal models demonstrate that there is yet to be a setting where complete absence of a specific cytokine or its cognate receptor entirely ablates IV induced cytokine storm. As TNFα and IFNαβ correlate well with disease severity in both clinical and experimental IV infection and are potent immunomodulators, known to be upstream of proinflammatory cytokine and chemokine secretion from many cell types, multiple studies have proposed treatment with these cytokines to promote viral clearance, or blockade of these cytokines to minimize host mediated tissue damage (12, 15, 94–101).

TNFα drives the activation of multiple intracellular signaling pathways through the activation of NF-κB (102). In response to IV infection TNFα promotes the secretion of the antiviral cytokine families: type I, II, and III IFNs through upregulating RIG-I and toll-like receptor 3, Myeloid differentiation primary response 88 (MyD88), TIR-domain-containing adapter-inducing interferon-β (TRIF), and IRF7 genes. TNFα drives IV clearance via induction of apoptosis, stimulation of reactive oxygen species and activation of Nicotinamide Adenine Dinucleotide Phosphate Hydrogen (NADPH) oxidases in neutrophils and macrophages, such as NADPH oxidase 2 (NOX2), resulting in the generation of superoxide (103). Yet, TNFα is dispensable for control and clearance of IV, TNF deficient mice exhibited comparable mortality to controls upon H5N1 infection (104). Anti-TNF therapy in a murine H1N1 infection model reduced pulmonary recruitment of inflammatory cells, cytokine production by T cells and the severity of IV induced disease without preventing virus clearance (96). Similarly, treatment of mice lethally infected with H1N1 IAV with etanercept (**Table 1**), a soluble TNF receptor decoy, significantly reduced inflammatory cell infiltration, production of inflammatory cytokines and downregulated NFκB signaling, yet enhanced host control of virus replication, resulting in a 30% increase in host survival (105).

Interestingly, etanercept is used to treat a range of inflammatory conditions such as Rheumatoid Arthritis (RA). While patients with RA do exhibit an increased risk of IAV infection, treatment with etanercept does not contribute to this. In a retrospective cohort study Blumentals et al. found that etanercept or use of other biologics did not significantly affect the rate of influenza infection or its complications in RA patients (106). Yet whether or not etanercept lowered IV induced disease burden in treated patients compared to controls could not be assessed, as this data was not consistently recorded. Conversely, there is also evidence that TNFα is required for controlling the extent of IV induced immunopathology and tissue injury. In a mouse model of H1N1 infection Damjanovic et al. found that TNF-/- mice exhibited prolonged expression of inflammatory chemokines such as CCL2 leading to an exaggerated immune response and consequent damage to pulmonary epithelial cells (107). Further investigation by DeBerge et al. revealed that it is soluble, and not membrane bound, TNFα that is required to limit the IV induced immune response and tissue damage (108). Therefore, it is unclear if TNFα blockade is a suitable treatment for severe IV induced disease, however given the multiple components of the TNFα signaling system, TNFR1 vs. TNFR2 and the differing activities of membrane bound and soluble TNFα, there is the possibility to specifically inhibit certain aspects of TNFα signaling while not interfering with others.

IFNαβ are the canonical antiviral cytokine family in fact, they were discovered in the context of IV. IFNαβ induces the expression of hundreds of genes, such as MX dynamin like GTPase 1 (Mx1) and interferon induced transmembrane protein 3 (IFITM3) which have direct anti-IV activity. As such, IFNαβ has been periodically suggested as a therapy for IV (94, 97, 100, 101). Prophylactic or very early on treatment with IFNαβ in rhesus macaques, ferrets, guinea pigs and mice experimentally infected with IAV controls virus replication and spread thereby protecting against severe IV induced disease (101, 109–114). However, it appears the therapeutic window is short, later treatment with IFNαβ during infection still controls viral load but exacerbates disease by driving the cytokine storm and TRAIL mediated airway epithelial cell death (101, 109, 115). While there have been no studies directly assessing the effectiveness of IFNαβ blockade during IV infection in humans, IFNαβR deficient mice exhibit a range of susceptibility to IV induced disease depending on the virulence of the infecting IV strain and the genetic background of the mice (86, 115–118), demonstrating that the activity of IFNαβ on host immune response to IV is too complex to extract the immunopathogenic from the protective effects on the host.

Due to the pleiotropic actions of TNFα and IFNαβ direct targeting of these cytokines may not be the most suitable approach. Instead, a general dampening on the immune response may be more effective. Recently, chemical agonism of the sphingosine-1-phosphate (S1P) receptor (S1PR) pathway has been shown to blunt IV induced inflammation. The sphingosine analog: AAL-R (**Table 1**) agonizes S1P receptors 1, 3, 4, and 5. Treatment of IV infected mice with AAL-R during infection resulted in reduced release of proinflammatory cytokines and chemokines including IFNαβ and inhibited inflammatory cell infiltration and thereby decreased damage to pulmonary tissue. AAL-R treatment did not affect antibody responses and pulmonary viral load was comparable between treatment and control groups, however AAL-R did suppress dendritic cell maturation and inhibited IV specific T-cell responses (119, 120). Although the IV T cell response is dispensable for clearance of IV, it provides the host with herterosubtypic immunity, thus AAL-R is too immunosuppressive to be applied as an anti-IV therapy. But based on the promise of AAL-R, two agonists specific S1P1R: CYM-5442 and RP-002 (**Table 1**) were tested. Like AAL-R, CYM-5442 and RP-002 significantly reduced cytokine and chemokine responses associated with IV induced lung injury without effecting viral load. Yet, unlike AAL-R, neither CYM-5442 and RP-002 effected dendritic cell and T-cell responses (120, 121). Teijaro et al. proposed that agonism of S1PRs on endothelial cells was responsible for the blunted proinflammatory cytokine levels in the lung (121, 122). However, in follow up studies this group also found that S1P1R agonists act directly on plasmacytoid dendritic cells to block their secretion of IFNα (123, 124). Furthermore, these results defined signaling downstream of MyD88 in multiple cell types to be a key amplifier of IAV induced cytokine storm which could be inhibited by S1P1R agonism. Further characterization of S1PR agonists as IV-therapeutics is ongoing in mouse and ferret models (123).

Cyclooxygenase enzymes (COX) catalyze the conversion of arachidonic acid to prostaglandins, which can modulate the inflammatory response (125). Interestingly, there are two isoforms of COX: the constitutively expressed COX-1 and the inducible COX-2 which have divergent roles in influenza infection. Carey et al. demonstrated that in H3N2 IAV infection COX-2 deficient mice, compared to wild type controls, had lower levels of proinflammatory cytokines (IL-6, TNFα, IL-1β, and IFNγ) and inflammatory cells recruited to the lung during infection, and this correlated to a moderate increase in survival. While in contrast, COX-1 deficient mice in the same study exhibited a higher pulmonary inflammatory burden compared to wild type controls. The cost of this blunted inflammation in COX-2-/- mice was a higher viral burden early in infection, however by day six all three mouse strains had comparably low pulmonary titres of H3N2 IAV (126). In another study, COX-2 deficiency correlated to higher levels of the prostaglandin: PGE_2 which has an inhibitory effect on proinflammatory cytokine expression, the adaptive immune response and macrophage apoptosis in mice infected with H1N1 (127). Furthermore, COX-2 expression is elevated in autopsy tissue samples from patients infected by H5N1 IAV and induction of proinflammatory cytokines such as IL-6, TNFα, IFNα, and IFNβ by H5N1 in monocyte derived macrophages could be blocked by a COX-2 inhibitor (nimesulide) (128). Thus, there is strong evidence that COX-2 is an upstream driver of IV induced inflammation, however, the specific mechanism of action remains to be determined. In a follow up study, Carey et al. found that treatment of wild type mice with COX-1 inhibitor (SC-560) or a COX-2 inhibitor [celecoxib (**Table 1**)] prior to and during IAV infection resulted in the same pattern of susceptibility

(COX-2 inhibition being protective and COX-1 inhibition being detrimental) yet, neither treatment drastically altered pulmonary cytokine profiles, viral load or inflammatory cell recruitment (129). Furthermore, another *in vivo* study found that celecoxib alone did not protect H5N1 infected mice from mortality, although the authors did observe a protective effect of celecoxib administration when used in combination with zanamvir and mesalazine (a PPARγ agonist, see below) in mice challenged with H5N1 IAV. Significantly, combination treatment was administered post IAV infection. This protection did correlate to a moderate decrease in proinflammatory cytokine concentrations and a modest elevation PGE_2 in the lung late in infection however, it also correlated to decreased viral loads at this time point which may explain the change in pulmonary cytokine profile (130).

Currently, a phase III clinical trial is running to assess efficacy and safety of celecoxib used in combination with oseltamivir in patients with severe IAV infection (NCT02108366). While this is an exciting development for the use of immunomodulating drugs in the treatment of IV, in high concentrations celecoxib can also inhibit COX-1 (131), which may prove problematic. As demonstrated by Carey et al. COX-1 plays an anti-inflammatory and protective role in IV infection (126). Moreover, treatment with nonselective COX inhibitors such as aspirin and diclofenac confer an increased risk of mortality in animal models of infection and it has been proposed that an increase in aspirin use during the 1918 pandemic contributed to the October death spike (132, 133).

In 2006 Fedson proposed the use of statins to modulate IV induced cytokine storm (134). Statins (**Table 1**) block cholesterol synthesis by competitively inhibiting the enzyme 3-hydroxy-3-methylglutaryl coenzyme A (HMG-CoA) reductase (135). Commonly employed to reduce the risk of cardiovascular disease by lowering cholesterol levels, statins are inexpensive and widely available, therefore making them an attractive candidate for IV treatment. Statins can inhibit IV induced disease through multiple mechanisms, *in vitro* studies have shown that statins can interfere with viral replication (136, 137), block the induction of proinflammatory cytokines and chemokine such as IL-6 and TNFα and inhibit the activation of key signaling molecules including Signal transducer and activator of transcription 3 (STAT3) (138, 139). Animal studies have shown promise, Haidari et al. demonstrated statin treatment lowered pulmonary viral load and host mortality in murine H3N2 and H1N1 IAV infection models and An et al. demonstrated combination treatment with a statin, a NAI and a fibrate, protected mice from H5N1 mediated mortality (136, 140). In an intriguing study Liu et al. combined statins with another readily available drug: caffeine, and found that combination therapy lowered pulmonary viral load and ameliorated lung damage in H5N1-, H3N2-, and H1N1-infected mice (141). However, other studies conducted in mice have reported little to no effect of statins on IV clearance or cytokine profile (142, 143).

As statins are so widely used in the human population, there is a substantial amount of data on their use in the context of IV infection. Five retrospective studies conducted in four separate countries (Netherlands, United Kingdom, USA and Mexico) reported that to varying degrees, statin treatment associated with reduced IV-related pneumonia and a lower IV induced mortality rate (144–147). In contrast, Fleming et al. and Kwong et al. conducted retrospective studies over a 6 and 10 year periods (respectively) and found no association between statin treatment and decrease IV induced disease burden (148, 149). There are many caveats to these studies, including what other treatments patients were on during the study period and a lack of defined IV specific outcomes. Furthermore, the use of different statins and strains of infecting IVs likely contributes to the varied results. Overall, there is evidence that statins can ameliorate severe IV induced disease, and the availability of this class of drugs certainly makes it an attractive therapeutic option. Further study is required to delineate the specific actions of statins which block viral replication and inhibit over activation of the innate immune response, thereby allowing us to capitalize on these properties. Excitingly, a phase II trial has begun to test the effectivity of atorvastatin in minimizing IV induced disease severity in patients infected with seasonal IV (NCT02056340).

Peroxisome proliferator-activated receptors (PPARs) are nuclear receptors and ligand-activated transcription factors that control a number of target genes upon assembly of a transcriptional complex. PPARs regulate energy balance, including glucose homeostasis, fatty acid oxidation, and lipid metabolism (150). PPAR agonists are commonly used to treat patients with cardiovascular diseases and diabetes mellitus. Drugs which specifically antagonize PPARγ appear to be the most promising as therapeutics for IV. Treatment of mice, prior to and during IAV infection, with PPARγ agonist: pioglitazone (**Table 1**) was shown to temper recruitment of $Ly6C^{high}$ myeloid cells termed: TNF-α/inducible nitric oxide synthase (iNOS)-producing DCs (tipDCs), although likely these are comparable to what other studies have reported as inflammatory monocytes or exudate macrophages (20, 115, 151). Pioglitazone lowered pulmonary concentrations of chemokines known to attract tipDCs to the lung (CCL2 and CCL7) and this associated with a decrease in IAV induced morbidity and mortality. Importantly, pioglitazone treatment did not alter the rate of IAV clearance from the lung, as was observed when tipDC recruitment was entirely ablated through the genetic deletion of CCR2 (152). In a follow up study, this group also demonstrated that rosiglitazone (another PPARγ agonist) mediated better protection than pioglitazone (or vehicle control) in mice infected with H1N1 IAV (153). Finally, treatment of mice with 15-deoxy-Δ12,14-prostaglandin J2 (15d-PGJ2), 1 day post infection blunted IV induced proinflammatory cytokine secretion in the lung and increased host survival in a PPARγ dependent manner (154). As with statins, PPARγ agonists could be easily employed an adjunct therapy for IV induced disease, however human studies must be performed. Indeed, there is a somewhat surprisingly little amount of data about immunomodulating agents and IV infections. Although imperfect, retrospective studies on patients treated with immunomodulating agents such as IFNαβ for multiple sclerosis or hepatitis C, or any number of anti-inflammatory agents for heart disease may provide informative preliminary data in terms of effectivity and safety.

TARGETING THE EPITHELIUM

In general, productive IV replication is restricted to airway epithelial cells, as these cells exclusively express proteases required for HA maturation (155). Damage to the respiratory tract in the form of virally induced necrosis, immune mediated apoptosis or other forms of cell death leads to ARDS. Finding a way to directly target the cells which support IV replication is highly desirable in anti IV treatment design. As such, many of the treatments discussed in this review are delivered via inhalation. However, by focusing on features relatively specific to the epithelial cells therapies can directly protect the epithelium during infection or promote healing post viral clearance. For example, Fludase (**Table 1**), is a recombinant fusion protein consisting of a sialidase catalytic domain derived from *Actinomyces viscosus* fused with the epithelial anchoring domain of human amphiregulin. Fludase is effectively a neuraminidase mimic, it tethers to, and cleaves both α(2,6)-linked and α(2,3)-linked sialic acid receptors, thereby removing IV's entry point into epithelial cells (156). This drug is administered as an inhaled dry powder with microparticles of 5–10 μm in size, enabling the drug to access the upper and central, but not the lower respiratory tract. *In vitro* studies on human airway epithelial cells have shown that Fludase removed approximately 90% of sialic acid receptors within 15 min of treatment and desialylation lasted at least 2 days (157). Serial passage of IAV and IBV under increasing selective pressure of Fludase selected for several mutations in HA (G137R, S136T, S186I) and NA (W438L, L38P) which resulted in IVs with increased receptor binding, coupled with significantly reduced NA on the cell surface. These mutations lead to an attenuated phenotype *in vitro* and no change in virulence in a mouse model of IV infection. Furthermore, the resistance phenotype was unstable and was reversed after withdrawal of Fludase (158).

As it targets the common entry point of IVs Fludase has been shown to be effective at inhibiting a broad range of IAV and IBV strains *in vitro* (159–161). Prophylactic treatment of mice with Fludase inhibited establishment of infection by IAV strains H1N1, H5N1, H7N9 and therefore protected against host mortality. Furthermore, these studies reported that Fludase inhibited IV replication and therefore host mortality when given up to 3 days post infection, albeit with less effectivity than prophylactic treatment (156, 162, 163). Malakhov et al. also demonstrated effectivity of Fludase in a ferret model of H1N1 infection (156). Fludase has begun clinical trials and was generally well tolerated in phase I trial (164). A phase II trial performed over three influenza seasons (2009–2011) in otherwise healthy IV-infected participants demonstrated that Fludase was well tolerated and patients under a multi-dose treatment regime exhibited a significant decrease viral load and viral shedding (165).

While Fludase is a promising anti-IV therapy there are potential pitfalls to broad use. Sialic acid is catabolized by *S. pneumonia*, IV-mediated release of this metabolite is thought to facilitate bacterial colonization and consequent pneumonia (166). In a preclinical study Hedlund et al. demonstrated that Fludase treatment did not alter *S. pneumonia* colonization in an *in vitro* model of a human lung cell line (A549) or in healthy mice. This study also reported that Fludase treatment 24 h post infection with H1N1 or H3N2 strains of IAV protected mice from *S. pneumonia* colonization and therefore morbidity and mortality (167). However, it is important to note that Hedlund et al. administered the secondary bacterial infection 2 days after a single dose of Fludase in IAV infected mice, which, given that airway epithelial cells begin to recover sialylation by 2 days post treatment (157) may be too late to see direct effects of Fludase treatment on bacterial colonization in the context of IV infection. Furthermore, the authors employed a lethal dose of IV, with all vehicle control mice exhibiting highly similar morbidity and mortality regardless of secondary *S. pneumonia* infection. It is therefore unclear whether or not the inoculum of *S. pneumonia* used in this study actually increases disease burden (167). Further studies are required to understand if Fludase alters host susceptibility to secondary bacterial infection.

IFNαβ signal to all cell types in the body and, as discussed, are therefore too inflammatory to be used as anti-influenza therapeutics. However, type III IFNs (IFNλ) (**Table 1**) are an intriguing alternative. Discovered in 2003, IFNλ are induced during IV infection via the same pathways as IFNαβ and utilize an almost identical signaling cascade to activate transcription of ISGs (168–170). However, IFNλ engages a separate receptor complex with a limited tissue distribution, compared to the ubiquitously expressed IFNαβR. IFNλ receptor expression is predominantly restricted to mucosal surfaces, such as that of the lung, and only select immune cells, primarily neutrophils (86, 169, 171, 172). There is some evidence to suggest IFNλ may be more critical for protection against IV infection than IFNαβ. *In vitro* and *in vivo* analysis has revealed that IFNλ is produced more rapidly and in higher concentrations than IFNαβ by epithelial cells in response to IV infection (101, 170, 172), however this could be attributed to the sensitivity of the assays employed to detect various IFNs. More convincingly, Klinkhammer et al. have recently demonstrated in mice that prophylactic treatment with IFNλ, but not IFNα, confers sustained antiviral protection in the upper airways and blocks IV transmission to uninfected animals (173). In terms of employing IFNλ as in anti-IV therapy, IFNλ treatment consistently administered from 48 to 120 h post infection did not enhance proinflammatory cytokine signaling in the lung but did inhibit IV replication, lowered airway epithelial cell death and consequently promoted host survival (101). Kim et al. reported similar findings and Galani et al. further demonstrated IFNλ signaling to neutrophils also promotes IV clearance (172, 174). Pegylated recombinant IFNλ (PEG-IFNλ) was originally developed to treat Hepatitis C infection, however it was superseded by more specialized treatment options for the disease. Yet during development, PEG-IFNλ passed Phase I and II clinical trials, demonstrating desirable pharmacological properties and a safer drug profile than IFNαβ (175). PEG-IFNλ therefore constitutes a highly promising new broad-spectrum candidate for the treatment IV.

Apoptosis is an important process for resolution of IV infection, not only for elimination of infected cells but also for removing inflammatory cells such as CD8+ T cells, from the pulmonary environment once IV has been cleared.

Death-inducing members of the TNF superfamily, including TRAIL and first apoptosis signal (Fas) ligand (FasL) have been shown to induce apoptosis of cells during IV infection (176–180). DNA microarray analysis performed by Kash et al. found that FasL/Fas signaling related genes in the lung are associated with IAV induced mortality in mice (181). Additionally, *ex vivo* assessment of human macrophages has shown that TRAIL expression and secretion is enhanced in severe IV induced disease and human peripheral blood mononuclear cells upregulate TRAIL upon IV infection. Furthermore, IAV infection of a human lung epithelial cell line increases cell susceptibility to TRAIL mediated apoptosis (182, 183). Blocking extrinsic apoptosis by inhibition of Fas/FasL interaction though treatment with a recombinant decoy receptor for FasL or interruption of TRAIL signaling, either by genomic deletion or monoclonal antibody (mAb) blockade (**Table 1**) during IAV infection can increase the survival rate of mice after IV infection (115, 151, 179, 182–184). Furthermore, mAb blockade of TRAIL signaling protects against secondary bacterial infection (20). Protecting airway epithelial cells from death during IV infection associates with better prognosis. However, it is a fine balance, as mentioned FasL and TRAIL are also used to control inflammatory cells in the lung. Indeed, in severe IAV infection TRAIL deficient mice are more susceptible to IAV induced disease due to accumulation of cytotoxic CD8+ T cells in the lung (180). As yet, blockade of apoptosis in human IV infection has not been assessed.

An alternative approach to entirely blocking apoptosis is to try to target it specifically to infected cells. B-cell lymphoma 2 (Bcl-2) family members such as Bcl-xL, are key regulators of apoptosis and as such Bcl-2 inhibitors have been developed to treat cancer. It was recently proposed that Bcl-2 inhibitors could also be repurposed for antiviral drug development (185). A series of compounds (ABT-737, ABT-263, ABT-199, WEHI-539, A-1331852) have been show to induce premature death of IAV-infected cells at concentrations that were not toxic for non-infected cells *in vitro* (186). Furthermore, Bulanova et al. showed that A-1155463 (**Table 1**) limited viral spread (186). The authors hypothesize that recognition of IV infection by the cell causes the release of proapoptotic proteins from Bcl-xL to initiate mitochondrial membrane permeabilization, ATP degradation, and caspase-3 activation. Subsequent addition of Bcl-2 inhibitors in low concentrations acts synergistically, further driving apoptosis of IV infected cells. It appears this phenomenon is not specific to IV, as transfection with plasmid DNA elicited similar effects (186, 187). As ABT-199 (as known as Venetoclax) is approved for use in humans for treatment of chronic lymphocytic leukemia, this class of drugs may have potential to be used as anti-IV therapeutics. However, Kakkola et al. did report that ABT-263 treatment of IV-infected mice resulted in an altered pro-inflammatory cytokine profile in the lung and a slightly higher viral load, which associated with decreased host survival, indicating that these treatments may need to be supplemented with other therapeutics which modulate the inflammatory response or promote viral clearance (187).

CONCLUDING REMARKS

Globalisation and the continual growth of the world population means that we are living closer together and traveling further distances with greater ease and speed. Emerging strains of IV can transverse the globe in a matter of days. Furthermore, increased demand of fowl and swine products has enlarged the interface between humans and animal reservoirs of IAV, elevating the likelihood of zoonotic transmission. Under these circumstances it is not a case of "if" another IV pandemic emerges but "when." To combat future IV pandemics we need therapeutics to supplement or replace oseltamivir and other NAIs. Of trials registered on clinicaltrials.gov assessing combination therapies to treat IV (25 results, July 2018), all involve a NAI (primarily oseltamivir) and another therapeutic targeted to IV, with the exception of a single celecoxib/oseltamivir trial (NCT02108366). Combinations of antivirals which inhibit different aspects of IV's replication cycle such as inhibitors for PB and PA (NCT02888327) may have synergistic effects and reduce the likelihood of resistant strains developing. However, trials combining anti-HA stem antibodies and NAIs (NCT02293863 and NCT02603952) have reported no decrease in symptom severity and duration compared to monotherapies. As discussed, severity of IV induced disease is a function of the host immune response, therefore combining antivirals with immunomodulatory drugs will likely prove more effective in treating IV infection. Host directed therapies are less likely to drive drug resistance, are more apt for protecting the delicate epithelium from immune mediated cell death and consequently, may be superior at decreasing disease burden. Repurposing of clinically approved immunomodulators is a simple solution. More trials are needed to assess the feasibility of other immunomodulatory drugs to be used as adjuncts to oseltamivir or other antivirals. Selection of appropriate candidates should be based on *in vivo* models and retrospective studies. Furthermore, taking advantage of inhalers to deliver drugs directly to the site of infection and tailoring therapeutics to epithelial cells, where IV replication occurs will also improve effectivity of treatment while minimizing harmful side effects.

AUTHOR CONTRIBUTIONS

The author confirms being the sole contributor of this work and approved it for publication.

ACKNOWLEDGMENTS

SD thanks members of the Wack (Francis Crick Insitute for Medical research) Masters (Walter and Eliza Hall Institute) and Kile (Monash University) laboratories for advice and discussion on this review.

REFERENCES

1. Stohr K. Influenza–WHO cares. *Lancet Infect Dis.* (2002) 2:517. doi: 10.1016/S1473-3099(02)00366-3
2. Girard MP, Cherian T, Pervikov Y, Kieny MP. A review of vaccine research and development: human acute respiratory infections. *Vaccine* (2005) 23:5708–24. doi: 10.1016/j.vaccine.2005.07.046
3. Kreijtz JH, Fouchier RA, Rimmelzwaan GF. Immune responses to influenza virus infection. *Virus Res.* (2011) 162:19–30. doi: 10.1016/j.virusres.2011.09.022
4. Tong S, Zhu X, Li Y, Shi M, Zhang J, Bourgeois M, et al. New world bats harbor diverse influenza A viruses. *PLoS Pathog.* (2013) 9:e1003657. doi: 10.1371/journal.ppat.1003657
5. Olsen B, Munster VJ, Wallensten A, Waldenstrom J, Osterhaus AD, Fouchier RA. Global patterns of influenza a virus in wild birds. *Science* (2006) 312:384–8. doi: 10.1126/science.1122438
6. Wang Z, Loh L, Kedzierski L, Kedzierska K. Avian influenza viruses, inflammation, and CD8(+) T cell immunity. *Front Immunol.* (2016) 7:60. doi: 10.3389/fimmu.2016.00060
7. Robinson JL, Lee BE, Patel J, Bastien N, Grimsrud K, Seal RF, et al. Swine influenza (H3N2) infection in a child and possible community transmission, Canada. *Emerg Infect Dis.* (2007) 13:1865–70. doi: 10.3201/eid1312.070615
8. Kucharski AJ, Lessler J, Read JM, Zhu H, Jiang CQ, Guan Y, et al. Estimating the life course of influenza A(H3N2) antibody responses from cross-sectional data. *PLoS Biol.* (2015) 13:e1002082. doi: 10.1371/journal.pbio.1002082
9. Hensley SE, Das SR, Bailey AL, Schmidt LM, Hickman HD, Jayaraman A, et al. Hemagglutinin receptor binding avidity drives influenza A virus antigenic drift. *Science* (2009) 326:734–6. doi: 10.1126/science.1178258
10. Taubenberger JK. The origin and virulence of the 1918 "Spanish" influenza virus. *Proc Am Philos Soc.* (2006) 150:86–112.
11. Short KR, Kroeze E, Fouchier RM, Kuiken T. Pathogenesis of influenza-induced acute respiratory distress syndrome. *Lancet Infect Dis.* (2014). 14:57–69. doi: 10.1016/S1473-3099(13)70286-X
12. Hayden FG, Fritz R, Lobo MC, Alvord W, Strober W, Straus SE. Local and systemic cytokine responses during experimental human influenza A virus infection. Relation to symptom formation and host defense. *J Clin Invest.* (1998) 101:643–9. doi: 10.1172/JCI1355
13. Kaiser L, Fritz RS, Straus SE, Gubareva L, Hayden FG. Symptom pathogenesis during acute influenza: interleukin-6 and other cytokine responses. *J Med Virol.* (2001) 64:262–8. doi: 10.1002/jmv.1045
14. Peiris JS, Yu WC, Leung CW, Cheung CY, Ng WF, Nicholls JM, et al. Re-emergence of fatal human influenza A subtype H5N1 disease. *Lancet* (2004) 363:617–9. doi: 10.1016/S0140-6736(04)15595-5
15. De Jong MD, Simmons CP, Thanh TT, Hien VM, Smith GJ, Chau TN, et al. Fatal outcome of human influenza A (H5N1) is associated with high viral load and hypercytokinemia. *Nat Med.* (2006) 12:1203–7. doi: 10.1038/nm1477
16. Louie JK, Acosta M, Winter K, Jean C, Gavali S, Schechter R, et al. Factors associated with death or hospitalization due to pandemic 2009 influenza A(H1N1) infection in California. *JAMA* (2009) 302:1896–902. doi: 10.1001/jama.2009.1583
17. Arankalle VA, Lole KS, Arya RP, Tripathy AS, Ramdasi AY, Chadha MS, et al. Role of host immune response and viral load in the differential outcome of pandemic H1N1 (2009) influenza virus infection in Indian patients. *PLoS ONE* (2010) 5:e13099. doi: 10.1371/journal.pone.0013099
18. Mccullers JA. The co-pathogenesis of influenza viruses with bacteria in the lung. *Nat Rev Microbiol.* (2014) 12:252–62. doi: 10.1038/nrmicro3231
19. Shahangian A, Chow EK, Tian X, Kang JR, Ghaffari A, Liu SY, et al. Type I IFNs mediate development of postinfluenza bacterial pneumonia in mice. *J Clin Invest.* (2009) 119:1910–20. doi: 10.1172/JCI35412
20. Ellis GT, Davidson S, Crotta S, Branzk N, Papayannopoulos V, Wack A. TRAIL+ monocytes and monocyte-related cells cause lung damage and thereby increase susceptibility to influenza-Streptococcus pneumoniae coinfection. *EMBO Rep.* (2015) 16:1203–18. doi: 10.15252/embr.201540473
21. Rajao DS, Perez DR. Universal vaccines and vaccine platforms to protect against influenza viruses in humans and agriculture. *Front Microbiol.* (2018) 9:123. doi: 10.3389/fmicb.2018.00123
22. Shtyrya YA, Mochalova LV, Bovin NV. Influenza virus neuraminidase: structure and function. *Acta Naturae* (2009) 1:26–32.
23. Cohen M, Zhang XQ, Senaati HP, Chen HW, Varki NM, Schooley RT, et al. Influenza A penetrates host mucus by cleaving sialic acids with neuraminidase. *Virol J.* (2013) 10:321. doi: 10.1186/1743-422X-10-321
24. Colman PM, Hoyne PA, Lawrence MC. Sequence and structure alignment of paramyxovirus hemagglutinin-neuraminidase with influenza virus neuraminidase. *J Virol.* (1993) 67:2972–80.
25. Kamali A, Holodniy M. Influenza treatment and prophylaxis with neuraminidase inhibitors: a review. *Infect Drug Resist.* (2013) 6:187–98. doi: 10.2147/IDR.S36601
26. Ison MG. Antiviral treatments. *Clin Chest Med.* (2017) 38:139–53. doi: 10.1016/j.ccm.2016.11.008
27. Mendel DB, Roberts NA. *In-vitro* and *in-vivo* efficacy of influenza neuraminidase inhibitors. *Curr Opin Infect Dis.* (1998) 11:727–32. doi: 10.1097/00001432-199812000-00013
28. Dharan NJ, Gubareva LV, Meyer JJ, Okomo-Adhiambo M, Mcclinton RC, Marshall SA, et al. Infections with oseltamivir-resistant influenza A(H1N1) virus in the United States. *JAMA* (2009) 301:1034–41. doi: 10.1001/jama.2009.294
29. Hurt AC, Ernest J, Deng YM, Iannello P, Besselaar TG, Birch C, et al. Emergence and spread of oseltamivir-resistant A(H1N1) influenza viruses in Oceania, South East Asia and South Africa. *Antiviral Res.* (2009a) 83:90–3. doi: 10.1016/j.antiviral.2009.03.003
30. Hurt AC, Holien JK, Parker MW, Barr IG. Oseltamivir resistance and the H274Y neuraminidase mutation in seasonal, pandemic and highly pathogenic influenza viruses. *Drugs* (2009b) 69:2523–31. doi: 10.2165/11531450-000000000-00000
31. Meijer A, Lackenby A, Hungnes O, Lina B, Van-Der-Werf S, Schweiger B, et al. Oseltamivir-resistant influenza virus A (H1N1), Europe, 2007-08 season. *Emerg Infect Dis.* (2009) 15:552–60. doi: 10.3201/eid1504.181280
32. Collins PJ, Haire LF, Lin YP, Liu J, Russell RJ, Walker PA, et al. Crystal structures of oseltamivir-resistant influenza virus neuraminidase mutants. *Nature* (2008) 453:1258–61. doi: 10.1038/nature06956
33. Malaisree M, Rungrotmongkol T, Nunthaboot N, Aruksakunwong O, Intharathep P, Decha P, et al. Source of oseltamivir resistance in avian influenza H5N1 virus with the H274Y mutation. *Amino Acids* (2009) 37:725–32. doi: 10.1007/s00726-008-0201-z
34. Wang MZ, Tai CY, Mendel DB. Mechanism by which mutations at his274 alter sensitivity of influenza a virus n1 neuraminidase to oseltamivir carboxylate and zanamivir. *Antimicrob Agents Chemother.* (2002) 46:3809–16. doi: 10.1128/AAC.46.12.3809-3816.2002
35. Moscona A. Global transmission of oseltamivir-resistant influenza. *N Engl J Med.* (2009) 360:953–6. doi: 10.1056/NEJMp0900648
36. Weinstock DM, Zuccotti G. The evolution of influenza resistance and treatment. *JAMA* (2009) 301:1066–9. doi: 10.1001/jama.2009.324
37. Hurt AC, Hardie K, Wilson NJ, Deng YM, Osbourn M, Gehrig N, et al. Community transmission of oseltamivir-resistant A(H1N1)pdm09 influenza. *N Engl J Med.* (2011) 365:2541–2. doi: 10.1056/NEJMc1111078
38. Wang D, Sleeman K, Huang W, Nguyen HT, Levine M, Cheng Y, et al. Neuraminidase inhibitor susceptibility testing of influenza type B viruses in China during 2010 and 2011 identifies viruses with reduced susceptibility to oseltamivir and zanamivir. *Antiviral Res.* (2013) 97:240–4. doi: 10.1016/j.antiviral.2012.12.013
39. Ebell MH, Call M, Shinholser J. Effectiveness of oseltamivir in adults: a meta-analysis of published and unpublished clinical trials. *Fam Pract.* (2013) 30:125–33. doi: 10.1093/fampra/cms059
40. Michiels B, Van Puyenbroeck K, Verhoeven V, Vermeire E, Coenen S. The value of neuraminidase inhibitors for the prevention and treatment of seasonal influenza: a systematic review of systematic reviews. *PLoS ONE* (2013) 8:e60348. doi: 10.1371/journal.pone.0060348
41. Jefferson T, Jones M, Doshi P, Spencer EA, Onakpoya I, Heneghan CJ. Oseltamivir for influenza in adults and children: systematic review of clinical study reports and summary of regulatory comments. *BMJ* (2014) 348:g2545. doi: 10.1136/bmj.g2545
42. Jefferson T, Jones MA, Doshi P, Del Mar CB, Hama R, Thompson,MJ, et al. Neuraminidase inhibitors for preventing and treating influenza in

healthy adults and children. *Cochrane Database Syst Rev.* (2014) CD008965. doi: 10.1002/14651858.CD008965.pub3
43. Okoli GN, Otete HE, Beck CR, Nguyen-Van-Tam JS. Use of neuraminidase inhibitors for rapid containment of influenza: a systematic review and meta-analysis of individual and household transmission studies. *PLoS ONE* (2014) 9:e113633. doi: 10.1371/journal.pone.0113633
44. Skehel JJ, Wiley DC. Receptor binding and membrane fusion in virus entry: the influenza hemagglutinin. *Annu Rev Biochem.* (2000) 69:531–69. doi: 10.1146/annurev.biochem.69.1.531
45. Russell RJ, Kerry PS, Stevens DJ, Steinhauer DA, Martin SR, Gamblin SJ, et al. Structure of influenza hemagglutinin in complex with an inhibitor of membrane fusion. *Proc Natl Acad Sci USA.* (2008) 105:17736–41. doi: 10.1073/pnas.0807142105
46. Fleury D, Barrere B, Bizebard T, Daniels RS, Skehel JJ, Knossow M. A complex of influenza hemagglutinin with a neutralizing antibody that binds outside the virus receptor binding site. *Nat Struct Biol.* (1999) 6:530–4. doi: 10.1038/9299
47. Knossow M, Skehel JJ. Variation and infectivity neutralization in influenza. *Immunology* (2006) 119:1–7. doi: 10.1111/j.1365-2567.2006.02421.x
48. Xiong X, Corti D, Liu J, Pinna D, Foglierini M, Calder LJ, et al. Structures of complexes formed by H5 influenza hemagglutinin with a potent broadly neutralizing human monoclonal antibody. *Proc Natl Acad Sci USA.* (2015) 112:9430–5. doi: 10.1073/pnas.1510816112
49. Das SR, Puigbo P, Hensley SE, Hurt DE, Bennink JR, Yewdell JW. Glycosylation focuses sequence variation in the influenza A virus H1 hemagglutinin globular domain. *PLoS Pathog.* (2010) 6:e1001211. doi: 10.1371/journal.ppat.1001211
50. Medina RA, Stertz S, Manicassamy B, Zimmermann P, Sun X, Albrecht R A, et al. Glycosylations in the globular head of the hemagglutinin protein modulate the virulence and antigenic properties of the H1N1 influenza viruses. *Sci Transl Med.* (2013) 5:187ra170. doi: 10.1126/scitranslmed.3005996
51. Corti D, Voss J, Gamblin SJ, Codoni G, Macagno A, Jarrossay D, et al. A neutralizing antibody selected from plasma cells that binds to group 1 and group 2 influenza A hemagglutinins. *Science* (2011) 333:850–6. doi: 10.1126/science.1205669
52. Dilillo DJ, Tan GS, Palese P, Ravetch JV. Broadly neutralizing hemagglutinin stalk-specific antibodies require FcgammaR interactions for protection against influenza virus *in vivo*. *Nat Med.* (2014) 20:143–51. doi: 10.1038/nm.3443
53. Dilillo DJ, Palese P, Wilson PC, Ravetch JV. Broadly neutralizing anti-influenza antibodies require Fc receptor engagement for *in vivo* protection. *J Clin Invest.* (2016) 126:605–10. doi: 10.1172/JCI84428
54. Tharakaraman K, Subramanian V, Cain D, Sasisekharan V, Sasisekharan R. Broadly neutralizing influenza hemagglutinin stem-specific antibody CR8020 targets residues that are prone to escape due to host selection pressure. *Cell Host Microbe* (2014) 15:644–51. doi: 10.1016/j.chom.2014.04.009
55. Gupta P, Kamath AV, Park S, Chiu H, Lutman J, Maia M, et al. Preclinical pharmacokinetics of MHAA4549A, a human monoclonal antibody to influenza A virus, and the prediction of its efficacious clinical dose for the treatment of patients hospitalized with influenza A. *MAbs* (2016) 8:991–7. doi: 10.1080/19420862.2016.1167294
56. Kallewaard NL Corti D, Collins PJ, Neu U, Mcauliffe JM, Benjamin E, et al. Structure and function analysis of an antibody recognizing all influenza A subtypes. *Cell* (2016) 166:596–608. doi: 10.1016/j.cell.2016.05.073
57. Baranovich T, Jones JC, Russier M, Vogel P, Szretter KJ, Sloan SE, et al. The hemagglutinin stem-binding monoclonal antibody VIS410 controls influenza virus-induced acute respiratory distress syndrome. *Antimicrob Agents Chemother.* (2016) 60:2118–31. doi: 10.1128/AAC.02457-15
58. Mcbride JM, Lim JJ, Burgess T, Deng R, Derby MA, Maia M, et al. Phase 2 randomized trial of the safety and efficacy of MHAA4549A, a broadly neutralizing monoclonal antibody, in a human influenza A virus challenge model. *Antimicrob Agents Chemother.* (2017) 61:e01154-17. doi: 10.1128/AAC.01154-17
59. Omar Ali TT, Andrew C, Nyborg KM, Jensen FD, Raburn M. A phase 2a study to evaluate the safety of MEDI8852 in outpatient adults with acute, uncomplicated influenza A. *Open Forum Infect Dis.* (2017) 4:S519. doi: 10.1093/ofid/ofx163.1352
60. Wollacott AM, Boni MF, Szretter KJ, Sloan SE, Yousofshahi M, Viswanathan K, et al. Safety and upper respiratory pharmacokinetics of the hemagglutinin stalk-binding antibody VIS410 support treatment and prophylaxis based on population modeling of seasonal influenza A outbreaks. *EBioMedicine* (2016) 5:147–55. doi: 10.1016/j.ebiom.2016.02.021
61. Rayner CR, Bulik CC, Kamal MA, Reynolds DK, Toovey S, Hammel JP, et al. Pharmacokinetic-pharmacodynamic determinants of oseltamivir efficacy using data from phase 2 inoculation studies. *Antimicrob Agents Chemother.* (2013) 57:3478–87. doi: 10.1128/AAC.02440-12
62. Martin-Benito J, Ortin J. Influenza virus transcription and replication. *Adv Virus Res.* (2013) 87:113–37. doi: 10.1016/B978-0-12-407698-3.00004-1
63. Fu Y, Gaelings L, Soderholm S, Belanov S, Nandania J, Nyman TA, et al. JNJ872 inhibits influenza A virus replication without altering cellular antiviral responses. *Antiviral Res.* (2016) 133:23–31. doi: 10.1016/j.antiviral.2016.07.008
64. Smee DF, Barnard DL, Jones SM. Activities of JNJ63623872 and oseltamivir against influenza A H1N1pdm and H3N2 virus infections in mice. *Antiviral Res.* (2016) 136:45–50. doi: 10.1016/j.antiviral.2016.10.009
65. VRTX-GEN. *VX-787 Showed Significant Antiviral Activity and Reduced the Severity and Duration of Influenza Symptoms in Phase 2 Challenge Study.* Boston, MA (2016).
66. Clark MP, Ledeboer MW, Davies I, Byrn RA, Jones SM, Perola E, et al. Discovery of a novel, first-in-class, orally bioavailable azaindole inhibitor (VX-787) of influenza PB2. *J Med Chem.* (2014) 57:6668–78. doi: 10.1021/jm5007275
67. Baranovich T, Wong SS, Armstrong J, Marjuki H, Webby RJ, Webster RG, et al. T-705 (favipiravir) induces lethal mutagenesis in influenza A H1N1 viruses *in vitro*. *J Virol.* (2013) 87:3741–51. doi: 10.1128/JVI.02346-12
68. Furuta Y, Takahashi K, Fukuda Y, Kuno M, Kamiyama T, Kozaki K, et al. *In vitro* and *in vivo* activities of anti-influenza virus compound T-705. *Antimicrob Agents Chemother.* (2002) 46:977–81. doi: 10.1128/AAC.46.4.977-981.2002
69. Sidwell RW, Barnard DL, Day CW, Smee DF, Bailey KW, Wong MH, et al. Efficacy of orally administered T-705 on lethal avian influenza A (H5N1) virus infections in mice. *Antimicrob Agents Chemother.* (2007) 51:845–51. doi: 10.1128/AAC.01051-06
70. Kiso M, Takahashi K, Sakai-Tagawa Y, Shinya K, Sakabe S, Le QM, et al. T-705 (favipiravir) activity against lethal H5N1 influenza A viruses. *Proc Natl Acad Sci USA.* (2010) 107:882–7. doi: 10.1073/pnas.0909603107
71. Furuta Y, Gowen BB, Takahashi K, Shiraki K, Smee DF, Barnard DL. Favipiravir (T-705), a novel viral RNA polymerase inhibitor. *Antiviral Res.* (2013) 100:446–54. doi: 10.1016/j.antiviral.2013.09.015
72. Furuta Y, Takahashi K, Kuno-Maekawa M, Sangawa H, Uehara S, Kozaki K, et al. Mechanism of action of T-705 against influenza virus. *Antimicrob Agents Chemother.* (2005) 49:981–6. doi: 10.1128/AAC.49.3.981-986.2005
73. Cheung PP, Watson SJ, Choy KT, Fun Sia S, Wong DD, Poon LL, et al. Generation and characterization of influenza A viruses with altered polymerase fidelity. *Nat Commun.* (2014) 5:4794. doi: 10.1038/ncomms5794
74. Talon J, Horvath CM, Polley R, Basler CF, Muster T, Palese P, et al. Activation of interferon regulatory factor 3 is inhibited by the influenza A virus NS1 protein. *J Virol.* (2000) 74:7989–96. doi: 10.1128/JVI.74.17.7989-7996.2000
75. Wang X, Li M, Zheng H, Muster T, Palese P, Beg AA, et al. Influenza A virus NS1 protein prevents activation of NF-kappaB and induction of alpha/beta interferon. *J Virol.* (2000) 74:11566–73. doi: 10.1128/JVI.74.24.11566-11573.2000
76. Ludwig S, Wang X, Ehrhardt C, Zheng H, Donelan N, Planz O, et al. The influenza A virus NS1 protein inhibits activation of Jun N-terminal kinase and AP-1 transcription factors. *J Virol.* (2002) 76:11166–71. doi: 10.1128/JVI.76.21.11166-11171.2002
77. Donelan NR, Basler CF, Garcia-Sastre A. A recombinant influenza A virus expressing an RNA-binding-defective NS1 protein induces high levels of beta interferon and is attenuated in mice. *J Virol.* (2003) 77:13257–66. doi: 10.1128/JVI.77.24.13257-13266.2003
78. Pichlmair A, Schulz O, Tan CP, Naslund TI, Liljestrom P, Weber F, et al. RIG-I-mediated antiviral responses to single-stranded RNA

bearing 5'-phosphates. *Science* (2006) 314:997–1001. doi: 10.1126/science.1132998
79. Gack MU, Shin YC, Joo CH, Urano T, Liang C, Sun L, et al. TRIM25 RING-finger E3 ubiquitin ligase is essential for RIG-I-mediated antiviral activity. *Nature* (2007) 446:916–20. doi: 10.1038/nature05732
80. Guo Z, Chen LM, Zeng H, Gomez JA, Plowden J, Fujita T, et al. NS1 protein of influenza A virus inhibits the function of intracytoplasmic pathogen sensor, RIG-I. *Am J Respir Cell Mol Biol.* (2007) 36:263–9. doi: 10.1165/rcmb.2006-0283RC
81. Mibayashi M, Martinez-Sobrido L, Loo YM, Cardenas WB, Gale M Jr, Garcia-Sastre A. Inhibition of retinoic acid-inducible gene I-mediated induction of beta interferon by the NS1 protein of influenza A virus. *J Virol.* (2007) 81:514–24. doi: 10.1128/JVI.01265-06
82. Opitz B, Rejaibi A, Dauber B, Eckhard J, Vinzing M, Schmeck B, et al. IFNbeta induction by influenza A virus is mediated by RIG-I which is regulated by the viral NS1 protein. *Cell Microbiol.* (2007) 9:930–8. doi: 10.1111/j.1462-5822.2006.00841.x
83. Steidle S, Martinez-Sobrido L, Mordstein M, Lienenklaus S, Garcia-Sastre A, Staheli P, et al. Glycine 184 in nonstructural protein NS1 determines the virulence of influenza A virus strain PR8 without affecting the host interferon response. *J Virol.* (2010) 84:12761–70. doi: 10.1128/JVI.00701-10
84. Garcia-Sastre A, Egorov A, Matassov D, Brandt S, Levy DE, Durbin JE, et al. Influenza A virus lacking the NS1 gene replicates in interferon-deficient systems. *Virology* (1998) 252:324–30. doi: 10.1006/viro.1998.9508
85. Diebold SS, Montoya M, Unger H, Alexopoulou L, Roy P, Haswell LE, et al. Viral infection switches non-plasmacytoid dendritic cells into high interferon producers. *Nature* (2003) 424:324–8. doi: 10.1038/nature01783
86. Mordstein M, Kochs G, Dumoutier L, Renauld JC, Paludan SR, Klucher K, et al. Interferon-lambda contributes to innate immunity of mice against influenza A virus but not against hepatotropic viruses. *PLoS Pathog.* (2008) 4:e1000151. doi: 10.1371/journal.ppat.1000151
87. Kallfass C, Lienenklaus S, Weiss S, Staeheli P. Visualizing the beta interferon response in mice during infection with influenza A viruses expressing or lacking nonstructural protein 1. *J Virol.* (2013) 87:6925–30. doi: 10.1128/JVI.00283-13
88. Walkiewicz MP, Basu D, Jablonski JJ, Geysen HM, Engel DA. Novel inhibitor of influenza non-structural protein 1 blocks multi-cycle replication in an RNase L-dependent manner. *J Gen Virol.* (2011) 92:60–70. doi: 10.1099/vir.0.025015-0
89. Jablonski JJ, Basu D, Engel DA, Geysen HM. Design, synthesis, and evaluation of novel small molecule inhibitors of the influenza virus protein NS1. *Bioorg Med Chem.* (2012) 20:487–97. doi: 10.1016/j.bmc.2011.10.026
90. Zhang S, Tian H, Cui J, Xiao J, Wang M, Hu Y. The c-Jun N-terminal kinase (JNK) is involved in H5N1 influenza A virus RNA and protein synthesis. *Arch Virol.* (2016) 161:345–51. doi: 10.1007/s00705-015-2668-8
91. Monod A, Swale C, Tarus B, Tissot A, Delmas B, Ruigrok RW, et al. Learning from structure-based drug design and new antivirals targeting the ribonucleoprotein complex for the treatment of influenza. *Expert Opin Drug Discov.* (2015) 10:345–71. doi: 10.1517/17460441.2015.1019859
92. Beigel JH, Farrar J, Han AM, Hayden FG, Hyer R, De Jong MD, et al. Avian influenza A (H5N1) infection in humans. *N Engl J Med.* (2005) 353:1374–85. doi: 10.1056/NEJMra052211
93. Lichtner M, Mastroianni CM, Rossi R, Russo G, Belvisi V, Marocco R, et al. Severe and persistent depletion of circulating plasmacytoid dendritic cells in patients with 2009 pandemic H1N1 infection. *PLoS ONE* (2011) 6:e19872. doi: 10.1371/journal.pone.0019872
94. Finter NB, Chapman S, Dowd P, Johnston JM, Manna V, Sarantis N, et al. The use of interferon-alpha in virus infections. *Drugs* (1991) 42:749–65. doi: 10.2165/00003495-199142050-00003
95. Fritz RS, Hayden FG, Calfee DP, Cass LM, Peng AW, Alvord WG, et al. Nasal cytokine and chemokine responses in experimental influenza A virus infection: results of a placebo-controlled trial of intravenous zanamivir treatment. *J Infect Dis.* (1999) 180:586–93. doi: 10.1086/314938
96. Hussell T, Pennycook A, Openshaw PJ. Inhibition of tumor necrosis factor reduces the severity of virus-specific lung immunopathology. *Eur J Immunol.* (2001) 31:2566–573. doi: 10.1002/1521-4141(200109)31:9<2566::AID-IMMU2566>3.0.CO;2-L
97. Mckinlay MA. Recent advances in the treatment of rhinovirus infections. *Curr Opin Pharmacol.* (2001) 1:477–81. doi: 10.1016/S1471-4892(01)00083-2
98. Kim B, Ahn KK, Ha Y, Lee YH, Kim D, Lim JH, et al. Association of tumor necrosis factor-alpha with fever and pulmonary lesion score in pigs experimentally infected with swine influenza virus subtype H1N2. *J Vet Med Sci.* (2009) 71:611–6. doi: 10.1292/jvms.71.611
99. Shale M, Czub M, Kaplan GG, Panaccione R, Ghosh S. Anti-tumor necrosis factor therapy and influenza: keeping it in perspective. *Therap Adv Gastroenterol.* (2010) 3:173–7. doi: 10.1177/1756283X10366368
100. Wang Z, Zhang A, Wan Y, Liu X, Qiu C, Xi X, et al. Early hypercytokinemia is associated with interferon-induced transmembrane protein-3 dysfunction and predictive of fatal H7N9 infection. *Proc Natl Acad Sci USA.* (2014) 111:769–74. doi: 10.1073/pnas.1321748111
101. Davidson S, Mccabe TM, Crotta S, Gad HH, Hessel EM, Beinke S, et al. IFNlambda is a potent anti-influenza therapeutic without the inflammatory side effects of IFNalpha treatment. *EMBO Mol Med.* (2016) 8:1099–112. doi: 10.15252/emmm.201606413
102. Sethu S, Melendez AJ. New developments on the TNFalpha-mediated signalling pathways. *Biosci Rep.* (2011) 31:63–76. doi: 10.1042/BSR20100040
103. Matikainen S, Siren J, Tissari J, Veckman V, Pirhonen J, Severa M, et al. Tumor necrosis factor alpha enhances influenza A virus-induced expression of antiviral cytokines by activating RIG-I gene expression. *J Virol.* (2006) 80:3515–22. doi: 10.1128/JVI.80.7.3515-3522.2006
104. Szretter KJ, Gangappa S, Lu X, Smith C, Shieh WJ, Zaki SR, et al. Role of host cytokine responses in the pathogenesis of avian H5N1 influenza viruses in mice. *J Virol.* (2007) 81:2736–44. doi: 10.1128/JVI.02336-06
105. Shi X, Zhou W, Huang H, Zhu H, Zhou P, Zhu H, et al. Inhibition of the inflammatory cytokine tumor necrosis factor-alpha with etanercept provides protection against lethal H1N1 influenza infection in mice. *Crit Care* (2013) 17:R301. doi: 10.1186/cc13171
106. Blumentals WA, Arreglado A, Napalkov P, Toovey S. Rheumatoid arthritis and the incidence of influenza and influenza-related complications: a retrospective cohort study. *BMC Musculoskelet Disord.* (2012) 13:158. doi: 10.1186/1471-2474-13-158
107. Damjanovic D, Divangahi M, Kugathasan K, Small CL, Zganiacz A, Brown EG, et al. Negative regulation of lung inflammation and immunopathology by TNF-alpha during acute influenza infection. *Am J Pathol.* (2011) 179:2963–76. doi: 10.1016/j.ajpath.2011.09.003
108. Deberge MP, Ely KH, Enelow RI. Soluble, but not transmembrane, TNF-alpha is required during influenza infection to limit the magnitude of immune responses and the extent of immunopathology. *J Immunol.* (2014) 192:5839–51. doi: 10.4049/jimmunol.1302729
109. Beilharz MW, Cummins JM, Bennett AL. Protection from lethal influenza virus challenge by oral type 1 interferon. *Biochem Biophys Res Commun.* (2007) 355:740–4. doi: 10.1016/j.bbrc.2007.02.019
110. Tumpey TM, Szretter KJ, Van Hoeven N, Katz JM, Kochs G, Haller O, et al. The Mx1 gene protects mice against the pandemic 1918 and highly lethal human H5N1 influenza viruses. *J Virol.* (2007) 81:10818–21. doi: 10.1128/JVI.01116-07
111. Kugel D, Kochs G, Obojes K, Roth J, Kobinger GP, Kobasa D, et al. Intranasal administration of alpha interferon reduces seasonal influenza A virus morbidity in ferrets. *J Virol.* (2009) 83:3843–51. doi: 10.1128/JVI.02453-08
112. Van Hoeven N, Belser JA, Szretter KJ, Zeng H, Staeheli P, Swayne DE, et al. Pathogenesis of 1918 pandemic and H5N1 influenza virus infections in a guinea pig model: antiviral potential of exogenous alpha interferon to reduce virus shedding. *J Virol.* (2009) 83:2851–61. doi: 10.1128/JVI.02174-08
113. Matzinger SR, Carroll TD, Fritts L, Mcchesney MB, Miller CJ. Exogenous IFN-alpha administration reduces influenza A virus replication in the lower respiratory tract of rhesus macaques. *PLoS ONE* (2011) 6:e29255. doi: 10.1371/journal.pone.0029255
114. Cilloniz C, Pantin-Jackwood MJ, Ni C, Carter VS, Korth MJ, Swayne DE, et al. Molecular signatures associated with Mx1-mediated resistance to highly pathogenic influenza virus infection: mechanisms of survival. *J Virol.* (2012) 86:2437–46. doi: 10.1128/JVI.06156-11
115. Davidson S, Crotta S, Mccabe TM, Wack A. Pathogenic potential of interferon alphabeta in acute influenza infection. *Nat Commun.* (2014) 5:3864. doi: 10.1038/ncomms4864

116. Price GE, Gaszewska-Mastarlarz A, Moskophidis D. The role of alpha/beta and gamma interferons in development of immunity to influenza A virus in mice. *J Virol.* (2000) 74:3996–4003. doi: 10.1128/JVI.74.9.3996-4003.2000
117. Koerner I, Kochs G, Kalinke U, Weiss S, Staeheli P. Protective role of beta interferon in host defense against influenza A virus. *J Virol.* (2007) 81:2025–30. doi: 10.1128/JVI.01718-06
118. Szretter KJ, Gangappa S, Belser JA, Zeng H, Chen H, Matsuoka Y, et al. Early control of H5N1 influenza virus replication by the type I interferon response in mice. *J Virol.* (2009) 83:5825–34. doi: 10.1128/JVI.02144-08
119. Marsolais D, Rosen H. Chemical modulators of sphingosine-1-phosphate receptors as barrier-oriented therapeutic molecules. *Nat Rev Drug Discov.* (2009) 8:297–307. doi: 10.1038/nrd2356
120. Walsh KB, Teijaro JR, Wilker PR, Jatzek A, Fremgen DM, Das SC, et al. Suppression of cytokine storm with a sphingosine analog provides protection against pathogenic influenza virus. *Proc Natl Acad Sci USA.* (2011) 108:12018–23. doi: 10.1073/pnas.1107024108
121. Teijaro JR, Walsh KB, Cahalan S, Fremgen DM, Roberts E, Scott F, et al. Endothelial cells are central orchestrators of cytokine amplification during influenza virus infection. *Cell* (2011) 146:980–91. doi: 10.1016/j.cell.2011.08.015
122. Matheu MP, Teijaro JR, Walsh KB, Greenberg ML, Marsolais D, Parker I, et al. Three phases of CD8 T cell response in the lung following H1N1 influenza infection and sphingosine 1 phosphate agonist therapy. *PLoS ONE* (2013) 8:e58033. doi: 10.1371/journal.pone.0058033
123. Teijaro JR, Walsh KB, Rice S, Rosen H, Oldstone MB. Mapping the innate signaling cascade essential for cytokine storm during influenza virus infection. *Proc Natl Acad Sci USA.* (2014) 111:3799–804. doi: 10.1073/pnas.1400593111
124. Teijaro JR, Studer S, Leaf N, Kiosses WB, Nguyen N, Matsuki K, et al. S1PR1-mediated IFNAR1 degradation modulates plasmacytoid dendritic cell interferon-alpha autoamplification. *Proc Natl Acad Sci USA.* (2016) 113:1351–6. doi: 10.1073/pnas.1525356113
125. Ricciotti E, Fitzgerald GA. Prostaglandins and inflammation. *Arterioscler Thromb Vasc Biol.* (2011) 31:986–1000. doi: 10.1161/ATVBAHA.110.207449
126. Carey MA, Bradbury JA, Seubert JM, Langenbach R, Zeldin DC, Germolec DR. Contrasting effects of cyclooxygenase-1 (COX-1) and COX-2 deficiency on the host response to influenza A viral infection. *J Immunol.* (2005) 175:6878–84. doi: 10.4049/jimmunol.175.10.6878
127. Coulombe F, Jaworska J, Verway M, Tzelepis F, Massoud A, Gillard J, et al. Targeted prostaglandin E2 inhibition enhances antiviral immunity through induction of type I interferon and apoptosis in macrophages. *Immunity* (2014) 40:554–68. doi: 10.1016/j.immuni.2014.02.013
128. Lee SM, Cheung CY, Nicholls JM, Hui KP, Leung CY, Uiprasertkul M, et al. Hyperinduction of cyclooxygenase-2-mediated proinflammatory cascade: a mechanism for the pathogenesis of avian influenza H5N1 infection. *J Infect Dis.* (2008) 198:525–35. doi: 10.1086/590499
129. Carey MA, Bradbury JA, Rebolloso YD, Graves JP, Zeldin DC, Germolec DR. Pharmacologic inhibition of COX-1 and COX-2 in influenza A viral infection in mice. *PLoS ONE* (2010) 5:e11610. doi: 10.1371/journal.pone.0011610
130. Zheng BJ, Chan KW, Lin YP, Zhao GY, Chan C, Zhang HJ, et al. Delayed antiviral plus immunomodulator treatment still reduces mortality in mice infected by high inoculum of influenza A/H5N1 virus. *Proc Natl Acad Sci USA.* (2008) 105:8091–6. doi: 10.1073/pnas.0711942105
131. Tacconelli S, Capone ML, Sciulli MG, Ricciotti E, Patrignani P. The biochemical selectivity of novel COX-2 inhibitors in whole blood assays of COX-isozyme activity. *Curr Med Res Opin.* (2002) 18:503–11. doi: 10.1185/030079902125001335
132. Starko KM. Salicylates and pandemic influenza mortality, 1918-1919 pharmacology, pathology, and historic evidence. *Clin Infect Dis.* (2009) 49:1405–10. doi: 10.1086/606060
133. Eyers S, Weatherall M, Shirtcliffe P, Perrin K, Beasley R. The effect on mortality of antipyretics in the treatment of influenza infection: systematic review and meta-analysis. *J R Soc Med.* (2010) 103:403–11. doi: 10.1258/jrsm.2010.090441
134. Fedson DS. Pandemic influenza: a potential role for statins in treatment and prophylaxis. *Clin Infect Dis.* (2006) 43:199–205. doi: 10.1086/505116
135. Mohammad S, Nguyen H, Nguyen M, Abdel-Rasoul M, Nguyen V, Nguyen CD, et al. Pleotropic Effects of Statins: untapped potential for statin pharmacotherapy. *Curr Vasc Pharmacol.* (2018). doi: 10.2174/1570161116666180723120608. [Epub ahead of print].
136. Haidari M, Ali M, Casscells SW, Madjid M. Statins block influenza infection by down-regulating rho/rho kinase pathway. *Circulation* (2007) 116:116–7. doi: 10.1161/circ.116.suppl_16.II_7
137. Mehrbod P, Omar AR, Hair-Bejo M, Haghani A, Ideris A. Mechanisms of action and efficacy of statins against influenza. *Biomed Res Int.* (2014) 2014:872370. doi: 10.1155/2014/872370
138. Mehrbod P, El Zowalaty M, Omar AR, Hair-Bejo M, Ideris A. Statins reduce the expression of proinflammatory cytokines in influenza A virus infected CrFK cells. *Acta Virol.* (2012) 56:353–5. doi: 10.4149/av_2012_04_353
139. Lee CS, Yi EH, Lee JK, Won C, Lee YJ, Shin MK, et al. Simvastatin suppresses RANTES-mediated neutrophilia in polyinosinic-polycytidylic acid-induced pneumonia. *Eur Respir J.* (2013) 41:1147–56. doi: 10.1183/09031936.00050612
140. An SC, Xu LL, Li FD, Bao LL, Qin C, Gao ZC. Triple combinations of neuraminidase inhibitors, statins and fibrates benefit the survival of patients with lethal avian influenza pandemic. *Med Hypotheses* (2011) 77:1054–7. doi: 10.1016/j.mehy.2011.09.001
141. Liu Z, Guo Z, Wang G, Zhang D, He H, Li G, et al. Evaluation of the efficacy and safety of a statin/caffeine combination against H5N1, H3N2 and H1N1 virus infection in BALB/c mice. *Eur J Pharm Sci.* (2009) 38:215–23. doi: 10.1016/j.ejps.2009.07.004
142. Kumaki Y, Morrey JD, Barnard DL. Effect of statin treatments on highly pathogenic avian influenza H5N1, seasonal and H1N1pdm09 virus infections in BALB/c mice. *Future Virol.* (2012) 7:801–18. doi: 10.2217/fvl.12.71
143. Radigan KA, Urich D, Misharin AV, Chiarella SE, Soberanes S, Gonzalez A, et al. The effect of rosuvastatin in a murine model of influenza A infection. *PLoS ONE* (2012) 7:e35788. doi: 10.1371/journal.pone.0035788
144. Enserink M. Infectious disease. Old drugs losing effectiveness against flu; could statins fill gap? *Science* (2005) 309:1976–7. doi: 10.1126/science.309.5743.1976a
145. Frost FJ, Petersen H, Tollestrup K, Skipper B. Influenza and COPD mortality protection as pleiotropic, dose-dependent effects of statins. *Chest* (2007) 131:1006–12. doi: 10.1378/chest.06-1997
146. Carrillo-Esper R, Sosa-Garcia JO, Arch-Tirado E. Experience in the management of the severe form of human influenza A H1N1 pneumonia in an intensive care unit. *Cir Cir.* (2011) 79:409–16.
147. Vandermeer ML, Thomas AR, Kamimoto L, Reingold A, Gershman K, Meek J, et al. Association between use of statins and mortality among patients hospitalized with laboratory-confirmed influenza virus infections: a multistate study. *J Infect Dis.* (2012) 205:13–9. doi: 10.1093/infdis/jir695
148. Kwong JC, Li P, Redelmeier DA. Influenza morbidity and mortality in elderly patients receiving statins: a cohort study. *PLoS ONE* (2009) 4:e8087. doi: 10.1371/journal.pone.0008087
149. Fleming DM, Verlander NQ, Elliot AJ, Zhao H, Gelb D, Jehring D, et al. An assessment of the effect of statin use on the incidence of acute respiratory infections in England during winters 1998-1999 to 2005-2006. *Epidemiol Infect.* (2010) 138:1281–8. doi: 10.1017/S0950268810000105
150. Grygiel-Gorniak B. Peroxisome proliferator-activated receptors and their ligands: nutritional and clinical implications–a review. *Nutr J.* (2014) 13:17. doi: 10.1186/1475-2891-13-17
151. Herold S, Steinmueller M, Von Wulffen W, Cakarova L, Pinto R, Pleschka S, et al. Lung epithelial apoptosis in influenza virus pneumonia: the role of macrophage-expressed TNF-related apoptosis-inducing ligand. *J Exp Med.* (2008) 205:3065–77. doi: 10.1084/jem.20080201
152. Aldridge JRJr, Moseley CE, Boltz DA, Negovetich NJ, Reynolds C, Franks J, et al. TNF/iNOS-producing dendritic cells are the necessary evil of lethal influenza virus infection. *Proc Natl Acad Sci USA.* (2009) 106:5306–11. doi: 10.1073/pnas.0900655106
153. Moseley CE, Webster RG, Aldridge JR. Peroxisome proliferator-activated receptor and AMP-activated protein kinase agonists protect against lethal influenza virus challenge in mice. *Influenza Other Respir Viruses* (2010) 4:307–11. doi: 10.1111/j.1750-2659.2010.00155.x

154. Cloutier A, Marois I, Cloutier D, Verreault C, Cantin AM, Richter MV. The prostanoid 15-deoxy-Delta12,14-prostaglandin-j2 reduces lung inflammation and protects mice against lethal influenza infection. *J Infect Dis.* (2012) 205:621–30. doi: 10.1093/infdis/jir804
155. Bottcher-Friebertshauser E, Freuer C, Sielaff F, Schmidt S, Eickmann M, Uhlendorff J, et al. Cleavage of influenza virus hemagglutinin by airway proteases TMPRSS2 and HAT differs in subcellular localization and susceptibility to protease inhibitors. *J Virol.* (2010) 84:5605–14. doi: 10.1128/JVI.00140-10
156. Malakhov MP, Aschenbrenner LM, Smee DF, Wandersee MK, Sidwell RW, Gubareva LV, et al. Sialidase fusion protein as a novel broad-spectrum inhibitor of influenza virus infection. *Antimicrob Agents Chemother.* (2006) 50:1470–9. doi: 10.1128/AAC.50.4.1470-1479.2006
157. Triana-Baltzer GB, Babizki M, Chan MC, Wong AC, Aschenbrenner LM, Campbell ER, et al. DAS181, a sialidase fusion protein, protects human airway epithelium against influenza virus infection: an *in vitro* pharmacodynamic analysis. *J Antimicrob Chemother.* (2010) 65:275–84. doi: 10.1093/jac/dkp421
158. Triana-Baltzer GB, Sanders RL, Hedlund M, Jensen KA, Aschenbrenner LM, Larson JL, et al. Phenotypic and genotypic characterization of influenza virus mutants selected with the sialidase fusion protein DAS181. *J Antimicrob Chemother.* (2011) 66:15–28. doi: 10.1093/jac/dkq387
159. Chan RW, Chan MC, Wong AC, Karamanska R, Dell A, Haslam SM, et al. DAS181 inhibits H5N1 influenza virus infection of human lung tissues. *Antimicrob Agents Chemother* (2009) 53:3935–41. doi: 10.1128/AAC.00389-09
160. Triana-Baltzer GB, Gubareva LV, Klimov AI, Wurtman DF, Moss RB, Hedlund M, et al. Inhibition of neuraminidase inhibitor-resistant influenza virus by DAS181, a novel sialidase fusion protein. *PLoS ONE* (2009a) 4:e7838. doi: 10.1371/journal.pone.0007838
161. Triana-Baltzer GB, Gubareva LV, Nicholls JM, Pearce MB, Mishin VP, Belser JA, et al. Novel pandemic influenza A(H1N1) viruses are potently inhibited by DAS181, a sialidase fusion protein. *PLoS ONE* (2009b) 4:e7788. doi: 10.1371/journal.pone.0007788
162. Belser JA, Lu X, Szretter KJ, Jin X, Aschenbrenner LM, Lee A, et al. DAS181, a novel sialidase fusion protein, protects mice from lethal avian influenza H5N1 virus infection. *J Infect Dis.* (2007) 196:1493–9. doi: 10.1086/522609
163. Marjuki H, Mishin VP, Chesnokov AP, De La Cruz JA, Fry AM, Villanueva J, et al. An investigational antiviral drug, DAS181, effectively inhibits replication of zoonotic influenza A virus subtype H7N9 and protects mice from lethality. *J Infect Dis.* (2014) 210:435–40. doi: 10.1093/infdis/jiu105
164. Zenilman JM, Fuchs EJ, Hendrix CW, Radebaugh C, Jurao R, Nayak SU, et al. Phase 1 clinical trials of DAS181, an inhaled sialidase, in healthy adults. *Antiviral Res.* (2015) 123:114–9. doi: 10.1016/j.antiviral.2015.09.008
165. Moss RB, Hansen C, Sanders RL, Hawley S, Li T, Steigbigel RT. A phase II study of DAS181, a novel host directed antiviral for the treatment of influenza infection. *J Infect Dis.* (2012) 206:1844–51. doi: 10.1093/infdis/jis622
166. Siegel SJ, Roche AM, Weiser JN. Influenza promotes pneumococcal growth during coinfection by providing host sialylated substrates as a nutrient source. *Cell Host Microbe* (2014) 16:55–67. doi: 10.1016/j.chom.2014.06.005
167. Hedlund M, Aschenbrenner LM, Jensen K, Larson JL, Fang F. Sialidase-based anti-influenza virus therapy protects against secondary pneumococcal infection. *J Infect Dis.* (2010) 201:1007–15. doi: 10.1086/651170
168. Kotenko SV, Gallagher G, Baurin VV, Lewis-Antes A, Shen M, Shah NK, et al. IFN-lambdas mediate antiviral protection through a distinct class II cytokine receptor complex. *Nat Immunol.* (2003) 4:69–77. doi: 10.1038/ni875
169. Sheppard P, Kindsvogel W, Xu W, Henderson K, Schlutsmeyer S, Whitmore TE, et al. IL-28, IL-29 and their class II cytokine receptor IL-28R. *Nat Immunol.* (2003) 4:63–8. doi: 10.1038/ni873
170. Crotta S, Davidson S, Mahlakoiv T, Desmet CJ, Buckwalter MR, Albert ML, et al. Type I and type III interferons drive redundant amplification loops to induce a transcriptional signature in influenza-infected airway epithelia. *PLoS Pathog.* (2013) 9:e1003773. doi: 10.1371/journal.ppat.1003773
171. Sommereyns C, Paul S, Staeheli P, Michiels T. IFN-lambda (IFN-lambda) is expressed in a tissue-dependent fashion and primarily acts on epithelial cells *in vivo*. *PLoS Pathog.* (2008) 4:e1000017. doi: 10.1371/journal.ppat.1000017
172. Galani IE, Triantafyllia V, Eleminiadou EE, Koltsida O, Stavropoulos A, Manioudaki M, et al. Interferon-lambda mediates non-redundant front-line antiviral protection against influenza virus infection without compromising host fitness. *Immunity* (2017). 46:875–90.e6. doi: 10.1016/j.immuni.2017.04.025
173. Klinkhammer J, Schnepf D, Ye L, Schwaderlapp M, Gad HH, Hartmann R, et al. IFN-lambda prevents influenza virus spread from the upper airways to the lungs and limits virus transmission. *Elife* (2018) 7:e33354. doi: 10.7554/eLife.33354
174. Kim S, Kim MJ, Kim CH, Kang JW, Shin HK, Kim DY, et al. The superiority of IFN-lambda as a therapeutic candidate to control acute influenza viral lung infection. *Am J Respir Cell Mol Biol.* (2017) 56:202–12. doi: 10.1165/rcmb.2016-0174OC
175. Muir AJ, Arora S, Everson G, Flisiak R, George J, Ghalib R, et al. A randomized phase 2b study of peginterferon lambda-1a for the treatment of chronic HCV infection. *J Hepatol.* (2014) 61:1238–46. doi: 10.1016/j.jhep.2014.07.022
176. Topham DJ, Tripp RA, Doherty PC. CD8+ T cells clear influenza virus by perforin or Fas-dependent processes. *J Immunol.* (1997) 159:5197–200.
177. Fujimoto I, Takizawa T, Ohba Y, Nakanishi Y. Co-expression of Fas and Fas-ligand on the surface of influenza virus-infected cells. *Cell Death Differ.* (1998) 5:426–31. doi: 10.1038/sj.cdd.4400362
178. Ishikawa E, Nakazawa M, Yoshinari M, Minami M. Role of tumor necrosis factor-related apoptosis-inducing ligand in immune response to influenza virus infection in mice. *J Virol.* (2005) 79:7658–63. doi: 10.1128/JVI.79.12.7658-7663.2005
179. Brincks EL, Katewa A, Kucaba TA, Griffith TS, Legge KL. CD8 T cells utilize TRAIL to control influenza virus infection. *J Immunol.* (2008a) 181:4918–25. doi: 10.4049/jimmunol.181.7.4918
180. Brincks EL, Gurung P, Langlois RA, Hemann EA, Legge KL, Griffith TS. The magnitude of the T cell response to a clinically significant dose of influenza virus is regulated by TRAIL. *J Immunol.* (2011) 187:4581–8. doi: 10.4049/jimmunol.1002241
181. Kash JC, Tumpey TM, Proll SC, Carter V, Perwitasari O, Thomas MJ, et al. Genomic analysis of increased host immune and cell death responses induced by 1918 influenza virus. *Nature* (2006) 443:578–81. doi: 10.1038/nature05181
182. Brincks EL, Kucaba TA, Legge KL, Griffith TS. Influenza-induced expression of functional tumor necrosis factor-related apoptosis-inducing ligand on human peripheral blood mononuclear cells. *Hum Immunol.* (2008b) 69:634–46. doi: 10.1016/j.humimm.2008.07.012
183. Hogner K, Wolff T, Pleschka S, Plog S, Gruber AD, Kalinke U, et al. Macrophage-expressed IFN-beta contributes to apoptotic alveolar epithelial cell injury in severe influenza virus pneumonia. *PLoS Pathog.* (2013) 9:e1003188. doi: 10.1371/journal.ppat.1003188
184. Fujikura D, Chiba S, Muramatsu D, Kazumata M, Nakayama Y, Kawai T, et al. Type-I interferon is critical for FasL expression on lung cells to determine the severity of influenza. *PLoS ONE* (2013) 8:e55321. doi: 10.1371/journal.pone.0055321
185. Shim JM, Kim J, Tenson T, Min JY, Kainov DE. Influenza virus infection, interferon response, viral counter-response, and apoptosis. *Viruses* (2017) 9:223. doi: 10.3390/v9080223
186. Bulanova D, Ianevski A, Bugai A, Akimov Y, Kuivanen S, Paavilainen H, et al. Antiviral Properties of chemical inhibitors of cellular anti-apoptotic Bcl-2 proteins. *Viruses* (2017) 9:271. doi: 10.3390/v9100271
187. Kakkola L, Denisova OV, Tynell J, Viiliainen J, Ysenbaert T, Matos RC, et al. Anticancer compound ABT-263 accelerates apoptosis in virus-infected cells and imbalances cytokine production and lowers survival rates of infected mice. *Cell Death Dis.* (2013) 4:e742. doi: 10.1038/cddis.2013.267

2

Advancements in Host-Based Interventions for Influenza Treatment

*Tsz-Fung Yip[1], Aisha Sami Mohammed Selim[1], Ida Lian[2] and Suki Man-Yan Lee[1]**

[1] HKU-Pasteur Research Pole, School of Public Health, The University of Hong Kong, Hong Kong,
[2] School of Life Sciences and Chemical Technology, Ngee Ann Polytechnic, Singapore

Correspondence:
Suki Man-Yan Lee
suki@hku.hk,
myleesuki01@gmail.com

Influenza is a major acute respiratory infection that causes mortality and morbidity worldwide. Two classes of conventional antivirals, M2 ion channel blockers and neuraminidase inhibitors, are mainstays in managing influenza disease to lessen symptoms while minimizing hospitalization and death in patients with severe influenza. However, the development of viral resistance to both drug classes has become a major public health concern. Vaccines are prophylaxis mainstays but are limited in efficacy due to the difficulty in matching predicted dominant viral strains to circulating strains. As such, other potential interventions are being explored. Since viruses rely on host cellular functions to replicate, recent therapeutic developments focus on targeting host factors involved in virus replication. Besides controlling virus replication, potential targets for drug development include controlling virus-induced host immune responses such as the recently suggested involvement of innate lymphoid cells and NADPH oxidases in influenza virus pathogenesis and immune cell metabolism. In this review, we will discuss the advancements in novel host-based interventions for treating influenza disease.

Keywords: host factors, influenza, cytokines, metabolism, immunomodulation

INTRODUCTION

Influenza remains a source of public health concern. Influenza A virus (IAV) has been the cause of historical noxious pandemics, such as the Spanish flu 1918 H1N1, Asian flu H2N2 1957, Hong Kong H3N2 flu 1968, and more recently the pandemic of H1N1 2009 (Swine flu). Influenza also causes seasonal epidemics and outbreaks with high morbidity and mortality rates such as the 2015 H1N1 outbreak in India (1, 2). The error-prone nature of the viral RNA polymerase (RdRP) and virus' capacity for genetic re-assortment (antigenic drift and shift) result in the viral components' susceptibility to mutations, allowing the viruses to evade the immune system and increases their resistance to control strategies.

Currently, influenza vaccination and two classes of antiviral drugs—M2 ion channel blockers (amantadine and rimantadine) and neuraminidase (NA) inhibitor (oseltamivir, zanamivir, and peramivir)—and the novel treatment option using polymerase inhibitor (favipiravir) are considered as mainstays in influenza infection treatment and control. The use of influenza vaccinations remains challenging due to antigenic drifts and shifts, with seasonal variation of new circulating species. Production of vaccine is time consuming with efficacy concerns, especially in the case of pandemic. Variations in vaccine efficacy caused by age should be aware, with studies suggesting that vaccine-conferred protection may not be optimal in certain age groups (3).

The disadvantages of using the conventional antiviral drugs have also been a concern. Significant levels of resistance to both classes of drugs have been repeatedly reported (4, 5). High level of resistance (up to 91%) to M2 blockers has been reported in H3N2 virus strain in American isolates (6). Resistance has also been reported in H5N1 virus (7). IAV resistance to NA inhibitors has also become an increasingly prevalent concern, with the recent highly fatal outbreak of influenza A(H1N1)pdm09 in India 2015 associated with oseltamivir drug resistance (8, 9). In addition, a large cluster of influenza A(H1N1)pdm09 viruses in Japan was found to have increased oseltamivir and peramivir drug resistance (5). There is an urgent need to search for alternative targets to treat influenza virus infections, including non-viral targets such as host cellular factors; which are promising as viruses rely on the host machinery for replication. While host immune response is intended to confer a degree of protection against the infection, an impaired or exaggerated host immune response could be detrimental—IAV H5N1 and H7N9 virus infection was reported to exaggerate aberrant cytokine release, resulting in a cytokine storm that caused accelerated host death (10–12).

Many recent studies have focused on the investigation of targeting host factors to control virus replication as well as modulate immune response, which we have previously evaluated (13). In this review, we will discuss the latest studies (in the past 5 years) on the investigation of novel host-based approaches with potential for influenza treatment.

STRATEGIES TARGETING HOST CELL MACHINERY

The replication cycle of IAV can be grossly divided into four different stages: (1) entry, (2) genome nuclear import, (3) replication and protein synthesis, and (4) genome nuclear export, apical transport, assembly, and budding. As an obligate intracellular pathogen, IAVs are heavily dependent on host machinery for replication and propagation. To this extent, studies employing genome-wide RNA interference (RNAi) to screen for host factors involved in IAV replication cycle have been performed (14, 15) and an increasing number of approaches targeting these host factors to control IAV replication have been investigated.

Entry of IAV

Entry of IAV into the host cell is divided into several steps (16, 17). First, hemagglutinin (HA) on the surface of IAV binds to the terminal α-sialic acid on the host cell receptor. This induces the internalization of the viral particle by clathrin-dependent, caveolin-, and clathrin-independent endocytosis (18). Macropinocytosis was revealed as an alternative entry pathway for IAV (19), which subsequently enters the canonical endocytic pathway (20, 21). The vesicle-containing viral particle forms an early endosome (also known as sorting endosome), which matures into a late endosome as the endocytic pathway progresses. A gradual decrease in intraluminal pH from pH 6.5 to 5.0, mediated by V-ATPase proton pump (22), takes place as the endosome matures (23, 24). This pH drop in the endosomal lumen induces a conformational change in HA, which is activated by proteolytic cleavage to generate HA1 and HA2 from precursor molecule HA0 (25, 26). This conformational change triggers the fusion of the viral envelope with the endosomal membrane, releasing the viral genome into the cytoplasm.

Acidification of the endosome causes the subsequent acidification of viral lumen *via* the IAV M2 proton channel (27), which in turn promotes the dissociation of M1 layer from both the viral envelope (24) and the viral ribonucleoprotein (vRNP) complex (28). Interestingly, a sharp decrease in pH from neutral to an acidic pH of 5.0 as utilized by acid bypass has been observed to be sub-optimal for viral replication. It is hence proposed that a gradual decrease in endosomal pH is necessary for sequential reduction in viral stiffness, dissociation of M1 from the NP in the vRNP complex, destabilization of M1 layer from the viral envelope, and the eventual conformational change of the HA for the release of viral genome and proteins to the cytoplasm from late endosome (24).

Inhibition of Proteolytic Cleavage of HA

Proteolytic cleavage of HA0 to HA1/HA2 is an important step in IAV replication. This cleavage relocates HA2, converting previously uncleaved HA0 to a metastable conformation that induces membrane fusion at acidic pH (29). Inefficient cleavage and activation of HA leads to low infectivity (30). As identified proteins encoded by the viral genome do not possess proteolytic properties, the virus is dependent on host protease for the cleavage of HA. This provides a potential target to control IAV infection. HA is commonly cleaved by trypsin-like proteases at the single arginine residue at position 329. Human airway epithelium serine proteases HAT and TMPRSS2 were identified as the host factors for cleavage at this residue (31).

Aprotinin, purified from bovine lung (32), is a protease inhibitor with a long history of clinical use as an antifibrinolytic agent in cardiac surgery (33). Its potential as an anti-IAV drug has been recognized for over a decade (34) and has been shown to reduce the infectivity of a broad spectrum of IAV strains (34, 35) both *in vitro* (26) and *in vivo* (36). Once withdrawn from the Western drug market due to its association with mortality (33), aprotinin has been approved as a locally administered, small-particle aerosol drug for the treatment of IAV infection in Russia (36). However, side-effects associated with the systemic administration of aprotinin raises the need for an alternative protease inhibitor for use in treatment of IAV infections.

Camostat, a serine protease inhibitor, was reported to demonstrate anti-IAV potential in mice dating back to 1996 (37), but little to no research has been conducted to develop it into an anti-IAV treatment. It was revisited and proven to be one of the most efficient serine protease inhibitors for the inhibition of IAV replication in primary human tracheal epithelial cells *in vitro* when tested compounds were used at similar molarities (35). At present, camostat is widely administered for the treatment of liver fibrosis, chronic pancreatitis, and cancer (38, 39), making it a highly promising candidate for drug repurposing. Despite the lack of association between camostat and increased mortality (as with aprotinin), reports of camostat potentially inducing acute eosinophilic pneumonia (38) warrants the need for careful consideration and further research into the repositioning of drugs from the same class.

Highly pathogenic IAV, such as the H5 and H7 subtypes, are reported to have HA cleavage sites rich in basic residues (30). The polybasic nature of the cleavage sites provides multiple targets for a broad spectrum of proteases, including the more ubiquitously expressed intracellular proteases such as furin (40). This increased protease spectrum could be utilized by these viruses for the activation of HA prior to viral budding, allowing for evasion of potential inhibition by exogenously administered serine protease inhibitors. Furthermore, an *in vivo* study utilizing mice treated with a single protease inhibitor prior to infection with H7 virus bearing a polybasic cleavage site showed poor efficacy despite good results were obtained for infection with H1N1 virus bearing single cleavage site (41), suggesting strain specificity in using serine protease inhibitors to treat IAV infections.

Inhibition of Endosomal Acidification

Endosomal acidification is required for the release of IAV genome (in the form of a vRNP complex) into the cytoplasm (24). Research has shown that an increase in endosomal pH during the early phases of infection could inhibit IAV infection *in vitro* (42), bringing to light the possibility of controlling IAV infection through the prevention of endosomal acidification.

The V-ATPase inhibitor bafilomycin A1, when used at high concentrations (10–100 nM) has been proven to inhibit IAV replication through the efficient suppression of V-ATPase (43, 44). However, prominent cytotoxicity to host cells was also observed at such concentrations (44). Interestingly, lower concentrations (0.1 nM) of bafilomycin A1 lack inhibitory effects on V-ATPase attenuated IAV replication due to disruption of endosomal trafficking. Thus, bafilomycin A1 is suggested to exert its antiviral function *via* distinct mechanisms at differing concentrations.

Diphyllin, isolated from the plant *Cleistanthus collinus*, is a natural compound able to induce a V-ATPase inhibitory effect (45). In contrast to bafilomycin A1, diphyllin is well-tolerated *in vitro* without inducing obvious cytotoxic effects (46). Most notably, diphyllin is found to effectively inhibit replication of viral strains resistant to amantadine and/or oseltamivir (46). Since drug resistance to these widely administered antivirals is of major public health concern (13), diphyllin is regarded as a promising antiviral against drug-resistant IAV strains.

Controlling Cholesterol Homeostasis

The release of IAV genomic material during replication requires the fusion of the endosomal membrane with the viral envelope. Since cholesterol plays a major role in controlling the fluidity of the lipid bilayer in cells, it is hence suspected to have a role in the infection cycle of IAV.

Interferon-induced transmembrane proteins (IFITMs) are proteins expressed in many vertebrates (including humans) and are found on the plasma membrane, the membranes of early and late endosomes, as well as on lysosomes (47, 48). While humans express IFITM1, IFITM2, IFITM3, IFITM5, and IFITM10, only IFITM 1, 2, and 3 are both immune-related as well as interferon (IFN)-inducible (48), and have been observed to restrict the replication of different viruses, including IAV (49). Studies suggest that IFITMs limit viral infection by reducing membrane fluidity and hence restrict the hemifusion (the mixing of lipid bilayer without the release of viral content) of viral and endosomal membranes (50), probably *via* the disruption of cholesterol homeostasis of late endosomes, where viral fusion and genome release conventionally take place (51). A recent study using RNAi also demonstrated that cholesterol homeostasis can be regulated *via* acid phosphatase 2 (ACP2)-mediated Niemann–Pick C2 activity and impaired the membrane fusion of IAV and influenza B virus (IBV) (52), further suggesting the importance of controlling cholesterol homeostasis in the release of viral genome to cytoplasm.

On the contrary, later studies suggest that IFITM3 exerts its antiviral activity in a cholesterol-independent manner, showing that an increase in cholesterol composition of late endosomal membranes fail to inhibit viral membrane fusion (53). In addition, studies suggested the accumulation of cholesterol level in the late endosome does not inhibit the IAV genome release into cytoplasm (54, 55).

With the modulation of cholesterol levels in host endosomal membrane as a mean to inhibit IAV host cell entry is still under debate, further studies are required before clear conclusions can be drawn.

Other Possible Targets for IAV Entry Inhibition

By comparing the miRNA profiles of the IAV-permissive HEK 293T cells and (less permissive) HeLa cells, miRNA-33a has been identified as a negative regulator for IAV infection *via* the inhibition of archain 1 (ARCN1, also known as δ-COPI) (56). ARCN1 is a subunit of the COPI complex that is required for intracellular trafficking and endosome function (57), depletion of which has been reported to inhibit IAV infection (14). Despite impaired IAV internalization caused by ARCN1 depletion *via* siRNA (56, 58), it was not able to recapitulate through acute inhibition of COPI complex by pharmaceutical means (58). It is hypothesized that the long-term (lasting days) perturbation on ARCN1 by RNAi affected the general endosomal trafficking network, a phenomena which cannot be recapitulated by acute pharmaceutical inhibition to block IAV infection (58). The potential of targeting ARCN1 for IAV treatment deserves further investigation, despite the favorable results from RNAi studies.

Blocking the Nuclear Import of vRNP Complex

Nuclear import of vRNP complexes from the cytoplasm following fusion of the viral and the endosomal membrane is required for replication to take place (59). An early study suggested that vRNP complexes could be transported to the periphery of the nucleus (60), while recent studies report that vRNP complexes utilize the importin-α-importin-β1 (IMPα-IMPβ1) system for nuclear import (59, 61) and lacking of importin-α7, in an importin-α7 knockout mouse model were found to be resistant to IAV infection (62).

Ivermectin has long been clinically administered for the treatment of parasitosis (63), but has recently come to attention as a potential inhibitor of IMPα/β (64). Ivermectin inhibition of IMPα/β has shown to inhibit the replication of RNA viruses such as dengue virus and HIV-1 (64). Ivermectin was recently tested for the inhibition of IAV *in vitro*, with nuclear import of vRNP complex (of both wild-type and antiviral MxA escape mutant) efficiently inhibited (65). Given ivermectin's longstanding record of clinical applications and FDA-approved status, repurposing of this drug for the treatment of IAV should be considered, especially while under threat of pandemic IAV outbreak.

Genomic Replication and Protein Synthesis

Following the import of the vRNP complex into the nucleus of the host cell, RdRP uses the vRNA as a template to synthesize mRNA or cRNA. Synthesized cRNA remains in the nucleus for new vRNA generation, while mRNA is exported out of the nucleus for translation. Viral protein products are either transported to the cell surface *via* Golgi (in case of HA and NA) or imported back into the nucleus to bind with vRNA, forming new vRNP complex (59). Numerous host factors are involved in this process and hence could be possible targets for therapeutic intervention.

Regulation of the Splicing of Pre-mRNA

Out of the eight genome segments of IAV, the M and NS segments are well known for undergoing splicing to generate at least two different mRNAs per individual segment (66, 67). Cdc2-like kinase 1 (CLK1) is a kinase which regulates alternative splicing of pre-mRNA (68). Inhibition of CLK1 by the chemical TG003 or knockdown of CLK1 is shown to cause a decrease in M2 mRNA generation and disrupt downstream M2 protein expression, prominently reduced IAV propagation (15).

Clypearin and corilagin were both found to be potent anti-IAV compounds, with a higher therapeutic index than TG003 *in vitro* (69). Clypearin is isolated from herbs used by Chinese medicine practitioners for treating respiratory tract diseases (69), while corilagin is isolated from medicinal plants and herbs. The identification of effective compounds and the systemic investigation of the use of traditional Chinese medicine (TCM) in the treatment of IAV infection open new frontiers in research and therapeutics.

Inhibition of mRNA Export

During replication, viral mRNA is exported from the nucleus to cytoplasm, where protein synthesis takes place. Human RNA polymerase II activity is found to be correlated with IAV replication through the inhibition of nuclear export of certain viral mRNAs, such as M1 mRNA (70).

Cyclosporine A (CsA) is a FDA-approved drug with immunomodulatory functions (71) that has been found to have an anti-IAV effect in both cyclophilin A (CypA)-dependent and -independent manners (72). The CypA-dependent effect was found to correlate with nuclear export of vRNP complex (see Targeting Nuclear Export Complex). The CypA-independent effect caused inhibition of host RNA polymerase II. CsA is a prospective drug candidate for treatment of IAV infections with a relatively high barrier for development of intrinsic drug resistance, as opposed to commonly used antivirals (73).

Nuclear RNA export factor 1 (NXF1) is a host factor that has been identified to be involved in the nuclear export of IAV mRNA. The knockdown of NXF1 in HEK 293T cells revealed prominent viral mRNA nuclear retention in host cell nucleus (74). Protectin D1 (PD1), an endogenously produced lipid in the respiratory tract, has been identified to have potent anti-inflammatory and antiviral effects (75). PD1 production was notably found to be reduced in the lungs of IAV-infected mice. Therapeutic administration of PD1 was shown to significantly reduce IAV mRNA expression, lower lung viral titer, as well as improve survival of IAV-infected mice. Mechanistic studies revealed attenuated cytoplasmic translocation of viral mRNA with such treatment. A decrease in recruitment of viral transcripts to NXF1 was observed while nuclear export of host RNA remained largely unaffected, suggesting a role of PD1 in regulating NXF1 in nuclear export of viral RNA. Natural PD1 expression in the human airway makes this an ideal candidate for novel therapeutics in the treatment of IAV infection.

Inhibition of mRNA Translation

The eukaryotic initiation factor-4A (eIF4A) family plays an important role in protein translation (76, 77). eIF4A impairment has been proven to be related to antiviral activity in a broad spectrum of RNA viruses *in vitro* (78), with inhibition of IAV mRNA translation (79). The eIF4A inhibitors, silvestrol and pateamine A were demonstrated to arrest viral protein synthesis, thus blocking viral genome replication *in vitro* (80). Although both silvestrol and pateamine A caused high cytotoxicity at the concentration required effective for IAV inhibition, drugs targeting mRNA translation for various diseases have been approved by FDA or are under active development (81). As such, inhibition of IAV infections by disrupting mRNA translation may well be a therapeutic approach in the future.

Inhibition of HA Maturation

Post-translational modifications during protein maturation ensure proper function of proteins, with proteins of IAV no exception. Nitazoxanide, a FDA-licensed drug used to treat enteritis, was found to be effective in controlling IAV infection by interfering with HA N-glycosylation as well as intracellular trafficking in host cell and eventually led to a reduction in viral budding (82). Despite the mechanism of nitazoxanide being presently unknown, its ability to inhibit replication of numerous viruses [IAV, respiratory syncytial virus, coronavirus, hepatitis B virus, and many others (83)] suggests that it may act on host machinery. The drug has also been proven *in vitro* to inhibit the propagation of many circulating strains of human IAV, including those resistant to oseltamivir or zanamivir (84). Nitazoxanide has a high barrier of resistance to IAV (83) and other viral strains resistance to neuraminidase inhibitors (85), making it a very promising therapeutic target for IAV treatment. The drug is currently under phase III clinical trials (83).

Nuclear Export, Assembly, Apical Transport, and Viral Budding

In the later stage of viral replication, viral RNAs of IAV packed with RdRP and NP (known as vRNP complexes) are exported from the nucleus (59), assembled (86), and transported to the plasma membrane [apical in polarized cells (87)] for budding.

Inhibition of Nuclear Export

Targeting Nuclear Export Complex

Exportin 1 (XPO1, also known as CRM1) is well known for its function in the nuclear export of protein (88) and RNA, including viral RNA (89). Similar to HIV (89, 90), IAV viral RNA does not directly bind to XPO1 but is instead held together by several viral proteins. The viral nuclear export protein (NEP, or previously known as NS2) and the vRNP complex have been proposed as the nuclear export complex (91). Cellular XPO1 has been proven to be crucial in the nuclear export of the vRNP complex, with early studies using leptomycin B (LMB), a potent XPO1 inhibitor, revealing that *in vitro* inhibition of XPO1 led to nuclear retention of vRNP complex (92, 93). However, LMB was deemed unsuitable for development as a potential drug in the phase I clinical trial due to observed cytotoxic effects (94).

Verdinexor (also known as KPT-355) is a new bioavailable selective inhibitor of XPO1. It has been shown to be effective against different strains of IAVs both *in vitro* and *in vivo* as prophylactic and therapeutic treatments (95, 96). It is worth mentioning that delayed administration of verdinexor at day 4 post-infection was still deemed beneficial, with reduced viral load *in vivo* (96). This suggests a prolonged therapeutic time window when compared to the mainstay antiviral drugs such as oseltamivir, where recommended administration is at the early stage of infection (within 48 h of symptom onset) (97). Currently, verdinexor has passed the phase I clinical study trials, suggesting that it does not pose severe cytotoxic effects as LMB does.

In addition, a recent report demonstrated that a new drug, DP2392-E10, which binds and inhibits the function of XPO1, can suppress IAV replication *in vitro* (98) further strengthens the concept of IAV intervention by targeting XPO1.

Viral M1 protein is crucial in assisting the nuclear export of vRNP complex. It was commonly suggested that M1 protein links vRNP complex to viral nuclear export protein NEP which interacts with XPO1 for nuclear export (59). Thus, viral M1 protein may serve as a target to inhibit nuclear export of vRNP. As previously mentioned (see Inhibition of mRNA Export), CsA inhibits IAV replication *via* both CypA-dependent and -independent mechanisms. A recent study using a transgenic mice overexpressing CypA showed greater resistance to IAV challenge (99). In the CypA-dependent mechanism, CsA enhances the binding of CypA to M1 protein (72), increases the self-association of M1, and hinders M1 nuclear import (100). CsA also promotes the CypA-dependent degradation of viral M1 protein (72, 101). CsA seems to be a promising drug to inhibit the nuclear export of vRNP complex by inhibiting viral M1 protein stability and function.

Recently, CD151, a tetraspanin (defined by four transmembrane domains with conserved residues) that is expressed abundantly in lungs and interacts with integrins has been implicated in the regulation of IAV replication *in vitro* and *in vivo* (102). Knockdown of CD151 in primary human nasal epithelial cells resulted in the nuclear retention of host XPO1, viral NP, NEP, and M1 proteins, with an increased survival rate observed in IAV-infected CD151 knockout mice. Co-immunoprecipitation assays suggest that CD151 interacts with viral NP, M1, and NEP proteins (102); however, the exact domains involved in interaction and the mechanism of CD151 function in nuclear export remain unclear. Given that a small molecule inhibitor for CD151 is now under development (103), more data revealing the role of CD151 in IAV infection and subsequent use in targeting CD151 as anti-IAV therapy is anticipated.

Targeting the Raf/MEK/ERK Pathway

During IAV infection, Raf/MEK/ERK signaling cascade is activated, while the inhibition of MEK by U0126, probably mediated *via* myosin (light chain) (104), a known motor protein, impairs the nuclear export of vRNP complexes (105). Suppressing IAV replication by inhibition of Raf/MEK/ERK signaling cascade has been illustrated both *in vivo* (106) and *in vitro* (105). The replication of IBV (107) as well as Borna disease virus (108) was shown to be inhibited by U0126, suggesting the versatility of this approach in controlling infection by different viruses. Despite being effective when administered locally to lungs *via* aerosol, U0126 has little effect when administered orally (106).

Another MEK inhibitor, CI-1040 (also known as PD184352) was shown to have high potency against IAV *in vitro* (106). CI-1040 has completed phase II clinical trials as an anti-tumor drug, with the application of CI-1040 as a potential anti-IAV drug candidate recently revisited. Unlike U0126, CI-1040 is orally bioavailable and oral administration of CI-1040 at 48 h post-infection protected 60% of the IAV-infected mice, while the oseltamivir-treated group experienced a 100% death rate (109). Oseltamivir is known to be effective only when administered in the early stages of IAV infection. This suggests the potential use of CI-1040 as an agent used in IAV treatment due to its potentially longer therapeutic time window than mainstay antivirals.

Formyl peptide receptor 2 (FPR2) located at the host cell surface was identified as an ERK stimulator (110). Antagonizing FPR2 promoted the survival of IAV-infected mice (110). Furthermore, FPR2 antagonists have been described to possess antiviral activity against not only IAV but also IBV infection (111), promoting the idea that antagonizing FPR2 to suppress Raf/MEK/ERK signaling cascade could potentially be a novel approach for the treatment of a broad spectrum of influenza viruses.

Apical Transport of Viral Components

After the nuclear export of the vRNP complexes, host cell's intracellular transport mechanism is required to deliver vRNP complexes to the host plasma membrane for the assembly of viral RNAs and proteins at the final stage of viral replication. Among the various vesicular compartments found in a cell, the Rab11A$^+$ endosomes are known to recycle endocytosed membrane proteins and lipids to the plasma membrane for membrane homeostasis (112), a property utilized by many RNA viruses, including IAV (87, 113–115). IAV progeny virus production was found to be significantly reduced in Rab11A$^+$ knockdown human cell lines (116). Furthermore, vRNP complex plasma membrane transport perturbation was observed in *Rab11A* knockdown cells (114, 115); in cells expressing deletion mutant of Rab11 family interacting proteins (87); as well as cells treated with chemicals to interfere microtubule (114). Direct interaction of vRNP complex with Rab11A has also been verified (114, 115), demonstrating the dependence of vRNA complex transport on Rab11A$^+$ vesicles and the microtubule network during viral replication. Since Rab11A proteins do not confer any mobile properties to the vesicle, molecular motors such as kinesins are required for the active transportation of vesicles through cytoskeletons.

KIF13A, a kinesin-3 family member, was recently identified as a molecular motor for plasma membrane transportation of vRNP-loaded Rab11A+ vesicles (117). KIF13A knockdown was found to reduce progeny virus production. Overexpression of a mutant form of KIF13A lacking in motor capacity resulted in disruption of the plasma membrane distribution of vRNP complex during later stages of infection. This data suggest that the apical transport of viral components *via* Rab11A or KIF13A could potentially serve as therapeutic targets against IAV infection. Further examination is merited.

Tubulin acetylation and deacetylation affects microtubule stability (118). Histone deacetylase 6 (HDAC6) was found to deacetylate α-tubulin, one of the subunits of microtubule (119). A study has demonstrated that HDAC6 is involved in IAV replication (120). Inhibition of HDAC6 by tubacin or knockdown of HDAC6 gene resulted in an increase of progeny virus production with vRNP complex redistributed toward the periphery of infected cells. In addition, transportation of HA to the plasma membrane for viral budding was also found to be inhibited by HDAC6. This data suggests that activation of HDAC6 by its stimulant could be a potential approach to anti-IAV therapy, despite HDAC6 stimulants still being under development.

Interference of Viral Budding

While several studies have suggested IAV transmission between cells through apical membranes (121) and intercellular connections (122), virus budding from cell membranes remains the major route for transmission of viruses to uninfected cells. NA is responsible for the cleavage of sialic acid to prevent the interaction between HA and the host cell during viral budding. Besides, viral NA, viral HA, M1 as well as M2, are also suggested to play an important role in the initiation of the budding process (123, 124).

In Section "Controlling Cholesterol Homeostasis," we discussed the involvement of host cholesterol in viral membrane fusion and viral genome release to cytoplasm. Recent studies have demonstrated that host cholesterol may also play an important role in viral budding. It was demonstrated that overexpression of annexin A6 (AnxA6), a phospholipid binding protein, could lead to a decrease in cholesterol levels within the Golgi apparatus and plasma membrane (55), ultimately causing a reduction in egression of progeny virion from infected cells (54). This reduction could be reversed by the addition of exogenous cholesterol (55). Similar to AnxA6 overexpression, addition of a hydrophobic polyamine, U18666A, could reduce cholesterol level in plasma membrane, also inhibited viral replication (55). Since IAV is assumed to bud from lipid rafts (cholesterol-rich plasma membrane domains) (123), it was demonstrated that AnxA6 overexpression or U18666A treatment could hinder progeny virus production by lowering the cholesterol content in the plasma membrane. This hypothesis was strengthened through recent studies resolving the cholesterol-binding site of viral M2 protein, suggesting that IAV M2 clustering (which provides membrane curvature for scission) is mediated by cholesterol (125). A recent report utilizing two different FDA-approved cholesterol-lowering drugs, gemfibrozil and lovastatin, stated that there was reduction in stability and infectivity of progeny virus compared to that replicating within cholesterol-sufficient host cells (126). Taken together, this data suggests that controlling cellular cholesterol content would be an effective alternative with drugs available for repurposing IAV treatment. Further *in vivo* works are needed to confirm this hypothesis.

The Gi-type G-protein coupled receptor α2-adrenergic receptors (α2-ARs) have been recently identified as a key host factor involved in IAV replication (127). Apical transport of the viral protein HA is inhibited by low intracellular cAMP level after stimulating the α2-AR-mediated signaling. *In vitro* stimulation of α2-AR by its agonist clonidine inhibits IAV replication. Therapeutic administration of clonidine reduced pulmonary edema and improved survival rate of IAV-infected mice. Development of a new antiviral targeting the α2-AR-mediated signaling seems promising and deserves further investigation.

Interrupting the Virus Replication Cycle by Combinatory Use Targeting Both Virus and Host Factors

Although targeting host factors for viral interventions generally provides a better resistance barrier, emergence of resistance may still arise (61). Therefore, combined use of interventions targeting both virus and host factors have been recommended to reduce opportunities for viral development of resistance. One such example would be the combined administration of NA inhibitor (oseltamivir) alongside an anti-host factor [such as V-ATPase inhibitor diphyllin (46), HA maturation inhibitor nitazoxanide (85), FPR2 antagonists (111), and XPO1 inhibitor verdinexor (96)]. While further direct assessment for the ease of emergence of escape mutants between single and combinatory use of drugs is required, the synergistic effects of a combined, multi-drug approach observed thus far highly suggest an increased effectiveness over a single-drug approach.

Table 1 summarizes novel host targets regulating IAV replication. Compared to RNAi, small molecular chemicals remain the best choice as drug candidates due to their fast acting and easy-to-deliver properties. Although small molecular chemicals targeting certain host factors aforementioned have yet to be developed, their RNAi-identified involvement in the IAV replication cycle provide leads for the development of new IAV interventions.

REGULATION OF ABERRANT IMMUNE RESPONSES IN IAV INFECTION

The immune system aims to protect the host from infection and clear the pathogen once an infection occurs. In addition, the complex networks formed between the host physiology and the immune system co-operatively shape the disease outcome; modulations on the networks could alleviate disease severity in IAV infections.

The immunological responses elicited by IAV infection has been reviewed in detail (128–130). At the initial stage of IAV

TABLE 1 | Advancements on targeting host factors for antivirals.

Cellular target	New potential therapeutic approach	Suggested function	Reference
Viral entry			
Serine proteases	Camostat	Inhibits HA0 cleavage	Yamaya et al. (35)
V-ATPase	Diphyllin	Inhibits endosomal acidification	Chen et al. (46)
Acid phosphatase 2	siRNA	Indirectly disrupts cholesterol homeostasis	Lee et al. (52)
Nuclear import			
Importins	Ivermectin	Inhibits nuclear import of viral ribonucleoprotein (vRNP) complex	Gotz et al. (65)
Genomic replication and protein synthesis			
Cdc2-like kinase 1	Clypearin	Attenuates M2 splicing	Zu et al. (69)
RNA polymerase II	Cyclosporine A	Inhibits viral mRNA export	Ma et al. (73)
Nuclear RNA export factor 1	PD1	Inhibits viral RNA export	Morita et al. (75)
Eukaryotic initiation factor-4A	a. Silvestrol b. Pateamine A	Inhibits mRNA translation	Slaine et al. (80)
vRNP complex nuclear export			
XPO1	a. Verdinexor b. DP2392-E10	Inhibit vRNP complex nuclear export	a. Perwitasari et al. (95, 96) b. Chutiwitoonchai et al. (98)
CypA	Cyclosporine A	Promotes M1 degradation	Liu et al. (72, 101)
CD151	siRNA	Inhibits vRNP complex nuclear export	Qiao Y. et al. (102)
MEK	CI-1040	Inhibits MEK to suppress phosphorylation of myosin light chain leading to nuclear retention of vRNP complex	Haasbach et al. (109)
Formyl peptide receptor 2 (FPR2)	WRW4	Inhibits activation of Raf/MEK/ERK by the ligation of AnxA1 to FPR2	Courtin et al. (111)
Viral component apical transport			
KIF13A	To be determined	Blocks vRNP apical transport	Ramos-Nascimento et al. (117)
Histone deacetylase 6	To be determined	Regulates microtubule stability	Husain et al. (120)
AnxA6	To be determined	Reduces plasma membrane cholesterol level and decreases virion egress or stability	Musiol et al. (55)
Cholesterol	U18666A	Reduces plasma membrane cholesterol level and decreases virion egress	Musiol et al. (55)
α2-adrenergic receptors	Clonidine	Reduces intracellular cAMP to impair Influenza A virus HA plasma membrane transport	Matsui et al. (127)
Other			
Cholesterol	a. Gemfibrozil b. lovastatin	Reduces progeny virus stability and infectivity	Bajimaya et al. (126)

infection, the respiratory epithelial cells are the primary target for infection. Once the infection is initiated, the recognition of infection is accomplished *via* the detection of pathogen-associated molecular patterns (PAMPs) by pattern recognition receptors (PRRs) (see Toll-Like Receptors), and lead to the expression and secretion of different cytokines and chemokines, such as IL-6, IL-8, tumor necrosis factor (TNF)-α, and CCL2 as well as type I and III IFNs. As sentinel cells, alveolar macrophages could also be infected, inducing cytokines and is the main source of type I IFNs (128, 129). Type I IFNs are known inducer for the upregulation of death receptor 5, which is the receptor for TNF-related apoptosis-inducing ligand (TRAIL), in lung pneumocytes (128). IL-8 and CCL2 produced by both epithelial cells and macrophages act as chemoattractants for neutrophils and monocytes, respectively. Neutrophils are one of the earliest immune cells being recruited to the site of infection (131) with transmigration of neutrophils carry out by adhesion molecules, such as CD11a, CD11b, and CD18 (132). In addition to the antiviral activity of neutrophil-released reactive oxygen species (ROS), defensin and pentraxin (132), uptaking IAV by neutrophils could also help in controlling viral propagation as these cells do not support replication of IAV (133). Besides controlling viral replication, neutrophils also play an important role in guiding the migration of IAV-specific CD8^{+} T-cells in the infection site by secreting and leaving a trail of CXCL12 (134). Infiltrated monocytes will, however, differentiate into macrophages or dendritic cells (DCs).

The monocytes-derived macrophages are reported to be a permissive host for IAV production (135), sustaining inflammation by producing cytokines in a magnitude larger than that of the resident alveolar macrophages. The monocyte-derived DC as well as the resident airway CD11c^{low}B220^{+} plasmacytoid DC (pDC) and two types of conventional DCs (CD103^{+}CD11b^{low} and CD103^{-}CD11b^{hi}) acquire the antigen of the invading pathogen through either direct infection or up-taking infected dead cells (129). In the presence of type I IFNs, DCs mature when encountering PAMPs from invading pathogen (129). Depending on the sub-cellular localization of the antigen, cytosolic and endosomal antigen will be loaded onto major histocompatibility complex (MHC) class I and II molecules respectively (130). Once mature, DCs migrate from the infection site to the draining lymph nodes *via* the interaction of CCR7 and CCL19/CCL21 (130, 136) for antigen presentation *via* MHC class I and II to naïve CD8^{+} and CD4^{+} T-cells, respectively (137–140). Interestingly, monocytes-derived DCs that engulfed the infected dead cells are poor antigen presenters for CD8^{+} T-cells and require the transfer of intact MHC class I/peptide complex to lymph node-resident CD8α^{+} DCs which are the most efficient antigen-presenting cells to CD8^{+} T-cells (137). In addition to antigen presentation, pDC are well known for their high ability in type I IFNs production to limit viral propagation (141).

Within the lymph node, naïve CD8^{+} T-cells are activated by the DCs, differentiate and clonal expand into cytotoxic T-lymphocytes (CTLs) with the aid of various cytokines, including IFN-γ, IL-12, type I IFNs, and IL2 (142, 143), and the help from activated CD4^{+} T helper cells (144). Differentiated CTLs downregulate their lymph node homing receptor CCR7 and upregulate CCR4 and CXCR3 for the migration to the site of infection. Within the site of infection, CTLs control viral replication by targeting and inducing apoptosis of virus-infected cells *via* the secretion of perforin and granzymes as well as the ligation of death receptors on the infected cells by TNF, Fas ligand, and TRAIL. On the other hand, CD4^{+} T-cells are activated by the presentation of MHC class II/antigen complex by DCs, with co-stimulatory receptors such as CD28 expressed on the T-cells and the ligand for CD28 (CD80 and CD86) expressed on DCs playing an important role (144). Activation of CD4^{+} T-cells lead to differentiation into different effector cells subsets, including the classical Th1 and Th2, and the more recently identified regulatory T cells, follicular T helper cells, Th9, and Th17 subsets (144). Th1 cells regulate to the differentiation of CTLs as mentioned whereas Th2 cells contributes to the activation of B-cells through CD40L. Within the pregerminal center of the lymph node, the follicular T helper cells interact with antigen-primed B-cells and promote their proliferation. Antigen-primed B-cells differentiates into plasmablast and undergo antibody class-switching in the germinal center (145). Detailed functions of regulatory T cells, follicular T cells, Th9, and Th17 cells are discussed elsewhere (144, 145). Plasmablasts enter the blood-stream, are recruited to the inflamed tissue, and terminally differentiate into plasma B cells which specialize in the production of antibody for pathogen neutralization, opsonization, and antibody-dependent cell-mediated cytotoxicity, etc. Memory T- and B-cells are also developed during the maturation process, and has been discussed and reviewed elsewhere (146–149). A schematic diagram showing a summary of the immune response after IAV infection has been illustrated in **Figure 1**.

The Yin and Yang theory is always used to describe the importance in balancing the host immune response. In the light of this theory, the treatment strategy aims to suppress the overwhelming activation of the host immune response and in reverse to compensate any unfavorable suppression.

Although adaptive immune responses are important in viral clearance, the immediate innate immunity play an important role in the early control of an infection, and conversely, is a major factor for disease severity due to immunopathology. Dysregulated immune responses caused by viral infections have been implicated in severe disease development (150, 151), such as acute lung injury (ALI). ALI in its most severe form, known as acute respiratory distress syndrome (ARDS), is reported to be the most prevalent cause of mortality in IAV-infected patients (152).

Studies suggested that IAV strains could be associated with either over-activating (human infection by avian H5N1 and H7N9) (153, 154) or suppressing (H1N1, H3N2) (155) immune response.

Regulation of Neutrophil Infiltration and Neutrophil Extracellular Trap

Recent history has seen the outbreak of IAV pandemics of varying severity takes place at the cost of millions of lives. One such example would be the deadly Spanish flu of 1918, which claimed the lives of 20–50 million of the 500 million people infected worldwide.

The pathological examination of lung sections from mice infected with reconstituted 1918 IAV virus revealed necrotizing bronchiolitis and severe alveolitis in tissue, with neutrophils observed as the predominant inflammatory cell type present (156), suggesting neutrophil involvement in the pathogenesis of IAV infection.

The majority of immune cells in blood circulation are neutrophils; of which they are among the first innate immune cells recruited to the site of infection (131). Neutrophils characteristically control microbial infections by generating bactericidal (157) neutrophil extracellular traps (NETs), consisting of granule proteins, histones, and decondensed chromatin (131). Both protective and destructive role of neutrophils in IAV infections have been described. The contrasting role of neutrophils could be explained by factors such as viral strain and viral dose used in different experimental setup, etc.

The protective role of neutrophils was observed when mice infected with a low, non-lethal dose of IAV H3N2 strain HKx31 displayed neutrophil-mediated viral clearance *via* phagocytosis (132, 158). Depletion of neutrophils has found to enhance viral load in the IAV-infected animals (158).

On the contrary, this protective nature is disputed due to the association of neutrophil-generated NETs. Extensive NET formation was observed in mice infected with PR8, an IAV strain highly pathogenic to mice (159). Histones and myeloperoxidase within the NET induce cell death of lung epithelium and endothelium (157), leading to the loss of integrity of the alveolar-capillary barrier, a characteristic of ALI. Yet, while histones have

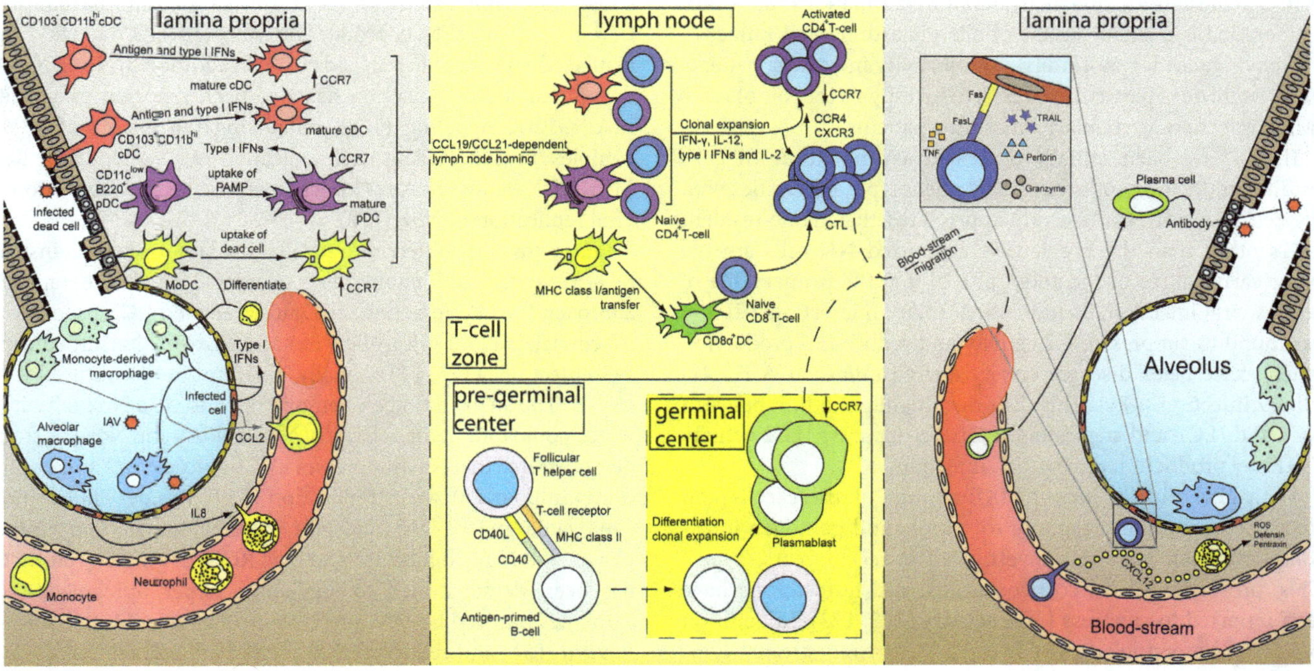

FIGURE 1 | Immune responses of primary influenza A virus (IAV) infection. At the initial stage of infection (left), airway epithelial cells and pneumocytes are major targets for IAV. Various cytokines are secreted by these cells as well as alveolar macrophages to induce inflammation and recruits blood immune cells. Infiltrated neutrophils secrete different antimicrobial products to control viral replication. Besides, CXCL12 is secreted by neutrophils to guide the cytotoxic T-lymphocytes (CTLs) in the later stage of infection. Infiltrated monocytes will further differentiate into monocyte-derived macrophages and monocyte-derived dendritic cells (MoDC). Constant surveying of the airway and uptake of virus-infected dead cells by DCs lead to their maturation. Upregulation of CCR7 results in a CCL19/CCL21-dependent lymph node homing of DCs. Within the lymph node (middle), MoDCs cross-dress CD8α⁺ DC. CD4⁺ and CD8⁺ T-cells are activated by DCs in the presence of cytokines and undergo clonal expansion. Antigen-primed B-cells mature with the aid from follicular T helper cells and further differentiate into plasmablasts in the germinal center. Differential expression of receptors upon maturation of T- and B-cells prompt them to leave the lymph node, enter the blood-stream and recruited to the lung. In the inflamed lung (right), neutrophils leave a trail of CXCL12 to guide CTLs migration. Measures utilized by CTLs for killing infected cells are depicted in inset. Plasmablasts further terminally differentiate into plasma cells and increase antibody production for IAV neutralization.

been shown to suppress IAV replication *in vitro* (160), *in vivo* study demonstrated that there was increase in lung inflammation and damage in IAV-infected mice treated with histones (161). Interestingly, co-treatment of lethally infected mice with anti-histone antibody and oseltamivir resulted in an increase in animal survival when compared to infected mice groups treated solely with oseltamivir (161).

In agreement with the *in vitro* and *in vivo* data, it has been reported that NET produced by cultured neutrophils from patient with H7N9 and severe H1N1 infection increased alveolar epithelial cell permeability (162) leading to ALI. More importantly, plasma NET level positively correlated with the disease severity index (including higher acute physiology and chronic health evaluation II score) and multiple organ dysfunction syndrome (162), further demonstrating the detrimental role of NET in the pathogenesis of severe IAV infections.

Studies have demonstrated the involvement of superoxide dismutase and myeloperoxidase in NETosis, the formation of NET (159). The presence of anti-myeloperoxidase antibody as well as the superoxide dismutase inhibitor (DETC) significantly reduced NETosis. Finally, tetrahydroisoquinolines (163) and a pan-peptidylarginine deiminase (PAD) inhibitor, named Cl-amidine (164) have been suggested to inhibit NETosis. Despite it has been reported that during IAV H1N1 infection, PAD4 knockout mice displayed only slight improvement in weight loss and a slight prolonged but no end-point survival advantage was observed compared to WT mice (165), based on the extensive findings presented above, targeting NET to prevent ALI in the severe case of IAV infection, including the highly pathogenic avian IAV, remain promising and may warrant further investigation.

Innate Lymphoid Cells (ILCs)

Innate lymphoid cells are cells of lymphoid lineages that do not express antigen-specific B- or T-cell receptors (166). Similar to T-helper cells, they are classified into subsets by their ability to produce type 1 (Th1), type 2 (Th2), and type 3 (Th17 and Th22) cytokines.

Previous studies confirmed the involvement of ILCs of group 2 linage (ILC2) in IAV infection and airway inflammation (166, 167). On the positive side, during the recovery phase of IAV infection, ILC2 expresses amphiregulin which promote airway epithelium repair (166, 168), thus facilitating the recovery of the infected lung.

On the other hand, in response to IL-33 produced by macrophages, DCs, and NKT cells, ILC2 secretes IL-5 and IL-13 and induce airway hyper-responsiveness. Recruitment of eosinophils by IL-5 to the lung also mediates airway inflammation (166). Since eosinophilia is a characteristic of allergic asthma and influenza is a major cause for morbidity and mortality in asthma patients (166), it will be of particular interest to investigate the role of ILC2 in IAV infection, particularly in asthma patients.

ILC1s have been initially described as immature NK cells residing in the liver and share many phenotypic similarities with NK cells (169). It was recently appreciated that tissue-resident ILC1s other than the previously recognized NK cells are the major early source of the antiviral IFN-γ at the primary site of various viral infection, including IAV (170). Interestingly, IFN-γ was found to suppress ILC2 activity and reduce IL5 production which exacerbates disease severity during influenza A(H1N1) pdm09 infection (171). This data may highlight a link between ILC1 and ILC2 and suggesting ILC1 can suppress ILC2 activity *via* IFN-γ production during IAV infection.

With ILCs finally identified, functions of these cells and their role in immune response to tumors and pathogen infections have been massively investigated in recent years. Type I IFNs, prostaglandin I_2, corticosteroids, and testosterone have been reported to suppress ILC2 activity (172, 173). In addition to IL-33, the epithelial cytokines IL-25, thymic stromal lymphopoietin, as well as the lipid mediator prostaglandin D_2 were found to activate ILC2 (173). The therapeutic potential of these ILC2 activators and suppressors is yet to be deduced. With more and more studies demonstrating the involvement of ILC in IAV infection, the interplay between different ILC subtypes in IAV infection would, therefore, be an interesting area to explore and modulate the ILC activity may be a future approach to combat IAV infection.

Reactive Oxygen Species

Reactive oxygen species, generated by specialized enzymes such as NADPH oxidases, are released during IAV infection (174). The NADPH oxidase family consists of enzymes containing different catalytic subunit named Nox1–5 and dual oxidase (Duox) 1 and 2. ROS have been reported to display both beneficial (limiting viral replication) and detrimental (promoting ALI) effects in the course of IAV infection. Interestingly, the protective or destructive effect of ROS is dependent on the enzyme of which the ROS is generated (174).

Dual oxidase1 and 2 are found to be host-protective (174, 175). *In vitro*, ROS generated by nuclear Duox indirectly regulates the splicing of IAV mRNAs *via* the nuclear speckle-associated splicing complex (175). In addition to altering viral mRNA splicing, ROS generated by Doux2 has been attributed to the production of IFN-λ, an important anti-IAV IFN. In response to IAV infection, increased viral mRNA replication was observed when *Duox2* was silenced *in vitro* (176). Increased viral replication was also observed in mice with *Doux* silenced (175), further depicting the protective role of Doux in IAV infection.

Unlike Doux, Nox2 activation could be harmful to host. IAV infection was reported to induce Nox2-dependent endosomal ROS production (177). ROS could target the conserved Cys98 on Toll-like receptor (TLR) 7, and inhibit TLR7-mediated type I IFN expression during a mild IAV H3N2 infection *in vivo* (177). IAV-infected mice treated with specific Nox2 inhibitor, cholestanol-conjugated gp91ds-TAT, were found to have reduction in endosomal ROS production, restored TLR7 activity, and displayed a decreased viral load (177). In addition to Nox2, Nox4-dependent ROS production has also been reported to activate MAPK/ERK signaling (178), enhancing the export of vRNP complex, thus increasing viral replication (see Targeting the Raf/MEK/ERK Pathway). *Nox4* knockdown resulted in a reduction of viral replication *in vitro* (178).

Targeting the different NADPH oxidase isoforms, instead of scavenging ROS should be considered as the therapeutic approach for IAV infection, as Doux-mediated ROS production is beneficial (175, 176), while Nox2 and Nox4 are harmful during IAV infections (177, 178). Finally, NS1 (not to be confused with IAV NS1 protein) has been demonstrated to be a Nox inhibitor, which could inhibit the activity of Nox1, Nox2, and Nox4. A study demonstrated that NS1 suppresses IAV-induced Nox2 and significantly inhibits IAV virus replication (179). Besides cholestanol-conjugated gp91ds-TAT and NS1 aforementioned, apocynin, a phagocytic Nox2 inhibitor as well as ROS scavenger (180–182), has been demonstrated to ameliorate hyper upregulation of cytokines induced by IAV infection through SOCS1 and SOCS3 *in vitro* (154) and reduce peri-bronchial inflammation and viral titer *in vivo* (183). Interestingly, ebselen, another Nox2 inhibitor and glutathione peroxidase mimetic, could reduce inflammatory status measured in bronchoalveolar lavage fluid (BALF) of mice pre-exposed to cigarette smoke and subsequently infected with IAV (184). Taken together, these reports highlight the potential use of NADPH oxidases inhibitors and ROS scavengers to treat IAV infections.

Soluble Mediators and Receptor-Based Immunomodulation

Dysregulated cytokine production has been associated with the elevated mortality rate observed in severe IAV infections (185, 186). As such, the immunomodulation of cytokines are regarded as promising therapeutic tactics. Recent advancements developed with this approach will be highlighted in the following section.

Tumor Necrosis Factor

Tumor necrosis factor has two main functions during viral infection—it activates NF-κB, inducing the expression of cytokines responsible for the host immune response; and induces apoptosis through activation of a signaling cascade involving TRADD, FADD, and caspase 3, 7, 8, and 10 (187–189). TNF is known to be highly upregulated in IAV-infected hosts, especially in hosts infected with highly pathogenic IAV (153, 190). However, it is both protective and counter-protective functions associated with TNF that makes it a target in the treatment of IAV.

The protective role of TNF is observed during infection by low pathogenic IAV, where extrinsically derived TNF is responsible for attenuating tissue-damaging $CD8^+$ T-cell response (191). In addition to recruiting monocytic cells to the infection site, $CD8^+$ T-cells response was observed to deteriorate lung pathology (192) and damage healthy, non-infected lung epithelial cells (193) upon IAV infection. Furthermore, TNF deficiency has been associated with an increased detection of IL-15 and IL-6 in BALF (192), which promote the survival of and proliferation of $CD8^+$ T-cells (194, 195) and subsequent tissue damage. Exacerbated lung pathology caused by the upregulation of the monocyte chemoattractant protein-1 was observed in $TNF^{-/-}$ mice infected with sub-lethal dose of IAV (196). In addition, decreased $CD8^+$ T-cell contraction due to enhanced expression of the anti-apoptotic protein Bcl-2 was observed in sub-lethally IAV-infected TNF-deficient mice when compared to WT mice (192). As a whole, there is substantial evidence supporting the protective role of TNF in IAV infection.

On the other hand, the correlation of TNF with pulmonary edema has been well-documented (197). TNF has been observed to stimulate the expression of CXCL2 in alveolar epithelial cells in a transgenic mice model resembling extensive IAV infection in lung tissue, causing alveolar damage, lung edema, and hemorrhage (198). In addition to lung edema, TNF has also been reported to correlate with IAV-associated encephalopathy (199, 200). However, it is notable that despite IAV-associated encephalopathy, direct invasion of the central nervous system is rare (201), suggesting that IAV-associated encephalopathy could instead be a result of peripheral infection. Furthermore, TNF has been shown to increase the permeability of the blood–brain barrier (BBB) (202, 203), contributing to neural damage (204). These studies further support an anti-TNF approach as a potential therapy for severe IAV infection.

At present, etanercept, an anti-TNF drug administered in the treatment of rheumatoid arthritis, is the only TNF inhibitor (or even TNF directed treatment) tested for IAV treatment. Etanercept has been shown to protect against the *in vivo* lethal infection of mice with a highly virulent, mouse-adapted IAV strain (205), with observations made of an increased survival rate with decreased morbidity, expression of the proinflammatory cytokine IL-6, lung injury, and edema (205).

IL-6 and IL-27

The protective role of IL-6 was demonstrated in mice challenged with sub-lethal IAV infection. IL-6-deficient mice displayed exacerbated pulmonary damage (206, 207) and lung injury due to an observed decline in the survival of alveolar type II cells and alveolar epithelial cells (207). IAV suppresses the anti-apoptotic Mcl-1 and $Bcl\text{-}X_L$ expression, causing cell death of neutrophils which are critical in viral clearance (206). Addition of IL-6 restored the expression of Mcl-1 and $Bcl\text{-}X_L$ *in vitro* and is considered as the underlying mechanism for the observed survival advantage of WT mice over *IL-6* knockout mice during mild IAV infection.

IL-6 has also been shown to induce the proliferation of lung $IL\text{-}10^+$ regulatory T cells and IL-27, which act to limit excessive proliferation of $CD8^+$ T-cells and subsequent $CD8^+$-inflicted damage. This would hence prevent the tissue damage observed in lung immunopathology (208).

Despite the apparent protective role of IL-6, high levels of IL-6 in serum or cerebrospinal fluid have been reported in severe neurologically complicated IAV cases, with IL-6 used as a marker for prognosis (199–201, 209, 210). The role of IL-6 in regulation of BBB permeability was reported (211), with potentially detrimental neurological complications. As such, the suppression of hyper-induced IL-6 as a form of therapy in severe IAV infection should be considered. One such option is the anti-IL6 antibody-based drug tocilizumab, which is currently administered clinically for the treatment of rheumatoid arthritis. However, study on the usage of this drug to treat hyper upregulation of IL-6 due to severe IAV infection has yet to be conducted. On the other hand, in a case of H1N1 virus-induced ARDS, the use of an extracorporeal cytokine hemoadsorption device to remove cytokines including TNF and IL-6 from the bloodstream (212) has showed beneficial to the patient (213). More research is required to confirm whether the removal or neutralization of IL-6 could be a potential therapy for severe IAV infections.

The activation of $CD8^+$ T-cell is crucial for viral clearance. It should, however, be tightly regulated to limit $CD8^+$ T-cell inflicted host cell damage. IL-6 mediates IL-27 induction (208). IL-27 acts to suppress $CD8^+$ T-cells and reduce morbidity through IL-10 and regulatory T-cells (208). Much like other immunomodulatory approaches, the timing for applying IL-27 should be carefully assessed. Compared to placebo-treated IAV-infected group, early administration of IL-27 to IAV-infected mice in fact led to poorer viral clearance, increased morbidity, and deteriorated lung histopathology, while IL-27 administration during the recovery phase (5–10 days post-infection) accelerated recovery and improve lung immunopathology (214). Notably, IL-27 could also suppress Th17 responses and increases susceptibility to secondary *S. aureus* infection (215). Therefore, co-administration of antibiotics should be considered when utilizing IL-27 as potential IAV treatment.

Type I and III Interferons

Both type I and III IFNs have antiviral properties, with viruses counteract IFNs to gain an advantage for their propagation. The IAV viral protein NS1 inhibits the production of IFNs by antagonizing IRF-3, a key transcriptional factor for IFNs. This prevents the processing of cellular pre-mRNAs (including those for IFNs) and directly interacts with retinoic acid-inducible gene (RIG)-I receptors, which are critical in innate sensing, to suppress IFN production during infection (216, 217). In addition to inhibiting IFN expression, the induction of SOCS3 inhibits IFNs signaling by suppressing cytokine signaling has been documented (155).

The recognition of 5′ triphosphate on viral RNA by RIG-I receptor is shown to induce the expression of SOCS3, which in turn represses type I IFNs expression (155). Due to IFNs being a key contributor to antiviral immune response, an impairment of type I or III IFN production may cause the escalation of otherwise mildly pathogenic IAV infection into a life-threatening one (218).

While type I IFN has been demonstrated to inhibit IAV replication *in vitro* (219); the *in vivo* administration of type I IFN in animal models only displayed effectiveness in a prophylactic capacity. A lowered viral titer was detected in the nasal wash of test animals. However, host susceptibility to IAV infection remained unchanged (219). Notably, this protective effect is only conferred by an optimal dose of type I IFN of low to moderate amounts (10–100 units per mice daily); with higher dosages (1,000–10,000 units per mice daily) shown to increase morbidity (220). In addition, clinical trials demonstrated that prophylactic administration of type I IFN reduced disease severity and lowered susceptibility to IAV in males and participants aged 50 or above (221).

Despite relatively successful results seen in the prophylactic use of IFNs, its therapeutic use is of greater clinical relevance. Mice treated with type I IFN post-IAV infection showed a successful reduction in lung IAV titer but displayed increased morbidity and mortality in comparison to vehicle-treated mice (222). A possible explanation for this phenomenon is the induction of excessive inflammatory response and TRAIL-DR5-mediated epithelial cell death by type I IFN (223), which accounts for the observed lung pathology in IAV-infected animals treated with type I IFN (224). In addition, downregulation of γδ T-cells by type I IFN has been correlated with increased susceptibility to secondary *S. pneumoniae* infection (225), further arguing against the potential use of type I IFNs for the treatment of IAV infection.

In comparison to type I IFNs, the administration of type III IFNs may provide advantages in the control of IAV replication (176, 222, 224) without the risk of previously reported type I IFNs-mediated immunopathologic side-effects (222, 224, 226). However, a recent study aiming to stimulate IFNs signaling through the systematic administration of RIG-I ligand post-IAV infection demonstrated that type I, but not type III IFNs signaling is important in conferring protection during fatal IAV infection *in vivo* (227). Though, this study did not measure the production of type I and III IFNs as well as any changes in viral load with respect to *Ifnar* or *Ifnlr* knockout. In addition, while human immune cells are not primary targets in IAV infection, they could be susceptible to IAV and become efficient host cells for virus replication. They are reported to possess a subpar response to type III IFNs (222); leading to the preliminary conclusion that solely using type III IFN as treatment may not be feasible. As such, reports suggesting the use of type III IFNs over type I IFNs as a front-line therapeutic agent to counter IAV infections may require further investigation.

Prostaglandin E_2

The inhibition of COX-2 by selective inhibitors, nimesulide and celecoxib, was previously demonstrated to suppress the hyper upregulation of pro-inflammatory cytokines induced by highly pathogenic avian IAV (228–230). In addition, the use of zanamivir in tandem with a specific COX-2 inhibitor was shown to increase the survival rate of mice lethally infected with avian H7N9 IAV, when compared to mice treated solely with zanamivir (229).

Activated COX-2 regulates downstream prostaglandin production. One such example is PGE_2, a major type of prostaglandin recently demonstrated to play an important role during IAV infection. PGE_2 was significantly upregulated in response to IAV infection, leading to the inhibition of antiviral type I IFN production in macrophages and the subsequent increase in virus replication (231). The use of chemicals AH6809 and GW627368X to antagonize PGE_2 downstream signaling molecules EP2 and EP4 respectively, was shown to induce antiviral type I IFN production. The *in vivo* treatment of mice lethally challenged IAV with both EP2 and EP4 antagonists significantly improved the survival rate.

A recent study demonstrated the ability of a modified TCM decoction to reduce PEG_2 production and subsequent morbidity in mice lethally challenged with IAV. Improved lung pathology was observed (232). The long history of clinical TCM use supports the clinical feasibility of PEG_2 inhibition as an option to treat severe IAV infections.

Toll-Like Receptors (TLRs)

Pattern recognition receptors on host cells sense specific PAMPs present on the viral surface or generated during replication. PRRs can be broadly divided into two classes by their function or location. When defined by location, PRRs are classified into 3 groups—membrane-bound (TLRs and C-type lectin receptors), cytosolic (RIG-I-like and NOD-like receptors), and secreted (collectins and pentraxins) (233).

Significant research has been conducted on PRRs with regards to IAV infection. TLRs and RIG-I receptors have been extensively studied for their major roles in eliciting host immune responses (cytokine and IFN expression) during IAV infection (234–236). RIG-I receptors have been investigated for their functional relevance to IAV infection and targeting these receptors as a form of IAV treatment has been extensively reviewed (237–239). This section will cover recent research on TLRs and the targeting of different TLRs to treat IAV infection.

Humans have been identified to express TLR1–10, while mice have been identified to express functional TLR1–9 as well as TLR11–13 (240). Most TLRs—with the exception of TLR3—utilize MyD88 as an adaptor protein during signal transduction. TLR3 utilizes TRIF as an adaptor. TLR4 is known for its ability to utilize either MyD88 or TRIF, with the choice of adaptor dependent on its sub-cellular location (241). Different TLRs, such as TLR3, 7, and 8 (240) as well as TLR2, TLR4, and most recently TLR10 (235), have been revealed to play a role in the orchestration of host immune responses contributing to IAV pathogenesis.

With TLR10 being an exception (242–244), TLR activation largely causes the release of pro-inflammatory cytokines, with hypercytokinemia leading to ALI as a major cause of mortality in severe IAV infections. In addition to dysregulated cytokine release, excessive production of ROS has been associated with ALI development. In fact, lung injury during severe pulmonary infections, such as IAV and SARS, could be caused by oxidative stress (245). IAV infection activates NADPH oxidase that subsequently produces oxidized PAPC, an endogenous phospholipid. The oxidized PAPC serves as an agonist for TLR4, activating a TLR4-TRIF-TRAF6-NF-κB signaling cascade to eventually trigger the release of IL-6, ultimately inducing the onset of ALI. In addition to oxidized PAPC, the induction of endogenous protein S100A9 upon intracellular PRR DDX21 recognition of IAV subsequently induces the activation of TLR4, further contributing to IAV-induced mortality (246). Since TLR4 has been proven to be important in ALI induction (and hence IAV-related mortality), manipulating the stimulation and antagonism of TLR4 could potentially reduce the severity of IAV infections.

Eritoran (E5564) is a specific TLR4 antagonist initially purposed for the treatment of sepsis, but a failed a phase III clinical trial due to improved patient care in the placebo group prevented its eventual use in sepsis treatment (247). *In vivo* administration of eritoran in mice lethally infected with IAV resulted in improved clinical score, lung pathology results, and reduced viral titer. Delayed administration of eritoran, at day 6 after infection beyond the recommended therapeutic time window (within 48 h after the first display of clinical symptom) for use of oseltamivir (248), also demonstrated a significant benefit to infected mice compared to non-treated group, suggesting a prolonged therapeutic time window for IAV treatment when compared to mainstay antiviral drug treatment. A newer and structurally simpler specific TLR4 antagonist, FP7 (249), alongside a newly developed decoy peptide 2R9 that has been shown to disrupt TLR2, 4, 7, and 9 signaling *via* TIRAP, has been shown to protect mice from lethal IAV infection (250). These results support the potential use of TLR4 antagonism as a means to treat severe IAV infection.

The suppression of other TLR signaling pathways—such as blocking TLR2-mediated signaling through the use of an anti-TLR2 antibody, significantly protected against lethality when administered on day 2 and 4 post-IAV infection (251).

A study also demonstrated that H5N1-infected TLR3 knock-out mice had better survival than H5N1-infected wild-type mice, which is evident through the significantly faster regaining of body weight post-infection, lower viral titer in the lung, and fewer pathological changes in the lung (252).

An increasing number of TLR antagonists are now under development (253, 254), alongside several other agents also shown to have effects on TLRs. Polysaccharides isolated from *R. isatidis*, a traditional Chinese medicinal herb used to treat IAV infection, have recently been shown to inhibit pro-inflammatory cytokines such as IL-6 and CCL-5 *in vitro* by down-regulating upstream TLR3 expression (255). MENK, an endogenous protein expressed in the adrenal medulla, was shown to both prophylactically and therapeutically increase the survival rate while reducing viral-caused lung pathology and viral titer in mice lethally challenged with IAV (256). This was determined to be caused by the downregulation of TLR7. These results suggest the potential of down-regulating TLR expression in the treatment of IAV infection.

The above-mentioned data suggest modulation of TLR signaling or expression as a promising approach in treating severe influenza disease and deserves immediate investigation. **Table 2** summarizes new immunomodulatory approaches to combat IAV infections.

MODULATION OF METABOLISM

It is well documented that patients with diabetes mellitus have a greater tendency to develop severe IAV infection than healthy patients (257). Hyperglycemia increases susceptibility of the

TABLE 2 | New immunomodulatory approaches to treat influenza A virus (IAV) infection.

Potential target/ approach	Possible intervention	Effect	Reference
Histones	Anti-histone antibodies	Prevents lung inflammation and damage induced by histones	Ashar et al. (161)
NETosis	a. Cl-amidine b. Tetrahydroisoquinolines (both tested on NETosis, effect on IAV yet to be determined)	Prevents lung injury mediated by NET	a. Kusunoki et al. (164) b. Martinez et al. (163)
ILC2	To be determined	Promotes airway epithelium repair	Califano et al. (171)
Nox2	a. Cholestanol-conjugated gp91ds-TAT b. Apocynin [also as reactive oxygen species (ROS) scavenger] c. Ebselen (also as ROS scavenger and glutathione peroxidase mimetic)	Inhibits Nox2 activity	a. To et al. (177) b. Ye et al. (154) c. Oostwoud et al. (184)
Tumor necrosis factor (TNF)	Etanercept	Prevents TNF-mediated lung injury and edema	Shi et al. (205)
IL-6	Administration of IL-6	Inhibits cell death of neutrophils; limits $CD8^+$ T-cell-induced lung injury	Dienz et al. (206); Pyle et al. (208)
IL-27	Administration of IL-27 at recovery phase (5–10 days post-infection)	Promotes recovery and improves lung immunopathology	Liu et al. (214)
Type III IFN	Administration of type III IFN	Controls IAV replication by type III IFN signaling pathways	Davidson et al. (222); Kim et al. (224)
PGE_2 signaling	a. AH6809 (EP2 antagonist) b. GW627368X (EP4 antagonist)	Restores type I IFNs induction which are suppressed by PGE_2 in macrophages	Coulombe et al. (231)
TLR4 signaling	TLR4 antagonists (a. Eritoran and b. FP7)	Ameliorates TLR4-mediated lung injury	a. Shirey et al. (248) b. Perrin-Cocon et al. (249)
TIRAP antagonism	Peptide 2R9	Inhibits multiple TLR signaling	Piao et al. (250)
TLR2 signaling	Anti-TLR2 antibody	Inhibits TLR2 signaling mediated lethality	Shirey et al. (251)
TLR3 signaling	Polysaccharides isolated from *R. isatidis*	Down regulates TLR3 expression to inhibit hypercytokinemia	Li et al. (255)
TLR7 signaling	MENK	Down regulates TLR7 expression and reduces lung pathology	Tian et al. (256)

host to IAV infection *via* viral uptake, through the promotion of V-ATPase assembly (258) and immunosuppression (257). In addition, viruses rely on host metabolism to perform essential functions during replication (259–262). These processes exert a large energy demand on the host within a very short period of time (263); energy of which is supplied by and is dependent on host metabolism. IAV viruses have been reported to modify the metabolic state of the host. For example, increased c-Myc-dependent glycolysis and glutaminolysis has been demonstrated in infected cells (264). The changes in glucose and glutamine metabolism were reversed upon the addition of BEZ235, which inhibited the IAV-mediated c-Myc induction. Administration of BEZ235 2 days prior to infection and up to 4 days post-infection was shown to decrease lung viral titer and improve the survival rate in IAV-infected mice. Small molecules such as clotrimazole and α-mangostin that target lipid metabolism have also been demonstrated to suppress IAV replication *in vitro* (264).

In addition to being important for generating energy and biosynthesis, recent research demonstrates that cellular metabolism affects immune cell function. Dysregulated immune responses observed in many diseases are associated with specific metabolic configurations. Viruses, influenza inclusive (265), were found to induce drastic alterations in metabolic levels and programs (263). Macrophages in infected hosts were observed to have marked differences in the Krebs cycle, a key metabolic pathway. This is of significance due to the role of macrophages, which are immune cells critical in the pathogenesis of many inflammatory diseases (263, 265, 266).

In activated macrophages, succinate, a Krebs cycle intermediate, was found to possess inflammatory signal. Accumulation of succinate generates ROS, leading to subsequent activation of hypoxia-inducible factor 1α and the induction of cytokines such as IL-1β (267). A recent study identified the ability of itaconate, another Krebs cycle-derived metabolite, to block the production of inflammatory factors. This prevented inflammation, protecting mice from lethal levels of inflammation that can occur during infection (268). This data suggest the critical roles of Krebs cycle intermediates in regulating cytokine profiles and inflammation. Metabolites generated by innate immune cells in distinct configurations could have different roles beyond that of bioenergetics, with functions in signaling regulation, transcription, and orchestrating innate immune responses.

Despite the lack of research conducted thus far on the application of immunometabolic approaches to influenza treatment, the prospect of manipulating immune responses by modulating immune cell metabolic state is promising. Further research should focus on the identification of metabolites for modulation of immune cell function with substantial improvement of therapeutic strategies to treat IAV disease.

Latest advancements in high-throughput technologies, e.g., metabolomics is a useful approach to systematically investigate the changes of metabolic mechanisms during IAV infections. Identification of important metabolites involved during IAV infection should be a new approach by modulating the host metabolism for interventions.

CONCLUDING REMARKS

Multiple host-based intervention strategies against influenza have been developed or are under development. While approaches targeting host machinery required for virus replication seem to be promising thus far, additional research is needed to determine the effect of modulating host immune response on influenza treatment. This is increasingly important, since targeted host factors may play distinct roles in response to infection by different influenza viral strains (252), making the management of influenza through solely targeting a single specific host factor is difficult.

Host-based interventions offer obvious advantages over conventional antivirals, such as a higher barrier to drug resistance (73, 83, 107) due to greater genetic stability of host factors than the mutation-prone nature of viral components. In addition, administration feasibility is a key factor to consider the usage of drugs. The mainstays of antivirals for IAV infections, the NA inhibitors, and M2 blockers, are recommended to be administered within 48 h of symptom onset for optimal antiviral activity. This short treatment window may not be fully fulfilled in a clinical setting. Novel host-based interventions were reported to have therapeutic time windows longer than this conventional timeframe (96, 109, 214, 251), even up to 6 days post-infection (248), providing a clear clinical advantage over NA inhibitors and M2 blockers. In addition, hypercytokinemia and ARDS could contribute to disease severity and mortality in instances of severe influenza infection, with virus-targeting antivirals providing little to no alleviation of such complications.

Since host immune response is indispensable in host defense against invading pathogens, the use of immune-modulators to suppress detrimental effects while retaining beneficial protection of the host remains challenging. The timing and dosage of medication administration would be critical in determining the drug effectiveness in influenza treatment.

Targeting virus-induced metabolic changes to restore host normal metabolism may be a new direction to combat influenza disease. Further research in the immunometabolism field, alongside studies on modulating immune response to infectious disease by altering host metabolic processes; would create a new direction for future research and is expected to yield significant discoveries that may provide new therapeutic options in the treatment of IAV infections.

AUTHOR CONTRIBUTIONS

SMYL conceptualized the work. IL and ASMS drafted some review sections and TFY and SMYL wrote the manuscript.

REFERENCES

1. Gurav YK, Chadha MS, Tandale BV, Potdar VA, Pawar SD, Shil P, et al. Influenza A(H1N1)pdm09 outbreak detected in inter-seasonal months during the surveillance of influenza-like illness in Pune, India, 2012-2015. *Epidemiol Infect* (2017) 145(9):1898–909. doi:10.1017/S0950268817000553
2. Hui DSC, Lee N, Chan PKS. Avian influenza A (H7N9) virus infections in humans across five epidemics in mainland China, 2013-2017. *J Thorac Dis* (2017) 9(12):4808–11. doi:10.21037/jtd.2017.11.17
3. Olafsdottir TA, Alexandersson KF, Sveinbjornsson G, Lapini G, Palladino L, Montomoli E, et al. Age and influenza-specific pre-vaccination antibodies strongly affect influenza vaccine responses in the Icelandic population whereas disease and medication have small effects. *Front Immunol* (2017) 8:1872. doi:10.3389/fimmu.2017.01872
4. Moscona A. Global transmission of oseltamivir-resistant influenza. *N Engl J Med* (2009) 360(10):953–6. doi:10.1056/NEJMp0900648
5. Takashita E, Fujisaki S, Shirakura M, Nakamura K, Kishida N, Kuwahara T, et al. Influenza A(H1N1)pdm09 virus exhibiting enhanced cross-resistance to oseltamivir and peramivir due to a dual H275Y/G147R substitution, Japan, March 2016. *Euro Surveill* (2016) 21(24):30258. doi:10.2807/1560-7917.ES.2016.21.24.30258
6. Centers for Disease Control and Prevention. High levels of adamantane resistance among influenza A (H3N2) viruses and interim guidelines for use of antiviral agents – United States, 2005-06 influenza season. *MMWR Morb Mortal Wkly Rep* (2006) 55(2):44–6.
7. Schaduangrat N, Phanich J, Rungrotmongkol T, Lerdsamran H, Puthavathana P, Ubol S. The significance of naturally occurring neuraminidase quasispecies of H5N1 avian influenza virus on resistance to oseltamivir: a point of concern. *J Gen Virol* (2016) 97(6):1311–23. doi:10.1099/jgv.0.000444
8. Lina B, Boucher C, Osterhaus A, Monto AS, Schutten M, Whitley RJ, et al. Five years of monitoring for the emergence of oseltamivir resistance in patients with influenza A infections in the Influenza Resistance Information Study. *Influenza Other Respi Viruses* (2018) 12(2):267–78. doi:10.1111/irv.12534
9. Tandel K, Sharma S, Dash PK, Parida M. Oseltamivir-resistant influenza A(H1N1)pdm09 virus associated with high case fatality, India 2015. *J Med Virol* (2018) 90(5):836–43. doi:10.1002/jmv.25013
10. Szretter KJ, Gangappa S, Lu X, Smith C, Shieh WJ, Zaki SR, et al. Role of host cytokine responses in the pathogenesis of avian H5N1 influenza viruses in mice. *J Virol* (2007) 81(6):2736–44. doi:10.1128/JVI.02336-06
11. Short KR, Veeris R, Leijten LM, van den Brand JM, Jong VL, Stittelaar K, et al. Proinflammatory cytokine responses in extra-respiratory tissues during severe influenza. *J Infect Dis* (2017) 216(7):829–33. doi:10.1093/infdis/jix281
12. Chi Y, Zhu Y, Wen T, Cui L, Ge Y, Jiao Y, et al. Cytokine and chemokine levels in patients infected with the novel avian influenza A (H7N9) virus in China. *J Infect Dis* (2013) 208(12):1962–7. doi:10.1093/infdis/jit440
13. Lee SM, Yen HL. Targeting the host or the virus: current and novel concepts for antiviral approaches against influenza virus infection. *Antiviral Res* (2012) 96(3):391–404. doi:10.1016/j.antiviral.2012.09.013
14. Konig R, Stertz S, Zhou Y, Inoue A, Hoffmann HH, Bhattacharyya S, et al. Human host factors required for influenza virus replication. *Nature* (2010) 463(7282):813–7 doi:10.1038/nature08699
15. Karlas A, Machuy N, Shin Y, Pleissner KP, Artarini A, Heuer D, et al. Genome-wide RNAi screen identifies human host factors crucial for influenza virus replication. *Nature* (2010) 463(7282):818–22. doi:10.1038/nature08760
16. Edinger TO, Pohl MO, Stertz S. Entry of influenza A virus: host factors and antiviral targets. *J Gen Virol* (2014) 95(Pt 2):263–77. doi:10.1099/vir.0.059477-0
17. Luo M. Influenza virus entry. *Adv Exp Med Biol* (2012) 726:201–21. doi:10.1007/978-1-4614-0980-9_9
18. Rust MJ, Lakadamyali M, Zhang F, Zhuang X. Assembly of endocytic machinery around individual influenza viruses during viral entry. *Nat Struct Mol Biol* (2004) 11(6):567–73. doi:10.1038/nsmb769
19. de Vries E, Tscherne DM, Wienholts MJ, Cobos-Jimenez V, Scholte F, Garcia-Sastre A, et al. Dissection of the influenza A virus endocytic routes reveals macropinocytosis as an alternative entry pathway. *PLoS Pathog* (2011) 7(3):e1001329. doi:10.1371/journal.ppat.1001329
20. Yasuda S, Morishita S, Fujita A, Nanao T, Wada N, Waguri S, et al. Mon1-Ccz1 activates Rab7 only on late endosomes and dissociates from the lysosome in mammalian cells. *J Cell Sci* (2016) 129(2):329–40. doi:10.1242/jcs.178095
21. Rossman JS, Leser GP, Lamb RA. Filamentous influenza virus enters cells via macropinocytosis. *J Virol* (2012) 86(20):10950–60. doi:10.1128/JVI.05992-11
22. Huotari J, Helenius A. Endosome maturation. *EMBO J* (2011) 30(17):3481–500. doi:10.1038/emboj.2011.286
23. Hu YB, Dammer EB, Ren RJ, Wang G. The endosomal-lysosomal system: from acidification and cargo sorting to neurodegeneration. *Transl Neurodegener* (2015) 4:18. doi:10.1186/s40035-015-0041-1
24. Li S, Sieben C, Ludwig K, Hofer CT, Chiantia S, Herrmann A, et al. pH-Controlled two-step uncoating of influenza virus. *Biophys J* (2014) 106(7):1447–56. doi:10.1016/j.bpj.2014.02.018
25. Steinhauer DA. Role of hemagglutinin cleavage for the pathogenicity of influenza virus. *Virology* (1999) 258(1):1–20. doi:10.1006/viro.1999.9716
26. Zhirnov OP, Ikizler MR, Wright PF. Cleavage of influenza a virus hemagglutinin in human respiratory epithelium is cell associated and sensitive to exogenous antiproteases. *J Virol* (2002) 76(17):8682–9. doi:10.1128/JVI.76.17.8682-8689.2002
27. Pielak RM, Chou JJ. Influenza M2 proton channels. *Biochim Biophys Acta* (2011) 1808(2):522–9. doi:10.1016/j.bbamem.2010.04.015
28. Ye Z, Liu T, Offringa DP, McInnis J, Levandowski RA. Association of influenza virus matrix protein with ribonucleoproteins. *J Virol* (1999) 73(9):7467–73.
29. Byrd-Leotis L, Galloway SE, Agbogu E, Steinhauer DA. Influenza hemagglutinin (HA) stem region mutations that stabilize or destabilize the structure of multiple HA subtypes. *J Virol* (2015) 89(8):4504–16. doi:10.1128/JVI.00057-15
30. Lu X, Shi Y, Gao F, Xiao H, Wang M, Qi J, et al. Insights into avian influenza virus pathogenicity: the hemagglutinin precursor HA0 of subtype H16 has an alpha-helix structure in its cleavage site with inefficient HA1/HA2 cleavage. *J Virol* (2012) 86(23):12861–70. doi:10.1128/JVI.01606-12
31. Bottcher E, Matrosovich T, Beyerle M, Klenk HD, Garten W, Matrosovich M. Proteolytic activation of influenza viruses by serine proteases TMPRSS2 and HAT from human airway epithelium. *J Virol* (2006) 80(19):9896–8. doi:10.1128/JVI.01118-06
32. Xin Y, Liu L, Chen B, Zhang L, Tong Y. Affinity purification of aprotinin from bovine lung. *J Sep Sci* (2015) 38(9):1441–8. doi:10.1002/jssc.201401188
33. Swaminathan M, Stuart M, Hughes GC, Jaggers J, Hill SE, Milano CA, et al. Institutional response to FDA warning on aprotinin and impact on outcomes. *HSR Proc Intensive Care Cardiovasc Anesth* (2009) 1(1):30–6.
34. Ovcharenko AV, Zhirnov OP. Aprotinin aerosol treatment of influenza and paramyxovirus bronchopneumonia of mice. *Antiviral Res* (1994) 23(2):107–18. doi:10.1016/0166-3542(94)90038-8
35. Yamaya M, Shimotai Y, Hatachi Y, Lusamba Kalonji N, Tando Y, Kitajima Y, et al. The serine protease inhibitor camostat inhibits influenza virus replication and cytokine production in primary cultures of human tracheal epithelial cells. *Pulm Pharmacol Ther* (2015) 33:66–74. doi:10.1016/j.pupt.2015.07.001
36. Zhirnov OP, Klenk HD, Wright PF. Aprotinin and similar protease inhibitors as drugs against influenza. *Antiviral Res* (2011) 92(1):27–36. doi:10.1016/j.antiviral.2011.07.014
37. Lee MG, Kim KH, Park KY, Kim JS. Evaluation of anti-influenza effects of camostat in mice infected with non-adapted human influenza viruses. *Arch Virol* (1996) 141(10):1979–89. doi:10.1007/BF01718208
38. Ota S, Hara Y, Kanoh S, Shinoda M, Kawano S, Fujikura Y, et al. Acute eosinophilic pneumonia caused by camostat mesilate: the first case report. *Respir Med Case Rep* (2016) 19:21–3. doi:10.1016/j.rmcr.2016.06.005
39. Shen LW, Mao HJ, Wu YL, Tanaka Y, Zhang W. TMPRSS2: a potential target for treatment of influenza virus and coronavirus infections. *Biochimie* (2017) 142:1–10. doi:10.1016/j.biochi.2017.07.016
40. Stieneke-Grober A, Vey M, Angliker H, Shaw E, Thomas G, Roberts C, et al. Influenza virus hemagglutinin with multibasic cleavage site is activated by furin, a subtilisin-like endoprotease. *EMBO J* (1992) 11(7):2407–14.
41. Bahgat MM, Blazejewska P, Schughart K. Inhibition of lung serine proteases in mice: a potentially new approach to control influenza infection. *Virol J* (2011) 8:27. doi:10.1186/1743-422X-8-27
42. Matlin KS, Reggio H, Helenius A, Simons K. Infectious entry pathway of influenza virus in a canine kidney cell line. *J Cell Biol* (1981) 91(3 Pt 1):601–13. doi:10.1083/jcb.91.3.601

43. Ochiai H, Sakai S, Hirabayashi T, Shimizu Y, Terasawa K. Inhibitory effect of bafilomycin A1, a specific inhibitor of vacuolar-type proton pump, on the growth of influenza A and B viruses in MDCK cells. *Antiviral Res* (1995) 27(4):425–30. doi:10.1016/0166-3542(95)00040-S
44. Yeganeh B, Ghavami S, Kroeker AL, Mahood TH, Stelmack GL, Klonisch T, et al. Suppression of influenza A virus replication in human lung epithelial cells by noncytotoxic concentrations bafilomycin A1. *Am J Physiol Lung Cell Mol Physiol* (2015) 308(3):L270–86. doi:10.1152/ajplung.00011.2014
45. Sorensen MG, Henriksen K, Neutzsky-Wulff AV, Dziegiel MH, Karsdal MA. Diphyllin, a novel and naturally potent V-ATPase inhibitor, abrogates acidification of the osteoclastic resorption lacunae and bone resorption. *J Bone Miner Res* (2007) 22(10):1640–8. doi:10.1359/jbmr.070613
46. Chen HW, Cheng JX, Liu MT, King K, Peng JY, Zhang XQ, et al. Inhibitory and combinatorial effect of diphyllin, a v-ATPase blocker, on influenza viruses. *Antiviral Res* (2013) 99(3):371–82. doi:10.1016/j.antiviral.2013.06.014
47. Diamond MS, Farzan M. The broad-spectrum antiviral functions of IFIT and IFITM proteins. *Nat Rev Immunol* (2013) 13(1):46–57. doi:10.1038/nri3344
48. Shi G, Schwartz O, Compton AA. More than meets the I: the diverse antiviral and cellular functions of interferon-induced transmembrane proteins. *Retrovirology* (2017) 14(1):53. doi:10.1186/s12977-017-0377-y
49. Perreira JM, Chin CR, Feeley EM, Brass AL. IFITMs restrict the replication of multiple pathogenic viruses. *J Mol Biol* (2013) 425(24):4937–55. doi:10.1016/j.jmb.2013.09.024
50. Li K, Markosyan RM, Zheng YM, Golfetto O, Bungart B, Li M, et al. IFITM proteins restrict viral membrane hemifusion. *PLoS Pathog* (2013) 9(1):e1003124. doi:10.1371/journal.ppat.1003124
51. Amini-Bavil-Olyaee S, Choi YJ, Lee JH, Shi M, Huang IC, Farzan M, et al. The antiviral effector IFITM3 disrupts intracellular cholesterol homeostasis to block viral entry. *Cell Host Microbe* (2013) 13(4):452–64. doi:10.1016/j.chom.2013.03.006
52. Lee J, Kim J, Son K, d'Alexandry d'Orengiani AP, Min JY. Acid phosphatase 2 (ACP2) is required for membrane fusion during influenza virus entry. *Sci Rep* (2017) 7:43893. doi:10.1038/srep43893
53. Desai TM, Marin M, Chin CR, Savidis G, Brass AL, Melikyan GB. IFITM3 restricts influenza A virus entry by blocking the formation of fusion pores following virus-endosome hemifusion. *PLoS Pathog* (2014) 10(4):e1004048. doi:10.1371/journal.ppat.1004048
54. Ma H, Kien F, Maniere M, Zhang Y, Lagarde N, Tse KS, et al. Human annexin A6 interacts with influenza a virus protein M2 and negatively modulates infection. *J Virol* (2012) 86(3):1789–801. doi:10.1128/JVI.06003-11
55. Musiol A, Gran S, Ehrhardt C, Ludwig S, Grewal T, Gerke V, et al. Annexin A6-balanced late endosomal cholesterol controls influenza A replication and propagation. *MBio* (2013) 4(6):e608–13. doi:10.1128/mBio.00608-13
56. Hu Y, Jiang L, Lai W, Qin Y, Zhang T, Wang S, et al. MicroRNA-33a disturbs influenza A virus replication by targeting ARCN1 and inhibiting viral ribonucleoprotein activity. *J Gen Virol* (2016) 97(1):27–38. doi:10.1099/jgv.0.000311
57. Xu X, Kedlaya R, Higuchi H, Ikeda S, Justice MJ, Setaluri V, et al. Mutation in archain 1, a subunit of COPI coatomer complex, causes diluted coat color and Purkinje cell degeneration. *PLoS Genet* (2010) 6(5):e1000956. doi:10.1371/journal.pgen.1000956
58. Sun E, He J, Zhuang X. Dissecting the role of COPI complexes in influenza virus infection. *J Virol* (2013) 87(5):2673–85. doi:10.1128/JVI.02277-12
59. Eisfeld AJ, Neumann G, Kawaoka Y. At the centre: influenza A virus ribonucleoproteins. *Nat Rev Microbiol* (2015) 13(1):28–41. doi:10.1038/nrmicro3367
60. Babcock HP, Chen C, Zhuang X. Using single-particle tracking to study nuclear trafficking of viral genes. *Biophys J* (2004) 87(4):2749–58. doi:10.1529/biophysj.104.042234
61. Resa-Infante P, Paterson D, Bonet J, Otte A, Oliva B, Fodor E, et al. Targeting importin-alpha7 as a therapeutic approach against pandemic influenza viruses. *J Virol* (2015) 89(17):9010–20. doi:10.1128/JVI.00583-15
62. Gabriel G, Klingel K, Otte A, Thiele S, Hudjetz B, Arman-Kalcek G, et al. Differential use of importin-alpha isoforms governs cell tropism and host adaptation of influenza virus. *Nat Commun* (2011) 2:156. doi:10.1038/ncomms1158
63. Rosenblatt JE. Antiparasitic agents. *Mayo Clin Proc* (1992) 67(3):276–87. doi:10.1016/S0025-6196(12)60105-0
64. Wagstaff KM, Sivakumaran H, Heaton SM, Harrich D, Jans DA. Ivermectin is a specific inhibitor of importin alpha/beta-mediated nuclear import able to inhibit replication of HIV-1 and dengue virus. *Biochem J* (2012) 443(3):851–6. doi:10.1042/BJ20120150
65. Gotz V, Magar L, Dornfeld D, Giese S, Pohlmann A, Hoper D, et al. Influenza A viruses escape from MxA restriction at the expense of efficient nuclear vRNP import. *Sci Rep* (2016) 6:23138. doi:10.1038/srep23138
66. Mor A, White A, Zhang K, Thompson M, Esparza M, Munoz-Moreno R, et al. Influenza virus mRNA trafficking through host nuclear speckles. *Nat Microbiol* (2016) 1(7):16069. doi:10.1038/nmicrobiol.2016.69
67. Dubois J, Terrier O, Rosa-Calatrava M. Influenza viruses and mRNA splicing: doing more with less. *MBio* (2014) 5(3):e70–14. doi:10.1128/mBio.00070-14
68. Bullock AN, Das S, Debreczeni JE, Rellos P, Fedorov O, Niesen FH, et al. Kinase domain insertions define distinct roles of CLK kinases in SR protein phosphorylation. *Structure* (2009) 17(3):352–62. doi:10.1016/j.str.2008.12.023
69. Zu M, Li C, Fang JS, Lian WW, Liu AL, Zheng LS, et al. Drug discovery of host CLK1 inhibitors for influenza treatment. *Molecules* (2015) 20(11):19735–47. doi:10.3390/molecules201119653
70. Amorim MJ, Read EK, Dalton RM, Medcalf L, Digard P. Nuclear export of influenza A virus mRNAs requires ongoing RNA polymerase II activity. *Traffic* (2007) 8(1):1–11. doi:10.1111/j.1600-0854.2006.00507.x
71. Utine CA, Stern M, Akpek EK. Clinical review: topical ophthalmic use of cyclosporin A. *Ocul Immunol Inflamm* (2010) 18(5):352–61. doi:10.3109/09273948.2010.498657
72. Liu X, Zhao Z, Li Z, Xu C, Sun L, Chen J, et al. Cyclosporin A inhibits the influenza virus replication through cyclophilin A-dependent and -independent pathways. *PLoS One* (2012) 7(5):e37277. doi:10.1371/journal.pone.0037277
73. Ma C, Li F, Musharrafieh RG, Wang J. Discovery of cyclosporine A and its analogs as broad-spectrum anti-influenza drugs with a high in vitro genetic barrier of drug resistance. *Antiviral Res* (2016) 133:62–72. doi:10.1016/j.antiviral.2016.07.019
74. Read EK, Digard P. Individual influenza A virus mRNAs show differential dependence on cellular NXF1/TAP for their nuclear export. *J Gen Virol* (2010) 91(Pt 5):1290–301. doi:10.1099/vir.0.018564-0
75. Morita M, Kuba K, Ichikawa A, Nakayama M, Katahira J, Iwamoto R, et al. The lipid mediator protectin D1 inhibits influenza virus replication and improves severe influenza. *Cell* (2013) 153(1):112–25. doi:10.1016/j.cell.2013.02.027
76. Cencic R, Pelletier J. Hippuristanol – a potent steroid inhibitor of eukaryotic initiation factor 4A. *Translation (Austin)* (2016) 4(1):e1137381. doi:10.1080/21690731.2015.1137381
77. Sokabe M, Fraser CS. A helicase-independent activity of eIF4A in promoting mRNA recruitment to the human ribosome. *Proc Natl Acad Sci U S A* (2017) 114(24):6304–9. doi:10.1073/pnas.1620426114
78. Muller C, Schulte FW, Lange-Grunweller K, Obermann W, Madhugiri R, Pleschka S, et al. Broad-spectrum antiviral activity of the eIF4A inhibitor silvestrol against corona- and picornaviruses. *Antiviral Res* (2017) 150:123–9. doi:10.1016/j.antiviral.2017.12.010
79. Yanguez E, Castello A, Welnowska E, Carrasco L, Goodfellow I, Nieto A. Functional impairment of eIF4A and eIF4G factors correlates with inhibition of influenza virus mRNA translation. *Virology* (2011) 413(1):93–102. doi:10.1016/j.virol.2011.02.012
80. Slaine PD, Kleer M, Smith NK, Khaperskyy DA, McCormick C. Stress granule-inducing eukaryotic translation initiation factor 4A inhibitors block influenza A virus replication. *Viruses* (2017) 9(12):E388. doi:10.3390/v9120388
81. Malina A, Mills JR, Pelletier J. Emerging therapeutics targeting mRNA translation. *Cold Spring Harb Perspect Biol* (2012) 4(4):a012377. doi:10.1101/cshperspect.a012377
82. Rossignol JF, La Frazia S, Chiappa L, Ciucci A, Santoro MG. Thiazolides, a new class of anti-influenza molecules targeting viral hemagglutinin at the post-translational level. *J Biol Chem* (2009) 284(43):29798–808. doi:10.1074/jbc.M109.029470
83. Rossignol JF. Nitazoxanide: a first-in-class broad-spectrum antiviral agent. *Antiviral Res* (2014) 110:94–103. doi:10.1016/j.antiviral.2014.07.014
84. Tilmanis D, van Baalen C, Oh DY, Rossignol JF, Hurt AC. The susceptibility of circulating human influenza viruses to tizoxanide, the active

metabolite of nitazoxanide. *Antiviral Res* (2017) 147:142–8. doi:10.1016/j.antiviral.2017.10.002
85. Belardo G, Cenciarelli O, La Frazia S, Rossignol JF, Santoro MG. Synergistic effect of nitazoxanide with neuraminidase inhibitors against influenza A viruses in vitro. *Antimicrob Agents Chemother* (2015) 59(2):1061–9. doi:10.1128/AAC.03947-14
86. Lakdawala SS, Wu Y, Wawrzusin P, Kabat J, Broadbent AJ, Lamirande EW, et al. Influenza a virus assembly intermediates fuse in the cytoplasm. *PLoS Pathog* (2014) 10(3):e1003971. doi:10.1371/journal.ppat.1003971
87. Momose F, Sekimoto T, Ohkura T, Jo S, Kawaguchi A, Nagata K, et al. Apical transport of influenza A virus ribonucleoprotein requires Rab11-positive recycling endosome. *PLoS One* (2011) 6(6):e21123. doi:10.1371/journal.pone.0021123
88. Kudo N, Khochbin S, Nishi K, Kitano K, Yanagida M, Yoshida M, et al. Molecular cloning and cell cycle-dependent expression of mammalian CRM1, a protein involved in nuclear export of proteins. *J Biol Chem* (1997) 272(47):29742–51. doi:10.1074/jbc.272.47.29742
89. Kohler A, Hurt E. Exporting RNA from the nucleus to the cytoplasm. *Nat Rev Mol Cell Biol* (2007) 8(10):761–73. doi:10.1038/nrm2255
90. Fischer U, Huber J, Boelens WC, Mattaj IW, Luhrmann R. The HIV-1 Rev activation domain is a nuclear export signal that accesses an export pathway used by specific cellular RNAs. *Cell* (1995) 82(3):475–83. doi:10.1016/0092-8674(95)90436-0
91. Brunotte L, Flies J, Bolte H, Reuther P, Vreede F, Schwemmle M. The nuclear export protein of H5N1 influenza A viruses recruits Matrix 1 (M1) protein to the viral ribonucleoprotein to mediate nuclear export. *J Biol Chem* (2014) 289(29):20067–77. doi:10.1074/jbc.M114.569178
92. Elton D, Simpson-Holley M, Archer K, Medcalf L, Hallam R, McCauley J, et al. Interaction of the influenza virus nucleoprotein with the cellular CRM1-mediated nuclear export pathway. *J Virol* (2001) 75(1):408–19. doi:10.1128/JVI.75.1.408-419.2001
93. Watanabe K, Takizawa N, Katoh M, Hoshida K, Kobayashi N, Nagata K. Inhibition of nuclear export of ribonucleoprotein complexes of influenza virus by leptomycin B. *Virus Res* (2001) 77(1):31–42. doi:10.1016/S0168-1702(01)00263-5
94. Newlands ES, Rustin GJ, Brampton MH. Phase I trial of elactocin. *Br J Cancer* (1996) 74(4):648–9. doi:10.1038/bjc.1996.415
95. Perwitasari O, Johnson S, Yan X, Howerth E, Shacham S, Landesman Y, et al. Verdinexor, a novel selective inhibitor of nuclear export, reduces influenza a virus replication in vitro and in vivo. *J Virol* (2014) 88(17):10228–43. doi:10.1128/JVI.01774-14
96. Perwitasari O, Johnson S, Yan X, Register E, Crabtree J, Gabbard J, et al. Antiviral efficacy of verdinexor in vivo in two animal models of influenza A virus infection. *PLoS One* (2016) 11(11):e0167221. doi:10.1371/journal.pone.0167221
97. Muthuri SG, Venkatesan S, Myles PR, Leonardi-Bee J, Al Khuwaitir TS, Al Mamun A, et al. Effectiveness of neuraminidase inhibitors in reducing mortality in patients admitted to hospital with influenza A H1N1pdm09 virus infection: a meta-analysis of individual participant data. *Lancet Respir Med* (2014) 2(5):395–404. doi:10.1016/S2213-2600(14)70041-4
98. Chutiwitoonchai N, Mano T, Kakisaka M, Sato H, Kondoh Y, Osada H, et al. Inhibition of CRM1-mediated nuclear export of influenza A nucleoprotein and nuclear export protein as a novel target for antiviral drug development. *Virology* (2017) 507:32–9. doi:10.1016/j.virol.2017.04.001
99. Li J, Chen C, Wong G, Dong W, Zheng W, Li Y, et al. Cyclophilin A protects mice against infection by influenza A virus. *Sci Rep* (2016) 6:28978. doi:10.1038/srep28978
100. Liu X, Sun L, Yu M, Wang Z, Xu C, Xue Q, et al. Cyclophilin A interacts with influenza A virus M1 protein and impairs the early stage of the viral replication. *Cell Microbiol* (2009) 11(5):730–41. doi:10.1111/j.1462-5822.2009.01286.x
101. Liu X, Zhao Z, Xu C, Sun L, Chen J, Zhang L, et al. Cyclophilin A restricts influenza A virus replication through degradation of the M1 protein. *PLoS One* (2012) 7(2):e31063. doi:10.1371/journal.pone.0031063
102. Qiao Y, Yan Y, Tan KS, Tan SS, Seet JE, Arumugam TV, et al. CD151, a novel host factor of nuclear export signaling in influenza virus infection. *J Allergy Clin Immunol* (2018) 141(5):1799–817. doi:10.1016/j.jaci.2017.11.032
103. Gavara MM, Zaveri K, Badana AK, Gugalavath S, Amajala KC, Patnala K, et al. A novel small molecule inhibitor of CD151 inhibits proliferation of metastatic triple negative breast cancer cell lines. *Proc Biochem* (2018) 66:254–62. doi:10.1016/j.procbio.2017.12.004
104. Haidari M, Zhang W, Ganjehei L, Ali M, Chen Z. Inhibition of MLC phosphorylation restricts replication of influenza virus – a mechanism of action for anti-influenza agents. *PLoS One* (2011) 6(6):e21444. doi:10.1371/journal.pone.0021444
105. Pleschka S, Wolff T, Ehrhardt C, Hobom G, Planz O, Rapp UR, et al. Influenza virus propagation is impaired by inhibition of the Raf/MEK/ERK signalling cascade. *Nat Cell Biol* (2001) 3(3):301–5. doi:10.1038/35060098
106. Droebner K, Pleschka S, Ludwig S, Planz O. Antiviral activity of the MEK-inhibitor U0126 against pandemic H1N1v and highly pathogenic avian influenza virus in vitro and in vivo. *Antiviral Res* (2011) 92(2):195–203. doi:10.1016/j.antiviral.2011.08.002
107. Ludwig S, Wolff T, Ehrhardt C, Wurzer WJ, Reinhardt J, Planz O, et al. MEK inhibition impairs influenza B virus propagation without emergence of resistant variants. *FEBS Lett* (2004) 561(1–3):37–43. doi:10.1016/S0014-5793(04)00108-5
108. Planz O, Pleschka S, Ludwig S. MEK-specific inhibitor U0126 blocks spread of Borna disease virus in cultured cells. *J Virol* (2001) 75(10):4871–7. doi:10.1128/JVI.75.10.4871-4877.2001
109. Haasbach E, Muller C, Ehrhardt C, Schreiber A, Pleschka S, Ludwig S, et al. The MEK-inhibitor CI-1040 displays a broad anti-influenza virus activity in vitro and provides a prolonged treatment window compared to standard of care in vivo. *Antiviral Res* (2017) 142:178–84. doi:10.1016/j.antiviral.2017.03.024
110. Tcherniuk S, Cenac N, Comte M, Frouard J, Errazuriz-Cerda E, Galabov A, et al. Formyl peptide receptor 2 plays a deleterious role during influenza A virus infections. *J Infect Dis* (2016) 214(2):237–47. doi:10.1093/infdis/jiw127
111. Courtin N, Fotso AF, Fautrad P, Mas F, Alessi MC, Riteau B. Antiviral activity of formyl peptide receptor 2 antagonists against influenza viruses. *Antiviral Res* (2017) 143:252–61. doi:10.1016/j.antiviral.2017.05.001
112. Grant BD, Donaldson JG. Pathways and mechanisms of endocytic recycling. *Nat Rev Mol Cell Biol* (2009) 10(9):597–608. doi:10.1038/nrm2755
113. Bruce EA, Stuart A, McCaffrey MW, Digard P. Role of the Rab11 pathway in negative-strand virus assembly. *Biochem Soc Trans* (2012) 40(6):1409–15. doi:10.1042/BST20120166
114. Amorim MJ, Bruce EA, Read EK, Foeglein A, Mahen R, Stuart AD, et al. A Rab11- and microtubule-dependent mechanism for cytoplasmic transport of influenza A virus viral RNA. *J Virol* (2011) 85(9):4143–56. doi:10.1128/JVI.02606-10
115. Eisfeld AJ, Kawakami E, Watanabe T, Neumann G, Kawaoka Y. RAB11A is essential for transport of the influenza virus genome to the plasma membrane. *J Virol* (2011) 85(13):6117–26. doi:10.1128/JVI.00378-11
116. Bruce EA, Digard P, Stuart AD. The Rab11 pathway is required for influenza A virus budding and filament formation. *J Virol* (2010) 84(12):5848–59. doi:10.1128/JVI.00307-10
117. Ramos-Nascimento A, Kellen B, Ferreira F, Alenquer M, Vale-Costa S, Raposo G, et al. KIF13A mediates trafficking of influenza A virus ribonucleoproteins. *J Cell Sci* (2017) 130(23):4038–50. doi:10.1242/jcs.210807
118. Portran D, Schaedel L, Xu Z, Thery M, Nachury MV. Tubulin acetylation protects long-lived microtubules against mechanical ageing. *Nat Cell Biol* (2017) 19(4):391–8. doi:10.1038/ncb3481
119. Hubbert C, Guardiola A, Shao R, Kawaguchi Y, Ito A, Nixon A, et al. HDAC6 is a microtubule-associated deacetylase. *Nature* (2002) 417(6887):455–8. doi:10.1038/417455a
120. Husain M, Cheung CY. Histone deacetylase 6 inhibits influenza A virus release by downregulating the trafficking of viral components to the plasma membrane via its substrate, acetylated microtubules. *J Virol* (2014) 88(19):11229–39. doi:10.1128/JVI.00727-14
121. Mori K, Haruyama T, Nagata K. Tamiflu-resistant but HA-mediated cell-to-cell transmission through apical membranes of cell-associated influenza viruses. *PLoS One* (2011) 6(11):e28178. doi:10.1371/journal.pone.0028178
122. Roberts KL, Manicassamy B, Lamb RA. Influenza A virus uses intercellular connections to spread to neighboring cells. *J Virol* (2015) 89(3):1537–49. doi:10.1128/JVI.03306-14
123. Rossman JS, Lamb RA. Influenza virus assembly and budding. *Virology* (2011) 411(2):229–36. doi:10.1016/j.virol.2010.12.003

124. Martyna A, Rossman J. Alterations of membrane curvature during influenza virus budding. *Biochem Soc Trans* (2014) 42(5):1425–8. doi:10.1042/BST20140136
125. Elkins MR, Williams JK, Gelenter MD, Dai P, Kwon B, Sergeyev IV, et al. Cholesterol-binding site of the influenza M2 protein in lipid bilayers from solid-state NMR. *Proc Natl Acad Sci U S A* (2017) 114(49):12946–51. doi:10.1073/pnas.1715127114
126. Bajimaya S, Frankl T, Hayashi T, Takimoto T. Cholesterol is required for stability and infectivity of influenza A and respiratory syncytial viruses. *Virology* (2017) 510:234–41. doi:10.1016/j.virol.2017.07.024
127. Matsui K, Ozawa M, Kiso M, Yamashita M, Maekawa T, Kubota M, et al. Stimulation of alpha2-adrenergic receptors impairs influenza virus infection. *Sci Rep* (2018) 8(1):4631. doi:10.1038/s41598-018-22927-0
128. Herold S, Becker C, Ridge KM, Budinger GR. Influenza virus-induced lung injury: pathogenesis and implications for treatment. *Eur Respir J* (2015) 45(5):1463–78. doi:10.1183/09031936.00186214
129. Pulendran B, Maddur MS. Innate immune sensing and response to influenza. *Curr Top Microbiol Immunol* (2015) 386:23–71. doi:10.1007/82_2014_405
130. Chen X, Liu S, Goraya MU, Maarouf M, Huang S, Chen JL. Host immune response to influenza A virus infection. *Front Immunol* (2018) 9:320. doi:10.3389/fimmu.2018.00320
131. Kruger P, Saffarzadeh M, Weber AN, Rieber N, Radsak M, von Bernuth H, et al. Neutrophils: between host defence, immune modulation, and tissue injury. *PLoS Pathog* (2015) 11(3):e1004651. doi:10.1371/journal.ppat.1004651
132. Tate MD, Brooks AG, Reading PC. The role of neutrophils in the upper and lower respiratory tract during influenza virus infection of mice. *Respir Res* (2008) 9:57. doi:10.1186/1465-9921-9-57
133. Tate MD, Ioannidis LJ, Croker B, Brown LE, Brooks AG, Reading PC. The role of neutrophils during mild and severe influenza virus infections of mice. *PLoS One* (2011) 6(3):e17618. doi:10.1371/journal.pone.0017618
134. Lim K, Hyun YM, Lambert-Emo K, Capece T, Bae S, Miller R, et al. Neutrophil trails guide influenza-specific CD8(+) T cells in the airways. *Science* (2015) 349(6252):aaa4352. doi:10.1126/science.aaa4352
135. van Riel D, Leijten LM, van der Eerden M, Hoogsteden HC, Boven LA, Lambrecht BN, et al. Highly pathogenic avian influenza virus H5N1 infects alveolar macrophages without virus production or excessive TNF-alpha induction. *PLoS Pathog* (2011) 7(6):e1002099. doi:10.1371/journal.ppat.1002099
136. Seth S, Oberdorfer L, Hyde R, Hoff K, Thies V, Worbs T, et al. CCR7 essentially contributes to the homing of plasmacytoid dendritic cells to lymph nodes under steady-state as well as inflammatory conditions. *J Immunol* (2011) 186(6):3364–72. doi:10.4049/jimmunol.1002598
137. Qu C, Nguyen VA, Merad M, Randolph GJ. MHC class I/peptide transfer between dendritic cells overcomes poor cross-presentation by monocyte-derived APCs that engulf dying cells. *J Immunol* (2009) 182(6):3650–9. doi:10.4049/jimmunol.0801532
138. Allan RS, Waithman J, Bedoui S, Jones CM, Villadangos JA, Zhan Y, et al. Migratory dendritic cells transfer antigen to a lymph node-resident dendritic cell population for efficient CTL priming. *Immunity* (2006) 25(1):153–62. doi:10.1016/j.immuni.2006.04.017
139. Leon B, Ardavin C. Monocyte-derived dendritic cells in innate and adaptive immunity. *Immunol Cell Biol* (2008) 86(4):320–4. doi:10.1038/icb.2008.14
140. Qu C, Brinck-Jensen NS, Zang M, Chen K. Monocyte-derived dendritic cells: targets as potent antigen-presenting cells for the design of vaccines against infectious diseases. *Int J Infect Dis* (2014) 19:1–5. doi:10.1016/j.ijid.2013.09.023
141. Swiecki M, Gilfillan S, Vermi W, Wang Y, Colonna M. Plasmacytoid dendritic cell ablation impacts early interferon responses and antiviral NK and CD8(+) T cell accrual. *Immunity* (2010) 33(6):955–66. doi:10.1016/j.immuni.2010.11.020
142. Hochrein H, Shortman K, Vremec D, Scott B, Hertzog P, O'Keeffe M. Differential production of IL-12, IFN-alpha, and IFN-gamma by mouse dendritic cell subsets. *J Immunol* (2001) 166(9):5448–55. doi:10.4049/jimmunol.166.9.5448
143. Pipkin ME, Sacks JA, Cruz-Guilloty F, Lichtenheld MG, Bevan MJ, Rao A. Interleukin-2 and inflammation induce distinct transcriptional programs that promote the differentiation of effector cytolytic T cells. *Immunity* (2010) 32(1):79–90. doi:10.1016/j.immuni.2009.11.012
144. Luckheeram RV, Zhou R, Verma AD, Xia B. CD4(+)T cells: differentiation and functions. *Clin Dev Immunol* (2012) 2012:925135. doi:10.1155/2012/925135
145. Crotty S. T follicular helper cell differentiation, function, and roles in disease. *Immunity* (2014) 41(4):529–42. doi:10.1016/j.immuni.2014.10.004
146. Kurosaki T, Kometani K, Ise W. Memory B cells. *Nat Rev Immunol* (2015) 15(3):149–59. doi:10.1038/nri3802
147. Jameson SC, Masopust D. Understanding subset diversity in T cell memory. *Immunity* (2018) 48(2):214–26. doi:10.1016/j.immuni.2018.02.010
148. Obar JJ, Lefrancois L. Memory CD8+ T cell differentiation. *Ann N Y Acad Sci* (2010) 1183:251–66. doi:10.1111/j.1749-6632.2009.05126.x
149. MacLeod MK, Kappler JW, Marrack P. Memory CD4 T cells: generation, reactivation and re-assignment. *Immunology* (2010) 130(1):10–5. doi:10.1111/j.1365-2567.2010.03260.x
150. Kong KF, Delroux K, Wang X, Qian F, Arjona A, Malawista SE, et al. Dysregulation of TLR3 impairs the innate immune response to West Nile virus in the elderly. *J Virol* (2008) 82(15):7613–23. doi:10.1128/JVI.00618-08
151. Openshaw PJ, Chiu C. Protective and dysregulated T cell immunity in RSV infection. *Curr Opin Virol* (2013) 3(4):468–74. doi:10.1016/j.coviro.2013.05.005
152. Hendrickson CM, Matthay MA. Viral pathogens and acute lung injury: investigations inspired by the SARS epidemic and the 2009 H1N1 influenza pandemic. *Semin Respir Crit Care Med* (2013) 34(4):475–86. doi:10.1055/s-0033-1351122
153. Cheung CY, Poon LL, Lau AS, Luk W, Lau YL, Shortridge KF, et al. Induction of proinflammatory cytokines in human macrophages by influenza A (H5N1) viruses: a mechanism for the unusual severity of human disease? *Lancet* (2002) 360(9348):1831–7. doi:10.1016/S0140-6736(02)11772-7
154. Ye S, Lowther S, Stambas J. Inhibition of reactive oxygen species production ameliorates inflammation induced by influenza A viruses via upregulation of SOCS1 and SOCS3. *J Virol* (2015) 89(5):2672–83. doi:10.1128/JVI.03529-14
155. Pauli EK, Schmolke M, Wolff T, Viemann D, Roth J, Bode JG, et al. Influenza A virus inhibits type I IFN signaling via NF-kappaB-dependent induction of SOCS-3 expression. *PLoS Pathog* (2008) 4(11):e1000196. doi:10.1371/journal.ppat.1000196
156. Tumpey TM, Basler CF, Aguilar PV, Zeng H, Solorzano A, Swayne DE, et al. Characterization of the reconstructed 1918 Spanish influenza pandemic virus. *Science* (2005) 310(5745):77–80. doi:10.1126/science.1119392
157. Saffarzadeh M, Juenemann C, Queisser MA, Lochnit G, Barreto G, Galuska SP, et al. Neutrophil extracellular traps directly induce epithelial and endothelial cell death: a predominant role of histones. *PLoS One* (2012) 7(2):e32366. doi:10.1371/journal.pone.0032366
158. Tate MD, Deng YM, Jones JE, Anderson GP, Brooks AG, Reading PC. Neutrophils ameliorate lung injury and the development of severe disease during influenza infection. *J Immunol* (2009) 183(11):7441–50. doi:10.4049/jimmunol.0902497
159. Narasaraju T, Yang E, Samy RP, Ng HH, Poh WP, Liew AA, et al. Excessive neutrophils and neutrophil extracellular traps contribute to acute lung injury of influenza pneumonitis. *Am J Pathol* (2011) 179(1):199–210. doi:10.1016/j.ajpath.2011.03.013
160. Hoeksema M, Tripathi S, White M, Qi L, Taubenberger J, van Eijk M, et al. Arginine-rich histones have strong antiviral activity for influenza A viruses. *Innate Immun* (2015) 21(7):736–45. doi:10.1177/1753425915593794
161. Ashar HK, Mueller NC, Rudd JM, Snider TA, Achanta M, Prasanthi M, et al. The role of extracellular histones in influenza virus pathogenesis. *Am J Pathol* (2018) 188(1):135–48. doi:10.1016/j.ajpath.2017.09.014
162. Zhu L, Liu L, Zhang Y, Pu L, Liu J, Li X, et al. High level of neutrophil extracellular traps correlates with poor prognosis of severe influenza A infection. *J Infect Dis* (2018) 217(3):428–37. doi:10.1093/infdis/jix475
163. Martinez NE, Zimmermann TJ, Goosmann C, Alexander T, Hedberg C, Ziegler S, et al. Tetrahydroisoquinolines: new inhibitors of Neutrophil Extracellular Trap (NET) formation. *Chembiochem* (2017) 18(10):888–93. doi:10.1002/cbic.201600650
164. Kusunoki Y, Nakazawa D, Shida H, Hattanda F, Miyoshi A, Masuda S, et al. Peptidylarginine deiminase inhibitor suppresses neutrophil extracellular trap formation and MPO-ANCA production. *Front Immunol* (2016) 7:227. doi:10.3389/fimmu.2016.00227

165. Hemmers S, Teijaro JR, Arandjelovic S, Mowen KA. PAD4-mediated neutrophil extracellular trap formation is not required for immunity against influenza infection. *PLoS One* (2011) 6(7):e22043. doi:10.1371/journal.pone.0022043
166. Kim HY, Umetsu DT, Dekruyff RH. Innate lymphoid cells in asthma: will they take your breath away? *Eur J Immunol* (2016) 46(4):795–806. doi:10.1002/eji.201444557
167. Monticelli LA, Sonnenberg GF, Artis D. Innate lymphoid cells: critical regulators of allergic inflammation and tissue repair in the lung. *Curr Opin Immunol* (2012) 24(3):284–9. doi:10.1016/j.coi.2012.03.012
168. Monticelli LA, Sonnenberg GF, Abt MC, Alenghat T, Ziegler CG, Doering TA, et al. Innate lymphoid cells promote lung-tissue homeostasis after infection with influenza virus. *Nat Immunol* (2011) 12(11):1045–54. doi:10.1031/ni.2131
169. Jiao Y, Huntington ND, Belz GT, Seillet C. Type 1 innate lymphoid cell biology: lessons learnt from natural killer cells. *Front Immunol* (2016) 7:426. doi:10.3389/fimmu.2016.00426
170. Weizman OE, Adams NM, Schuster IS, Krishna C, Pritykin Y, Lau C, et al. ILC1 confer early host protection at initial sites of viral infection. *Cell* (2017) 171(4):795–808.e12. doi:10.1016/j.cell.2017.09.052
171. Califano D, Furuya Y, Roberts S, Avram D, McKenzie ANJ, Metzger DW. IFN-γ increases susceptibility to influenza A infection through suppression of group II innate lymphoid cells. *Mucosal Immunol* (2017) 11(1):209–19. doi:10.1038/mi.2017.41
172. Cephus JY, Stier MT, Fuseini H, Yung JA, Toki S, Bloodworth MH, et al. Testosterone attenuates Group 2 innate lymphoid cell-mediated airway inflammation. *Cell Rep* (2017) 21(9):2487–99. doi:10.1016/j.celrep.2017.10.110
173. Doherty TA, Broide DH. Pathways to limit group 2 innate lymphoid cell activation. *J Allergy Clin Immunol* (2017) 139(5):1465–7. doi:10.1016/j.jaci.2016.12.003
174. Vlahos R, Selemidis S. NADPH oxidases as novel pharmacologic targets against influenza A virus infection. *Mol Pharmacol* (2014) 86(6):747–59. doi:10.1124/mol.114.095216
175. Strengert M, Jennings R, Davanture S, Hayes P, Gabriel G, Knaus UG. Mucosal reactive oxygen species are required for antiviral response: role of Duox in influenza a virus infection. *Antioxid Redox Signal* (2014) 20(17):2695–709. doi:10.1089/ars.2013.5353
176. Kim HJ, Kim CH, Ryu JH, Kim MJ, Park CY, Lee JM, et al. Reactive oxygen species induce antiviral innate immune response through IFN-lambda regulation in human nasal epithelial cells. *Am J Respir Cell Mol Biol* (2013) 49(5):855–65. doi:10.1165/rcmb.2013-0003OC
177. To EE, Vlahos R, Luong R, Halls ML, Reading PC, King PT, et al. Endosomal NOX2 oxidase exacerbates virus pathogenicity and is a target for antiviral therapy. *Nat Commun* (2017) 8(1):69. doi:10.1038/s41467-017-00057-x
178. Amatore D, Sgarbanti R, Aquilano K, Baldelli S, Limongi D, Civitelli L, et al. Influenza virus replication in lung epithelial cells depends on redox-sensitive pathways activated by NOX4-derived ROS. *Cell Microbiol* (2015) 17(1):131–45. doi:10.1111/cmi.12343
179. Lejal N, Truchet S, Bechor E, Bouguyon E, Khedkar V, Bertho N, et al. Turning off NADPH oxidase-2 by impeding p67(phox) activation in infected mouse macrophages reduced viral entry and inflammation. *Biochim Biophys Acta* (2018) 1862(6):1263–75. doi:10.1016/j.bbagen.2018.03.004
180. Wind S, Beuerlein K, Eucker T, Muller H, Scheurer P, Armitage ME, et al. Comparative pharmacology of chemically distinct NADPH oxidase inhibitors. *Br J Pharmacol* (2010) 161(4):885–98. doi:10.1111/j.1476-5381.2010.00920.x
181. Altenhofer S, Kleikers PW, Radermacher KA, Scheurer P, Rob Hermans JJ, Schiffers P, et al. The NOX toolbox: validating the role of NADPH oxidases in physiology and disease. *Cell Mol Life Sci* (2012) 69(14):2327–43. doi:10.1007/s00018-012-1010-9
182. Heumuller S, Wind S, Barbosa-Sicard E, Schmidt HH, Busse R, Schroder K, et al. Apocynin is not an inhibitor of vascular NADPH oxidases but an antioxidant. *Hypertension* (2008) 51(2):211–7. doi:10.1161/HYPERTENSIONAHA.107.100214
183. Vlahos R, Stambas J, Bozinovski S, Broughton BR, Drummond GR, Selemidis S. Inhibition of Nox2 oxidase activity ameliorates influenza A virus-induced lung inflammation. *PLoS Pathog* (2011) 7(2):e1001271. doi:10.1371/journal.ppat.1001271
184. Oostwoud LC, Gunasinghe P, Seow HJ, Ye JM, Selemidis S, Bozinovski S, et al. Apocynin and ebselen reduce influenza A virus-induced lung inflammation in cigarette smoke-exposed mice. *Sci Rep* (2016) 6:20983. doi:10.1038/srep20983
185. Liu Q, Zhou YH, Yang ZQ. The cytokine storm of severe influenza and development of immunomodulatory therapy. *Cell Mol Immunol* (2016) 13(1):3–10. doi:10.1038/cmi.2015.74
186. Betakova T, Kostrabova A, Lachova V, Turianova L. Cytokines induced during influenza virus infection. *Curr Pharm Des* (2017) 23(18):2616–22. doi:10.2174/1381612823666170316123736
187. Julkunen I, Sareneva T, Pirhonen J, Ronni T, Melen K, Matikainen S. Molecular pathogenesis of influenza A virus infection and virus-induced regulation of cytokine gene expression. *Cytokine Growth Factor Rev* (2001) 12(2–3):171–80. doi:10.1016/S1359-6101(00)00026-5
188. Iwai A, Shiozaki T, Miyazaki T. Relevance of signaling molecules for apoptosis induction on influenza A virus replication. *Biochem Biophys Res Commun* (2013) 441(3):531–7. doi:10.1016/j.bbrc.2013.10.100
189. Zhou X, Jiang W, Liu Z, Liu S, Liang X. Virus infection and death receptor-mediated apoptosis. *Viruses* (2017) 9(11):E316. doi:10.3390/v9110316
190. To KK, Lau CC, Woo PC, Lau SK, Chan JF, Chan KH, et al. Human H7N9 virus induces a more pronounced pro-inflammatory cytokine but an attenuated interferon response in human bronchial epithelial cells when compared with an epidemiologically-linked chicken H7N9 virus. *Virol J* (2016) 13:42. doi:10.1186/s12985-016-0498-2
191. Quinn KM, Kan WT, Watson KA, Liddicoat BJ, Swan NG, McQuilten H, et al. Extrinsically derived TNF is primarily responsible for limiting antiviral CD8+ T cell response magnitude. *PLoS One* (2017) 12(9):e0184732. doi:10.1371/journal.pone.0184732
192. DeBerge MP, Ely KH, Enelow RI. Soluble, but not transmembrane, TNF-α is required during influenza infection to limit the magnitude of immune responses and the extent of immunopathology. *J Immunol* (2014) 192(12):5839–51. doi:10.4049/jimmunol.1302729
193. van de Sandt CE, Barcena M, Koster AJ, Kasper J, Kirkpatrick CJ, Scott DP, et al. Human CD8(+) T cells damage noninfected epithelial cells during influenza virus infection in vitro. *Am J Respir Cell Mol Biol* (2017) 57(5):536–46. doi:10.1165/rcmb.2016-0377OC
194. Brincks EL, Woodland DL. Novel roles for IL-15 in T cell survival. *F1000 Biol Rep* (2010) 2:67. doi:10.3410/B2-67
195. Gagnon J, Ramanathan S, Leblanc C, Cloutier A, McDonald PP, Ilangumaran S. IL-6, in synergy with IL-7 or IL-15, stimulates TCR-independent proliferation and functional differentiation of CD8+ T lymphocytes. *J Immunol* (2008) 180(12):7958–68. doi:10.4049/jimmunol.180.12.7958
196. Damjanovic D, Divangahi M, Kugathasan K, Small CL, Zganiacz A, Brown EG, et al. Negative regulation of lung inflammation and immunopathology by TNF-alpha during acute influenza infection. *Am J Pathol* (2011) 179(6):2963–76. doi:10.1016/j.ajpath.2011.09.003
197. Yang G, Hamacher J, Gorshkov B, White R, Sridhar S, Verin A, et al. The dual role of TNF in pulmonary edema. *J Cardiovas Dis Res* (2010) 1(1):29–36. doi:10.4103/0975-3583.59983
198. DeBerge MP, Ely KH, Cheng GS, Enelow RI. ADAM17-mediated processing of TNF-α expressed by antiviral effector CD8+ T cells is required for severe T-cell-mediated lung injury. *PLoS One* (2013) 8(11):e79340. doi:10.1371/journal.pone.0079340
199. Hasegawa S, Matsushige T, Inoue H, Shirabe K, Fukano R, Ichiyama T. Serum and cerebrospinal fluid cytokine profile of patients with 2009 pandemic H1N1 influenza virus-associated encephalopathy. *Cytokine* (2011) 54(2):167–72. doi:10.1016/j.cyto.2011.01.006
200. Ichiyama T, Nishikawa M, Yoshitomi T, Hayashi T, Furukawa S. Tumor necrosis factor-alpha, interleukin-1 beta, and interleukin-6 in cerebrospinal fluid from children with prolonged febrile seizures. Comparison with acute encephalitis/encephalopathy. *Neurology* (1998) 50(2):407–11. doi:10.1212/WNL.50.2.407
201. Ito Y, Ichiyama T, Kimura H, Shibata M, Ishiwada N, Kuroki H, et al. Detection of influenza virus RNA by reverse transcription-PCR and proinflammatory cytokines in influenza-virus-associated encephalopathy. *J Med Virol* (1999) 58(4):420–5. doi:10.1002/(SICI)1096-9071(199908)58:4<420::AID-JMV16>3.0.CO;2-T
202. Lv S, Song HL, Zhou Y, Li LX, Cui W, Wang W, et al. Tumour necrosis factor-alpha affects blood-brain barrier permeability and tight

junction-associated occludin in acute liver failure. *Liver Int* (2010) 30(8): 1198–210. doi:10.1111/j.1478-3231.2010.02211.x
203. Tsuge M, Yasui K, Ichiyawa T, Saito Y, Nagaoka Y, Yashiro M, et al. Increase of tumor necrosis factor-alpha in the blood induces early activation of matrix metalloproteinase-9 in the brain. *Microbiol Immunol* (2010) 54(7):417–24. doi:10.1111/j.1348-0421.2010.00226.x
204. Kuperberg SJ, Wadgaonkar R. Sepsis-associated encephalopathy: the blood-brain barrier and the sphingolipid rheostat. *Front Immunol* (2017) 8:597. doi:10.3389/fimmu.2017.00597
205. Shi X, Zhou W, Huang H, Zhu H, Zhou P, Zhu H, et al. Inhibition of the inflammatory cytokine tumor necrosis factor-alpha with etanercept provides protection against lethal H1N1 influenza infection in mice. *Crit Care* (2013) 17(6):R301. doi:10.1186/cc13171
206. Dienz O, Rud JG, Eaton SM, Lanthier PA, Burg E, Drew A, et al. Essential role of IL-6 in protection against H1N1 influenza virus by promoting neutrophil survival in the lung. *Mucosal Immunol* (2012) 5(3):258–66. doi:10.1038/mi.2012.2
207. Yang ML, Wang CT, Yang SJ, Leu CH, Chen SH, Wu CL, et al. IL-6 ameliorates acute lung injury in influenza virus infection. *Sci Rep* (2017) 7:43829. doi:10.1038/srep43829
208. Pyle CJ, Uwadiae FI, Swieboda DP, Harker JA. Early IL-6 signalling promotes IL-27 dependent maturation of regulatory T cells in the lungs and resolution of viral immunopathology. *PLoS Pathog* (2017) 13(9):e1006640. doi:10.1371/journal.ppat.1006640
209. Aiba H, Mochizuki M, Kimura M, Hojo H. Predictive value of serum interleukin-6 level in influenza virus-associated encephalopathy. *Neurology* (2001) 57(2):295–9. doi:10.1212/WNL.57.2.295
210. Fukumoto Y, Okumura A, Hayakawa F, Suzuki M, Kato T, Watanabe K, et al. Serum levels of cytokines and EEG findings in children with influenza associated with mild neurological complications. *Brain Dev* (2007) 29(7):425–30. doi:10.1016/j.braindev.2006.12.005
211. Cohen SS, Min M, Cummings EE, Chen X, Sadowska GB, Sharma S, et al. Effects of interleukin-6 on the expression of tight junction proteins in isolated cerebral microvessels from yearling and adult sheep. *Neuroimmunomodulation* (2013) 20(5):264–73. doi:10.1159/000350470
212. Song M, Winchester J, Albright RL, Capponi VJ, Choquette MD, Kellum JA. Cytokine removal with a novel adsorbent polymer. *Blood Purif* (2004) 22(5):428–34. doi:10.1159/000080235
213. Lees NJ, Rosenberg A, Hurtado-Doce AI, Jones J, Marczin N, Zeriouh M, et al. Combination of ECMO and cytokine adsorption therapy for severe sepsis with cardiogenic shock and ARDS due to Panton-Valentine leukocidin-positive *Staphylococcus aureus* pneumonia and H1N1. *J Artif Organs* (2016) 19(4):399–402. doi:10.1007/s10047-016-0915-8
214. Liu FD, Kenngott EE, Schroter MF, Kuhl A, Jennrich S, Watzlawick R, et al. Timed action of IL-27 protects from immunopathology while preserving defense in influenza. *PLoS Pathog* (2014) 10(5):e1004110. doi:10.1371/journal.ppat.1004110
215. Robinson KM, Lee B, Scheller EV, Mandalapu S, Enelow RI, Kolls JK, et al. The role of IL-27 in susceptibility to post-influenza *Staphylococcus aureus* pneumonia. *Respir Res* (2015) 16:10. doi:10.1186/s12931-015-0168-8
216. Krug RM. Functions of the influenza A virus NS1 protein in antiviral defense. *Curr Opin Virol* (2015) 12:1–6. doi:10.1016/j.coviro.2015.01.007
217. Jureka AS, Kleinpeter AB, Cornilescu G, Cornilescu CC, Petit CM. Structural basis for a novel interaction between the NS1 protein derived from the 1918 influenza virus and RIG-I. *Structure* (2015) 23(11):2001–10. doi:10.1016/j.str.2015.08.007
218. Ciancanelli MJ, Huang SX, Luthra P, Garner H, Itan Y, Volpi S, et al. Infectious disease. Life-threatening influenza and impaired interferon amplification in human IRF7 deficiency. *Science* (2015) 348(6233):448–53. doi:10.1126/science.aaa1578
219. Davidson S, Maini MK, Wack A. Disease-promoting effects of type I interferons in viral, bacterial, and coinfections. *J Interferon Cytokine Res* (2015) 35(4):252–64. doi:10.1089/jir.2014.0227
220. Beilharz MW, Cummins JM, Bennett AL. Protection from lethal influenza virus challenge by oral type 1 interferon. *Biochem Biophys Res Commun* (2007) 355(3):740–4. doi:10.1016/j.bbrc.2007.02.019
221. Bennett AL, Smith DW, Cummins MJ, Jacoby PA, Cummins JM, Beilharz MW. Low-dose oral interferon alpha as prophylaxis against viral respiratory illness: a double-blind, parallel controlled trial during an influenza pandemic year. *Influenza Other Respi Viruses* (2013) 7(5):854–62. doi:10.1111/irv.12094
222. Davidson S, McCabe TM, Crotta S, Gad HH, Hessel EM, Beinke S, et al. IFNlambda is a potent anti-influenza therapeutic without the inflammatory side effects of IFNalpha treatment. *EMBO Mol Med* (2016) 8(9):1099–112. doi:10.15252/emmm.201606413
223. Davidson S, Crotta S, McCabe TM, Wack A. Pathogenic potential of interferon alphabeta in acute influenza infection. *Nat Commun* (2014) 5:3864. doi:10.1038/ncomms4864
224. Kim S, Kim MJ, Kim CH, Kang JW, Shin HK, Kim DY, et al. The superiority of IFN-lambda as a therapeutic candidate to control acute influenza viral lung infection. *Am J Respir Cell Mol Biol* (2017) 56(2):202–12. doi:10.1165/rcmb.2016-0174OC
225. Li W, Moltedo B, Moran TM. Type I interferon induction during influenza virus infection increases susceptibility to secondary *Streptococcus pneumoniae* infection by negative regulation of gammadelta T cells. *J Virol* (2012) 86(22):12304–12. doi:10.1128/JVI.01269-12
226. Galani IE, Triantafyllia V, Eleminiadou EE, Koltsida O, Stavropoulos A, Manioudaki M, et al. Interferon-lambda mediates non-redundant front-line antiviral protection against influenza virus infection without compromising host fitness. *Immunity* (2017) 46(5):875–890.e6. doi:10.1016/j.immuni.2017.04.025
227. Coch C, Stumpel JP, Lilien-Waldau V, Wohlleber D, Kummerer BM, Bekeredjian-Ding I, et al. RIG-I activation protects and rescues from lethal influenza virus infection and bacterial superinfection. *Mol Ther* (2017) 25(9):2093–103. doi:10.1016/j.ymthe.2017.07.003
228. Lee SM, Gai WW, Cheung TK, Peiris JS. Antiviral effect of a selective COX-2 inhibitor on H5N1 infection in vitro. *Antiviral Res* (2011) 91(3):330–4. doi:10.1016/j.antiviral.2011.07.011
229. Li C, Li C, Zhang AJ, To KK, Lee AC, Zhu H, et al. Avian influenza A H7N9 virus induces severe pneumonia in mice without prior adaptation and responds to a combination of zanamivir and COX-2 inhibitor. *PLoS One* (2014) 9(9):e107966. doi:10.1371/journal.pone.0107966
230. Lee MY, Cheung CY, Peiris JS. Role of cyclooxygenase-2 in H5N1 viral pathogenesis and the potential use of its inhibitors. *Hong Kong Med J* (2013) 19(Suppl 4):S29–35.
231. Coulombe F, Jaworska J, Verway M, Tzelepis F, Massoud A, Gillard J, et al. Targeted prostaglandin E2 inhibition enhances antiviral immunity through induction of type I interferon and apoptosis in macrophages. *Immunity* (2014) 40(4):554–68. doi:10.1016/j.immuni.2014.02.013
232. Chen L, Fan J, Li Y, Shi X, Ju D, Yan Q, et al. Modified Jiu Wei Qiang Huo decoction improves dysfunctional metabolomics in influenza A pneumonia-infected mice. *Biomed Chromatogr* (2014) 28(4):468–74. doi:10.1002/bmc.3055
233. Takeuchi O, Akira S. Pattern recognition receptors and inflammation. *Cell* (2010) 140(6):805–20. doi:10.1016/j.cell.2010.01.022
234. Le Goffic R, Pothlichet J, Vitour D, Fujita T, Meurs E, Chignard M, et al. Cutting edge: influenza A virus activates TLR3-dependent inflammatory and RIG-I-dependent antiviral responses in human lung epithelial cells. *J Immunol* (2007) 178(6):3368–72. doi:10.4049/jimmunol.178.6.3368
235. Lee SM, Kok KH, Jaume M, Cheung TK, Yip TF, Lai JC, et al. Toll-like receptor 10 is involved in induction of innate immune responses to influenza virus infection. *Proc Natl Acad Sci U S A* (2014) 111(10):3793–8. doi:10.1073/pnas.1324266111
236. Wu W, Zhang W, Duggan ES, Booth JL, Zou MH, Metcalf JP. RIG-I and TLR3 are both required for maximum interferon induction by influenza virus in human lung alveolar epithelial cells. *Virology* (2015) 482:181–8. doi:10.1016/j.virol.2015.03.048
237. Patel JR, Garcia-Sastre A. Activation and regulation of pathogen sensor RIG-I. *Cytokine Growth Factor Rev* (2014) 25(5):513–23. doi:10.1016/j.cytogfr.2014.08.005
238. Weber-Gerlach M, Weber F. Standing on three legs: antiviral activities of RIG-I against influenza viruses. *Curr Opin Immunol* (2016) 42:71–5. doi:10.1016/j.coi.2016.05.016
239. Yoneyama M, Onomoto K, Jogi M, Akaboshi T, Fujita T. Viral RNA detection by RIG-I-like receptors. *Curr Opin Immunol* (2015) 32:48–53. doi:10.1016/j.coi.2014.12.012
240. De Nardo D. Toll-like receptors: activation, signalling and transcriptional modulation. *Cytokine* (2015) 74(2):181–9. doi:10.1016/j.cyto.2015.02.025

241. Kagan JC, Su T, Horng T, Chow A, Akira S, Medzhitov R. TRAM couples endocytosis of toll-like receptor 4 to the induction of interferon-beta. *Nat Immunol* (2008) 9(4):361–8. doi:10.1038/ni1569
242. Oosting M, Cheng SC, Bolscher JM, Vestering-Stenger R, Plantinga TS, Verschueren IC, et al. Human TLR10 is an anti-inflammatory pattern-recognition receptor. *Proc Natl Acad Sci U S A* (2014) 111(42):E4478–84. doi:10.1073/pnas.1410293111
243. Jiang S, Li X, Hess NJ, Guan Y, Tapping RI. TLR10 is a negative regulator of both MyD88-dependent and -independent TLR signaling. *J Immunol* (2016) 196(9):3834–41. doi:10.4049/jimmunol.1502599
244. Lee SMY, Yip TF, Yan S, Jin DY, Wei HL, Guo RT, et al. Recognition of double-stranded RNA and regulation of interferon pathway by toll-like receptor 10. *Front Immunol* (2018) 9:516. doi:10.3389/fimmu.2018.00516
245. Imai Y, Kuba K, Neely GG, Yaghubian-Malhami R, Perkmann T, van Loo G, et al. Identification of oxidative stress and toll-like receptor 4 signaling as a key pathway of acute lung injury. *Cell* (2008) 133(2):235–49. doi:10.1016/j.cell.2008.02.043
246. Tsai SY, Segovia JA, Chang TH, Morris IR, Berton MT, Tessier PA, et al. DAMP molecule S100A9 acts as a molecular pattern to enhance inflammation during influenza A virus infection: role of DDX21-TRIF-TLR4-MyD88 pathway. *PLoS Pathog* (2014) 10(1):e1003848. doi:10.1371/journal.ppat.1003848
247. Opal SM, Laterre PF, Francois B, LaRosa SP, Angus DC, Mira JP, et al. Effect of eritoran, an antagonist of MD2-TLR4, on mortality in patients with severe sepsis: the ACCESS randomized trial. *JAMA* (2013) 309(11):1154–62. doi:10.1001/jama.2013.2194
248. Shirey KA, Lai W, Scott AJ, Lipsky M, Mistry P, Pletneva LM, et al. The TLR4 antagonist eritoran protects mice from lethal influenza infection. *Nature* (2013) 497(7450):498–502. doi:10.1038/nature12118
249. Perrin-Cocon L, Aublin-Gex A, Sestito SE, Shirey KA, Patel MC, Andre P, et al. TLR4 antagonist FP7 inhibits LPS-induced cytokine production and glycolytic reprogramming in dendritic cells, and protects mice from lethal influenza infection. *Sci Rep* (2017) 7:40791. doi:10.1038/srep40791
250. Piao W, Shirey KA, Ru LW, Lai W, Szmacinski H, Snyder GA, et al. A decoy peptide that disrupts TIRAP recruitment to TLRs is protective in a murine model of influenza. *Cell Rep* (2015) 11(12):1941–52. doi:10.1016/j.celrep.2015.05.035
251. Shirey KA, Lai W, Patel MC, Pletneva LM, Pang C, Kurt-Jones E, et al. Novel strategies for targeting innate immune responses to influenza. *Mucosal Immunol* (2016) 9(5):1173–82. doi:10.1038/mi.2015.141
252. Leung YH, Nicholls JM, Ho CK, Sia SF, Mok CK, Valkenburg SA, et al. Highly pathogenic avian influenza A H5N1 and pandemic H1N1 virus infections have different phenotypes in toll-like receptor 3 knockout mice. *J Gen Virol* (2014) 95(Pt 9):1870–9. doi:10.1099/vir.0.066258-0
253. Gao W, Xiong Y, Li Q, Yang H. Inhibition of toll-like receptor signaling as a promising therapy for inflammatory diseases: a journey from molecular to nano therapeutics. *Front Physiol* (2017) 8:508. doi:10.3389/fphys.2017.00508
254. Cheng K, Wang X, Yin H. Small-molecule inhibitors of the TLR3/dsRNA complex. *J Am Chem Soc* (2011) 133(11):3764–7. doi:10.1021/ja111312h
255. Li Z, Li L, Zhou H, Zeng L, Chen T, Chen Q, et al. Radix isatidis polysaccharides inhibit influenza a virus and influenza A virus-induced inflammation via suppression of Host TLR3 signaling in vitro. *Molecules* (2017) 22(1):E116. doi:10.3390/molecules22010116
256. Tian J, Jiao X, Wang X, Geng J, Wang R, Liu N, et al. Novel effect of methionine enkephalin against influenza A virus infection through inhibiting TLR7-MyD88-TRAF6-NF-kappaB p65 signaling pathway. *Int Immunopharmacol* (2017) 55:38–48. doi:10.1016/j.intimp.2017.12.001
257. Hulme KD, Gallo LA, Short KR. Influenza virus and glycemic variability in diabetes: a killer combination? *Front Microbiol* (2017) 8:861. doi:10.3389/fmicb.2017.00861
258. Kohio HP, Adamson AL. Glycolytic control of vacuolar-type ATPase activity: a mechanism to regulate influenza viral infection. *Virology* (2013) 444(1–2):301–9. doi:10.1016/j.virol.2013.06.026
259. Miyake-Stoner SJ, O'Shea CC. Metabolism goes viral. *Cell Metab* (2014) 19(4):549–50. doi:10.1016/j.cmet.2014.03.022
260. Munger J, Bajad SU, Coller HA, Shenk T, Rabinowitz JD. Dynamics of the cellular metabolome during human cytomegalovirus infection. *PLoS Pathog* (2006) 2(12):e132. doi:10.1371/journal.ppat.0020132
261. Koyuncu E, Purdy JG, Rabinowitz JD, Shenk T. Saturated very long chain fatty acids are required for the production of infectious human cytomegalovirus progeny. *PLoS Pathog* (2013) 9(5):e1003333. doi:10.1371/journal.ppat.1003333
262. Goodwin CM, Xu S, Munger J. Stealing the keys to the kitchen: viral manipulation of the host cell metabolic network. *Trends Microbiol* (2015) 23(12):789–98. doi:10.1016/j.tim.2015.08.007
263. Sanchez EL, Lagunoff M. Viral activation of cellular metabolism. *Virology* (2015) 47(9–480):609–18. doi:10.1016/j.virol.2015.02.038
264. Smallwood HS, Duan S, Morfouace M, Rezinciuc S, Shulkin BL, Shelat A, et al. Targeting metabolic reprogramming by influenza infection for therapeutic intervention. *Cell Rep* (2017) 19(8):1640–53. doi:10.1016/j.celrep.2017.04.039
265. Ritter JB, Wahl AS, Freund S, Genzel Y, Reichl U. Metabolic effects of influenza virus infection in cultured animal cells: Intra- and extracellular metabolite profiling. *BMC Syst Biol* (2010) 4:61. doi:10.1186/1752-0509-4-61
266. Ryan DG, O'Neill LAJ. Krebs cycle rewired for macrophage and dendritic cell effector functions. *FEBS Lett* (2017) 591(19):2992–3006. doi:10.1002/1873-3468.12744
267. Tannahill GM, Curtis AM, Adamik J, Palsson-McDermott EM, McGettrick AF, Goel G, et al. Succinate is an inflammatory signal that induces IL-1beta through HIF-1alpha. *Nature* (2013) 496(7444):238–42. doi:10.1038/nature11986
268. Mills EL, Ryan DG, Prag HA, Dikovskaya D, Menon D, Zaslona Z, et al. Itaconate is an anti-inflammatory metabolite that activates Nrf2 via alkylation of KEAP1. *Nature* (2018) 556(7699):113–7. doi:10.1038/nature25986

3

Flavivirus Receptors: Diversity, Identity and Cell Entry

Mathilde Laureti [1,2†], Divya Narayanan [1,2†], Julio Rodriguez-Andres [1,2†], John K. Fazakerley [1,2] and Lukasz Kedzierski [1,2]*

[1] *Department of Microbiology and Immunology, Peter Doherty Institute for Infection and Immunity, University of Melbourne, Melbourne, VIC, Australia,* [2] *Faculty of Veterinary and Agricultural Sciences, University of Melbourne, Melbourne, VIC, Australia*

***Correspondence:**
Lukasz Kedzierski
lukaszk@unimelb.edu.au

† *These authors have contributed equally to this work*

Flaviviruses are emerging and re-emerging arthropod-borne pathogens responsible for significant mortality and morbidity worldwide. The genus comprises more than seventy small, positive-sense, single-stranded RNA viruses, which are responsible for a spectrum of human and animal diseases ranging in symptoms from mild, influenza-like infection to fatal encephalitis and haemorrhagic fever. Despite genomic and structural similarities across the genus, infections by different flaviviruses result in disparate clinical presentations. This review focusses on two haemorrhagic flaviviruses, dengue virus and yellow fever virus, and two neurotropic flaviviruses, Japanese encephalitis virus and Zika virus. We review current knowledge on host-pathogen interactions, virus entry strategies and tropism.

Keywords: flaviviruses, Japanese encephalitis virus, Zika virus (ZIKV), dengue virus, yellow fever virus, entry receptor

INTRODUCTION

The *Flavivirus* genus consists of more than 70 small, positive-sense, single-stranded RNA viruses transmitted by arthropods, in particular mosquitos and ticks. These include globally important human pathogens such as West Nile virus (WNV), Japanese encephalitis virus (JEV), dengue virus (DENV), Murray Valley encephalitis virus (MVE), tick-borne encephalitis virus (TBEV), Yellow Fever virus (YFV), and Zika virus (ZIKV). These viruses are responsible for some of the most severe arbovirus infections affecting humans, pose a serious threat to global health and have the potential to cause severe outbreaks. These are exemplified by the global distribution of DENV (1), the recent ZIKV outbreak in South America (2), YFV outbreaks in Africa (3), and Brazil (4) and the spread of WNV across North America (5). Flavivirus infections range from asymptomatic, through mild fever and arthralgia to life threatening haemorrhagic or encephalitic diseases (6). Flaviviruses are also able to persist in patients and can be responsible for long-term morbidities (7). There are no antiviral treatments for flavivirus infection currently in clinical use, and despite licensed vaccines against several of the viruses including YFV, JEV, TBEV, or DENV, outbreaks still occur highlighting challenges in implementing effective vaccination programs (8).

The flaviviral genome of ~11 kb contains a single open reading frame flanked by untranslated regions, and encodes 3 structural proteins (C, M, and E) and 7 non-structural proteins (NS). The mature virion features a surface densely covered with E glycoproteins and M proteins and a core consisting of capsid (C) protein and the RNA genome (9, 10). The entry into the target cell is dependent on E protein contact with its cognate receptor. E protein initially binds to attachment factors such as glycosaminoglycans. This effectively increases viral density on the cell surface, leading to high affinity receptor binding (11). The E protein ectodomain consists of three domains (E-DI, E-DII, E-DIII) of which E-DIII is thought to interact with attachment factors and receptors (12). E-DIII domain's importance is highlighted by the fact that a vast majority of potent, neutralizing antibodies has been mapped to this region. Nevertheless, anti-DI and DII antibodies, although less potent, show broader cross-reactivity and form a major pool of anti-E protein specific immonoglobulins (13). Receptor binding is followed by clathrin-mediated endocytosis (14), which is considered to be a major mechanism of flavivirus cell entry, although there are exceptions described below. This leads to formation of endosomes and low pH dependent changes in the E glycoprotein with subsequent membrane fusion and release of nucleocapsid into the cytosol (15). *In vitro,* flaviviruses are able to infect a plethora of cell lines originating from rodents, non-human primates, humans and mosquitos. However *in vivo,* fewer cell types seem able to support flavivirus replication (16). A wide range of cell surface receptors has been implicated in flavivirus entry into different cells types (11). Amongst the entry receptors postulated to be involved in flavivirus entry, the best characterized to date include $\alpha_V\beta_3$ integrins (17, 18), C-type lectin receptors (CLR) (19–23), phosphatidylserine receptors TIM (T-cell immunoglobulin and mucin domain) and TYRO3, AXL and MER (TAM) (24). Recent studies indicate that flaviviruses can produce a range of structurally different virions. This structural heterogeneity may expand tissue tropism and ability to infect different cell types both in invertebrate and vertebrate hosts (25).

Flaviviruses are deposited into the skin epidermis by a mosquito bite where they encounter cells permissive to infection such as keratinocytes and skin dendritic cells (Langerhans cells) (26). Dendritic cells in particular appear to be a common initial target for flaviviruses. When infected, dendritic cells migrate to lymphoid organs where viral replication takes place allowing for flavivirus dissemination into circulation and internal organs (12). Viruses such DENV (27), JEV (28), ZIKV (29) have been shown to infect skin dendritic cells, and although there are no reports on YFV infecting Langerhans cells, it can nevertheless infect other types of dendritic cells (30). This interaction is mediated by DC-SIGN for JEV (28) and ZIKV (29), but appears to be DC-SIGN independent in case of DENV (31) and YFV (30).

Many flaviviruses are neuroinvasive and neurovirulent and cause central nervous system (CNS) damage (32). Neuroinvasive infections are observed with JEV, TBEV, and WNV (33, 34), and occasionally with haemorrhagic viruses including DENV (35). There is a paucity of knowledge regarding factors involved in CNS cell entry. While CLRs and TIMs are expressed by cells of the CNS (36–38), they are not expressed by neurons (39–41). However, members of the TAM family of receptors are expressed by different neuronal subtypes (42), though they are dispensable for ZIKV infection as ZIKV was able to infect and replicate in TAM receptor knockout mice (43).

As natural vectors, mosquitos and ticks are highly permissive to flavivirus infection. The virus can replicate in a range of arthropod tissues and cells (44, 45). Given that flaviviruses have only one glycoprotein, it seems likely that the mechanism of entry into vertebrate and invertebrate cells is evolutionarily conserved. A number of the cellular receptors implicated in flavivirus entry into mosquito cell lines overlaps with those identified for mammalian cells (46). Some flaviviruses are more selective regarding their arthropod host than others. For example, DENV is spread mainly by *Aedes spp.* mosquitos (6), WNV by *Culex spp.* (47), whereas JEV is transmitted by *Aedes*, *Anopheles* and *Culex spp.* (48). There appears to be a more restricted receptor repertoire used by flaviviruses for insect cell entry compared to mammalian cell entry. The range of clinical manifestations of flaviviral infection in the mammalian host suggests that these viruses may use a wide range of receptors. Mammalian tissues in general offer much greater range of receptors compared to invertebrates.

Identification of flavivirus entry receptors, particularly those involved in CNS infection, could lead to identification of novel therapeutic targets. For this review we will focus on four major flaviviruses of humans—DENV, JEV, ZIKV, and YFV, and discuss the differences and similarities in their mechanisms of entry into arthropod and mammalian cells.

DENGUE VIRUS

DENV is one of the most common mosquito-borne viruses, mainly transmitted by *Aedes aegypti* mosquitoes, and occasionally by *Ae. albopictus.* Symptoms of DENV infection range from fever and muscle and joint pain (Dengue fever) to potentially life threatening haemorrhagic fever or shock syndrome. While DENV was endemic in <10 countries in the 1970's, it is presently a threat in over 128 countries and is responsible for almost 400 million human infections every year. About 24% of infections manifest in severe clinical symptoms. There is currently no treatment for DENV serotypes. There are four virus serotypes, and recovery from one serotype provides lifelong homologous immunity (49).

DENV is an icosahedral particle of 50 nm with a positive, single-stranded RNA genome of 10–11 kb (50). As in other flaviviruses, E protein is involved in receptor binding and fusion (51) and has the ability to bind to a wide range of cellular receptors to initiate DENV entry. The E-DIII domain has a role in cellular recognition (52) and has been suggested as a target for the development of a DENV vaccine (53).

Over the years, several cell membrane receptors involved in DENV entry have been identified. These include carbohydrate molecules (54–56), lectins (57, 58), and claudin-1 cell receptors (59). Carbohydrate molecules such as glycosaminoglycans (GAGs), sulphated polysaccharides, and glycosphingolipids (GSL) are widely expressed cell surface co-receptors for DENV entry and are believed to enhance viral entry efficiency. The highly sulphated form of GAGs, the heparan sulfates (HS) and heparan sulfates proteoglycans (HSPG), are essential for cellular adhesion to extracellular matrix and binding of polypeptide growth factors involved in intracellular signaling (56). It has been suggested that DENV first contacts HSPG, and that this weak interaction facilitates binding of virus to other receptors, which then results in virus internalization (55). Several studies have shown that pre-treatment with heparin can reduce or block DENV-2 infection (60, 61). However, the efficiency of inhibition of viral entry was dependent on numerous factors, such as the virus strains and the target cell (61). GSLs, a member of the same family of carbohydrate molecules as HS, are ubiquitous cellular components of eukaryotic plasma membranes that can also facilitate entry and binding of virus (54). However, GSLs are not required for DENV entry as the virus was able to enter GSL-deficient cells (62).

Cellular C-type lectin receptors (CLRs) are part of the host immune response to fungal, bacterial and viral infections (57). CLRs in mammalian cells include DC-SIGN/L-SIGN, mannose receptors (MR), and CLEC5A. DC-SIGN receptors are widely known because of their association with HIV. These receptors are also involved in DENV binding and internalization into dendritic cells (63). MR has been found to be the primary DENV cell receptor in macrophages. The CLEC5A receptor cooperates with DC-SIGN or MR to increase DENV binding and stability (58).

Other studies have suggested claudin-1 as a putative cell receptor for DENV entry through a direct interaction with the viral prM protein. Claudins are vital components of tight junction complexes and are essential for normal permeability of the epithelia (59, 64). DENV-2 entry was significantly reduced in claudin-1 deficient cells (59). Also, it has been demonstrated that caudin-1 is upregulated early in infection in order to facilitate entry and downregulated in late stage of infection (64).

Protein binding assays and mass spectrometry analysis have identified several additional potential flavivirus cellular receptors (65–67). Among them, the tubulin and tubulin-like proteins in C6/36 *Ae. albopictus* cell line (65). Heat shock proteins (HSPs) of ~70 kDa and 80 kDa were also identified as cellular receptors for all four DENV serotypes in C6/36 cell line (66, 68). HSPs are chaperone proteins involved in the regulation of folding and unfolding of cellular, and upon infection, viral proteins (69). The 70 kDa protein, also known as heat shock cognate protein (HSC70) or HSPA8, acts as a chaperone protein during DENV entry (70, 71). Modulation of HSC70 expression was observed during DENV-2 infection, with an increase on the cell membrane during infection, suggesting that DENV-2 utilizes HSC70 for entry into mosquito cells (67). In addition to its role in viral entry, HSP70 is involved in virion biogenesis and RNA replication (71). It appears that all four DENV serotypes are dependent on this chaperone protein family, which makes HSP70 proteins an interesting target for the design of a tetravalent DENV therapy or vaccine (71).

HSP90, another heat shock protein, can also act as chaperone. This protein interacts with six DENV proteins (69). While the involvement of HSP70 and HSP90 in DENV binding to host cells has been reported (70–72), these proteins are not involved in internalization of virus into the host cell (73).

As mentioned before, TIM/TAM family receptors have been implicated in flavivirus entry. DENV express on its surface phosphatidylserine (PS) and phosphatidylethanolamine (PE) molecules. Both PS and PE are known to directly interact with TIM/TAM receptors and DENV is able to enhance its entry by exploiting these interactions (74).

After binding to cellular receptors, internalization of viral particles occurs. For DENV, internalization occurs via pH-dependent endocytosis. Several endocytosis pathways are currently known, but clathrin-mediated endocytosis is the main pathway for DENV (75). The DENV use of clathrin-mediated endocytosis was demonstrated in C6/36 mosquito cells by biochemical inhibition of cell receptors (76), and in several human cell lines through siRNA silencing of genes associated with clathrin-mediated receptors (75, 77, 78). While this inhibition and specific gene silencing resulted in a decrease in viral load, a complete inhibition was not achieved, suggesting the existence of alternative entry pathways in mosquito and mammalian cells.

In addition to the exploitation of clathrin-mediated endocytosis, the host immune system can also promote viral entry (79). This phenomenon, known as antibody-dependent enhancement (ADE), was first described in 1964 by Hawkes (80) for WNV and JEV, and observed for DENV more than a decade later (81). Antibody-virus complexes are internalized by phagocytosis via Fc gamma receptors (FcγR) into macrophages, monocytes and dendritic cells (82) (**Figure 1**), thus facilitating virus entry (83). It has recently been shown that ADE increases membrane fusion activity, promoting DENV entry (79). Moreover, prM antibodies have the capacity to convert non-infectious, immature DENV particles into infectious particles and enhance their infectivity to levels comparable to wild-type

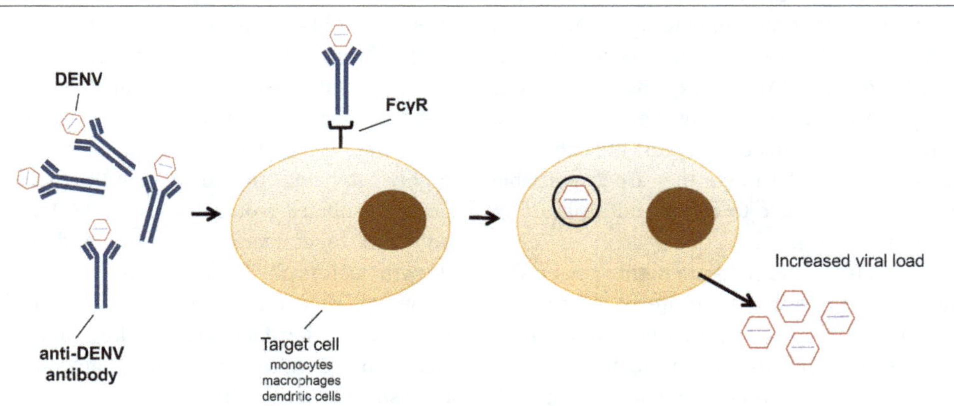

FIGURE 1 | Schematic representation of antibody dependent enhancement (ADE) entry into monocytes, macrophages and dendritic cells as employed by dengue virus.

virus (50). ADE has been linked to the observation that one flavivirus infection can enhance another (84). However, a recent study showed that ADE is dependent on the level of neutralizing antibodies, particularly IgG and IgM (85); only patients with a low level of neutralizing antibodies showed enhancement of DENV infection (85). Antibodies, even at low concentration, against the EDIII domain were able to block viral entry of the four DENV serotypes without inducing antibody-dependent enhancement (86). However, high IgG titres were observed in patients with ADE following DENV infection, in particular IgG1 levels were the highest in patients with dengue fever or shock syndrome (87). ADE has been recently identified as consequence of sensitisation with Dengvaxia quadrivalent vaccine, leading to severe vaccine-enhanced disease resulting in hospitalization (88).

JAPANESE ENCEPHALITIS VIRUS

Globally, Japanese encephalitis is the most clinically important arboviral encephalitis, with an estimated annual prevalence of up to 50,000 cases (89). As is the case with most arboviral encephalitic infections, humans are dead-end hosts unable to develop a sufficiently high viremia to transmit to feeding mosquitos. The majority of JEV infections are asymptomatic. Approximately a third of clinical cases are fatal and half of survivors have neurological or neuropsychiatric sequelae with symptoms resembling Parkinsonian movement disorders, poliomyelitis-like paralysis or impaired cognition (90). Disease is most common in children up to 14 years of age. JEV has been expanding its endemic areas in Asia (91) and poses an unpredictable and emerging global threat.

In humans, JEV has been found in different anatomical compartments and a variety of cell types is able to support its replication. These include endothelial cells, granulocytes, dendritic cells, macrophages and cells of the CNS including astrocytes, neurons and microglia (92). The virus spreads from dermal tissues (93) to lymphoid organs (94) and during the acute stage of infection can be found in blood (95). Although highly neuroinvasive, the mechanism of JEV entry into the CNS is unclear. Transport along the olfactory nerve and across the blood brain barrier have been implicated in JEV invasion of the CNS (96, 97). Studies in rodent models indicate that the blood brain barrier is disrupted following neuroinvasion (98), and might be a consequence of invasion rather than an entry route. Once in the brain, JEV can infect pericytes (99), astrocytes (100) and microglia (101), and has a predilection for developing neurons and neuronal progenitors (102, 103). As described below, a number of receptors mediate entry into different cells types. The distinctive neuronal tropism suggests the existence of JEV-specific receptors in the CNS, but their nature remains elusive (104).

In vitro studies on mouse neuroblastoma cells indicate heat shock protein (HSP) 70 as a putative entry receptor present on neuronal cells (105). This has not been corroborated by *in vivo* experiments, but in human hepatoma Huh7 cells, HSP70 is required for entry (106). Recently, a member of the HSP70 family, glucose-regulated protein (GRP) 78, has been implicated in JEV entry into Neuro2a and BHK-21 cells (107, 108). In addition to HSP70 and GRP78, HSP90β also interacts with E protein and may be used by JEV to enter mammalian cells (109). Another member of the HSP70 family is heat shock cognate (HSC) protein 70. HSC70 has been suggested to be a receptor for entry into mosquito cells (110). HSC70 isoform D is essential for clathrin-dependent endocytosis of JEV into C6/36 cells (111). Clathrin dependence seems to be critical for JEV entry into mammalian cells with the exception of neuronal cells (112), where JEV internalization into rodent neuroblastoma cell lines has been shown to be clathrin-independent (113, 114) and independent of HSP70 family proteins. JEV can enter human neuronal cells by caveolin-mediated endocytosis (115), a process that is receptor-independent (116). Interestingly, JEV has been shown to utilize the dopaminergic signal transduction pathway to increase neuronal susceptibility to infection (117). Infection of human dopaminergic neuroblastoma cells *in vitro* leads to increased levels of secreted dopamine and activation of the phospholipase C cascade. The latter enhances formation of structures known as focal adhesions on the cell surface and increases JEV binding and entry. One of the main components of focal adhesions is αvβ3 integrin that recruits vimentin to the cell surface (118), and is involved in JEV binding and infection of BHK-21 cells (18). Vimentin is a putative JEV receptor (119, 120). Thus, by signaling through dopamine D2 receptors and activating the phospholipase C cascade, JEV induces recruitment of surface molecules that enhance and propagate infection in adjacent cells. Enhanced infection of dopaminergic neurons also explains why JEV is predominantly found in brain areas rich in these cells including the thalamus and the midbrain (121, 122). Whereas JEV infection of neurons may be most directly relevant for disease, other cells types are also likely to have an important role in the disease process. Microglial cells may be a viral reservoir due to long-term, high level of virus production in these cells (123). CD4 has been identified as a major receptor for JEV entry into microglia (124). Presumably, CD4 can be used by JEV to enter other CD4 positive cells such as T cells, macrophages or dendritic cells. Published data are scarce, however, JEV productive infection of splenic macrophages and T cells has been reported in a mouse model of infection (125). T lymphocytes have also been reported as a reservoir of latent JEV in asymptomatic children following recovery from acute infection (126). The involvement of CD4 in microglial cell entry has not been reported for any other flavivirus, however CD4 is the main receptor for retroviral entry and is primarily localized in lipid rafts (127). As mentioned above, HSP70 in lipid rafts is involved in JEV entry into human cells and in general lipid rafts play a critical role in JEV entry (128, 129). Moreover, lipid rafts, as well as clathrin-coated pits and caveolae, contain sphingolipids such as sphingomyelin (SM) that is involved in JEV attachment and entry (130). Studies in SM synthase 1 deficient mice infected with JEV showed a reduction in disease, indicating a role for SM in JEV infection models (130).

Despite advances in identification of new receptors associated with JEV entry and its clear tropism for neuronal cells in the CNS, the identity of a specific neuronal receptor remains elusive. Notably, JEV has the ability to infect cells in the absence of above mentioned putative receptors although at a reduced rate (104). This suggests that the entry process involves multi protein interactions with high degree of redundancy and a single, specific entry receptor might not exist. Alternatively, the inability to identify such a receptor highlights the limitations of *in vitro* systems commonly used to investigate virus-cell interactions.

ZIKA VIRUS

ZIKV is a mosquito-borne emerging pathogen that poses significant public health concerns due to recent rapidly expanding outbreaks. ZIKV was relatively unknown until 2007, when an outbreak occurred in Yap Island (Micronesia) (131). The virus was first isolated in the Zika Forest in Uganda from a rhesus monkey in 1947. In 1948 a second isolate from *Ae. africanus* mosquitoes was obtained from the same forest (132). Prior to the recent serious outbreak in French Polynesia, New Caledonia, the Cook Islands and Easter Island in 2013 and 2014 (133), Zika has not been reported to cause significant disease. Data from French Polynesia during the ZIKV epidemic documented the occurrence of Guillain-Barre syndrome and other neurological complications (134). The pathogenesis of ZIKV infection is poorly understood and involves a multifaceted interaction between viral and host factors. ZIKV has shown a significant tropism to the CNS and causes neurodegeneration, particularly of neural progenitor cells (135–137). ZIKV is also the only flavivirus known to have teratogenic effects in humans, including microcephaly, intracranial calcification and fetal death (138). As a result, the World Health Organization announced in 2016 that the ZIKV outbreak was a health emergency of international concern (139). Like other flaviviruses, ZIKV likely enters host cells through endocytosis instigated by an interaction of E glycoprotein with cell surface receptors. Identification of the entry receptor(s) for ZIKV is essential to understanding viral tropism and pathogenesis, and could lead to the development of novel therapeutics to treat the infection.

The first barrier for the virus to enter the host cell is the skin epidermis. ZIKV is transmitted by *Aedes* spp. mosquitoes, which deposit virus in the epidermis and dermis during the blood meal. Both dermal fibroblast and epidermal keratinocytes are permissive to ZIKV infection as are skin dendritic cells. Several entry receptors including the innate immune receptor DC-SIGN, transmembrane protein TIM-1 and TAM receptors (TYRO3, AXL, MER), have been shown to facilitate entry and enhance ZIKV infection (29). RNA silencing of TIM-1 and AXL in subsets of human skin cells showed a significant reduction in ZIKV titre in AXL knockdown, and in double AXL and TIM-1 knockdown, indicating that AXL is a major receptor for ZIKV entry at least in human skin cells. However, a recent study (43) investigating different infection routes of ZIKV, including subcutaneous, transplacental, vaginal, and intracranial infections in wild-type and TAM receptor null mice, showed no difference in viral titres. TAM receptors, at least in mice, are therefore not essential for ZIKV infection. Interestingly, WNV infection of neurons can be enhanced in mice lacking AXL and MER. This increase in infectivity was associated with changes in blood brain barrier permeability (140), suggesting that AXL and MER do not serve exclusively as receptors and might have other roles in WNV infection of the brain.

To reach the fetal brain, ZIKV must first be transported to the fetal circulation, and cross the placental barrier. The placental barrier is composed of placental barrier cells, trophoblasts and fetal endothelial cells, which separate the fetal blood in capillaries from maternal blood. ZIKV has been reported in the amniotic fluid of fetuses in Brazil (141). This observation strengthened the association of ZIKV with microcephaly in neonates. Moreover, it has been shown that microcephaly caused by maternal viral infection in mice could result from direct viral infection of the fetus via the trans-placental route as well as from a placental inflammatory response that affects fetal development (142). ZIKV can efficiently infect fetal endothelial cells, whereas WNV and DENV do not, highlighting ZIKV unique tropism among flaviviruses (143). These differences between flaviviruses are due to ZIKV ability to efficiently use AXL receptor to enter fetal endothelial cells (143).

TIM-1 was also observed to have an important role in placental entry of ZIKV (144). ZIKV was able to infect different human primary placental cell types and explants from chorionic villi. AXL, TYRO3, and TIM-1 were present in the primary placental cells and are found at the uterine-placental interface. Particularly high expression of TIM-1 has been observed in cells where maternal blood perfused placenta including basal decidua and neighboring chorionic villi. Expression of AXL and TYRO3 varied with explant donor, gestational age and cell type. Specific pharmacological inhibition of TIM-1 by duramycin (145) could inhibit ZIKV infection at the uterine-placental interface, indicating that TIM-1 is a putative receptor for ZIKV placental cell entry. However, the role of AXL, variation in the expression of AXL and TYRO3 in pregnant women and whether TIM-1 is the sole receptor for ZIKV infection of the placenta need further study.

Numerous studies on ZIKV infection in mice having defective interferon signaling, including IFNα/β knockout mice (146, 147), double knockout of IFNα/β and IFNγ (148), and triple knockout of IRF-3,-5,-7 (136, 149) showed viremia, microcephaly and death in young mice and viremia with recovery in adult mice. However, cell death and reduced proliferation was observed for adult neural stem cells (136) suggesting possible long term effects in adult brain followin ZIKV infection. ZIKV also infects other cell types, especially in the eye. ZIKV-inoculated mice develop ocular defects including conjunctivitis, pan uveitis, and infection of the optic nerve, cornea, iris, and ganglion and bipolar cells in the retina (150). AXL is expressed at high levels in retinal progenitor cells (151) suggesting a possible role in ZIKV infection of ocular cells. However, the ocular abnormalities were shown to be independent of AXL or MER, given that AXL$^{-/-}$, MER$^{-/-}$, and AXL$^{-/-}$ MER$^{-/-}$ double knockout mice sustained levels of infection similar to those of control animals. Nevertheless, AXL might have a role in ZIKV infection of glial cells via Gas6 mediated activation of AXL kinase (152).

In vitro and *in vivo* systems to study ZIKV infection of neural cells have been developed. ZIKV neuro-infection models using cultured neural precursor cells (NPCs), cortical organoids, mouse brains, and human fetal brain materials have been studied (153). Microcephaly in these models is associated with inflammation, reduced proliferation of NPCs and neuronal cell death. ZIKV-BR can infect mouse fetuses and infection of pregnant mice also causes disease in embryos with intrauterine growth restriction, including signs of microcephaly (154). This study also demonstrated that ZIKV-BR infects human cortical progenitor cells, increasing the rate of cell death. ZIKV was found to directly infect human NPCs with high efficiency providing a plausible explanation for the observed developmental phenotypes and associated teratogenicity in the neonatal brains (137). Based on previous studies (29, 151, 152), AXL is a strong candidate receptor for the entry of ZIKV into cells of the developing brain. The potential role of AXL to facilitate ZIKV infection of the neonatal brain was explored by determining, at a single cell level, RNA expression profiles in the developing human cerebral cortex (151). The study revealed a higher expression of AXL in the radial cells and neural stem cells of the developing brain throughout neurogenesis and in capillaries and astrocytes. However, loss of AXL expression following CRISPR/Cas9 gene editing, did not affect ZIKV infectivity into hNPCs or cerebral organoids (155).

As is the case with JEV, the identity of the receptors involved in ZIKV receptor mediated endocytosis remains to be elucidated. There might be tissue specificity in receptor mediated viral entry, with variation in receptor repertoire in the skin, placenta, neurons, and other cell types. Alternatively, given ZIKV unique ability to cross the placenta and infect developing neurons in the fetal brain, there might be some as yet unidentified receptors facilitating this process.

YELLOW FEVER VIRUS

YFV is the prototype and namesake virus of the *Flavivirus* genus; *flavi* means yellow in Latin. When infecting humans YFV replicates in liver, heart, kidneys, and lungs causing a broad spectrum of clinical symptoms. These vary from asymptomatic infection to renal and hepatic failures with severe haemorrhagic disease (156). A live attenuated YFV vaccine 17D was created over 70 years ago and has been used safely in over 500 million people. The parent strain of 17D is the virulent Asibi strain (157) isolated in Africa in 1927. 17D was passaged more than 230 times in mouse and chicken embryonic tissue. The adaptation of 17D to grow in tissue culture resulted in loss of viscerotropism, neurotropism, and mosquito tropism (156), making it an ideal candidate for a vaccine. The genome of both strains has been sequenced (158). The extensive passage history gave rise to 68 nucleotide mutations and 32 amino acid substitutions. Most of the genetic differences occur in the envelope (E) protein gene (157). Interestingly, the molecular determinants and mechanisms of this attenuation remain largely unknown. It has been suggested that the differences in the E protein and its involvement in cell entry are determinants of the difference in pathogenicity between the 17D and Asibi strains (159, 160). Mutations in the E gene have been suggested to allow the 17D strain to bind and enter hosts cells more efficiently.

YFV shares genome organization and entry by clarithin-mediated endocytosis (CME) with most of the other flaviviruses. During YFV infection, the E protein binds to an unknown entry receptor that traffics the virion to endosomes. Similarly to other flaviviruses, increase in acidification of the endosome results in conformational changes in the E protein, membrane fusion and nucleocapsid release into the cytoplasm (156). The vaccine strain uses a clathrin- and caveolin-independent, but dynamin-2-dependent, pathway for infection (160). Dynamin-2 is a GTPase involved in cleaving off endocytic vesicles from the plasma membrane (161). The entry pathway of the 17D strain was further characterized as Rac1, Pak1, and cortactin independent (160). Clarithin-independent entry has been reported to mediate the internalization of a variety of viruses, such as rotavirus, human rhinovirus, influenza, and interestingly, JEV vaccine strain in neuronal cells (114, 162–164). Cells infected with 17D have been found to produce more viral RNA and INF-β, IL-29, ISG56, CCL5, and CXCL10 mRNA than those infected with the parental Asibi strain. In addition, 17D infected cells secrete INF-β, whereas cells infected with the Asibi strain do not. Virus entry through a clathrin-independent pathway allows for more efficient virion delivery into endosomes or protection from degradation, relative to entry via the classical clathrin-mediated route. This former entry route has been suggested to allow for a higher amount of viral RNA released into the cytoplasm (160). Viral RNA in the cytoplasm is detected by RIG-I, MDA5 and TLR7 (165), triggering strong innate immune responses. The Asibi strain on other hand, replicates at lower levels and inhibits the innate immune system. This difference in entry mechanism has been suggested to account for the differences in cytokine response between the two YFV strains, though further mutations in other proteins, such as NS2A could also be involved.

CONCLUSIONS

Glycoprotein E is responsible for receptor-mediated attachment of flaviviruses to the host cell and membrane fusion. Although E protein of different flaviviruses share approximately 40% sequence identity (e.g., DENV and TBEV), their overall structural features are almost identical and this is assumed to apply to all flaviviruses (166). Cell entry is facilitated by a conserved peptide of 16 amino acids, located in E-DII region of the envelope glycoprotein (167). This conservation, coupled with highly organized conformational changes upon exposure to low pH (168), suggests evolutionary constraints allowing flaviviruses to enter both mammalian and arthropod cells. Yet, flavivirus receptors show diversity and significant cell type specificity. It is not unusual that a single molecule can bind to variety of targets as exemplified by immunoglobulins. However, their diversity and specificity are governed by V(D)J recombination, while the flaviviral glycoprotein E is conserved. The flavivirus infection is a consequence of multiple complex interactions between the virus and the target cell. It is clear that the flavivirus can exploit different endocytic routes that can be either clathrin or caveolae dependent or independent. The neurotropism of specific flaviviruses raises the question, is there a single specific neuronal receptor? What is the identity of this receptor and is the same receptor being used by all encephalitic flaviviruses? Another unresolved question is whether all flaviviruses share the same features of infection in the developing brain, or whether viruses such as microcephaly-causing ZIKV, exhibit a different infection pattern. It is also relevant to note that the expression of entry receptors (e.g., CLRs or TAM) does not account for flavivirus tropism and cellular models lacking those receptors are still permissive to infection. Identifying the relevant entry receptors is essential to deciphering the mechanisms of pathogenesis, tropism and viral biology. A better understanding of those processes will uncover new strategies for designing therapeutics and vaccines against flaviviruses.

AUTHOR CONTRIBUTIONS

ML, DN, JR-A, and LK wrote sections of the manuscript, JF and LK edited and critically evaluated the manuscript.

REFERENCES

1. Messina JP, Brady OJ, Scott TW, Zou C, Pigott DM, Duda KA, et al. Global spread of dengue virus types: mapping the 70 year history. *Trends Microbiol.* (2014) 2:138–46. doi: 10.1016/j.tim.2013.12.011
2. Weaver SC, Costa F, Garcia-Blanco MA, Ko AI, Ribeiro GS, Saade G, et al. Zika virus: History, emergence, biology, and prospects for control. *Antiviral Res.* (2016) 30:69–80. doi: 10.1016/j.antiviral.2016.03.010
3. Kraemer MUG, Faria NR, Reiner RC Jr, Golding N, Nikolay B, Stasse S, et al. Spread of yellow fever virus outbreak in angola and the democratic republic of the Congo 2015-16: a modelling study. *Lancet Infect Dis.* (2017) 7:330–8. doi: 10.1016/S1473-3099(16)30513-8
4. Hamer DH, Angelo K, Caumes E, van Genderen PJJ, Florescu SA, Popescu CP, et al. Fatal Yellow Fever in Travelers to Brazil, 2018. *MMWR Morb Mortal Wkly Rep.* (2018) 67:340–1. doi: 10.15585/mmwr.mm6711e1
5. Hayes EB, Gubler DJ. West Nile virus: epidemiology and clinical features of an emerging epidemic in the United States. *Annu Rev Med.* (2006) 7:181–94. doi: 10.1146/annurev.med.57.121304.131418
6. Gould EA, Solomon, T. Pathogenic flaviviruses. *Lancet* (2008) 71:500–9. doi: 10.1016/S0140-6736(08)60238-X
7. Mlera L, Melik W, Bloom M, E. The role of viral persistence in flavivirus biology. *Pathog Dis.* (2014) 1:137–63. doi: 10.1111/2049-632X.12178
8. Collins MH, Metz S, W. Progress and works in progress: update on flavivirus vaccine development. *Clin Ther.* (2017) 9:1519–36. doi: 10.1016/j.clinthera.2017.07.001
9. Sirohi D, Chen Z, Sun L, Klose T, Pierson TC, Rossmann MG, et al. The 3.8 A resolution cryo-EM structure of Zika virus. *Science* (2016) 52:467–70. doi: 10.1126/science.aaf5316
10. Zhang X, Ge P, Yu X, Brannan JM, Bi G, Zhang Q, et al. Cryo-EM structure of the mature dengue virus at 3.5-A resolution. *Nat Struct Mol Biol.* (2013) 20:105–10. doi: 10.1038/nsmb.2463
11. Perera-Lecoin M, Meertens L, Carnec X, Amara, A. Flavivirus entry receptors: an update. *Viruses* (2013) 6:69–88. doi: 10.3390/v6010069
12. Pierson TC, Kielian, M. Flaviviruses: braking the entering. *Curr Opin Virol.* (2013) 3:3–12. doi: 10.1016/j.coviro.2012.12.001
13. Sun H, Chen Q, Lai, H. Development of antibody therapeutics against flaviviruses. *Int J Mol Sci.* (2017) 19:E54. doi: 10.3390/ijms19010054
14. Smit JM, Moesker B, Rodenhuis-Zybert I, Wilschut, J. Flavivirus cell entry and membrane fusion. *Viruses* (2011) 3:160–71. doi: 10.3390/v3020160
15. Stiasny K, Fritz R, Pangerl K, Heinz F, X. Molecular mechanisms of flavivirus membrane fusion. *Amino Acids* (2011) 1:1159–63. doi: 10.1007/s00726-009-0370-4
16. Noisakran S, Onlamoon N, Songprakhon P, Hsiao H M, Chokephaibulkit K, Perng G, C. Cells in dengue virus infection *in vivo*. *Adv Virol.* (2010) 2010:164878. doi: 10.1155/2010/164878
17. Chu JJ, Ng M, L. Interaction of West Nile virus with alpha v beta 3 integrin mediates virus entry into cells. *J Biol Chem.* (2004) 79:54533–41. doi: 10.1074/jbc.M410208200
18. Fan W, Qian P, Wang D, Zhi X, Wei Y, Chen H, et al. Integrin alphavbeta3 promotes infection by Japanese encephalitis virus. *Res Vet Sci.* (2017) 11:67–74. doi: 10.1016/j.rvsc.2016.12.007
19. Davis CW, Nguyen HY, Hanna SL, Sanchez MD, Doms RW, Pierson T, C. West Nile virus discriminates between DC-SIGN and DC-SIGNR for cellular attachment and infection. *J Virol.* (2006) 80:1290–301. doi: 10.1128/JVI.80.3.1290-1301.2006
20. Davis CW, Mattei LM, Nguyen HY, Ansarah-Sobrinho C, Doms RW, Pierson T, C. The location of asparagine-linked glycans on West Nile virions controls their interactions with CD209 (dendritic cell-specific ICAM-3 grabbing nonintegrin). *J Biol Chem.* (2006) 81:37183–94. doi: 10.1074/jbc.M605429200
21. Miller JL, de Wet BJ, Martinez-Pomares L, Radcliffe CM, Dwek RA, Rudd PM, et al. The mannose receptor mediates dengue virus infection of macrophages. *PLoS Pathog* (2008) 4:e17. doi: 10.1371/journal.ppat.0040017
22. Chen ST, Liu RS, Wu MF, Lin YL, Chen SY, Tan DT, et al. CLEC5A regulates Japanese encephalitis virus-induced neuroinflammation and lethality. *PLoS Pathog* (2012) 8:e1002655. doi: 10.1371/journal.ppat.1002655
23. Cheng G, Cox J, Wang P, Krishnan MN, Dai J, Qian F, et al. AC-type lectin collaborates with a CD45 phosphatase homolog to facilitate West Nile virus infection of mosquitoes. *Cell* (2010) 42:714–25. doi: 10.1016/j.cell.2010.07.038
24. Meertens L, Carnec X, Lecoin MP, Ramdasi R, Guivel-Benhassine F, Lew E, et al. The TIM and TAM families of phosphatidylserine receptors mediate dengue virus entry. *Cell Host Microbe* (2012) 2:544–57. doi: 10.1016/j.chom.2012.08.009
25. Rey FA, Stiasny K, Heinz F, X. Flavivirus structural heterogeneity: implications for cell entry. *Curr Opin Virol.* (2017) 4:132–9. doi: 10.1016/j.coviro.2017.06.009
26. Briant L, Despres P, Choumet V, Misse, D. Role of skin immune cells on the host susceptibility to mosquito-borne viruses. *Virology* (2014) 4:64–465, 26–32. doi: 10.1016/j.virol.2014.06.023
27. Wu SJ, Grouard-Vogel G, Sun W, Mascola JR, Brachtel E, Putvatana R, et al. Human skin Langerhans cells are targets of dengue virus infection. *Nat Med.* (2000) 6:816–20. doi: 10.1038/77553
28. Wang P, Hu K, Luo S, Zhang M, Deng X, Li C, et al. DC-SIGN as an attachment factor mediates Japanese encephalitis virus infection of human dendritic cells via interaction with a single high-mannose residue of viral E glycoprotein. *Virology* (2016) 88:108–19. doi: 10.1016/j.virol.2015.11.006
29. Hamel R, Dejarnac O, Wichit S, Ekchariyawat P, Neyret A, Luplertlop N, et al. Biology of Zika Virus Infection in Human Skin Cells. *J Virol.* (2015) 9:8880–96. doi: 10.1128/JVI.00354-15
30. Barba-Spaeth G, Longman RS, Albert ML, Rice C, M. Live attenuated yellow fever 17D infects human DCs and allows for presentation of endogenous and recombinant T cell epitopes. *J Exp Med.* (2005) 02:1179–84. doi: 10.1084/jem.20051352
31. Lozach PY, Burleigh L, Staropoli I, Navarro-Sanchez E, Harriague J, Virelizier JL, et al. Dendritic cell-specific intercellular adhesion molecule 3-grabbing non-integrin (DC-SIGN)-mediated enhancement of dengue virus infection is independent of DC-SIGN internalization signals. *J Biol Chem.* (2005) 80:23698–708. doi: 10.1074/jbc.M504337200
32. Neal J, W. Flaviviruses are neurotropic, but how do they invade the CNS? *J Infect.* (2014) 9:203–15. doi: 10.1016/j.jinf.2014.05.010
33. Solomon, T. Flavivirus encephalitis. *N Engl J Med.* (2004) 51:370–8. doi: 10.1056/NEJMra030476
34. Kramer LD, Li J, Shi P, Y. West Nile virus. *Lancet Neurol.* (2007) 6:171–81. doi: 10.1016/S1474-4422(07)70030-3

35. Domingues RB, Fuster GW, Onuki-Castro FL, Souza VA, Levi JE, Pannuti C, S. Involvement of the central nervous system in patients with dengue virus infection. *J Neurol Sci.* (2008) 2:67:36–40. doi: 10.1016/j.jns.2007.09.040
36. Linehan SA, Martinez-Pomares L, Stahl PD, Gordon, S. Mannose receptor and its putative ligands in normal murine lymphoid and nonlymphoid organs: *In situ* expression of mannose receptor by selected macrophages, endothelial cells perivascular microglia, and mesangial cells, but not dendritic cells. *J Exp Med.* (1999) 89:1961–72.
37. Burudi EM, Riese S, Stahl PD, A. Regnier-Vigouroux: Identification and functional characterization of the mannose receptor in astrocytes. *Glia* (1999) 5:44–55.
38. Mukhtar M, Harley S, Chen P, BouHamdan M, Patel C, Acheampong E, et al. Primary isolated human brain microvascular endothelial cells express diverse HIV/SIV-associated chemokine coreceptors and DC-SIGN and L-SIGN. *Virology* (2002) 297:78–88. doi: 10.1006/viro.2002.1376
39. Galea I, Palin E, Newman TA, Van Rooijen N, Perry VH, Boche, D. Mannose receptor expression specifically reveals perivascular macrophages in normal, injured, and diseased mouse brain. *Glia* (2005) 9:375–84. doi: 10.1002/glia.20124
40. Prodinger C, Bunse J, Kruger M, Schiefenhovel F, Brandt C, Laman JD, et al. CD11c-expressing cells reside in the juxtavascular parenchyma and extend processes into the glia limitans of the mouse nervous system. *Acta Neuropathol.* (2011) 21:445–58. doi: 10.1007/s00401-010-0774-y
41. Todorich B, Zhang X, Slagle-Webb B, Seaman WE, Connor J, R. Tim-2 is the receptor for H-ferritin on oligodendrocytes. *J Neurochem.* (2008) 107:1495–505. doi: 10.1111/j.1471-4159.2008.05678.x
42. Prieto AL, Weber JL, Lai, C. Expression of the receptor protein-tyrosine kinases Tyro-3, Axl, and mer in the developing rat central nervous system. *J Comp Neurol.* (2000) 25:295–314. doi: 10.1002/1096-9861(20000918)425:2<295::AID-CNE11>3.0.CO;2-G
43. Hastings AK, Yockey LJ, Jagger BW, Hwang J, Uraki R, Gaitsch HF, et al. TAM receptors are not required for zika virus infection in Mice. *Cell Rep.* (2017) 9:558–68 doi: 10.1016/j.celrep.2017.03.058
44. Girard YA, Klingler KA, Higgs, S. West Nile virus dissemination and tissue tropisms in orally infected Culex pipiens quinquefasciatus. *Vector Borne Zoonotic Dis* (2004) 4:109–22. doi: 10.1089/1530366041210729
45. Salazar MI, Richardson JH, Sanchez-Vargas I, Olson KE, Beaty B, J. Dengue virus type 2: replication and tropisms in orally infected Aedes aegypti mosquitoes. *BMC Microbiol.* (2007) 7:9. doi: 10.1186/1471-2180-7-9
46. Vega-Almeida TO, Salas-Benito M, M. A. De Nova-Ocampo, Del Angel RM, Salas-Benito J. S. Surface proteins of C6/36 cells involved in dengue virus 4 binding and entry. *Arch Virol.* (2013) 58:1189–207. doi: 10.1007/s00705-012-1596-0
47. Lima-Camara TN. Emerging arboviruses and public health challenges in Brazil. *Rev Saude Publica* (2016) 50:S0034-89102016000100602. doi: 10.1590/S1518-8787.2016050006791
48. Sucharit S, Surathin K, Shrestha S, R. Vectors of Japanese encephalitis virus (JEV): species complexes of the vectors. *Southeast Asian J Trop Med Public Health* (1989) 20:611–21.
49. WHO. *Dengue and Severe Dengue.* Geneva: WHO (2018).
50. Rodenhuis-Zybert IA, Wilschut J, Smit J, M. Dengue virus life cycle: Viral and host factors modulating infectivity. *Cell Mol Life Sci.* (2010) 67:2773–86. doi: 10.1007/s00018-010-0357-z
51. Watterson D, Kobe B, Young P, R. Residues in domain III of the dengue virus envelope glycoprotein involved in cell-surface glycosaminoglycan binding. *J Gen Virol.* (2012) 3:72–82. doi: 10.1099/vir.0.037317-0
52. Tripathi NK, Shrivastava A, Biswal KC, Rao PV, L. Recombinant dengue virus type 3 envelope domain III protein from *Escherichia coli. Biotechnol J.* (2011) 6:604–8. doi: 10.1002/biot.201000399
53. Chiang CY, Pan CH, Chen MY, Hsieh CH, Tsai JP, Liu HH, et al. Immunogenicity of a novel tetravalent vaccine formulation with four recombinant lipidated dengue envelope protein domain IIIs in mice. *Sci Rep.* (2016) 6:30648. doi: 10.1038/srep30648
54. Aoki C, Hidari KIPJ, Itonori S, Yamada A, Takahashi N, Kasama T, et al. Identification and characterization of carbohydrate molecules in mammalian cells recognized by dengue virus type 2. *J Biochem.* (2006) 139:607–14. doi: 10.1093/jb/mvj067
55. Hilgard P, Stockert, R. Heparan sulfate proteoglycans initiate dengue virus infection of hepatocytes. *Hepatology* (2000) 2:1069–77. doi: 10.1053/jhep.2000.18713
56. Kato D, Era S, Watanabe I, Arihara M, Sugiura N, Kimata K, et al. Antiviral activity of chondroitin sulphate E targeting dengue virus envelope protein. *Antiviral Res.* (2010) 8:236–43. doi: 10.1016/j.antiviral.2010.09.002
57. Hoving JC, Wilson GJ, Brown G, D. Signalling C-type lectin receptors, microbial recognition and immunity. *Cell Microbiol.* (2014) 6:185–94. doi: 10.1111/cmi.12249
58. Lo YL, Liou GG, Lyu JH, Hsiao M, Hsu TL, Wong CH. Dengue virus infection is through a cooperative interaction between a mannose receptor and CLEC5A on macrophage as a multivalent hetero-complex. *PLoS ONE* (2016) 1:e0166474. doi: 10.1371/journal.pone.0166474
59. Che P, Tang H, Li, Q. The interaction between claudin-1 and dengue viral prM/M protein for its entry. *Virology* (2013) 46:303–13. doi: 10.1016/J.VIROL.2013.08.009
60. Dalrymple N, Mackow E, R. Productive dengue virus infection of human endothelial cells is directed by heparan sulfate-containing proteoglycan receptors. *J Virol.* (2011) 5:9478–85. doi: 10.1128/JVI.05008-11
61. Germi R, Crance JM, Garin D, Guimet J, Lortat-Jacob H, Ruigrok RW, et al. Heparan sulfate-mediated binding of infectious dengue virus type 2 and yellow fever virus. *Virology* (2002) 92:162–8. doi: 10.1006/viro.2001.1232
62. Wang K, Wang J, Sun T, Bian G, Pan W, Feng T, et al. Glycosphingolipid GM3 is Indispensable for Dengue Virus Genome Replication. *Int J Biol Sci.* (2016) 2:872–83. doi: 10.7150/ijbs.15641
63. Liu P, Ridilla M, Patel P, Betts L, Gallichotte E, Shahidi L, et al. Beyond attachment: Roles of DC-SIGN in dengue virus infection. *Traffic* (2017) 8:218–31. doi: 10.1111/tra.12469
64. Gao F, Duan X, Lu X, Liu Y, Zheng L, Ding Z, et al. Novel binding between pre-membrane protein and claudin-1 is required for efficient dengue virus entry. *Biochem Biophys Res Commun.* (2010) 91:952–7. doi: 10.1016/J.BBRC.2009.11.172
65. H.-Chee Y, AbuBakar, S. Identification of a 48kDa tubulin or tubulin-like C6/36 mosquito cells protein that binds dengue virus 2 using mass spectrometry. *Biochem Biophys Res Commun.* (2004) 20:11–17. doi: 10.1016/j.bbrc.2004.05.124
66. Mercado-Curiel RF, Esquinca-Avilés HA, Tovar R, Díaz-Badillo A, Camacho-Nuez M, M. d. L. Muñoz: The four serotypes of dengue recognize the same putative receptors in Aedes aegypti midgut and Ae. albopictus cells. *BMC Microbiol.* (2006) 6:85. doi: 10.1186/1471-2180-6-85
67. Paingankar MS, Gokhale MD, Deobagkar D, N. Dengue-2-virus-interacting polypeptides involved in mosquito cell infection. *Arch Virol.* (2010) 55:1453–61. doi: 10.1007/s00705-010-0728-7
68. Cao-Lormeau VM. Dengue viruses binding proteins from Aedes aegypti and Aedes polynesiensis salivary glands. *Virol J.* (2009) 6:35. doi: 10.1186/1743-422X-6-35
69. Srisutthisamphan K, Jirakanwisal K, Ramphan S, Tongluan N, Kuadkitkan A, Smith D, R. Hsp90 interacts with multiple dengue virus 2 proteins. *Sci Rep.* (2018) 8:4308. doi: 10.1038/s41598-018-22639-5
70. Salas-Benito J, Reyes-Del Valle J, Salas-Benito M, Ceballos-Olvera I, Mosso C, del Angel RM. Evidence that the 45-kD Glycoprotein, part of a putative dengue virus receptor complex in the mosquito cell line C6/36, is a heat-shock-related protein. *Am J Trop Med Hygiene* (2007) 7:283–90. doi: 10.4269/ajtmh.2007.77.283
71. Taguwa S, Maringer K, Li X, Bernal-Rubio D, Rauch JN, Gestwicki JE, et al. Defining Hsp70 subnetworks in dengue virus replication reveals key vulnerability in flavivirus infection HHS public access. *Cell* (2015) 9:1108–23. doi: 10.1016/j.cell.2015.10.046
72. Reyes-Del Valle J, Chávez-Salinas S, Medina F, Del Angel RM. Heat shock protein 90 and heat shock protein 70 are components of dengue virus receptor complex in human cells. *J Virol.* (2005) 9:4557–67. doi: 10.1128/JVI.79.8.4557-4567.2005
73. Cabrera-Hernandez A, Thepparit C, Suksanpaisan L, Smith DR. Dengue virus entry into liver (HepG2) cells is independent of hsp90 and hsp70. *J Med Virol.* (2007) 9:386–92. doi: 10.1002/jmv.20786
74. Dejarnac O, Hafirassou M L, Chazal M, Versapuech M, Gaillard J, Perera-Lecoin M, et al. TIM-1 ubiquitination mediates dengue virus Entry. *Cell Rep.* (2018) 3:1779–93. doi: 10.1016/j.celrep.2018.04.013

75. Alhoot MA, Wang SM, Sekaran SD. Inhibition of dengue virus entry and multiplication into monocytes using RNA interference. *PLoS Negl Trop Dis.* (2011) 5:e1410. doi: 10.1371/journal.pntd.0001410
76. Acosta EG, Castilla V, Damonte EB. Infectious dengue-1 virus entry into mosquito C6/36 cells. *Virus Res.* (2011) 60:173–9. doi: 10.1016/J.VIRUSRES.2011.06.008
77. Alhoot MA, Wang SM, Sekaran SD. RNA Interference mediated inhibition of dengue virus multiplication and entry in HepG2 Cells. *PLoS ONE* (2012) 7:e34060. doi: 10.1371/journal.pone.0034060
78. Acosta EG, Castilla V, Damonte EB. Alternative infectious entry pathways for dengue virus serotypes into mammalian cells. *Cell Microbiol.* (2009) 1:1533–49. doi: 10.1111/j.1462-5822.2009.01345.x
79. Flipse J, Diosa-Toro MA, Hoornweg TE, van de Pol DPI, Urcuqui-Inchima S, Smit JM. Antibody-dependent enhancement of dengue virus infection in primary human macrophages; balancing higher fusion against antiviral responses. *Sci Rep.* (2016) 6:29201. doi: 10.1038/srep29201
80. Hawkes RA. Enhancement of the infectivity of arboviruses by specific antisera produced in domestic fowls. *Aust J Exp Biol Med Sci.* (1964) 42:465–82.
81. Halstead SB, O'Rourke EJ. Dengue viruses and mononuclear phagocytes. I. Infection enhancement by non-neutralizing antibody. *J Exp Med.* (1977) 46:201–17.
82. Boonnak K, Dambach K M, Donofrio G C, Tassaneetrithep B, Marovich MA. Cell type specificity and host genetic polymorphisms influence antibody-dependent enhancement of dengue virus infection. *J Virol.* (2011) 5:1671–83. doi: 10.1128/JVI.00220-10
83. Gollins SW, Porterfield JS. Flavivirus infection enhancement in macrophages: radioactive and biological studies on the effect of antibody on viral fate. *J Gen Virol.* (1984) 65(Pt 8):1261–72.
84. Priyamvada L, Quicke KM, Hudson WH, Onlamoon N, Sewatanon J, Edupuganti S, et al. Human antibody responses after dengue virus infection are highly cross-reactive to Zika virus. *Proc Natl Acad Sci USA.* (2016) 13:7852–7. doi: 10.1073/pnas.1607931113
85. Ly MHP, Moi ML, Vu TBH, Tun MMN, Saunders T, Nguyen CN, et al. Dengue virus infection-enhancement activity in neutralizing antibodies of healthy adults before dengue season as determined by using FcγR-expressing cells. *BMC Infect Dis.* (2018) 8:31. doi: 10.1186/s12879-017-2894-7
86. Ramasamy V, Arora U, Shukla R, Poddar A, Shanmugam RK, White LJ, et al. A tetravalent virus-like particle vaccine designed to display domain III of dengue envelope proteins induces multi-serotype neutralizing antibodies in mice and macaques which confer protection against antibody dependent enhancement in AG129 mice. *PLoS Negl Trop Dis.* (2018) 2:e0006191. doi: 10.1371/journal.pntd.0006191
87. Thein S, Aaskov J, Myint TT, Shwe TN, Saw TT, Zaw A. Changes in levels of anti-dengue virus IgG subclasses in patients with disease of varying severity. *J Med Virol.* (1993) 106:102–6.
88. Halstead SB. Dengvaxia sensitizes seronegatives to vaccine enhanced disease regardless of age. *Vaccine* (2017) 5:6355–8. doi: 10.1016/j.vaccine.2017.09.089
89. Simon LV, Kruse B. Encephalitis, Japanese. In. *StatPearls.* Treasure Island (FL) (2018)
90. Mackenzie JS, Gubler DJ, Petersen LR. Emerging flaviviruses: the spread and resurgence of Japanese encephalitis, West Nile and dengue viruses. *Nat Med.* (2004) 10(12 Suppl):S98–109. doi: 10.1038/nm1144
91. Misra UK, Kalita J. Overview: Japanese encephalitis. *Prog Neurobiol.* (2010) 1:108–20. doi: 10.1016/j.pneurobio.2010.01.008
92. Lannes N, Summerfield A, Filgueira L. Regulation of inflammation in Japanese encephalitis. *J Neuroinflammation* (2017) 4:158. doi: 10.1186/s12974-017-0931-5
93. Agrawal T, Sharvani V, Nair D, Medigeshi GR. Japanese encephalitis virus disrupts cell-cell junctions and affects the epithelial permeability barrier functions. *PLoS ONE* (2013) 8:e69465. doi: 10.1371/journal.pone.0069465
94. Nagata N, Iwata-Yoshikawa N, Hayasaka D, Sato Y, Kojima A, Kariwa H, et al. The pathogenesis of 3 neurotropic flaviviruses in a mouse model depends on the route of neuroinvasion after viremia. *J Neuropathol Exp Neurol.* (2015) 4:250–60. doi: 10.1097/NEN.0000000000000166
95. Sapkal GN, Wairagkar NS, Ayachit VM, Bondre VP, Gore MM. Detection and isolation of Japanese encephalitis virus from blood clots collected during the acute phase of infection. *Am J Trop Med Hyg.* (2007) 7:1139-45. doi: 10.4269/ajtmh.2007.77.1139
96. Myint KS, Raengsakulrach B, Young G D, Gettayacamin M, Ferguson L M, Innis BL, et al. Production of lethal infection that resembles fatal human disease by intranasal inoculation of macaques with Japanese encephalitis virus. *Am J Trop Med Hyg* (1999) 60:338–42.
97. Liou ML, Hsu CY. Japanese encephalitis virus is transported across the cerebral blood vessels by endocytosis in mouse brain. *Cell Tissue Res.* (1998) 93:389–94.
98. Li F, Wang Y, Yu L, Cao S, Wang K, Yuan J, et al. Viral infection of the central nervous system and neuroinflammation precede blood-brain barrier disruption during japanese encephalitis virus infection. *J Virol.* (2015) 9:5602–14. doi: 10.1128/JVI.00143-15
99. Chen CJ, Ou YC, Li JR, Chang CY, Pan HC, Lai CY, et al. Infection of pericytes in vitro by Japanese encephalitis virus disrupts the integrity of the endothelial barrier. *J Virol.* (2014) 8:1150–61. doi: 10.1128/JVI.02738-13
100. Chang CY, Li JR, Chen WY, Ou YC, Lai CY, Hu YH, et al. Disruption of *in vitro* endothelial barrier integrity by Japanese encephalitis virus-Infected astrocytes. *Glia* (2015) 63:1915–32. doi: 10.1002/glia.22857
101. Myint KS, Kipar A, Jarman RG, Gibbons RV, Perng GC, Flanagan B, et al. Neuropathogenesis of Japanese encephalitis in a primate model. *PLoS Negl Trop Dis.* (2014) 8:e2980. doi: 10.1371/journal.pntd.0002980
102. Kimura-Kuroda J, Ichikawa M, Ogata A, Nagashima K, Yasui, K. Specific tropism of Japanese encephalitis virus for developing neurons in primary rat brain culture. *Arch Virol.* (1993) 130:477–84.
103. Das S, Basu, A. Japanese encephalitis virus infects neural progenitor cells and decreases their proliferation. *J Neurochem.* (2008) 6:1624–36. doi: 10.1111/j.1471-4159.2008.05511.x
104. Nain M, Abdin MZ, Kalia M, Vrati, S. Japanese encephalitis virus invasion of cell: allies and alleys. *Rev Med Virol.* (2016) 6:129–41. doi: 10.1002/rmv.1868
105. Das S, Laxminarayana SV, Chandra N, Ravi V, Desai, A. Heat shock protein 70 on Neuro2a cells is a putative receptor for Japanese encephalitis virus. *Virology* (2009) 85:47–57. doi: 10.1016/j.virol.2008.10.025
106. Zhu YZ, Cao MM, Wang WB, Wang W, Ren H, Zhao P, et al. Association of heat-shock protein 70 with lipid rafts is required for Japanese encephalitis virus infection in Huh7 cells. *J Gen Virol.* (2012) 93(Pt. 1):61–71. doi: 10.1099/vir.0.034637-0
107. Nain M, Mukherjee S, Karmakar SP, Paton AW, Paton JC, Abdin MZ, et al. GRP78 is an important host factor for Japanese Encephalitis virus entry and replication in mammalian cells. *J Virol.* (2017) 91:e02274-16. doi: 10.1128/JVI.02274-16
108. Wu YP, Chang CM, Hung CY, Tsai MC, Schuyler SC, Wang RY. Japanese encephalitis virus co-opts the ER-stress response protein GRP78 for viral infectivity. *Virol J.* (2011) 8:128. doi: 10.1186/1743-422X-8-128
109. Hung CY, Tsai MC, Wu YP, Wang RY. Identification of heat-shock protein 90 beta in Japanese encephalitis virus-induced secretion proteins. *J Gen Virol.* (2011) 92(Pt. 12):2803–9. doi: 10.1099/vir.0.033993-0
110. Ren J, Ding T, Zhang W, Song J, Ma, W. Does Japanese encephalitis virus share the same cellular receptor with other mosquito-borne flaviviruses on the C6/36 mosquito cells? *Virol J.* (2007) 4:83. doi: 10.1186/1743-422X-4-83
111. Chuang CK, Yang TH, Chen TH, Yang CF, Chen WJ. Heat shock cognate protein 70 isoform D is required for clathrin-dependent endocytosis of Japanese encephalitis virus in C6/36 cells. *J Gen Virol.* (2015) 96(Pt. 4):793–803. doi: 10.1099/jgv.0.000015
112. Liu CC, Zhang YN, Li ZY, Hou JX, Zhou J, Kan L, et al. Rab5 and Rab11 are required for clathrin-dependent endocytosis of Japanese Encephalitis virus in BHK-21 Cells. *J Virol.* (2017) 91:e01113-17. doi: 10.1128/JVI.01113-17
113. Zhu YZ, Xu QQ, Wu DG, Ren H, Zhao P, Lao WG, et al. Japanese encephalitis virus enters rat neuroblastoma cells via a pH-dependent, dynamin and caveola-mediated endocytosis pathway. *J Virol.* (2012) 6:13407-22. doi: 10.1128/JVI.00903-12
114. Kalia M, Khasa R, Sharma M, Nain M, Vrati, S. Japanese encephalitis virus infects neuronal cells through a clathrin-independent endocytic mechanism. *J Virol.* (2013) 7:148–62. doi: 10.1128/JVI.01399-12
115. Xu Q, Cao M, Song H, Chen S, Qian X, Zhao P, et al. Caveolin-1-mediated Japanese encephalitis virus entry requires a two-step

regulation of actin reorganization. *Future Microbiol.* (2016) 1:1227–48. doi: 10.2217/fmb-2016-0002
116. Liu P, Rudick M, Anderson RG. Multiple functions of caveolin-1. *J Biol Chem.* (2002) 77:41295–8. doi: 10.1074/jbc.R200020200
117. Simanjuntak Y, Liang JJ, Lee YL, Lin YL. Japanese Encephalitis virus exploits Dopamine D2 receptor-phospholipase C to target dopaminergic human neuronal cells. *Front Microbiol.* (2017) 8:651. doi: 10.3389/fmicb.2017.00651
118. Bhattacharya R, Gonzalez AM, Debiase PJ, Trejo HE, Goldman RD, Flitney FW, et al. Recruitment of vimentin to the cell surface by beta3 integrin and plectin mediates adhesion strength. *J Cell Sci.* (2009) 122(Pt. 9):1390–400. doi: 10.1242/jcs.043042
119. Das S, Ravi V, Desai, A. Japanese encephalitis virus interacts with vimentin to facilitate its entry into porcine kidney cell line. *Virus Res.* (2011) 160:404–8. doi: 10.1016/j.virusres.2011.06.001
120. Liang JJ, Yu CY, Liao CL, Lin YL. Vimentin binding is critical for infection by the virulent strain of Japanese encephalitis virus. *Cell Microbiol.* (2011) 3:1358–70. doi: 10.1111/j.1462-5822.2011.01624.x
121. Kalita J, Misra UK. Comparison of CT scan and MRI findings in the diagnosis of Japanese encephalitis. *J Neurol Sci.* (2000) 74:3–8. doi: 10.1016/S0022-510X(99)00318-4
122. Kumar S, Kalita J, Saxena V, Khan MY, Khanna VK, Sharma S, et al. Some observations on the tropism of Japanese encephalitis virus in rat brain. *Brain Res.* (2009) 268:135–41. doi: 10.1016/j.brainres.2009.02.051
123. Thongtan T, Cheepsunthorn P, Chaiworakul V, Rattanarungsan C, Wikan N, Smith DR. Highly permissive infection of microglial cells by Japanese encephalitis virus: a possible role as a viral reservoir. *Microbes Infect.* (2010) 2:37–45. doi: 10.1016/j.micinf.2009.09.013
124. Thongtan T, Wikan N, Wintachai P, Rattanarungsan C, Srisomsap C, Cheepsunthorn P, et al. Characterization of putative Japanese encephalitis virus receptor molecules on microglial cells. *J Med Virol.* (2012) 4:615–23. doi: 10.1002/jmv.23248
125. Mathur A, Bharadwaj M, Kulshreshtha R, Rawat S, Jain A, Chaturvedi UC. Immunopathological study of spleen during Japanese encephalitis virus infection in mice. *Br J Exp Pathol.* (1988) 9:423–32.
126. Sharma S, Mathur A, Prakash V, Kulshreshtha R, Kumar R, Chaturvedi UC. Japanese encephalitis virus latency in peripheral blood lymphocytes and recurrence of infection in children. *Clin Exp Immunol.* (1991) 5:85–9.
127. Popik W, Alce TM, Au WC. Human immunodeficiency virus type 1 uses lipid raft-colocalized CD4 and chemokine receptors for productive entry into CD4(+) T cells. *J Virol.* (2002) 6:4709–22. doi: 10.1128/JVI.76.10.4709-4722.2002
128. Lee C J, Lin HR, Liao CL, Lin YL. Cholesterol effectively blocks entry of flavivirus. *J Virol.* (2008) 2:6470–80. doi: 10.1128/JVI.00117-08
129. Das S, Chakraborty S, Basu, A. Critical role of lipid rafts in virus entry and activation of phosphoinositide 3' kinase/Akt signaling during early stages of Japanese encephalitis virus infection in neural stem/progenitor cells. *J Neurochem.* (2010) 15:537–49. doi: 10.1111/j.1471-4159.2010.06951.x
130. Taniguchi M, Tasaki T, Ninomiya H, Ueda Y, Kuremoto KI, Mitsutake S, et al. Sphingomyelin generated by sphingomyelin synthase 1 is involved in attachment and infection with Japanese encephalitis virus. *Sci Rep.* (2016) 6:37829. doi: 10.1038/srep37829
131. Duffy MR, Chen TH, Hancock WT, Powers AM, Kool JL, Lanciotti RS, et al. Zika virus outbreak on Yap Island, Federated States of Micronesia. *N Engl J Med.* (2009) 60:2536–43. doi: 10.1056/NEJMoa0805715
132. Dick GW, Kitchen SF, Haddow AJ. Zika virus. Isolations I, and serological specificity. *Trans R Soc Trop Med Hyg.* (1952) 6:509–20.
133. Petersen LR, Jamieson DJ, Powers AM, Honein MA. Zika Virus. *N Engl J Med.* (2016) 74:1552–63. doi: 10.1056/NEJMra1602113
134. Cao-Lormeau VM, Roche C, Teissier A, Robin E, Berry AL, Mallet HP, et al. Zika Virus, French Polynesia, South Pacific 2013. *Emerg Infect Dis.* (2014) 20:1085–6. doi: 10.3201/eid2006.140138
135. Dang J, Tiwari SK, Lichinchi G, Qin Y, Patil VS, Eroshkin AM, et al. Zika virus depletes neural progenitors in human cerebral organoids through activation of the innate immune receptor TLR3. *Cell Stem Cell* (2016) 9:258–65. doi: 10.1016/j.stem.2016.04.014
136. Li H, Saucedo-Cuevas L, Regla-Nava JA, Chai G, Sheets N, Tang W, et al. Zika virus infects neural progenitors in the adult mouse brain and alters proliferation. *Cell Stem Cell* (2016) 9:593–8. doi: 10.1016/j.stem.2016.08.005
137. Tang H, Hammack C, Ogden SC, Wen Z, Qian X, Li Y, et al. Zika virus infects human cortical neural progenitors and attenuates their growth. *Cell Stem Cell* (2016) 8:587–90. doi: 10.1016/j.stem.2016.02.016
138. Mlakar J, Korva M, Tul N, Popovic M, Poljsak-Prijatelj M, Mraz J, et al. Zika virus associated with microcephaly. *N Engl J Med.* (2016) 74:951–8. doi: 10.1056/NEJMoa1600651
139. Gulland, A. Zika virus is a global public health emergency, declares WHO. *BMJ* (2016) 52:i657. doi: 10.1136/bmj.i657
140. Miner JJ, Daniels BP, Shrestha B, Proenca-Modena JL, Lew ED, Lazear HM, et al. The TAM receptor Mertk protects against neuroinvasive viral infection by maintaining blood-brain barrier integrity. *Nat Med.* (2015) 1:1464–72. doi: 10.1038/nm.3974
141. Calvet G, Aguiar RS, Melo ASO, Sampaio SA, de Filippis I, Fabri A, et al. Detection and sequencing of Zika virus from amniotic fluid of fetuses with microcephaly in Brazil: a case study. *Lancet Infect Dis.* (2016) 6:653–60. doi: 10.1016/s1473-3099(16)00095-5
142. Adibi JJ, Marques ET A, Cartus A, and Beigi RH. Teratogenic effects of the Zika virus and the role of the placenta. *Lancet* (2016) 87:1587–90. doi: 10.1016/S0140-6736(16)00650-4
143. Richard AS, Shim BS, Kwon YC, Zhang R, Otsuka Y, Schmitt K, et al. AXL-dependent infection of human fetal endothelial cells distinguishes Zika virus from other pathogenic flaviviruses. *Proc Natl Acad Sci USA.* (2017) 14:2024–9. doi: 10.1073/pnas.1620558114
144. Tabata T, Petitt M, Puerta-Guardo H, Michlmayr D, Wang C, Fang-Hoover J, et al. Zika virus targets different primary human placental cells suggesting two routes for vertical transmission. *Cell Host Microb.* (2016) 20:155–66. doi: 10.1016/j.chom.2016.07.002
145. Richard AS, Zhang A, Park SJ, Farzan M, Zong M, Choe, H. Virion-associated phosphatidylethanolamine promotes TIM1-mediated infection by Ebola, dengue, and West Nile viruses. *Proc Natl Acad Sci USA.* (2015) 112:14682–7. doi: 10.1073/pnas.1508095112
146. Dowall SD, Graham VA, Rayner E, Atkinson B, Hall G, Watson RJ, et al. A susceptible mouse model for Zika virus infection. *PLoS Negl Trop Dis.* (2016) 10:e0004658. doi: 10.1371/journal.pntd.0004658
147. Rossi SL, Tesh RB, Azar SR, Muruato AE, Hanley KA, Auguste AJ, et al. Characterization of a novel murine model to study Zika virus. *Am J Trop Med Hyg.* (2016) 4:1362–9. doi: 10.4269/ajtmh.16-0111
148. Aliota MT, Caine EA, Walker EC, Larkin KE, Camacho E, Osorio JE. Characterization of Lethal Zika virus infection in AG129 mice. *PLoS Negl Trop Dis.* (2016) 10:e0004682. doi: 10.1371/journal.pntd.0004682
149. Lazear HM, Govero J, Smith AM, Platt DJ, Fernandez E, Miner JJ, et al. A mouse model of Zika virus pathogenesis. *Cell Host Microb.* (2016) 9:720–30. doi: 10.1016/j.chom.2016.03.010
150. Miner JJ, Sene A, Richner JM, Smith AM, Santeford A, Ban N, et al. Zika virus infection in mice causes panuveitis with shedding of virus in tears. *Cell Rep.* (2016) 6:3208–18. doi: 10.1016/j.celrep.2016.08.079
151. Nowakowski TJ, Pollen AA, Di Lullo E, Sandoval-Espinosa C, Bershteyn M, Kriegstein AR. Expression analysis highlights AXL as a Candidate Zika virus entry receptor in neural stem cells. *Cell Stem Cell* (2016) 8:591–6. doi: 10.1016/j.stem.2016.03.012
152. Meertens L, Labeau A, Dejarnac O, Cipriani S, Sinigaglia L, Bonnet-Madin L, et al. Axl Mediates ZIKA virus entry in human glial cells and modulates innate immune responses. *Cell Rep.* (2017) 8:324–33. doi: 10.1016/j.celrep.2016.12.045
153. Li H, Saucedo-Cuevas L, Shresta S, Gleeson JG. The neurobiology of Zika virus. *Neuron* (2016) 2:949–58. doi: 10.1016/j.neuron.2016.11.031
154. Cugola FR, Fernandes IR, Russo FB, Freitas BC, Dias JL, Guimaraes KP, et al. The Brazilian Zika virus strain causes birth defects in experimental models. *Nature* (2016) 34:267–71. doi: 10.1038/nature18296
155. Wells MF, Salick MR, Wiskow O, Ho DJ, Worringer KA, Ihry RJ, et al. Genetic ablation of AXL does not protect human neural progenitor cells and cerebral organoids from Zika Virus infection. *Cell Stem Cell* (2016) 9:703–08. doi: 10.1016/j.stem.2016.11.011
156. Monath TP, Barrett ADT. Pathogenesis and pathophysiology of yellow fever. *Adv Virus Res.* (2003) 60:343–95. doi: 10.1016/S0065-3527(03)60009-6

157. Hahn CS, Dalrymple JM, Strauss JH, Rice CM. Comparison of the virulent Asibi strain of yellow fever virus with the 17D vaccine strain derived from it. *Proc Natl Acad Sci USA.* (1987) 4:2019–23.
158. Rice C, Lenches E, Eddy, Shin S, Sheets R, Strauss, J. Nucleotide sequence of yellow fever virus: implications for flavivirus gene expression and evolution. *Science* (1985) 29:726–33. doi: 10.1126/science.4023707
159. Lee E, Lobigs, ME. Protein Domain III determinants of yellow fever virus 17D Vaccine strain enhance binding to Glycosaminoglycans, impede virus spread, and attenuate virulence. *J Virol.* (2008) 2:6024–33. doi: 10.1128/jvi.02509-07
160. Fernandez-Garcia MD, Meertens L, Chazal M, Hafirassou ML, Dejarnac O, Zamborlini A, et al. Vaccine and wild-type strains of yellow fever virus engage distinct entry mechanisms and differentially stimulate antiviral immune responses. *mBio* (2016) 7:e01956-1. doi: 10.1128/mBio.01956-15
161. Mayor S, Pagano RE. Pathways of clathrin-independent endocytosis. *Nat Rev Mol Cell Biol.* (2007) 8:603. doi: 10.1038/nrm2216
162. Sánchez-San Martín, C, López T, Arias CF, López, S. Characterization of rotavirus cell entry. *J Virol.* (2004) 8:2310–8. doi: 10.1128/jvi.78.5.2310-2318.2004
163. Khan AG, Pickl-Herk A, Gajdzik L, Marlovits TC, Fuchs R, Blaas, D. Human Rhinovirus 14 enters Rhabdomyosarcoma cells expressing ICAM-1 by a Clathrin-, Caveolin-, and Flotillin-independent pathway. *J Virol.* (2010) 4:3984–92. doi: 10.1128/jvi.01693-09
164. Sieczkarski SB, Whittaker GR. Influenza virus can enter and infect cells in the absence of clathrin-mediated endocytosis. *J Virol.* (2002) 6:10455–64. doi: 10.1128/jvi.76.20.10455-10464.2002
165. Mandl JN, Akondy R, Lawson B, Kozyr N, Staprans SI, Ahmed R, et al. Distinctive TLR7 signaling, type I IFN production, and attenuated innate and adaptive immune responses to yellow fever virus in a primate reservoir host. *J Immunol.* (2011) 86:6406–16. doi: 10.4049/jimmunol.1001191
166. Stiasny K, Heinz FX. Flavivirus membrane fusion. *J Gen Virol.* (2006) 87(Pt. 10):2755–66. doi: 10.1099/vir.0.82210-0
167. Seligman SJ. Constancy and diversity in the flavivirus fusion peptide. *Virol J.* (2008) 5:27. doi: 10.1186/1743-422X-5-27
168. Chao LH, Klein DE, Schmidt AG, Pena JM, Harrison SC. Sequential conformational rearrangements in flavivirus membrane fusion. *Elife* (2014) 3:e04389. doi: 10.7554/eLife.04389

4

Cell-Mediated Immune Responses and Immunopathogenesis of Human Tick-Borne Encephalitis Virus-Infection

Kim Blom [1], Angelica Cuapio [1], J. Tyler Sandberg [1], Renata Varnaite [1], Jakob Michaëlsson [1], Niklas K. Björkström [1], Johan K. Sandberg [1], Jonas Klingström [1], Lars Lindquist [2,3], Sara Gredmark Russ [1,2] and Hans-Gustaf Ljunggren [1]**

[1] Department of Medicine Huddinge, Center for Infectious Medicine, Karolinska Institutet, Karolinska University Hospital, Stockholm, Sweden, [2] Department of Infectious Diseases, Karolinska University Hospital, Stockholm, Sweden, [3] Unit of Infectious Diseases, Department of Medicine Huddinge, Karolinska Institutet, Karolinska University Hospital, Stockholm, Sweden

***Correspondence:**
Kim Blom
kim.blom@ki.se
Hans-Gustaf Ljunggren
hans-gustaf.ljunggren@ki.se

Tick-borne encephalitis virus (TBEV) is a flavivirus that belongs to the *Flaviviridae* family. TBEV is transmitted to humans primarily from infected ticks. The virus causes tick-borne encephalitis (TBE), an acute viral disease that affects the central nervous system (CNS). Infection can lead to acute neurological symptoms of significant severity due to meningitis or meningo(myelo)encephalitis. TBE can cause long-term suffering and has been recognized as an increasing public health problem. TBEV-affected areas currently include large parts of central and northern Europe as well as northern Asia. Infection with TBEV triggers a humoral as well as a cell-mediated immune response. In contrast to the well-characterized humoral antibody-mediated response, the cell-mediated immune responses elicited to natural TBEV-infection have been poorly characterized until recently. Here, we review recent progress in our understanding of the cell-mediated immune response to human TBEV-infection. A particular emphasis is devoted to studies of the response mediated by natural killer (NK) cells and CD8 T cells. The studies described include results revealing the temporal dynamics of the T cell- as well as NK cell-responses in relation to disease state and functional characterization of these cells. Additionally, we discuss specific immunopathological aspects of TBEV-infection in the CNS.

Keywords: cell-mediated immunity, flavivirus, NK cells, T cells, tick-borne encephalitis, tick-borne encephalitis virus, viral immunopathogenesis

INTRODUCTION

Tick-borne encephalitis virus (TBEV) is a flavivirus that belongs to the *Flaviviridae* family. Flaviviruses comprise many human pathogens including the commonly known Dengue virus (DENV), Japanese encephalitis virus (JEV), West Nile virus (WNV), Yellow fever virus (YFV), and Zika virus (ZIKV) (1). With respect to TBEV, three subtypes of the virus exist: European (TBEV-Eu), Siberian (TBEV-Sib), and Far Eastern (TBEV-FE) (2).

TBEV is transmitted to humans primarily from infected ticks, mainly from the *Ixodes* family. The virus can also be transmitted from unpasteurized dairy products from infected livestock (3–5). Infection with TBEV causes tick-borne encephalitis (TBE), an acute viral infection that affects the central nervous system (CNS) with often severe long-term neurological consequences (3, 4, 6, 7). The first TBE-like disease was described as early as in the eighteenth century in Scandinavian church records (8). Traditionally, the disease is described as a syndrome with a biphasic course beginning with an influenza-like illness followed by a second neuroinvasive phase with neurological symptoms of variable severity, ranging from meningitis to severe meningoencephalitis with or without myelitis (3, 4, 6) (**Figure 1**). It shall be noted, however, that also monophasic patterns of disease development have been described (9). Upon infection, virus is detected in serum in the first phase of the disease but rarely in the second phase (10).

Due to increased geographic distribution of TBEV as well as a marked increase in morbidity in many areas, TBEV-infection has more recently caught attention as a public health problem. TBE is now observed in large parts of Europe as well as in northern Asia (3, 4). The main risk areas for TBE in Europe are primarily parts of central and eastern Europe as well as the Baltic and Nordic countries. With respect to central Europe, risk areas extend from Switzerland in the west into northern Italy and the Balkan countries (11). The incidence of TBEV-infection in endemic countries varies from year to year (12–14), however, an overall upsurge has been reported in certain parts of Europe, including the borders between Austria, Slovenia, and Italy (15, 16). These changes have been related to climatic, ecological, environmental, and socioeconomic factors that all can lead to an increased risk of human exposure to infected ticks (17–20).

The total number of annual cases has been estimated to be up to 13,000, and as such the infection constitutes the most important tick-borne viral disease (4). More than 30% of patients with clinical symptoms from TBEV-infection develop prolonged sequelae, some of which may become life-long including neuropsychiatric symptoms, severe headaches, and a general decrease in quality of life (3, 4, 6, 7). The mortality rates differ between the strains. Infection with the Far Eastern strain (TBEV-FE) has a mortality rate of 5–35%, whereas the other two strains (TBEV-Eu and TBEV-Sib) have mortality rates of 1–3% (3, 4). There is no specific treatment (e.g., antivirals) for TBE; rather, symptomatic treatment is the only available option (3, 4, 9).

Of importance, TBE may be prevented by vaccination. There are in total four licensed vaccines to TBE. Two vaccines based on TBE-Eu subtype are licensed in Europe and two are licensed in Russia. Additionally, a TBEV-vaccine based on the Far Eastern subtype is produced and marketed in China. All vaccines are based on formalin-inactivated strains of TBEV (3, 4, 21, 22). In areas where the disease is highly endemic, WHO recommends that vaccination should be offered to all groups above 1 year of age (4, 23). Primary vaccination against TBE includes three doses of the vaccine within the first year, followed by revaccinations every third to fifth year to maintain immunity. Vaccination is generally considered effective and TBE incidence has decreased substantially in TBEV-endemic regions with successful vaccination-programs (24). Randomized controlled trials in large populations have shown high immunogenicity with often-strong antibody production and acceptable rates of adverse events following vaccination (25–28). Breakthrough TBE after vaccination is generally considered rare (4). However, over the last years, vaccine failures have been reported, in particular in middle-aged and elderly individuals, who have completed the primary vaccination (29–31).

Infection with TBEV triggers humoral and cell-mediated immune responses. A confirmed diagnosis of TBE is established by the detection of specific IgM and IgG in serum. IgM antibodies have been observed in sera very early in symptomatic TBE disease, whereas IgG antibodies peak in the convalescent phase of disease (32). IgG antibodies can persist over lifetime and prevent TBE (4, 33). Early after clinical disease onset, TBEV-specific antibodies can also be found in the cerebrospinal fluid (CSF) (32, 33). In contrast to the humoral immune response, the cell-mediated immune responses elicited to natural infection have been rather poorly studied until recently. The latter responses may contribute both to host resistance against infection as well as to pathological reactions affecting the target organ of the virus, i.e., primarily the CNS.

Here, we review recent progress in studies of the cell-mediated immune response to human TBEV infection. A particular emphasis is devoted to natural killer (NK) cell- and T cell-mediated responses. Responses to TBEV are discussed in context of cell-mediated immune responses toward other flavivirus infections. We also discuss some immunopathological aspects of TBE with a particular emphasis on cell-mediated immune reactions in the CNS. Cell-mediated immune reactions in the CNS may contribute to neural damage with severe consequences of brain function, and could in the worst cases lead to fatal outcome. First, however, some aspects of the TBEV itself are covered.

TBEV AND OTHER FLAVIVIRUSES

All flaviviruses are enveloped and have a positive-sense single stranded RNA genome, which *per se* acts as messenger RNA upon entrance in the host cell. The RNA encodes for a polyprotein, which is co- and post-translationally cleaved by viral and cellular proteases into three structural proteins; capsid (C), precursor membrane (prM) and envelope glycoproteins (E), and seven non-structural proteins including NS1, NS2A, NS2B, NS3, NS4A, NS4B, and NS5 (34). Flaviviruses enter the cell through clathrin-dependent endocytosis upon attachment of the E protein to a receptor. Heparan sulfate has been identified as such receptor for TBEV (35); however, there are most likely also other yet not identified receptors for the virus. Following cell entry, the flavivirus is delivered to endosomes (36), in which the low pH triggers the E protein to fuse with the endosomal membrane and the nucleocapsid is released into the cytosol. The assembly of immature flavivirus virions (36–38), including TBEV (39, 40), occurs in the ER, and the viral particles are transported to the

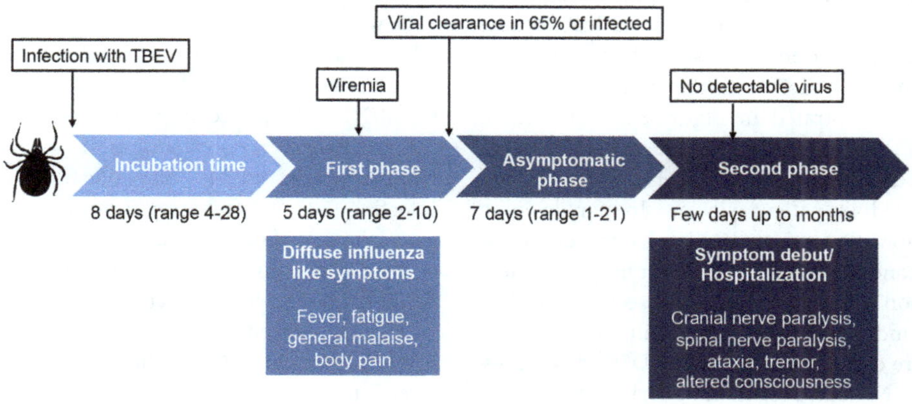

FIGURE 1 | Overview of the classic biphasic disease-pattern of human TBEV infection. The viremic first phase includes influenza-like symptoms and occurs around 1 week after virus transmission. It is estimated that 65–70% of infected individuals clear the virus after this phase, but for one third of the patients, an asymptomatic disease phase follows before the second phase of disease begins. In this phase, symptoms of meningitis or encephalitis occur, including fever, headache, tremor, nystagmus, altered state of consciousness, cranial nerve paralysis, and spinal nerve paralysis. Classically, no virus is detected in sera or plasma in the second phase of disease. Around 30% of patients that enter the second phase of disease will suffer from long lasting sequeale, with a decreased quality of life. Figure compiled from Lindquist and Vapalahti (3), Taba et al. (4), and Haglund and Gunther (6).

Golgi apparatus. The virion particles are immature until the envelope protein is rearranged and prM is cleaved by the host enzyme furin in the acidic environment in the Golgi apparatus. Immature particles are non-infectious and proteolytic cleavage of prM is a prerequisite for viral infectivity. However, studies have shown that complete cleavage of prM is not necessary for viral infectivity (41–43).

In general, species of flaviviruses have many similarities, but their preferred host cells differ. TBEV is shown to replicate 10,000-fold higher in human neuronal cells as compared with epithelial cells (44). A similar infection pattern has recently been shown for ZIKV (45).

NK CELLS

NK cells are innate lymphocytes, though recent studies have revealed "adaptive" features of these cells (46, 47). They are perhaps best known for their ability to kill virus-infected and tumor cells. NK cell cytotoxicity is regulated by the expression of numerous activating and inhibitory receptors that sense ligands on neighboring healthy and altered cells. Several activating receptors recognize molecules that are up-regulated on cells during conditions of cellular stress, such as viral infection and transformation [reviewed in (48, 49)] whereas many inhibitory receptors, e.g., human killer cell Ig-like receptors (KIR) bind to HLA class I molecules. Additionally, NK cells have an important role in producing cytokines and chemokines, as well as by other means interacting with other immune and non-immune cells.

Human NK cells are classically defined as $CD3^-$ (T cell receptor negative), $CD56^+$ cells and represent about 15% of peripheral blood lymphocytes. These cells have for long been divided into two main subsets; $CD56^{bright}$ and $CD56^{dim}$ cells (50). The $CD56^{bright}$ NK cells are thought to be less mature and are commonly known as primarily cytokine-producing cells with low cytotoxic ability, whereas $CD56^{dim}$ NK cells are best known for their potent cytotoxic activity upon target cell recognition (51). However, the latter are also ample cytokine producers upon interaction with target cells (51). Both "natural" and antibody-mediated NK cell cytotoxicity is mediated by exocytosis of cytoplasmic granules containing perforin and granzymes (52). Cytotoxic responses may also to various degrees involve TRAIL- and Fas-ligand-mediated induction of apoptosis (53, 54). $CD56^{dim}$ NK cells frequently express CD16 (FcγRIII), KIRs, and CD57, which regulate their function and define distinct stages of NK cell maturation (55), whereas $CD56^{bright}$ NK cells largely lack expression of these molecules.

THE ROLE OF NK CELLS IN HUMAN TBEV INFECTION

Direct evidence for a protective role of NK cells has been found in experimental models of several viral infections, including cytomegalovirus and influenza, and a number of studies have indicated that they play a role also in protection against viral infections in humans. For example, NK cell-deficiencies in humans result in severe herpes virus infections in childhood and adolescence (56). NK cells may also have a protective role in human TBEV-infection. At the same time, responses mediated by these cells may be associated with development of symptoms in the course of TBEV-infection. Although there is only little known about NK cells in TBE, NK cells have been detected in CSF of patients with TBE (57), an observation that indicates transmigration through the blood brain barrier (BBB).

To gain a better understanding of the NK cell response to human TBEV-infection, we recently performed a longitudinal study providing an in-depth analysis of the human NK cell response to acute TBEV-infection in a well-defined cohort of

TBE patients. The study had an emphasis on NK cell responses during the second stage of disease from which clinical samples were available. NK cell activation, as measured by expression of the proliferation marker Ki67, was apparent at the time of hospitalization (58) (illustrated in **Figure 2**). Concomitant with the increase in NK cell activation in the acute stage of disease, augmented levels of IL-12, IL-15, IL-18, IFN-γ, and TNF were detected in patient plasma. In parallel with high levels of activation, the activated NK cells expressed less perforin, granzyme B, and Bcl-2. By 3 weeks after hospitalization, the NK cell activation decreased to levels seen in healthy controls. This TBEV-induced NK cell activation was restricted predominantly to more differentiated $CD57^{+}CD56^{dim}$ NK cells. Functionally, $CD56^{dim}$ NK cells responded poorly to target cells at the time of hospitalization, but they recovered functional capacity to healthy control levels during the convalescent phase. The poor functionality of NK cell responses was exclusive for target cell recognition, since NK cell responses induced by IL-18 and IL-12 remained unchanged throughout the disease (58).

NK CELL RESPONSES TOWARD OTHER ACUTE FLAVIVIRUS INFECTIONS IN HUMANS

To be able to interpret the above-mentioned NK cell responses to acute TBEV infection, it is important to understand NK cell responses to other acute virus infections, including acute flavivirus infections. In this respect, NK cells have to various extent been studied *ex vivo* in other acute flavivirus infections, including DENV (60, 61) and WNV (62, 63) as well as hepatitis C virus (HCV), a distant relative within the *Flaviviridae* family (64, 65). NK cells have also been studied after vaccination with the live attenuated YFV 17D vaccine (66–68). They have been suggested to influence disease severity and outcome, and to contribute to viral control in these infections, even though underlying mechanisms are not well studied.

In this context, it was observed that the absolute number of NK cells in patients with a mild form of infection with DENV was higher as compared to patients with the more severe form of the infection, dengue hemorrhagic fever (DHF) (69). Reduced numbers of NK cells in the circulation may be indicative of migration toward peripheral target organs. Furthermore, a higher frequency of NK cells expressing CD69 early on during the infection in children developing severe DHF has been reported (70). In recent studies of DENV-infection, we found NK cells to be robustly activated during the first week after symptom debut. Here, the response seemed to be confined largely to the $CD56^{bright}$ subset of NK cells and less mature $CD56^{dim}$ NK cells (our own unpublished studies). Noteworthy in the context of acute TBEV infection, activation of NK cells may also occur very early, even before the onset of symptoms. This possibility is supported by the observation that the highest levels of NK cell activation in most TBEV infected patients were observed already at the time of hospitalization (58). This notion is corroborated in studies of YFV vaccinated individuals. An early response by NK cells was observed in study subjects vaccinated with YFV-17D, where expression of both Ki67 and CD69 was increased on NK cells as early as 1 week after vaccination (66). Accumulation of adaptive-like NK cells expressing the activating receptor CD94/NKG2C has been reported in some human viral infections (71–73); however, no expansion of $NKG2C^{+}$ NK cells in blood has been observed in TBEV-infection or any other flavivirus infection (58). It can, however, not be excluded that this type of expansion could occur locally, e.g., at the site of infection.

In addition to the observed activation of NK cells *in vivo* in different flavivirus infections, a protective role of NK cells is also supported by *in vitro* data. For example, primary activated human NK cells have been shown to inhibit WNV-infection of Vero cells (63) and IFNα-activated NK cells can kill HCV-infected hepatoma cells *in vitro* (65). In addition, flavivirus-infected target cells have been reported to display virus-mediated up-regulation of MHC class I (74), and could thereby theoretically evade lysis from NK cells by engaging inhibitory receptors. The dampened NK cell responses to target cells in acute TBEV-infection further support this notion (58). On the other hand, increased MHC class I expression could result in enhanced T cell responses. In such a scenario, one may speculate that flaviviruses may have been driven more toward escape from innate immunity rather than from adaptive T cell immunity (75).

T CELLS

In contrast to NK cells, CD8 and CD4 T cells recognize specific foreign peptide sequences presented by HLA class I and II molecules, respectively (76). Like NK cells, major functions of CD8 T cells are to kill infected cells through the release of perforin and granzymes, and to secrete cytokines such as IFN-γ, TNF, and IL-2. The cytotoxic T cell response to acute infection can typically be divided into three phases; priming and expansion, resolution and contraction, and memory formation. During the first phase, naïve CD8 T cells divide and differentiate into effector cells acquiring high cytotoxic ability (77). Following viral clearance, the effector T cell population contracts and the majority of the pathogen-specific T cells enter apoptosis. A small pool of pathogen specific T cells (5–10%) survives as memory cells in the third stage (78). Memory T cells are a principal component of immunity against intracellular pathogens such as viruses. They are distinguished by their capacity to survive long-term, and undergo rapid and robust proliferation and acquisition of effector function upon antigen re-exposure (78). Memory T cells can vary in their phenotype, localization, and function allowing them to protect the host against a broad array of potential insults.

Distinct stages of CD8 T cell differentiation are defined by the expression of specific surface markers such as the isoforms of CD45 and expression of the homing receptor CCR7. These stages of differentiation are useful in the characterization of responses to, e.g., anti-viral responses. The set stages define $CD45RA^{+}CCR7^{+}$ as naive (T_N), $CD45RA^{-}CCR7^{+}$ as central memory (T_{CM}), $CD45RA^{-}CCR7^{-}$ as effector memory (T_{EM}), and $CD45RA^{+}CCR7^{-}$ as effector memory RA (T_{EMRA})

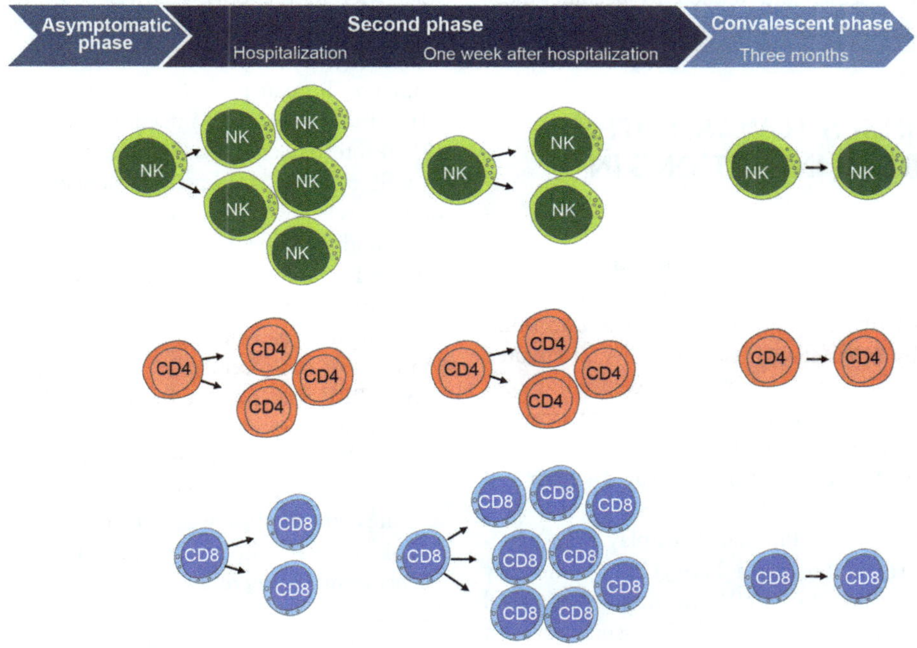

FIGURE 2 | Overview of the cell-mediated immune response to TBEV-infection. CD56^{dim} NK cells (mainly highly differentiated CD57^{+} cells) are highly activated at the time of hospitalization during the second phase of disease. They express significantly higher levels of Ki67, CD38, and produce less cytokines in response to target cells as compared to the convalescent phase. NK cells then become fully normalized, comparable to healthy control levels, at the convalescent phase as assessed 3 months after hospitalization. CD4 T cells show a similar pattern as the CD56^{dim} NK cells. They are activated at hospitalization and express significantly higher levels of Ki67, CD38, HLA-DR, and Granzyme B as compared to the convalescent phase. CD4 T cells have retracted to normal healthy control levels at the convalescent phase. CD8 T cells show a different pattern and peak in activation at 1 week after hospitalization. They express significantly higher levels of Ki67, CD38, HLA-DR, Granzyme B, Perforin, PD-1, T-bet, and Eomesodermin as compared CD8 T cells at the convalescent phase. The CD8 T cell activation subsequently return to normal healthy control levels at the convalescent phase, just as is the case for CD4 T cells and NK cells. Figure compiled from Blom et al. (58) and Blom et al. (59).

CD8 T cells (79, 80). T_{CM} cells primarily reside in secondary lymphoid organs, possess the greatest proliferative potential among the memory T cell subsets and can rapidly expand and differentiate following re-challenge. T_{CM} cells have higher sensitivity to antigenic stimulation, are less dependent on co-stimulation and provide better feedback to DCs and B cells compared to T_N cells. T_{EM} cells can migrate between tissues and secondary lymphoid organs and provide immune surveillance.

THE ROLE OF T CELLS IN HUMAN TBEV INFECTION

Due to difficulties in identifying the acute phase of viral infection in humans, T cell responses to viral infections have to a large extent been addressed in studies of pathogens causing chronic infections such as HIV-1, EBV, HCV, and CMV (81–85). Such responses can be very robust, as exemplified by the massive clonal expansion of antigen-specific CD8 T cells seen in many infections (83, 85). Based on these studies, it has also become clear that the resulting populations of human CD8 T cells display striking phenotypic differences, as determined by the expression profiles of surface markers (79–81). In contrast to many other infections, including some flavivirus infections (86–89), there are only few studies of T cell responses to TBEV-infection in humans. This hold true for acute as well as cases with prolonged TBE disease. Noteworthy, however, one report has shown that TBEV-specific CD4 T cells from naturally infected patients show a higher level of polyfunctionality in response to antigen in the convalescent phase of disease, as compared to TBE-vaccine specific T cells (90).

The general lack of studies more systematically characterizing the human T cell response to TBEV-infection prompted us to study the primary T cell-mediated immune response in patients diagnosed with TBE with a particular emphasis of CD8 T cells (59). Similar to our study on NK cells (58), the T cell study focused on responses during the second stage of disease from which clinical samples were available. During this phase, CD8 T cells were strongly activated, as detected by increased expression of Ki67, within 1 week of hospitalization (illustrated in **Figure 2**). A large part of these CD8 T cells expressed high levels of perforin and granzyme B, and low levels of the anti-apoptotic protein Bcl-2. In contrast to CD8 T cells, CD4 T cells showed only low or at most moderate levels of activation. The TBEV-antigen specific CD8 T cells had a T_{EM} PD-1^{+} phenotype throughout the course of disease. TBEV-specific CD8 T cells were predominantly Eomes^{+}Ki67^{+}T-bet^{+} in the acute stage of disease. This pattern was replaced by an Eomes^{-}Ki67^{-}T-bet^{+} profile in the convalescent phase of disease. TBEV-specific CD8 T cells were mainly monofunctional in the acute stage of disease, and tended to become more polyfunctional in the convalescent phase when clinical symptoms retracted (59).

T CELL RESPONSES TOWARD OTHER ACUTE FLAVIVIRUS INFECTIONS IN HUMANS

To be able to better interpret the above-mentioned T cell responses to acute TBEV infection, we compared the present results with T cell responses to other acute virus infections, including infections by other flaviviruses. The live attenuated YFV-vaccine strain can replicate after vaccination leading to a detectable viral load similar to a mild infection. Thus, this vaccine can be utilized as a controlled model to study mild acute viral infection in humans. CD8 T cells become activated within 1–2 weeks after vaccination with the YFV vaccine (86, 91, 92). YFV antigen-specific CD8 T cells predominantly display a T_{EM} PD-1^+ phenotype, which transition into a T_{EMRA} PD-1^- memory phenotype (86). With respect to DENV-infection, a high level of functionality of DENV-specific T cells is associated with a better disease outcome (93). Similarly, patients hospitalized with (severe) TBE show a low level of T cell functionality in the acute stage of disease (59), indicating the importance of high function among virus-specific T cells for beneficial disease outcome. CD8 T cells have been shown primarily to respond with IFN-γ to JEV in asymptomatic JEV-exposed donors (87).

Activation of CD4 T cells with an optimal magnitude, specificity and kinetics may be a requirement for viral clearance and protective immunity. In the immune response induced by the YFV vaccine, activation of CD4 T cells (peak at 10 days after vaccination) precedes that of CD8 T cells, and this may be of importance to elicit strong immunological memory (86). Furthermore, CD4 T cell release of IFN-γ may have an impact on disease outcome since CD4 T cells, and not CD8 T cells, were shown to dominate the IFN-γ response in recovered Japanese encephalitis (JE) patients. In addition, a high quality polyfunctional CD4 T cell response can be associated with better disease outcome in JE patients (87). In murine models, a perforin-dependent mechanism by the CD8 T cells has been shown to clear WNV from infected neurons, thereby suggesting an immunopathological role of T cells in mice (88). In this context, it is of interest to note that TBEV-specific T cells have a high content of both perforin and granzyme B (59), but whether the same perforin-dependent mechanism is causing immunopathogenesis in acute infection with TBEV remains to be investigated.

CROSS-REACTIVITY WITHIN THE FAMILY OF FLAVIVIRUSES

Immunological cross-reactivity between TBEV and other species within the flavivirus family may also contribute to disease (94, 95). Antibody-dependent enhancement (ADE) is a described phenomenon that can occur when non-neutralizing antibodies facilitate virus entry into host cells, leading to increased infectivity in the cells. ADE is commonly observed *in vitro* in cell culture-based models (96), but it is questioned as to which degree this phenomenon occurs *in vivo*. A recent study from non-human primates *in vivo*, did not observe increased ZIKV titers after prior infection with heterologous flaviviruses (97). Protective cross-reactivity of flaviviruses has been reported as well, opposing increased pathogenesis upon pre-exposure to other species of flaviviruses (98). TBEV has been suggested to cause both pathogenic and protective cross-reactivity. Polyclonal sera against members of the TBE serocomplex (including TBEV, Kyasanur Forest disease virus, Omsk hemorrhagic fever virus, and Langat virus) enhance viral replication of TBEV *in vitro* (96). However, it has recently been shown that antibodies generated from TBEV infection or from the TBEV vaccine can mediate cross neutralization against other, if not most, of the members of the TBE virus complex (99). Furthermore, sera from some individuals vaccinated against TBEV and JEV neutralized WNV, and the neutralization was enhanced by YFV vaccination in some recipients (95), altogether indicating that previous flavivirus exposure may sometimes provide a degree of protection to new flaviviruses.

Cell-mediated immunity and cross-reactivity caused by TBEV and other flaviviruses has been less well studied. Recently, a study demonstrated that JEV- and JE vaccine-specific T cells cross-react with DENV (87, 100). In line with this, it was also recently shown that vaccination with YFV vaccine could induce ZIKA-specific T cells, thereby suggesting cross-protection of flavivirus-specific T cells (101). The latter phenomena opened up a discussion as to the possibility of utilizing the YFV vaccine to protect against Zika virus infection (101). In the present context, it remains to be investigated whether YFV vaccination elicits protective cross-reactive immunity also toward TBEV.

IMMUNOPATHOLOGICAL ASPECTS OF TBEV INFECTION IN THE CNS

In contrast to the significant interest in emerging infections such as the recent Zika pandemic [reviewed in (45, 102, 103)], studies of the immune response toward TBEV-infection as such, and TBEV-induced immunopathology in particular, have been rather limited.

Immune and none-immune mechanisms have been proposed contribute to the crossing of TBEV over the BBB and invasion of the CNS [reviewed in (104)]. Cytokines may facilitate this process. Cytokines such as TNF-a and IL-6 have an impact on endothelial cell permeability that may induce a BBB disruption (105, 106), leading to crossover of the virus into the CNS. A distinct mechanism by which the TBEV could possibly cross the BBB is the *Trojan Horse* mechanism (107), by which TBEV-infected immune cells such as dendritic cells, neutrophils, monocytes, macrophages, and T cells would migrate into the parenchymal compartment causing infection of neurons or other cells in the brain and the spinal cord. Yet, an alternative route is invasion via the olfactory epithelium (108, 109).

After the landmark discovery of the lymphatic system present in the meninges that connects the CNS to the peripheral blood (110, 111), the classical concept of the CNS as an immune privileged site has been replaced by a view of an immune regulated site. Hence, under normal conditions a continuous transmigration of lymphocytes, monocytes, DCs and macrophages occurs. They may serve to detect any kind of infection or injury in the brain [reviewed in (112)]. Similar to other CNS infections, increased frequencies of T cells have been reported in CSF of TBE patients (57). Hence, activated T cells are crossing the BBB in TBE; however, the role of T cells at this site not well understood (113, 114). On one hand they could contribute toward clearing viral infection but on the other hand they may mediate immunopathology within the CNS. Corroborating the latter speculations are findings in which granzyme B^+ CD8 T cell infiltrates have been linked to cell-death in infected human neuronal tissue (113) and, in parallel, mice with CD8 T cell deficiency have been shown to have prolonged survival upon infection with TBEV compared to mice with adoptively transferred CD8 T cells to immuno-competent mice (114). Furthermore, studies of post-mortem tissue of TBE patients have shown a predominance of macrophages/microglia and $CD3^+$ T cells (both $CD4^+$ and $CD8^+$) in brain parenchyma (113). As seen in other flavivirus infections, macrophages and microglia also play a role in tissue destruction in human TBE.

In relation to NK cells and their possible role in causing immunopathogenesis, it is of interest to note that also these cells have been detected in the cerebrospinal fluid (CSF), albeit in low numbers, in patients with severe TBE meningitis or encephalitis (57). Activated NK cells may be protective, but they may also, like T cells, take part in immunopathological reactions as they are known to participate in direct killing of infected cells, indirect killing through cytokines or chemokines, or by the recruitment of inflammatory cells into the tissues (115, 116). Although recent results support a role for NK cells in clinical TBEV-infection, more studies are needed to provide a better understanding of the role NK cells play in pathogenic processes of human TBE infection.

Knowledge and experience gained in the field of the immunopathogenesis of other diseases affecting the CNS and its immunological compartments could be helpful in understanding TBE-specific diseases patterns. For example, in multiple sclerosis (MS), an inflammatory disease with pathology affecting the CNS (117), the concentration of the Sphingosine-1-Phosphate (S1P) in CSF is elevated and S1P-signaling is altered. In MS, binding of S1P to S1P1-receptors expressed on lymphocytes leads to invasion of autoreactive T cells into the CNS, the latter contributing to the hallmarks of the disease including demyelination and neurodegeneration (118). Interestingly, during the phase of acute infection in TBEV-infected patients, the levels of S1P in blood and CSF are highly elevated (119). This increase might promote a proinflammatory response. An increased production of extracellular S1P can be regulated by modulators of the S1P pathway, such as fingolimod, which is an immunomodulatory drug used in the treatment of MS (118). Therefore, therapeutic options used in other CNS diseases that share common immunopathogenic mechanisms with TBE could be used as models to aid in the development of new strategies for TBE treatment.

CONCLUDING REMARKS

In the present review, we have focused our attention to recent insights into the cell-mediated immune response to human TBEV infection, with an emphasis on studies of NK cell and CD8 T cell mediated responses. Until recently, the latter have been poorly studied. As yet, however, much more needs to be learnt with respect to these responses and research in this area should be encouraged. We have also addressed some aspects of TBEV CNS pathogenesis, a process still far from understood in detail. Clearly, however, cell-mediated immune responses likely play an important role in this process. As TBE continues to be an increasing global health problem and challenge, much more research is needed into this emerging disease. Several areas of research of the TBEV itself, and the clinical disease TBE merit further studies. Not the least, the specific organ pathogenesis caused by TBEV and the immune response, including infiltrating immune cells, needs more investigation. Furthermore, the possibility of antiviral treatment and other possible treatment modalities needs much more thorough investigation to prevent disease development and the often severe sequeale following infection of humans with TBEV.

AUTHOR CONTRIBUTIONS

KB, AC, and H-GL wrote the manuscript. All other authors provided valuable contributions and insights into the manuscript.

REFERENCES

1. Calisher CH. Antigenic classification and taxonomy of flaviviruses (family Flaviviridae) emphasizing a universal system for the taxonomy of viruses causing tick-borne encephalitis. *Acta Virol.* (1988) 32:469–78.
2. Heinz FX, Collett MS, Purcell RH, Gould EA, Howard CR, Houghton M, et al. *Family Flaviviridae*. San Diego, CA: Academic Press (2000).
3. Lindquist L, Vapalahti O. Tick-borne encephalitis. *Lancet* (2008) 371:1861–71. doi: 10.1016/S0140-6736(08)60800-4
4. Taba P, Schmutzhard E, Forsberg P, Lutsar I, Ljostad U, Mygland A, et al. EAN consensus review on prevention, diagnosis and management of tick-borne encephalitis. *Eur J Neurol.* (2017) 24:1214–e61. doi: 10.1111/ene.13356
5. Kohl I, Kozuch O, Eleckova E, Labuda M, Zaludko J. Family outbreak of alimentary tick-borne encephalitis in Slovakia associated with a natural

focus of infection. *Eur J Epidemiol.* (1996) 12:373–5. doi: 10.1007/BF00145300

6. Haglund M, Gunther G. Tick-borne encephalitis–pathogenesis, clinical course and long-term follow-up. *Vaccine* (2003) 21(Suppl. 1):S11–8. doi: 10.1016/S0264-410X(02)00811-3
7. Mansfield KL, Johnson N, Phipps LP, Stephenson JR, Fooks AR, Solomon T. Tick-borne encephalitis virus - a review of an emerging zoonosis. *J Gen Virol.* (2009) 90:1781–94. doi: 10.1099/vir.0.011437-0
8. Schneider H. On the epidemic acute serous meningitis. *Wien Klin Wochenschr.* (1931) 44:350–2.
9. Mickiene A, Laiskonis A, Gunther G, Vene S, Lundkvist A, Lindquist L. Tickborne encephalitis in an area of high endemicity in lithuania: disease severity and long-term prognosis. *Clin Infect Dis.* (2002) 35:650–8. doi: 10.1086/342059
10. Puchhammer-Stockl E, Kunz C, Mandl CW, Heinz FX. Identification of tick-borne encephalitis virus ribonucleic acid in tick suspensions and in clinical specimens by a reverse transcription-nested polymerase chain reaction assay. *Clin Diagn Virol.* (1995) 4:321–6. doi: 10.1016/0928-0197(95)00022-4
11. ECDC. Epidemiological situation of tick-borne encephalitis in the European Union and European Free Trade Association countries (2012).
12. Donoso Mantke O, Escadafal C, Niedrig M, Pfeffer M. Working Group For Tick-Borne Encephalitis Virus C. Tick-borne encephalitis in Europe, 2007 to 2009. *Euro Surveill.* (2011) 16.
13. Schuler M, Zimmermann H, Altpeter E, Heininger U. Epidemiology of tick-borne encephalitis in Switzerland, 2005 to 2011. *Euro Surveill.* (2014) 19. doi: 10.2807/1560-7917.ES2014.19.13.20756
14. Heinz FX, Stiasny K, Holzmann H, Grgic-Vitek M, Kriz B, Essl A, et al. Vaccination and tick-borne encephalitis, central Europe. *Emerg Infect Dis.* (2013) 19:69–76. doi: 10.3201/eid1901.120458
15. Amicizia D, Domnich A, Panatto D, Lai PL, Cristina ML, Avio U, et al. Epidemiology of tick-borne encephalitis (TBE) in Europe and its prevention by available vaccines. *Hum Vaccin Immunother.* (2013) 9:1163–71. doi: 10.4161/hv.23802
16. Heinz FX, Stiasny K, Holzmann H, Kundi M, Sixl W, Wenk M, et al. Emergence of tick-borne encephalitis in new endemic areas in Austria: 42 years of surveillance. *Euro Surveill.* (2015) 20:9–16. doi: 10.2807/1560-7917.ES2015.20.13.21077
17. Randolph SE, EDEN-TBD sub-project team. Human activities predominate in determining changing incidence of tick-borne encephalitis in Europe. *Euro Surveill.* (2010) 15:24–31. doi: 10.2807/ese.15.27.19606-en
18. Zeman P, Pazdiora P, Benes C. Spatio-temporal variation of tick-borne encephalitis (TBE) incidence in the Czech Republic: is the current explanation of the disease's rise satisfactory? *Ticks Tick Borne Dis.* (2010) 1:129–40. doi: 10.1016/j.ttbdis.2010.05.003
19. Gray JS, Dautel H, Estrada-Pena A, Kahl O, Lindgren E. Effects of climate change on ticks and tick-borne diseases in europe. *Interdiscip Perspect Infect Dis.* (2009) 2009:593232. doi: 10.1155/2009/593232
20. Sumilo D, Asokliene L, Bormane A, Vasilenko V, Golovljova I, Randolph SE. Climate change cannot explain the upsurge of tick-borne encephalitis in the Baltics. *PLoS ONE* (2007) 2:e500. doi: 10.1371/journal.pone.0000500
21. Lehrer AT, Holbrook MR. Tick-borne encephalitis vaccines. *J Bioterror Biodef.* (2011) 2011:3. doi: 10.4172/2157-2526.S1-003
22. Plotkin SA, Orenstein WA, Offit PA. *Vaccines.* Philadelphia, PA: Elsevier/Saunders (2012).
23. World Health Organization. *Tick-Borne Encephalitis* (2017).
24. Schondorf I, Beran J, Cizkova D, Lesna V, Banzhoff A, Zent O. Tick-borne encephalitis (TBE) vaccination: applying the most suitable vaccination schedule. *Vaccine* (2007) 25:1470–5. doi: 10.1016/j.vaccine.2006.10.028
25. Loew-Baselli A, Poellabauer EM, Pavlova BG, Fritsch S, Firth C, Petermann R, et al. Prevention of tick-borne encephalitis by FSME-IMMUN vaccines: review of a clinical development programme. *Vaccine* (2011) 29:7307–19. doi: 10.1016/j.vaccine.2011.07.089
26. Beran J, Xie F, Zent O. Five year follow-up after a first booster vaccination against tick-borne encephalitis following different primary vaccination schedules demonstrates long-term antibody persistence and safety. *Vaccine* (2014) 32:4275–80. doi: 10.1016/j.vaccine.2014.06.028
27. Loew-Baselli A, Konior R, Pavlova BG, Fritsch S, Poellabauer E, Maritsch F, et al. Safety and immunogenicity of the modified adult tick-borne encephalitis vaccine FSME-IMMUN: results of two large phase 3 clinical studies. *Vaccine* (2006) 24:5256–3. doi: 10.1016/j.vaccine.2006.03.061
28. Ehrlich HJ, Pavlova BG, Fritsch S, Poellabauer EM, Loew-Baselli A, Obermann-Slupetzky O, et al. Randomized, phase II dose-finding studies of a modified tick-borne encephalitis vaccine: evaluation of safety and immunogenicity. *Vaccine* (2003) 22:217–23. doi: 10.1016/S0264-410X(03)00563-2
29. Andersson CR, Vene S, Insulander M, Lindquist L, Lundkvist A, Gunther G. Vaccine failures after active immunisation against tick-borne encephalitis. *Vaccine* (2010) 28:2827–31. doi: 10.1016/j.vaccine.2010.02.001
30. Lotric-Furlan S, Bogovic P, Avsic-Zupanc T, Jelovsek M, Lusa L, Strle, F. Tick-borne encephalitis in patients vaccinated against this disease. *J Intern Med.* (2017) 282:142–55. doi: 10.1111/joim.12625
31. Stiasny K, Holzmann H, Heinz FX. Characteristics of antibody responses in tick-borne encephalitis vaccination breakthroughs. *Vaccine* (2009) 27:7021–6. doi: 10.1016/j.vaccine.2009.09.069
32. Gunther G, Haglund M, Lindquist L, Skoldenberg B, Forsgren M. Intrathecal IgM, IgA and IgG antibody response in tick-borne encephalitis. Long-term follow-up related to clinical course and outcome. *Clin Diagn Virol.* (1997) 8:17–29. doi: 10.1016/S0928-0197(97)00273-0
33. Holzmann, H. Diagnosis of tick-borne encephalitis. *Vaccine* (2003) 21(Suppl 1):S36–40. doi: 10.1016/S0264-410X(02)00819-8
34. Murray CL, Jones CT, Rice CM. Architects of assembly: roles of Flaviviridae non-structural proteins in virion morphogenesis. *Nat Rev Microbiol.* (2008) 6:699–708. doi: 10.1038/nrmicro1928
35. Kroschewski H, Allison SL, Heinz FX, Mandl CW. Role of heparan sulfate for attachment and entry of tick-borne encephalitis virus. *Virology* (2003) 308:92–100. doi: 10.1016/S0042-6822(02)00097-1
36. Smit JM, Moesker B, Rodenhuis-Zybert I, Wilschut J. Flavivirus cell entry and membrane fusion. *Viruses* (2011) 3:160–71. doi: 10.3390/v3020160
37. Mackenzie JM, Westaway EG. Assembly and maturation of the flavivirus Kunjin virus appear to occur in the rough endoplasmic reticulum and along the secretory pathway, respectively. *J Virol.* (2001) 75:10787–99. doi: 10.1128/JVI.75.22.10787-10799.2001
38. Welsch S, Miller S, Romero-Brey I, Merz A, Bleck CK, Walther P, et al. Composition and three-dimensional architecture of the dengue virus replication and assembly sites. *Cell Host Microbe* (2009) 5:365–75. doi: 10.1016/j.chom.2009.03.007
39. Miorin L, Romero-Brey I, Maiuri P, Hoppe S, Krijnse-Locker J, Bartenschlager R, et al. Three-dimensional architecture of tick-borne encephalitis virus replication sites and trafficking of the replicated RNA. *J Virol.* (2013) 87:6469–81. doi: 10.1128/JVI.03456-12
40. Bily T, Palus M, Eyer L, Elsterova J, Vancova M, Ruzek D. Electron tomography analysis of tick-borne encephalitis virus infection in human neurons. *Sci Rep.* (2015) 5:10745. doi: 10.1038/srep10745
41. Junjhon J, Lausumpao M, Supasa S, Noisakran S, Songjaeng A, Saraithong P, et al. Differential modulation of prM cleavage, extracellular particle distribution, and virus infectivity by conserved residues at nonfurin consensus positions of the dengue virus pr-M junction. *J Virol.* (2008) 82:10776–91. doi: 10.1128/JVI.01180-08
42. Stadler K, Allison SL, Schalich J, Heinz FX. Proteolytic activation of tick-borne encephalitis virus by furin. *J Virol.* (1997) 71:8475–81.
43. Yu IM, Zhang W, Holdaway HA, Li L, Kostyuchenko VA, Chipman PR, et al. Structure of the immature dengue virus at low pH primes proteolytic maturation. *Science* (2008) 319:1834–37. doi: 10.1126/science.1153264
44. Ruzek D, Vancova M, Tesarova M, Ahantarig A, Kopecky J, Grubhoffer L. Morphological changes in human neural cells following tick-borne encephalitis virus infection. *J Gen Virol.* (2009) 90:1649–58. doi: 10.1099/vir.0.010058-0
45. Miner JJ, Diamond MS. Zika virus pathogenesis and tissue tropism. *Cell Host Microbe* (2017) 21:134–42. doi: 10.1016/j.chom.2017.01.004
46. Paust S, Gill HS, Wang BZ, Flynn MP, Moseman EA, Senman B, et al. Critical role for the chemokine receptor CXCR6 in NK cell-mediated antigen-specific memory of haptens and viruses. *Nat Immunol.* (2010) 11:1127–35. doi: 10.1038/ni.1953
47. O'Sullivan TE, Sun JC, Lanier LL. Natural killer cell memory. *Immunity* (2015) 43:634–45. doi: 10.1016/j.immuni.2015.09.013

48. Bryceson YT, Chiang SC, Darmanin S, Fauriat C, Schlums H, Theorell J, et al. Molecular mechanisms of natural killer cell activation. *J Innate Immun.* (2011) 3:216–26. doi: 10.1159/000325265
49. Vivier E, Tomasello E, Baratin M, Walzer T, Ugolini S. Functions of natural killer cells. *Nat Immunol.* (2008) 9:503–10. doi: 10.1038/ni1582
50. Cooper MA, Fehniger TA, Caligiuri MA. The biology of human natural killer-cell subsets. *Trends Immunol.* (2001) 22:633–40. doi: 10.1016/S1471-4906(01)02060-9
51. Fauriat C, Long EO, Ljunggren HG, Bryceson YT. Regulation of human NK-cell cytokine and chemokine production by target cell recognition. *Blood* (2010) 115:2167–76. doi: 10.1182/blood-2009-08-238469
52. Cichicki F, Schlums H, Theorell J, Tesi B, Miller JS, Ljunggren HG, et al. Diversification and functional specialization of human NK cell subsets. *Curr Top Microbiol Immunol.* (2016) 395:63–94. doi: 10.1007/82_2015_487
53. Screpanti V, Wallin RP, Grandien A, Ljunggren HG. Impact of FASL-induced apoptosis in the elimination of tumor cells by NK cells. *Mol Immunol.* (2005) 42:495–9. doi: 10.1016/j.molimm.2004.07.033
54. Glassner A, Eisenhardt M, Kramer B, Korner C, Coenen M, Sauerbruch T, et al. NK cells from HCV-infected patients effectively induce apoptosis of activated primary human hepatic stellate cells in a TRAIL-, FasL- and NKG2D-dependent manner. *Lab Invest.* (2012) 92:967–77. doi: 10.1038/labinvest.2012.54
55. Bjorkstrom NK, Riese P, Heuts F, Andersson S, Fauriat C, Ivarsson MA, et al. Expression patterns of NKG2A, KIR, and CD57 define a process of CD56dim NK-cell differentiation uncoupled from NK-cell education. *Blood* (2010) 116:3853–64. doi: 10.1182/blood-2010-04-281675
56. Biron CA, Byron KS, Sullivan JL. Severe herpesvirus infections in an adolescent without natural killer cells. *N Engl J Med.* (1989) 320:1731–5. doi: 10.1056/NEJM198906293202605
57. Tomazic J, Ihan A. Flow cytometric analysis of lymphocytes in cerebrospinal fluid in patients with tick-borne encephalitis. *Acta Neurol Scand.* (1997) 95:29–33. doi: 10.1111/j.1600-0404.1997.tb00064.x
58. Blom K, Braun M, Pakalniene J, Lunemann S, Enqvist M, Dailidyte L, et al. NK cell responses to human tick-borne encephalitis virus infection. *J Immunol.* (2016) 197:2762–71. doi: 10.4049/jimmunol.1600950
59. Blom K, Braun M, Pakalniene J, Dailidyte L, Beziat V, Lampen MH, et al. Specificity and dynamics of effector and memory CD8 T cell responses in human tick-borne encephalitis virus infection. *PLoS Pathog.* (2015) 11:e1004622. doi: 10.1371/journal.ppat.1004622
60. Azeredo EL, De Oliveira-Pinto LM, Zagne SM, Cerqueira DI, Nogueira RM, Kubelka CF. NK cells, displaying early activation, cytotoxicity and adhesion molecules, are associated with mild dengue disease. *Clin Exp Immunol.* (2006) 143:345–56. doi: 10.1111/j.1365-2249.2006.02996.x
61. Lim DS, Yawata N, Selva KJ, Li N, Tsai CY, Yeong LH, et al. The combination of type I IFN, TNF-alpha, and cell surface receptor engagement with dendritic cells enables NK cells to overcome immune evasion by dengue virus. *J Immunol.* (2014) 193:5065–75. doi: 10.4049/jimmunol.1302240
62. Strauss-Albee DM, Fukuyama J, Liang EC, Yao Y, Jarrell JA, Drake AL, et al. Human NK cell repertoire diversity reflects immune experience and correlates with viral susceptibility. *Sci Transl Med.* (2015) 7:297ra115. doi: 10.1126/scitranslmed.aac5722
63. Zhang M, Daniel S, Huang Y, Chancey C, Huang Q, Lei YF, et al. Anti-West Nile virus activity of *in vitro* expanded human primary natural killer cells. *BMC Immunol.* (2010) 11:3. doi: 10.1186/1471-2172-11-3
64. Alter G, Jost S, Rihn S, Reyor LL, Nolan BE, Ghebremichael M, et al. Reduced frequencies of NKp30+NKp46+, CD161+, and NKG2D+ NK cells in acute HCV infection may predict viral clearance. *J Hepatol.* (2011) 55:278–88. doi: 10.1016/j.jhep.2010.11.030
65. Stegmann KA Bjorkstrom NK, Ciesek S, Lunemann S, Jaroszewicz J, Wiegand J, et al. Interferon alpha-stimulated natural killer cells from patients with acute hepatitis C virus (HCV) infection recognize HCV-infected and uninfected hepatoma cells via DNAX accessory molecule-1. *J Infect Dis.* (2012) 205:1351–62. doi: 10.1093/infdis/jis210
66. Marquardt N, Ivarsson MA, Blom K, Gonzalez VD, Braun M, Falconer K, et al. The human NK cell response to yellow fever virus 17D Is primarily governed by NK cell differentiation independently of NK cell education. *J Immunol.* (2015) 195:3262–72. doi: 10.4049/jimmunol.1401811
67. Nascimento Silva JR, Camacho LA, Siqueira MM, Freire Mde S, Castro YP, Maia Mde L, et al. Mutual interference on the immune response to yellow fever vaccine and a combined vaccine against measles, mumps and rubella. *Vaccine* (2011) 29:6327–34. doi: 10.1016/j.vaccine.2011.05.019
68. Neves PC, Matos DC, Marcovistz R, Galler R. TLR expression and NK cell activation after human yellow fever vaccination. *Vaccine* (2009) 27:5543–49. doi: 10.1016/j.vaccine.2009.07.028
69. Wahid SF, Sanusi S, Zawawi MM, Ali RA. A comparison of the pattern of liver involvement in dengue hemorrhagic fever with classic dengue fever. *Southeast Asian J Trop Med Public Health* (2000) 31:259–63.
70. Green S, Pichyangkul S, Vaughn DW, Kalayanarooj S, Nimmannitya S, Nisalak A, et al. Early CD69 expression on peripheral blood lymphocytes from children with dengue hemorrhagic fever. *J Infect Dis.* (1999) 180:1429–35. doi: 10.1086/315072
71. Bjorkstrom NK, Lindgren T, Stoltz M, Fauriat C, Braun M, Evander M, et al. Rapid expansion and long-term persistence of elevated NK cell numbers in humans infected with hantavirus. *J Exp Med.* (2011) 208:13–21. doi: 10.1084/jem.20100762
72. Guma M, Angulo A, Vilches C, Gomez-Lozano N, Malats N, Lopez-Botet M. Imprint of human cytomegalovirus infection on the NK cell receptor repertoire. *Blood* (2004) 104:3664–71. doi: 10.1182/blood-2004-05-2058
73. Petitdemange C, Becquart P, Wauquier N, Beziat V, Debre P, Leroy EM, et al. Unconventional repertoire profile is imprinted during acute chikungunya infection for natural killer cells polarization toward cytotoxicity. *PLoS Pathog.* (2011) 7:e1002268. doi: 10.1371/journal.ppat.1002268
74. Lobigs M, Mullbacher A, Regner M. MHC class I up-regulation by flaviviruses: immune interaction with unknown advantage to host or pathogen. *Immunol Cell Biol.* (2003) 81:217–23. doi: 10.1046/j.1440-1711.2003.01161.x
75. Fernandez-Garcia MD, Mazzon M, Jacobs M, Amara A. Pathogenesis of flavivirus infections: using and abusing the host cell. *Cell Host Microbe* (2009) 5:318–28. doi: 10.1016/j.chom.2009.04.001
76. Townsend A, Ohlen C, Bastin J, Ljunggren HG, Foster L, Karre K. Association of class I major histocompatibility heavy and light chains induced by viral peptides. *Nature* (1989) 340:443–8. doi: 10.1038/340443a0
77. Kaech SM, Ahmed R. Memory CD8+ T cell differentiation: initial antigen encounter triggers a developmental program in naive cells. *Nat Immunol.* (2001) 2:415–22. doi: 10.1038/87720
78. Ahmed R, Gray, D. Immunological memory and protective immunity: understanding their relation. *Science* (1996) 272:54–60. doi: 10.1126/science.272.5258.54
79. Champagne P, Ogg GS, King AS, Knabenhans C, Ellefsen K, Nobile M, et al. Skewed maturation of memory HIV-specific CD8 T lymphocytes. *Nature* (2001) 410:106–11. doi: 10.1038/35065118
80. Sallusto F, Lenig D, Forster R, Lipp M, Lanzavecchia A. Two subsets of memory T lymphocytes with distinct homing potentials and effector functions. *Nature* (1999) 401:708–12. doi: 10.1038/44385
81. Appay V, Dunbar PR, Callan M, Klenerman P, Gillespie GM, Papagno L, et al. Rowland-Jones. Memory CD8+ T cells vary in differentiation phenotype in different persistent virus infections. *Nat Med.* (2002) 8:379–85. doi: 10.1038/nm0402-379
82. Appay V, Rowland-Jones SL. Lessons from the study of T-cell differentiation in persistent human virus infection. *Semin Immunol.* (2004) 16:205–12. doi: 10.1016/j.smim.2004.02.007
83. Callan MF, Tan L, Annels N, Ogg GS, Wilson JD, O'Callaghan CA, et al. Direct visualization of antigen-specific CD8+ T cells during the primary immune response to Epstein-Barr virus *in vivo*. *J Exp Med.* (1998) 187:1395–402. doi: 10.1084/jem.187.9.1395
84. Lauer GM, Ouchi K, Chung RT, Nguyen TN, Day CL, Purkis DR, et al. Comprehensive analysis of CD8(+)-T-cell responses against hepatitis C virus reveals multiple unpredicted specificities. *J Virol.* (2002) 76:6104–13. doi: 10.1128/JVI.76.12.6104-6113.2002
85. Roos MT, van Lier RA, Hamann D, Knol GJ, Verhoofstad I, van Baarle D, et al. Changes in the composition of circulating CD8+ T cell subsets during acute epstein-barr and human immunodeficiency virus infections in humans. *J Infect Dis.* (2000) 182:451–8. doi: 10.1086/315737
86. Blom K, Braun M, Ivarsson MA, Gonzalez VD, Falconer K, Moll M, et al. Temporal dynamics of the primary human T cell response to yellow fever

virus 17D as it matures from an effector- to a memory-type response. *J Immunol.* (2013) 190:2150–8. doi: 10.4049/jimmunol.1202234

87. Turtle L, Bali T, Buxton G, Chib S, Chan S, Soni M, et al. Human T cell responses to Japanese encephalitis virus in health and disease. *J Exp Med.* (2016) 213:1331–52. doi: 10.1084/jem.20151517
88. Shrestha B, Samuel MA, Diamond MS. CD8+ T cells require perforin to clear West Nile virus from infected neurons. *J Virol.* (2006) 80:119–29. doi: 10.1128/JVI.80.1.119-129.2006
89. Hatch S, Endy TP, Thomas S, Mathew A, Potts J, Pazoles P, et al. Intracellular cytokine production by dengue virus-specific T cells correlates with subclinical secondary infection. *J Infect Dis.* (2011) 203:1282–91. doi: 10.1093/infdis/jir012
90. Aberle JH, Schwaiger J, Aberle SW, Stiasny K, Scheinost O, Kundi M, et al. Human CD4+ T helper cell responses after tick-borne encephalitis vaccination and infection. *PLoS ONE* (2015) 10:e0140545. doi: 10.1371/journal.pone.0140545
91. Miller JD, van der Most RG, Akondy RS, Glidewell JT, Albott S, Masopust D, et al. Human effector and memory CD8+ T cell responses to smallpox and yellow fever vaccines. *Immunity* (2008) 28:710–22. doi: 10.1016/j.immuni.2008.02.020
92. Akondy RS, Monson ND, Miller JD, Edupuganti S, Teuwen D, Wu H, et al. The yellow fever virus vaccine induces a broad and polyfunctional human memory CD8+ T cell response. *J Immunol.* (2009) 183:7919–30. doi: 10.4049/jimmunol.0803903
93. Jeewandara C, Adikari TN, Gomes L, Fernando S, Fernando RH, Perera MK, et al. Functionality of dengue virus specific memory T cell responses in individuals who were hospitalized or who had mild or subclinical dengue infection. *PLoS Negl Trop Dis.* (2015) 9:e0003673. doi: 10.1371/journal.pntd.0003673
94. Dejnirattisai W, Supasa P, Wongwiwat W, Rouvinski A, Barba-Spaeth G, Duangchinda T, et al. Dengue virus sero-cross-reactivity drives antibody-dependent enhancement of infection with zika virus. *Nat Immunol.* (2016) 17:1102–8. doi: 10.1038/ni.3515
95. Mansfield KL, Horton DL, Johnson N, Li L, Barrett AD, Smith DJ, et al. Flavivirus-induced antibody cross-reactivity. *J Gen Virol.* (2011) 92:2821–9. doi: 10.1099/vir.0.031641-0
96. Phillpotts RJ, Stephenson JR, Porterfield JS. Antibody-dependent enhancement of tick-borne encephalitis virus infectivity. *J Gen Virol.* (1985) 66 (Pt 8):1831–7.
97. McCracken MK, Gromowski GD, Friberg HL, Lin X, Abbink P, De La Barrera R, et al.Impact of prior flavivirus immunity on Zika virus infection in rhesus macaques. *PLoS Pathog.* (2017) 13:e1006487. doi: 10.1371/journal.ppat.1006487
98. Hoke CH, Nisalak A, Sangawhipa N, Jatanasen S, Laorakapongse T, Innis BL, et al. Protection against Japanese encephalitis by inactivated vaccines. *N Engl J Med.* (1988) 319:608–14. doi: 10.1056/NEJM198809083191004
99. McAuley AJ, Sawatsky B, Ksiazek T, Torres M, Korva M, Lotric-Furlan S, et al. Cross-neutralisation of viruses of the tick-borne encephalitis complex following tick-borne encephalitis vaccination and/or infection. *NPJ Vaccines* (2017) 2:5. doi: 10.1038/s41541-017-0009-5
100. Turtle L, Tatullo F, Bali T, Ravi V, Soni M, Chan S, et al. Cellular immune responses to live attenuated Japanese Encephalitis (JE) vaccine SA14-14-2 in adults in a JE/dengue co-endemic area. *PLoS Negl Trop Dis.* (2017) 11:e0005263. doi: 10.1371/journal.pntd.0005263
101. Blom K, Sandberg JT, Lore K, Ljunggren HG. Prospects for induction of CD8 T cell-mediated immunity to Zika virus infection by yellow fever virus vaccination. *J Intern Med.* (2017) 282:206–8. doi: 10.1111/joim.12638
102. Fauci AS, Morens DM. Zika virus in the Americas–yet another arbovirus threat. *N Engl J Med.* (2016) 374:601–4. doi: 10.1056/NEJMp1600297
103. Ferguson NM, Cucunuba ZM, Dorigatti I, Nedjati-Gilani GL, Donnelly CA, Basanez MG, et al. EPIDEMIOLOGY. Countering the Zika epidemic in Latin America. *Science* (2016) 353:353–4. doi: 10.1126/science.aag0219
104. Spindler KR, Hsu TH. Viral disruption of the blood-brain barrier. *Trends Microbiol.* (2012) 20:282–90. doi: 10.1016/j.tim.2012.03.009
105. de Vries HE, Blom-Roosemalen MC, van Oosten M, de Boer AG, van Berkel TJ, Breimer DD, et al. The influence of cytokines on the integrity of the blood-brain barrier *in vitro*. *J Neuroimmunol.* (1996) 64:37–43. doi: 10.1016/0165-5728(95)00148-4
106. Banks WA, Erickson MA. The blood-brain barrier and immune function and dysfunction. *Neurobiol Dis.* (2010) 37:26–32. doi: 10.1016/j.nbd.2009.07.031
107. Verma S, Lo Y, Chapagain M, Lum S, Kumar M, Gurjav U, et al. West Nile virus infection modulates human brain microvascular endothelial cells tight junction proteins and cell adhesion molecules: transmigration across the *in vitro* blood-brain barrier. *Virology* (2009) 385:425–33. doi: 10.1016/j.virol.2008.11.047
108. McMinn PC. The molecular basis of virulence of the encephalitogenic flaviviruses. *J Gen Virol.* (1997) 78 (Pt 11):2711–22.
109. Avsic-Zupanc T, Poljak M, Maticic M, Radsel-Medvescek A, LeDuc JW, Stiasny K, et al. Laboratory acquired tick-borne meningoencephalitis: characterisation of virus strains. *Clin Diagn Virol.* (1995) 4:51–9. doi: 10.1016/0928-0197(94)00062-Y
110. Louveau A, Smirnov I, Keyes TJ, Eccles JD, Rouhani SJ, Peske JD, et al. Structural and functional features of central nervous system lymphatic vessels. *Nature* (2015) 523:337–41. doi: 10.1038/nature14432
111. Aspelund A, Antila S, Proulx ST, Karlsen TV, Karaman S, Detmar M, et al. A dural lymphatic vascular system that drains brain interstitial fluid and macromolecules. *J Exp Med.* (2015) 212:991–9. doi: 10.1084/jem.20142290
112. Negi N, Das BK. CNS: not an immunoprivilaged site anymore but a virtual secondary lymphoid organ. *Int Rev Immunol.* (2018) 37:57–68. doi: 10.1080/08830185.2017.1357719
113. Gelpi E, Preusser M, Laggner U, Garzuly F, Holzmann H, Heinz FX, et al. Inflammatory response in human tick-borne encephalitis: analysis of postmortem brain tissue. *J Neurovirol.* (2006) 12:322–7. doi: 10.1080/13550280600848746
114. Ruzek D, Salat J, Palus M, Gritsun TS, Gould EA, Dykova I, et al. CD8+ T-cells mediate immunopathology in tick-borne encephalitis. *Virology* (2009) 384:1–6. doi: 10.1016/j.virol.2008.11.023
115. Biron CA, Nguyen KB, Pien GC, Cousens LP, Salazar-Mather TP. Natural killer cells in antiviral defense: function and regulation by innate cytokines. *Annu Rev Immunol.* (1999) 17:189–220. doi: 10.1146/annurev.immunol.17.1.189
116. Guidotti LG, Chisari FV. Immunobiology and pathogenesis of viral hepatitis. *Annu Rev Pathol.* (2006) 1:23–61. doi: 10.1146/annurev.pathol.1.110304.100230
117. Sospedra M, Martin, R. Immunology of multiple sclerosis. *Annu Rev Immunol.* (2005) 23:683–747. doi: 10.1146/annurev.immunol.23.021704.115707
118. Martin R, Sospedra, M. Sphingosine-1 phosphate and central nervous system. *Curr Top Microbiol Immunol.* (2014) 378:149–70. doi: 10.1007/978-3-319-05879-5_7
119. Kulakowska A, Byfield FJ, Zendzian-Piotrowska M, Zajkowska JM, Drozdowski W, Mroczko B, et al. Increased levels of sphingosine-1-phosphate in cerebrospinal fluid of patients diagnosed with tick-borne encephalitis. *J Neuroinflammation* (2014) 11:193. doi: 10.1186/s12974-014-0193-4

5

The Hurdles from Bench to Bedside in the Realization and Implementation of a Universal Influenza Vaccine

Sophie A. Valkenburg[1,2], Nancy H. L. Leung[2], Maireid B. Bull[1,2], Li-meng Yan[2], Athena P. Y. Li[1,2], Leo L. M. Poon[2] and Benjamin J. Cowling[2]*

[1] HKU Pasteur Research Pole, The University of Hong Kong, Pokfulam, Hong Kong, [2] WHO Collaborating Centre for Infectious Disease Epidemiology and Control, School of Public Health, The University of Hong Kong, Pokfulam, Hong Kong

***Correspondence:**
Sophie A. Valkenburg
sophiev@hku.hk

Influenza viruses circulate worldwide causing annual epidemics that have a substantial impact on public health. This is despite vaccines being in use for over 70 years and currently being administered to around 500 million people each year. Improvements in vaccine design are needed to increase the strength, breadth, and duration of immunity against diverse strains that circulate during regular epidemics, occasional pandemics, and from animal reservoirs. Universal vaccine strategies that target more conserved regions of the virus, such as the hemagglutinin (HA)-stalk, or recruit other cellular responses, such as T cells and NK cells, have the potential to provide broader immunity. Many pre-pandemic vaccines in clinical development do not utilize new vaccine platforms but use "tried and true" recombinant HA protein or inactivated virus strategies despite substantial leaps in fundamental research on universal vaccines. Significant hurdles exist for universal vaccine development from bench to bedside, so that promising preclinical data is not yet translating to human clinical trials. Few studies have assessed immune correlates derived from asymptomatic influenza virus infections, due to the scale of a study required to identity these cases. The realization and implementation of a universal influenza vaccine requires identification and standardization of set points of protective immune correlates, and consideration of dosage schedule to maximize vaccine uptake.

Keywords: influenza virus, universal vaccine, T cell, hemagglutinin-stalk, clinical trials

INTRODUCTION

Influenza A viruses have over 18 different hemagglutinin (HA) subtypes, and continual antigenic drift of seasonal H3N2 and H1N1 viruses generates new variants. In addition, there are distinct lineages of influenza B viruses that also exhibit antigenic drift, meaning there is a plethora of influenza viruses that pose a threat to public health (1). Reports of global influenza infection rates estimate that up to 18% of the population can be infected during annual influenza epidemics (2), causing excess morbidity and mortality resulting in projected economic losses of nearly US$87 billion (3). Influenza vaccines are the most widely used vaccines in the world due to annual updates on circulating strains and health authority recommendations for at risk groups (4). The groups most commonly targeted for influenza vaccination programs are children and elderly, pregnant women, immunocompromised, and healthcare workers (HCWs). Inactivated influenza vaccines (IIV) administered intramuscularly have been available since the 1940s and progressive developments have been made to increase breadth of immunity provided by the vaccine, from monovalent to bivalent and then trivalent, to most recently quadrivalent formulations (5). The use of split and subunit vaccines has provided a more purified formulation, and the use of improved adjuvants with reduced side effects in recent years, such as MF59 and AS03 has enabled antigen sparing and increased immunogenicity of vaccine antigens (5, 6). One important advance was the release of live-attenuated influenza vaccines (LAIV) by MedImmune to American markets in 2003, delivered as a nasal spray (7). The quadrivalent cell-grown recombinant HA protein vaccines, FluCelVax (Seqirus) available from 2012 (8) and FluBlok (Sanofi Pasteur) available from 2013 (9), provide an expedient pipeline for pandemic vaccine responsiveness and avoid egg adaptations generated during vaccine production.

A combination of issues exists for the current influenza vaccines (10), including egg adaptations (11), lag between strain selection and vaccine availability (10), and breadth and duration of immunity (12). Annual vaccine effectiveness (VE) is variable and contingent upon antigenic distance between vaccine and circulating strains and the individual's immune history (13). Shortcomings in VE for IIV and LAIV are repeatedly reported with a recent average VE found to be 78.4% and 30.7% against H1N1pdm09 infections, respectively, in 2- to 17-year olds in 2015/2016 in the UK, US, Canada, and Finland (14), while IIV VE reported by the CDC ranges from 10 to 60% from 2004 to 2016 (15). Therefore, current vaccines are not effective enough, with negative or low VE reported, and LAIV does not appear to improve upon VE over IIV consistently (16–18), hence, the need for universal vaccines. Furthermore, current IIV VE decreased over time by one-third from 3 to 6 months post vaccination (19), and reduced VE estimates over time were seen for LAIV (20, 21). Targeting the elderly for vaccination is a logical step as they are the demographic that have the highest morbidity and mortality risk from an influenza virus infection; however, current vaccines are even less effective at conferring protection within this susceptible age group (22).

CRITERIA FOR DESIGN OF NEXT-GENERATION UNIVERSAL INFLUENZA VACCINES

WHO published in 2017 the Preferred Product Characteristics for Next-Generation Influenza Vaccines which lays out the targets for influenza vaccine development over the next 5 and 10 years (23). In the first 5 years, the WHO encourages the evaluation of currently available vaccine and vaccine technologies to achieve greater protection against vaccine-matched or drifted influenza strains and protection against severe influenza for at least 1 year. In 10 years, by 2027, the WHO encourages research and development in next-generation vaccines to provide universal protection against severe influenza A illness for at least 5 years. In addition, a strategic work plan for the design of a universal vaccine has been outlined by the NIH NIAID (10, 24, 25). To achieve the goal of a universal influenza vaccine capable of providing protection beyond 1 year and with broader immunity against antigenically diverse strains, the work plan identified areas for expanded research efforts to address this goal, with an emphasis on research in the areas of (1) influenza transmission, natural history, and pathogenesis; (2) development of influenza immunity and correlates of protection; and (3) rational design of universal influenza vaccines.

Ultimately, an ideal universal influenza vaccine would provide protection (1) against seasonal influenza epidemics by drift variants between seasons or pan-influenza A and B viruses, (2) against influenza pandemics with limited prior population immunity, and (3) against zoonotic (e.g., avian) influenza infections with severe disease outcomes. However, this "ideal" vaccine is still stuck at the laboratory bench (26), with fundamental questions about immune correlates of protection required for universal protection against influenza viruses yet to be answered.

STRATEGIES TO INCREASE THE STRENGTH, DURATION, AND BREADTH OF VACCINE-INDUCED IMMUNE RESPONSES

Timing of Priming for T Cell Immunity

Existing inactivated virus-based vaccine technologies could be improved to increase the strength and duration of the vaccine-induced responses to overcome seasonal influenza epidemics of drifted variants. While natural infection may generate protective immunity for 2–10 years (2, 27), it has been reported that IIV sero-protection fell below 60% one year after vaccination (28). Therefore, bridging the gap between protection afforded by infection and vaccination, by defining immune correlates of protection (**Table 1**) associated with better outcomes of natural infection, severity of infection, and the protection afforded by current and other next-generation vaccines in clinical development (**Table 2**) is critical to future vaccine design.

Live-attenuated influenza vaccines have been shown to induce T cell responses in children but not adults (58), and in particular children under 10 years of age have greater T cell boosting (59). In mice, early-priming preserves optimal influenza-specific $CD8^+$ T cell function and diversity and protects against age-related immune decline (60), with similar age-associated effects of VE observed for LAIV (20). Furthermore, the thymus involutes during puberty greatly reducing naïve T cell output, while "inflammaging" impacts T cell priming (61). In another study, memory $CD8^+$ T cells have been observed and stable longitudinally for over more than a 10-year period, most likely due to multiple re-infections since childhood (27). It is likely that repeated boosting of T cell immunity to conserved, immunodominant epitopes of NP and M1 antigens (62) results in long-term maintenance of T cell responses associated with protection from symptomatic infection (2). In older adults, individuals who received 3–4 years of annual repeated IIV vaccination, rather than single vaccination, had higher response magnitude, long-term durability, and multifunctional quality cross-reactive memory $CD4^+$ T cells (63). Indeed, the T cell-based modified vaccinia virus Ankara (MVA) vector expressing NP + M1 influenza vaccine (MVA-NP + M1) could boost antigen-specific T cell memory responses in adults

TABLE 1 | Broadly reactive correlates of protection from symptomatic influenza virus infection from human studies.

Reference	Sample size	Age (years)	Time points	Infection/vaccination	Immune correlate	Findings
Infection studies						
Hayward et al. 2015 (2)	1,414 and 205 cases	0–65+	2006–2011, pre and post season	Natural infection (pdmH1N1)	CD8$^+$ and CD4$^+$ T cells	Prior T cell immunity correlates with reduced viral shedding
Sridhar et al. 2013 (29)	342, and 25 cases	18–64	2009–2011, recruitment, 6, 12, and 18 months	Natural infection (pdmH1N1)	CD8$^+$ T cells	Prior CD8$^+$ T cell immunity correlates with reduced viral shedding, 10-fold response increase results in 7-fold decrease risk of infection
Couch et al. 2013 (30)	1,509 and 226 cases	18–49	2009–2011, pre and post season	Natural infection (H1, H3, FluB)	Hemagglutination inhibition (HAI) and neuraminidase (NAI)	NAI and HAI are independent correlate of protection and NAI correlates with reduced symptoms
Johnstone et al. 2014 (31)	1,072 and 21 cases	>65	2009–2011, pre and post season	Natural infection	Treg	High Treg correlated with reduced infection, and high CMV + CD4$^+$ T cells correlated with increased risk of infection
Monto et al. 1973 (32)	274	<45	Recruitment, 6, and 12 months	Natural infection (H3N2)	NAI	No detectable NAI response correlates with increased infection
Aho et al. 1976 (33)	90	20–71	Pre and post season	Natural infection (H3N2)	Secreted IgA (sIgA)	IgA deficiency and lack of HAI serum rise correlated with increased symptoms scores
Savic et al. 2017 (34)	150 pregnant women	17–42	Recruitment	Natural infection (pdmH1N1)	CD8$^+$ and CD4$^+$ T cells, NK cells	Lower symptoms associated with higher late effector and naïve CD8$^+$ T cells, multifunctional CD4$^+$ T cells and lower NK cells
Oshansky et al. 2014 (35)	84	0–18+	0, 3, 7, 10, and 28 days	Natural infection (hospitalized vs non-hospitalized)	Monocytes and cytokines	Conventional monocytes vs patrolling monocytes and elevated IL-10, MCP3, IL-6 cytokines
Agrati et al. 2010 (36)	28	3–69	Acute and day 20–27 post admission	Natural infection (severe vs mild)	CD4$^+$ T cells	Lymphopenia resulted in severe infection, reduced CD4$^+$ T cells in circulation, increased TCM, TEM, reduced TN and apoptotic CD95$^+$
Fox et al. 2012 (37)	49	19–57	0, 2, 5, 10, 14, and 28 days post admission	Natural infection (severe vs mild)	NK cells, CD4$^+$, and CD8$^+$ T cells	Lymphopenia resulted in severe infection
Zhao et al. 2012 (38)	48	18–65	2–3 days post hospital admission	Natural infection (severe vs mild)	HAI, CD8$^+$ and CD4$^+$ T cells, monocytes, and cytokines	Severe infections had greater HAI titers and increase T cell response post-infection, reduced IL-17, increased GMCSF in severe group
Wong et al. 2018 (39)	52	12–78	Acute and day 14 post admission	Natural infection (severe vs mild)	HAI, CD8$^+$ and CD4$^+$ T cells, monocytes, and cytokines	Delay in T cell recruitment, prolonged activation, high pro-inflammatory cytokines and reduced regulation of T cell responses correlate with severe infection
Wang et al. 2015 (40)	16	47–88	10, 21, and 30 days	Natural infection (H7N9 survived vs fatal)	CD8$^+$ and CD4$^+$ T cells, NK cells	Delay in CD4$^+$ and CD8$^+$ T cell and NK cell recruitment in fatal cases
Vanderven et al. 2017 (41)	34	22–88	Admission and death/release	Natural infection (H7N9 vs seasonal)	ADCC	Fc effector functions (ADCC) precede nAb responses
Diao et al. 2014 (42)	23	18–65	Daily, 0–31 days post admission	Natural infection (H7N9 mild vs severe)	T cells, monocytes, cytokines	Lymphopenia resulted in severe infection and reduced T cells, monocytes and cytokines. HLA-DR$^+$ on CD14$^+$ negatively correlate with severity
McMichael et al. 1983 (43)	63	18–47	0, 5, and 14–21 days	Experimental infection	CD8$^+$ T cells	Prior T cell immunity (by birth year) and low HAI and NAI correlates with reduced viral shedding
Wilkinson et al. 2012 (44)	41	19–35	0, 7, and 28 days	Experimental infection	CD4$^+$ T cells	Prior CD4$^+$ T cell immunity correlates with reduced viral shedding
Memoli et al. 2016 (45)	65	NA	0–48 days	Experimental infection	NAI	NAI baseline > 1:40 correlates with reduced severity, duration and viral shedding
Park et al. 2018 (46)	65	18–50	0 and 8 weeks	Experimental infection (pdmH1N1)	NAI and hemagglutinin (HA)-stalk antibodies	HA-stalk antibodies reduce viral shedding (duration and load) and number of symptoms but not symptom severity and duration. Baseline NAI was a stronger correlate of reduced disease severity

(Continued)

TABLE 1 | Continued

Reference	Sample size	Age (years)	Time points	Infection/vaccination	Immune correlate	Findings
Gould et al. 2017 (47)	47	18–45	−1 and 29	Experimental infection (pdmH1N1)	IgA	Local sIgA not serum HAI correlates with protection from symptomatic infection
Vaccination studies						
McElhaney et al. 2006 (48)	100	60+	0, 4, and 10 weeks	Inactivated influenza vaccines (IIV) and natural infection	T cells	Increased T cell responses, not HAI, and IFNγ:IL-10 ratio correlated with reduced risk of infection in the elderly
Dunning et al. 2016 (49)	5,599, and 402 cases	>65	28 days	Phase III/IVb trial of IIV standard vs high dose, natural infection	NAI	HAI has limited value when viruses mismatched, NAI correlated with reduced infection cases
Clements et al. 1986 (50)	163	NA	NA	IIV, live-attenuated influenza vaccines (LAIV), experimental infection	NAI	IIV induced protective serum HAI and NAI, LAIV induced protective local HAI and NAI IgA
Jegaskanda et al. 2016 (51)	58 (IIV), 16 (LAIV), 9 (natural infection)	2–70	0, 28, and 56 days	IIV, LAIV, experimental infection	ADCC	ADCC Ab increased by IIV >1:320 reduced symptoms
Belshe et al. 2000 (52)	222	1.2–6	0–4 days	LAIV, natural and experimental infection	sIgA	LAIV was effective against natural H3N2 and FluB infection, and H1N1 challenge due to higher titers of strain-specific sIgA
Forrest et al. 2008 (20)	2,172	0.5–3	0, 7–10 days	LAIV, natural infection	T cells	>100 SFU/10^6 PBMC protected from symptomatic infection
Ambrose et al. 2012 (53)	1,340	0.5–3	0 and 1 month for 3 years	LAIV, natural infection	sIgA	LAIV variably induces strain-specific sIgA which correlates with reduced symptomatic infection
Lillie et al. 2012 (54)	22, and 7 cases	18–45	−1, 1, 4, 7, 66, 120, and 210 days	MVA-NP + M1, experimental infection	$CD8^+$ T cells	T cell activating vaccine reduced symptom severity and viral shedding
Lambkins et al. 2016 (55)	176	25 average	0, 28, 39 (post vacc.), E56, and 73 (post chall.) days	Proteasomal-IIV nasal, experimental infection	sIgA	2 dose P-IIV had 100% protection against symptomatic infection

TABLE 2 | Clinical trial phase, size, scale, and influenza vaccines in development.

Phase	Preclinical	I	II	III	IV (post-market)
Purpose	Method of action	Safety and dosage	Safety and Immunogenicity	Efficacy	Post marketing surveillance
Sample size (median, range)[a]	TC, animal, human studies	72 (12–780)	217 (8–4,560)	601 (20–43,695)	170 (7–31,989)
Total no. of studies (no. and % with industry funding)[a]	–	149 (92, 62%)	230 (177, 77%)	236 (216, 92%)	184 (99, 54%)
No. vaccines in development[b]	1,000+	61	189	52	237
e.g., influenza vaccines[b]	HA-signal VLP, HA-stem, Wyeth/IL-15/5flu	LAIV H7N9	MVA NP + M1, Biondvax conserved peptide with $Al(OH)_3$	IIV H5N1 with AS03	IIV H1N1 with adjuvant MF59; FluBlok

[a]*Included studies on 'Influenza' or 'Influenza vaccine' listed in ClinicalTrials.gov (56).*
[b]*Extracted from WHO Tables on clinical evaluation of influenza vaccines (57).*

over 65 years of age (64). The promising MVA-NP + M1, which is currently in phase II clinical trials (**Table 2**), has been proposed to be used in conjunction with current IIV (65) and shown to broaden both humoral and cellular immunity. Therefore, a window for priming optimal T cell immunity with longevity exists and could be considered for vaccine design to maintain effective T cell immunity.

In humans, the lungs are enriched with $CD8^+$ T resident memory (T_{RM}) that rapidly generate effector cytokines upon influenza infection (66). Furthermore, prime-pull strategies have been tested in mouse studies to seed local T_{RM} responses (67), whereby a vaccine is given first parentally, i.e., intramuscularly like traditional vaccination route, to prime the T cell responses; and then inflammatory or secondary vaccine is given locally, i.e., intranasally, to pull responses to the lung, but this has had limited effect in the lung where cognate antigen presentation is required to maintain T_{RM} (68).

However, the protective efficacy of localized T_{RM} responses vs. circulating responses can only be tested in animal models. A 7-month limitation of protection has been identified by lung-resident T_{RM} in mouse models (69), but may not reflect the decay of human peripheral T cell memory in labeling and tracking studies (70). Whether lung T_{RM} have a similar critical role in modulating disease outcome in humans is unknown, but it is essential to be understood for optimal vaccine design.

Stalling of the HA-Stalk

Development of next-generation vaccines that provide broader immune responses will be needed to protect against influenza pandemics and zoonotic influenza infections. A consensus on immune arms which are capable of providing broader immunity are split over a dichotomy, which are focused on either the anti-HA-stalk antibodies or T cell immunity. Theoretically, a HA-stalk vaccine has an exciting and promising potential, with subtype specific, multigroup, and even pan-influenza A and B antibodies being identified (71). Impressive *in vitro* and animal studies have shown the breadth of HA-stalk antibodies, yet passive transfer in human clinical trials have shown high concentrations are needed but with little therapeutic effect (72). While HA-stalk antibodies have been found to be enriched in some individuals infected with the 2009 H1N1 pandemic virus, these antibodies are notoriously low in frequency with universal antibodies such as F10 representing only 0.001% of circulating antibodies (73). There is a paucity of data on the protective role of HA-stalk antibodies in human infection studies (46) (**Table 1**). A human challenge study found that higher baseline level hemagglutination inhibition (HAI) antibodies were accompanied by increased HA-stalk-specific antibodies and reduced viral shedding but not symptom severity, while anti-neuraminidase (NAI) antibodies were the strongest correlate of protection (CoP) for symptomatic infection (46). Therefore, the independent role of HA-stalk antibodies remains to be defined separately from HAI and NAI antibodies. Ultimately, harnessing HA-stalk-specific B cells capable of universal immunity may also require repeated boosting to overcome immune waning, which limits the duration of current IIV.

Alternative Strategies in Development

There are a large number of universal vaccine strategies in development in animal models, and only 61 in phase I and 189 in phase II clinical trials (**Table 2**) which are designed for pandemic potential viruses (56), and in total only 12.8% of these are designed to be effectively T cell stimulating (74). Apart from HA, additional viral proteins including the NP, NA, M1, and M2, are proposed to be possible targets for universal vaccines (75). Cross-reactive antibodies against these viral proteins from different subtypes have been identified and they are shown to have heterosubtypic protective effects in animals and humans. Various strategies using recombinant proteins/peptides, recombinant DNA, recombinant RNA, virus-like particles, viral vectors, and synthetic viruses for inducing heterosubtypic protective effects have been reported. Some of these approaches do not only aim at inducing broadly reactive antibodies but also cross-reactive T cell immunity against influenza infections. Clinical trials of experimental vaccines, such as proteasomal adjuvanted IIV by nasal delivery and MVA-NP + M1 have been assessed by experimental challenge and immune correlates of protection evaluated (**Table 1**). Previous reports also show many experimental vaccines are not undergoing clinical trials or approved for human use, suggesting a bottleneck to preclinical development (76), which could be attributed to limitations of some animal models to show vaccine efficacy or support needed from industry funding for increasing scale of clinical studies (**Table 2**).

HURDLES IN EXTENDING EXPERIMENTAL FINDINGS TO COMMUNITY: IDENTIFICATION OF IMMUNE CORRELATES OF PROTECTION

Correlating Immune Responses to Infection and Illness Severity

Hemagglutination inhibition and single radial hemolysis assays are the only accepted serological methods used both in the US and Europe for accelerated licensure of seasonal IIV and only recognized immune CoPs for influenza currently (77–79). Other candidates of CoPs (**Table 1**) have been evaluated against experimental or natural human influenza virus infections and vaccine efficacy studies. The route of vaccination (intramuscular or intranasal) determines systemic vs. local immunity, and variability in sampling techniques at the mucosa may hinder the precise evaluation of mucosal antibody responses (53). Furthermore, different CoPs may be identified depending on the outcome measure that is used across the spectrum of severity, for example, from asymptomatic infection to severe illness leading to hospitalization. Therefore, the context under which each CoP was determined should be considered, and a comprehensive analytical approach is needed for clinical studies (80).

Cellular immunity is important for protection from clinical disease. For example, the Flu Watch study highlighted NP-specific $CD4^+$ and $CD8^+$ T cells correlated with lower nasal viral shedding (2). Other studies identified dysregulation of cytokines (namely, IL-10, MCP3, and IL-6) (35) and reduced cellular responses (including T, NK, and MAIT cells) (39, 40, 42) are associated with severe disease. The baseline presence and increasing titer of secreted IgA (33, 47) and NAI (30, 32, 45, 46) have also been identified across studies and appear as more effective correlates of protection from symptomatic infection than HAI. In addition, reports are emerging that HA-stalk (46) and antibody dependent cellular cytotoxicity (ADCC)-activating antibodies (51) have been associated with reduced viral titers upon infection. de Vries et al. showed HA-stalk-specific ADCC responses were boosted in children post-infection (81), while H7-cross-reactive ADCC antibodies were cumulative and detectable from 2 years of age but plateauing by 17 years of age (82). Early exposures to influenza boost ADCC antibodies, while older adults have limited rises in ADCC antibodies post-infection (83). A titer of HA-specific ADCC antibodies >320 correlated with reduced risk of infection, symptom scores, and viral shedding in a human challenge study (51).

While a HAI titer of 40 is believed to provide 50% protection from symptomatic infection (84), new thresholds are being defined for T cell immunity. IIV does not effectively boost T cell immunity, hence the need for new universal vaccines. The longevity derived from memory generated by natural infection is also limited, with repeated infection during our lifetime, estimated every 2–10 years (2, 27). Therefore, universal vaccines will need to do better than nature to provide longer duration immunity from symptomatic infection. From community cohort studies with baseline samples prior to symptomatic infection, Hayward et al. (2) defined the protective threshold for symptomatic infection as >20 SFU/10^6 PBMCs (by stimulation with overlapping peptides for NP/M1); and from a LAIV children cohort study Forrest et al. (20) defined protective T cell threshold for symptomatic influenza infection as evaluated by ELISPOT was >100 SFU/10^6 PBMCs. Inactivated vaccination from the study by Koutsakos et al. resulted in a modest boost of influenza-specific $CD4^+$ T cells, while $CD8^+$ T cells were not boosted (85). While $CD4^+$ T follicular helper cells (Tfh), correlate with greater antibody production and HAI titers (86), and are therefore important for current IIV efficacy. Future universal vaccines need to overcome limited immunogenicity of inactivated and LAIV vaccines by more immunogenic vaccine vectors (74). While universal vaccines, such as MVA-NP + M1, which uses systemic vaccination of a one-step replication vector encoding conserved NP and M1 proteins, boosted influenza-specific $CD8^+$ T cells in adults over >65 years of age (64), a notoriously difficult population for increased cellular immunity. Therefore, universal vaccines in development already show improved ability to establish T cell memory.

The immune correlates of protection from influenza are mostly derived from the comparison of infected subjects on a spectrum of severity (**Table 1**). However, there is a difference between correlates of protection against all infection vs. correlates of protection against symptomatic infection. Furthermore, studies of current IIV for boosting of T cell responses as correlates of protection are not ideal as IIV is not designed to stimulate cellular immunity and can impinge the cellular immunity that is being developed during natural infection (87). Rather, studies of uninfected but exposed and asymptomatic cases (low or no viral shedding) from naturally acquired infection could define immune correlates on a larger scale than possible with human challenge studies (**Table 1**) (2, 29, 30).

Limitations by Prior Immunity

Prior immunity may impact vaccine efficacy, original antigenic sin, and similarly "HA-imprinting" may skew antibody and $CD4^+$ T cell helper profiles by the viral subtype in the first exposure (88, 89). Furthermore, the level of neutralizing antibodies in a population will affect influenza transmission, and Bolton et al. proposed that T cell activating vaccines will have different efficacy depending on the population's prior immunity (90). For example, due to prior immunity to seasonal H3N2 viruses but not to avian H7N9 viruses, a T cell-activating vaccine would be more efficacious for H7N9 viruses. Vaccinating an immune population with biased prior immunity may reduce vaccine efficacy, and universal vaccine strategies may differ by age group due to HA imprinting and immunosenescence. Therefore, use of a universal vaccine in younger demographics could exploit immunological imprinting to their advantage. Previously, high-antibody titers generated from childhood influenza infections which were maintained have been seen to be cross-reactive to antigenically drifted strains (91, 92).

On the other hand, seasonal influenza vaccination history may not always play a positive role in heterologous protection against subsequent influenza infection. Bodewes et al. (87) have compared the influenza A virus-specific cellular and humoral responses between 14 annually immunized children with cystic fibrosis and 27 unvaccinated healthy control children during winter season 2009–2010. A similar level of influenza-specific $CD4^+$ T cell responses and neutralizing antibody titers were found between vaccinated and unvaccinated groups of children, but an age-dependent increase in the frequency of virus-specific $CD8^+$ T cells were only observed in unvaccinated children. These findings indicated repeated annual influenza vaccinations might hamper the development of influenza A virus-specific $CD8^+$ T cell immunity. One report in mice recently from Rowell et al. (93) also addressed such issue, which presented varied heterologous protection from a candidate universal influenza vaccine (A/NP + M2-rAd) following a history of conventional IIV vaccination. Interestingly, they found that humoral and cellular responses induced by universal vaccine could be enhanced, inhibited, or unaffected by selected prior vaccinations, and such variations may be affected by many factors including vaccine preparation and specific vaccine components.

Standardization of Assays and Findings Across Studies

Community cohort studies to identify natural influenza virus infections and measure immunity are established in the UK (2), US (94), Vietnam (95), Hong Kong (96, 97), China (98), and Nicaragua (99) with recruitment and experiments ongoing, making this area of research an exciting area to watch. The seasonality of influenza and year-to-year variation in infectivity of viruses requires these studies to span multiple years to generate robust data, for example, the Flu Watch study spanned 2006–2011 to capture 205 infections from baseline responses (2). Peripheral blood sampling will continue to be a proxy for cellular immune correlates for influenza virus infection, and simplified and standardized assays for immune signatures or biomarkers may aid future vaccine trials (**Table 2**).

One of the challenges in conducting studies to identify new correlates of protection is the sample size required. Typical community-based studies can follow up more than a thousand people over multiple years (2, 30, 97), measuring immune status before the season as baseline immunity and then identifying infections after influenza activity. Dunning et al. commented that data from 1,000 to 2,000 persons may be needed for a reasonably precise estimate of an influenza CoP (49). However, such sample size is logistically challenging, and the size scale of existing studies ranged from 16 to 226 infected individuals to stratify cases by severity to derive immune correlates (**Table 1**), and community cohort studies such as those by Sridhar et al. (25 cases from 342 participants) (29), Hayward et al. (205 cases from 1,414 participants) (2), and Couch et al. (226 cases from 1,509 participants) (30). The scale of vaccine efficacy trials precludes many vaccine studies, especially considering the need to show an improved standard of care from current IIV, which can be reasonable when well-matched viruses are in circulation but are limited for novel viruses.

The French Interior Milieu project (100) has provided baseline immune responses of 1,000 individuals over 2 time-points, sampled the individual's genetic background, skin biopsy, nasal swab, urine, and fecal samples, and uses 10 unique panels by flow cytometry, and 40 stimuli for characterizing adaptive and innate cellular responses. The panels measure in parallel innate cells and adaptive cells, including innate lymphoid cells, NK cells, mucosal associated invariant T cells, dendritic cells, neutrophils, B cells, and T cells (1, 2, 17, reg). Stimulation determines the individual's ability to respond to viral, microbial, agonists, and ligands, such as influenza and Sendai viruses, *Helicobacter pylori*, Poly I:C, Flagellin, TNFα, and CD3 + CD28 (101). The implementation of standardized assays, such as the stimulation of PBMCs with influenza viruses directly at blood collection by TruCulture tubes, was essential for multicenter experimental success (102). However, due to the use of an archetypal and outdated laboratory strain, A/Puerto Rico 8/1934, the results in regard to determining relevant baseline influenza virus-specific immunity were obsolete. The study protocols from the Interior Milieu project are now being extrapolated to other ethnicities and countries to provide a spectrum of a "healthy" baseline immune system and may provide a model for assays on a larger scale beyond HAI needed for universal vaccine design. The feasibility and scale of larger community cohort studies is beyond the capacity of a single research group for processing, storage, and experimental measures (80, 103) and needs commercial partners. Therefore, consensus and synergy with other established cohorts and network design to share expertise is essential to get past the bench to define quantifiable thresholds of immune correlates of protection.

MAXIMIZING THE USE AND EFFECTIVENESS OF INFLUENZA VACCINES IN THE COMMUNITY

Once a vaccine has been licensed to be truly effective within a population a certain coverage threshold must be reached. In 2009, the European Centre for Disease Prevention and Control set out to achieve 75% influenza vaccination coverage in the elderly and those suffering from chronic medical conditions by the winter season 2014/15. However, this target was only reached by one EU Member State in the 2013/14 season and during the 2014/15 influenza season no Member States were able to reach this coverage rate (104). Whereas the vaccination coverage rate for adults aged 18-64 years is even lower, reaching only 36.7% during 2013–2014 in the US (105). This demonstrates that current approach to vaccination, in the case of influenza, is insufficient and even with the development of novel vaccines, strategies for their implementation needs to be carefully considered.

Considerations and Strategies to Increase Accessibility and Uptake

The live-attenuated influenza vaccine only represents 8% of the vaccine market share (106), and production in the US has been threatened by low VE in recent years. Other enhanced influenza vaccines, such as QIV Fluzone by intradermal vaccination (107), have also been threatened by a dwindling market share. Combination and heterologous approaches may complicate adherence to vaccine schedules. Various methods have been developed to stimulate HA-stalk antibodies, such as HA-headless or chimeric HA, and combination strategies of prime boost for four doses (108). However, anti-HA-stalk antibody-stimulating vaccine regimes by heterologous prime boost used in mouse studies to elicit HA-stalk antibody responses may not be feasible in practice in the community, with each regime requiring separate licensure and multiple doses reducing vaccine adherence. The human papilloma virus (HPV) and hepatitis B virus (HBV) vaccines both require a homologous 3-dose regime within 2 years for optimal sero-protection, and HBV also requires a 10-year dose booster. Adherence to HPV vaccine 3-dose schedule is only 28% (109), and similarly 29% for HBV vaccination (110). A comprehensive vaccination record system will be instrumental for orderly vaccination schedules.

An increasingly difficult barrier to successful vaccination strategies is "vaccine hesitancy." The WHO Strategic Advisory Group of Experts (SAGE) on Immunization has defined vaccine hesitancy as a "delay in acceptance or refusal of vaccination despite availability of vaccination services" (111). Vaccine hesitancy can develop into refusal and the encouragement of others to refuse vaccination, leading to unvaccinated clusters within a community and severe public health consequences. One of the more concerning effects of vaccine hesitancy is the effect on vaccination coverage in HCWs. Vaccination for HCWs is recommended in most countries but mandatory vaccination programs vary. A survey of HCWs in China found a coverage rate of only 9.5% in the seasons of 2009/2010 to 2011/2012 (112). However, vaccination in HCWs in the US has increased since the 2010/2011 season, reaching 64.8% in 2014/2015 (113), demonstrating this issue varies greatly by country due to policy decisions and cultural factors. If HCWs themselves are hesitant about current vaccines, novel vaccines that utilize "non-traditional" approaches for universal immunity may require extensive explanation and promotion to HCWs to encourage self-vaccination and increase vaccine recommendations to patients.

Indirect Protection in the Community With Vaccine Uptake

Many studies have shown that increasing vaccination uptake in children and younger adults reduces influenza burden in older adults (114–116, 117). Older children and adolescents have been shown to be the key age groups affecting the initial spread of influenza infections within a community (118). Elderly individuals often come into contact with children and young adults in household and urban settings, public areas and transportation. One of the clearest examples of this was seen in Japan, when influenza vaccination of school children ceased in 1994, leading to an increase in elderly mortality rates (119). A study analyzing US vaccine data also found that in areas where there was ≥31% vaccine coverage in younger adults, the elderly had a 20.6% lower chance of being diagnosed with influenza than in areas with a ≤15% coverage rate (120). Vaccination of healthy

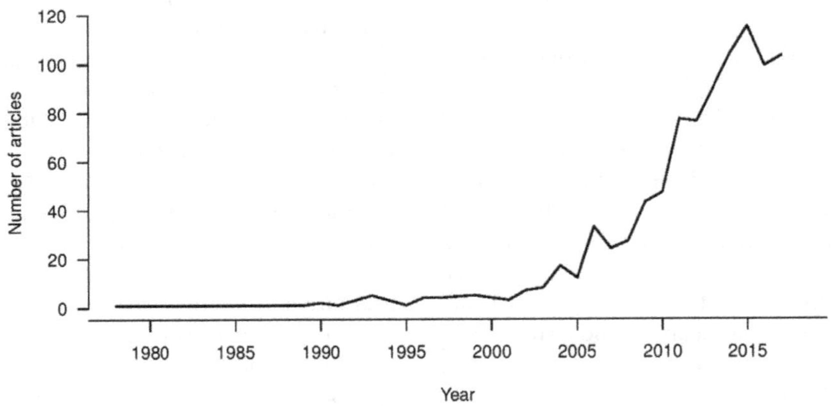

FIGURE 1 | Pubmed indexed publication trend for universal influenza vaccines.

children could also form the basis of establishing early T cell memory and broader HA imprinting from an immunological perspective.

CONCLUSION

Universal influenza vaccine research is a growing trend (**Figure 1**), with first reports in the 1970s of heterologous immunity in the absence of antibodies for recombinant vaccines being developed following the antigenic switch from H1N1 to H3N2 viruses (121). A large increase in the universal vaccine research field has been seen since 2003, coinciding with zoonotic infections from avian and equine sources and pandemic viruses becoming a real threat to public health. Therefore, the drive for increased breadth of coverage for influenza vaccine has been a long-term objective, and the recent NIAID push has been a "call to arms" to address this issue. An increasing number of immune biomarkers that are associated with protection against influenza virus infection and disease severity *in vitro* and *in vivo* have been identified, leading to vaccines designed to elicit these immune markers at different stages of clinical trials. Such a strategy assumes that these markers are correlates of protection in humans, but whether such assumptions hold is yet to be confirmed in large epidemiological studies. Ultimately, immune correlates should be compared in parallel and defined within a weighted hierarchy to drive vaccine design which can stimulate multiple immune arms effectively. Alternatively, despite measurable influenza-specific T and B cell immunity, all healthy adults experience repeat infections in their lifetime. Additionally the WHO goals to promote longevity of responses may also require a vaccine that elicits a "better than nature" response. With increased attention and funding for this area, particularly from the National Institutes of Health, there is real hope for the successful development of universal influenza vaccines.

AUTHOR CONTRIBUTIONS

SV, NL, MB, YLM, AL, LP and BC wrote and prepared the review. SV and NL prepared the figures and tables.

REFERENCES

1. Fauci AS. Pandemic influenza threat and preparedness. *Emerg Infect Dis* (2006) 12(1):73–7. doi:10.3201/eid1201.050983
2. Hayward AC, Wang L, Goonetilleke N, Fragaszy EB, Bermingham A, Copas A, et al. Natural T cell-mediated protection against seasonal and pandemic influenza. Results of the Flu Watch Cohort Study. *Am J Respir Crit Care Med* (2015) 191(12):1422–31. doi:10.1164/rccm.201411-1988OC
3. Molinari NA, Ortega-Sanchez IR, Messonnier ML, Thompson WW, Wortley PM, Weintraub E, et al. The annual impact of seasonal influenza in the US: measuring disease burden and costs. *Vaccine* (2007) 25(27):5086–96. doi:10.1016/j.vaccine.2007.03.046
4. Palache A, Abelin A, Hollingsworth R, Cracknell W, Jacobs C, Tsai T, et al. Survey of distribution of seasonal influenza vaccine doses in 201 countries (2004-2015): the 2003 World Health Assembly resolution on seasonal influenza vaccination coverage and the 2009 influenza pandemic have had very little impact on improving influenza control and pandemic preparedness. *Vaccine* (2017) 35(36):4681–6. doi:10.1016/j.vaccine.2017.07.053
5. Wong SS, Webby RJ. Traditional and new influenza vaccines. *Clin Microbiol Rev* (2013) 26(3):476–92. doi:10.1128/CMR.00097-12
6. Del Giudice G, Rappuoli R. Inactivated and adjuvanted influenza vaccines. *Curr Top Microbiol Immunol* (2015) 386:151–80. doi:10.1007/82_2014_406
7. Jin H, Subbarao K. Live attenuated influenza vaccine. *Curr Top Microbiol Immunol* (2015) 386:181–204. doi:10.1007/82_2014_410
8. Manini I, Domnich A, Amicizia D, Rossi S, Pozzi T, Gasparini R, et al. Flucelvax (Optaflu) for seasonal influenza. *Expert Rev Vaccines* (2015) 14(6):789–804. doi:10.1586/14760584.2015.1039520
9. Dunkle LM, Izikson R, Patriarca P, Goldenthal KL, Muse D, Callahan J, et al. Efficacy of recombinant influenza vaccine in adults 50 years of age or older. *N Engl J Med* (2017) 376(25):2427–36. doi:10.1056/NEJMoa1608862

10. Paules CI, Sullivan SG, Subbarao K, Fauci AS. Chasing seasonal influenza – the need for a universal influenza vaccine. *N Engl J Med* (2018) 378(1):7–9. doi:10.1056/NEJMp1714916
11. Manini I, Trombetta CM, Lazzeri G, Pozzi T, Rossi S, Montomoli E. Egg-independent influenza vaccines and vaccine candidates. *Vaccines (Basel)* (2017) 5(3):E18. doi:10.3390/vaccines5030018
12. Xu C, Thompson MG, Cowling BJ. Influenza vaccination in tropical and subtropical areas. *Lancet Respir Med* (2017) 5(12):920–2. doi:10.1016/S2213-2600(17)30377-6
13. Skowronski DM, Chambers C, Sabaiduc S, De Serres G, Winter AL, Dickinson JA, et al. Beyond antigenic match: possible agent-host and immuno-epidemiological influences on influenza vaccine effectiveness during the 2015-2016 season in Canada. *J Infect Dis* (2017) 216(12):1487–500. doi:10.1093/infdis/jix526
14. Pebody R, McMenamin J, Nohynek H. Live attenuated influenza vaccine (LAIV): recent effectiveness results from the USA and implications for LAIV programmes elsewhere. *Arch Dis Child* (2018) 103(1):101–5. doi:10.1136/archdischild-2016-312165
15. CDC. *Seasonal Influenza Vaccine Effectiveness, 2005-2018 [Online]*. (2018). Available from: https://www.cdc.gov/flu/professionals/vaccination/effectiveness-studies.htm (Accessed: February 24, 2018).
16. Caspard H, Mallory RM, Yu J, Ambrose CS. Live-attenuated influenza vaccine effectiveness in children from 2009 to 2015–2016: a systematic review and meta-analysis. *Open Forum Infect Dis* (2017) 4(3):ofx111. doi:10.1093/ofid/ofx111
17. McLean HQ, Caspard H, Griffin MR, Poehling KA, Gaglani M, Belongia EA, et al. Effectiveness of live attenuated influenza vaccine and inactivated influenza vaccine in children during the 2014-2015 season. *Vaccine* (2017) 35(20):2685–93. doi:10.1016/j.vaccine.2017.03.085
18. Poehling KA, Caspard H, Peters TR, Belongia EA, Congeni B, Gaglani M, et al. 2015-2016 vaccine effectiveness of live attenuated and inactivated influenza vaccines in children in the United States. *Clin Infect Dis* (2018) 66(5):665–72. doi:10.1093/cid/cix869
19. Young B, Sadarangani S, Jiang L, Wilder-Smith A, Chen MI. Duration of influenza vaccine effectiveness: a systematic review, meta-analysis, and meta-regression of test-negative design case-control studies. *J Infect Dis* (2018) 217(5):731–41. doi:10.1093/infdis/jix632
20. Forrest BD, Pride MW, Dunning AJ, Capeding MR, Chotpitayasunondh T, Tam JS, et al. Correlation of cellular immune responses with protection against culture-confirmed influenza virus in young children. *Clin Vaccine Immunol* (2008) 15(7):1042–53. doi:10.1128/CVI.00397-07
21. Petrie JG, Ohmit SE, Truscon R, Johnson E, Braun TM, Levine MZ, et al. Modest waning of influenza vaccine efficacy and antibody titers during the 2007–2008 influenza season. *J Infect Dis* (2016) 214(8):1142–9. doi:10.1093/infdis/jiw105
22. Beyer WE, McElhaney J, Smith DJ, Monto AS, Nguyen-Van-Tam JS, Osterhaus AD. Cochrane re-arranged: support for policies to vaccinate elderly people against influenza. *Vaccine* (2013) 31(50):6030–3. doi:10.1016/j.vaccine.2013.09.063
23. Ortiz JR, Hickling J, Jones R, Donabedian A, Engelhardt OG, Katz JM, et al. Report on eighth WHO meeting on development of influenza vaccines that induce broadly protective and long-lasting immune responses: Chicago, USA, 23-24 August 2016. *Vaccine* (2018) 36(7):932–8. doi:10.1016/j.vaccine.2017.11.061
24. Paules CI, Marston HD, Eisinger RW, Baltimore D, Fauci AS. The pathway to a universal influenza vaccine. *Immunity* (2017) 47(4):599–603. doi:10.1016/j.immuni.2017.09.007
25. Erbelding EJ, Post D, Stemmy E, Roberts PC, Augustine AD, Ferguson S, et al. A universal influenza vaccine: the strategic plan for the National Institute of Allergy and Infectious Diseases. *J Infect Dis* (2018). doi:10.1093/infdis/jiy103
26. Rajao DS, Perez DR. Universal vaccines and vaccine platforms to protect against influenza viruses in humans and agriculture. *Front Microbiol* (2018) 9:123. doi:10.3389/fmicb.2018.00123
27. van de Sandt CE, Hillaire ML, Geelhoed-Mieras MM, Osterhaus AD, Fouchier RA, Rimmelzwaan GF. Human influenza A virus-specific CD8+ T cell response is long-lived. *J Infect Dis* (2015) 212(1):81–5. doi:10.1093/infdis/jiv018
28. Young B, Zhao X, Cook AR, Parry CM, Wilder-Smith A, MC IC. Do antibody responses to the influenza vaccine persist year-round in the elderly? A systematic review and meta-analysis. *Vaccine* (2017) 35(2):212–21. doi:10.1016/j.vaccine.2016.11.013
29. Sridhar S, Begom S, Bermingham A, Hoschler K, Adamson W, Carman W, et al. Cellular immune correlates of protection against symptomatic pandemic influenza. *Nat Med* (2013) 19(10):1305–12. doi:10.1038/nm.3350
30. Couch RB, Atmar RL, Franco LM, Quarles JM, Wells J, Arden N, et al. Antibody correlates and predictors of immunity to naturally occurring influenza in humans and the importance of antibody to the neuraminidase. *J Infect Dis* (2013) 207(6):974–81. doi:10.1093/infdis/jis935
31. Johnstone J, Parsons R, Botelho F, Millar J, McNeil S, Fulop T, et al. Immune biomarkers predictive of respiratory viral infection in elderly nursing home residents. *PLoS One* (2014) 9(9):e108481. doi:10.1371/journal.pone.0108481
32. Monto AS, Kendal AP. Effect of neuraminidase antibody on Hong Kong influenza. *Lancet* (1973) 1(7804):623–5. doi:10.1016/S0140-6736(73)92196-X
33. Aho K, Pyhala R, Koistinen J. IgA deficiency and influenza infection. *Scand J Immunol* (1976) 5(10):1089–92. doi:10.1111/j.1365-3083.1976.tb00247.x
34. Savic M, Dembinski JL, Laake I, Hungnes O, Cox R, Oftung F, et al. Distinct T and NK cell populations may serve as immune correlates of protection against symptomatic pandemic influenza A(H1N1) virus infection during pregnancy. *PLoS One* (2017) 12(11):e0188055. doi:10.1371/journal.pone.0188055
35. Oshansky CM, Gartland AJ, Wong SS, Jeevan T, Wang D, Roddam PL, et al. Mucosal immune responses predict clinical outcomes during influenza infection independently of age and viral load. *Am J Respir Crit Care Med* (2014) 189(4):449–62. doi:10.1164/rccm.201309-1616OC
36. Agrati C, Gioia C, Lalle E, Cimini E, Castilletti C, Armignacco O, et al. Association of profoundly impaired immune competence in H1N1v-infected patients with a severe or fatal clinical course. *J Infect Dis* (2010) 202(5):681–9. doi:10.1086/655469
37. Fox A, Le NM, Horby P, van Doorn HR, Nguyen VT, Nguyen HH, et al. Severe pandemic H1N1 2009 infection is associated with transient NK and T deficiency and aberrant CD8 responses. *PLoS One* (2012) 7(2):e31535. doi:10.1371/journal.pone.0031535
38. Zhao Y, Zhang YH, Denney L, Young D, Powell TJ, Peng YC, et al. High levels of virus-specific CD4+ T cells predict severe pandemic influenza A virus infection. *Am J Respir Crit Care Med* (2012) 186(12):1292–7. doi:10.1164/rccm.201207-1245OC
39. Wong SS, Oshansky CM, Guo XJ, Ralston J, Wood T, Seeds R, et al. Severe influenza is characterized by prolonged immune activation: results from the SHIVERS Cohort Study. *J Infect Dis* (2018) 217(2):245–56. doi:10.1093/infdis/jix571
40. Wang Z, Wan Y, Qiu C, Quinones-Parra S, Zhu Z, Loh L, et al. Recovery from severe H7N9 disease is associated with diverse response mechanisms dominated by CD8(+) T cells. *Nat Commun* (2015) 6:6833. doi:10.1038/ncomms7833
41. Vanderven HA, Liu L, Ana-Sosa-Batiz F, Nguyen TH, Wan Y, Wines B, et al. Fc functional antibodies in humans with severe H7N9 and seasonal influenza. *JCI Insight* (2017) 2(13):92750. doi:10.1172/jci.insight.92750
42. Diao H, Cui G, Wei Y, Chen J, Zuo J, Cao H, et al. Severe H7N9 infection is associated with decreased antigen-presenting capacity of CD14+ cells. *PLoS One* (2014) 9(3):e92823. doi:10.1371/journal.pone.0092823
43. McMichael AJ, Gotch FM, Noble GR, Beare PA. Cytotoxic T-cell immunity to influenza. *N Engl J Med* (1983) 309(1):13–7. doi:10.1056/NEJM198307073090103
44. Wilkinson TM, Li CK, Chui CS, Huang AK, Perkins M, Liebner JC, et al. Preexisting influenza-specific CD4+ T cells correlate with disease protection against influenza challenge in humans. *Nat Med* (2012) 18(2):274–80. doi:10.1038/nm.2612
45. Memoli MJ, Shaw PA, Han A, Czajkowski L, Reed S, Athota R, et al. Evaluation of antihemagglutinin and antineuraminidase antibodies as correlates of protection in an influenza A/H1N1 virus healthy human challenge model. *MBio* (2016) 7(2):e417-416. doi:10.1128/mBio.00417-16
46. Park JK, Han A, Czajkowski L, Reed S, Athota R, Bristol T, et al. Evaluation of preexisting anti-hemagglutinin stalk antibody as a correlate of protection in a healthy volunteer challenge with influenza A/H1N1pdm virus. *MBio* (2018) 9(1):e02284-17. doi:10.1128/mBio.02284-17
47. Gould VMW, Francis JN, Anderson KJ, Georges B, Cope AV, Tregoning JS. Nasal IgA provides protection against human influenza challenge in volunteers with low serum influenza antibody titre. *Front Microbiol* (2017) 8:900. doi:10.3389/fmicb.2017.00900

48. McElhaney JE, Xie D, Hager WD, Barry MB, Wang Y, Kleppinger A, et al. T cell responses are better correlates of vaccine protection in the elderly. *J Immunol* (2006) 176(10):6333–9. doi:10.4049/jimmunol.176.10.6333
49. Dunning AJ, DiazGranados CA, Voloshen T, Hu B, Landolfi VA, Talbot HK. Correlates of protection against influenza in the elderly: results from an influenza vaccine efficacy trial. *Clin Vaccine Immunol* (2016) 23(3):228–35. doi:10.1128/CVI.00604-15
50. Clements ML, Betts RF, Tierney EL, Murphy BR. Serum and nasal wash antibodies associated with resistance to experimental challenge with influenza A wild-type virus. *J Clin Microbiol* (1986) 24(1):157–60.
51. Jegaskanda S, Luke C, Hickman HD, Sangster MY, Wieland-Alter WF, McBride JM, et al. Generation and protective ability of influenza virus-specific antibody-dependent cellular cytotoxicity in humans elicited by vaccination, natural infection, and experimental challenge. *J Infect Dis* (2016) 214(6):945–52. doi:10.1093/infdis/jiw262
52. Belshe RB, Gruber WC, Mendelman PM, Mehta HB, Mahmood K, Reisinger K, et al. Correlates of immune protection induced by live, attenuated, cold-adapted, trivalent, intranasal influenza virus vaccine. *J Infect Dis* (2000) 181(3):1133–7. doi:10.1086/315323
53. Ambrose CS, Wu X, Jones T, Mallory RM. The role of nasal IgA in children vaccinated with live attenuated influenza vaccine. *Vaccine* (2012) 30(48):6794–801. doi:10.1016/j.vaccine.2012.09.018
54. Lillie PJ, Berthoud TK, Powell TJ, Lambe T, Mullarkey C, Spencer AJ, et al. Preliminary assessment of the efficacy of a T-cell-based influenza vaccine, MVA-NP+M1, in humans. *Clin Infect Dis* (2012) 55(1):19–25. doi:10.1093/cid/cis327
55. Lambkin-Williams R, Gelder C, Broughton R, Mallett CP, Gilbert AS, Mann A, et al. An intranasal proteosome-adjuvanted trivalent influenza vaccine is safe, immunogenic & efficacious in the human viral influenza challenge model. Serum IgG & mucosal IgA are important correlates of protection against illness associated with infection. *PLoS One* (2016) 11(12): e0163089. doi:10.1371/journal.pone.0163089
56. WHO. *Tables on Clinical Evaluation of Influenza Vaccines*. (2017). Available from: http://www.who.int/immunization/diseases/influenza/clinical_evaluation_tables/en/
57. NIH, Clinical trials. (2018). Available from: ClinicalTrials.gov (Accessed: April 24, 2018).
58. Hoft DF, Babusis E, Worku S, Spencer CT, Lottenbach K, Truscott SM, et al. Live and inactivated influenza vaccines induce similar humoral responses, but only live vaccines induce diverse T-cell responses in young children. *J Infect Dis* (2011) 204(6):845–53. doi:10.1093/infdis/jir436
59. Mohn KGI, Zhou F, Brokstad KA, Sridhar S, Cox RJ. Boosting of cross-reactive and protection-associated T cells in children after live attenuated influenza vaccination. *J Infect Dis* (2017) 215(10):1527–35. doi:10.1093/infdis/jix165
60. Valkenburg SA, Venturi V, Dang TH, Bird NL, Doherty PC, Turner SJ, et al. Early priming minimizes the age-related immune compromise of CD8(+) T cell diversity and function. *PLoS Pathog* (2012) 8(2):e1002544. doi:10.1371/annotation/e142f9de-7f30-4759-bda1-a651e86d5ba6
61. Kedzierska K, Valkenburg SA, Doherty PC, Davenport MP, Venturi V. Use it or lose it: establishment and persistence of T cell memory. *Front Immunol* (2012) 3:357. doi:10.3389/fimmu.2012.00357
62. Lee LY, Ha, do LA, Simmons C, de Jong MD, Chau NV, et al. Memory T cells established by seasonal human influenza A infection cross-react with avian influenza A (H5N1) in healthy individuals. *J Clin Invest* (2008) 118(10):3478–90. doi:10.1172/JCI32460
63. Trieu MC, Zhou F, Lartey S, Jul-Larsen A, Mjaaland S, Sridhar S, et al. Long-term maintenance of the influenza-specific cross-reactive memory CD4+ T-cell responses following repeated annual influenza vaccination. *J Infect Dis* (2017) 215(5):740–9. doi:10.1093/infdis/jiw619
64. Antrobus RD, Lillie PJ, Berthoud TK, Spencer AJ, McLaren JE, Ladell K, et al. A T cell-inducing influenza vaccine for the elderly: safety and immunogenicity of MVA-NP+M1 in adults aged over 50 years. *PLoS One* (2012) 7(10):e48322. doi:10.1371/journal.pone.0048322
65. Antrobus RD, Berthoud TK, Mullarkey CE, Hoschler K, Coughlan L, Zambon M, et al. Coadministration of seasonal influenza vaccine and MVA-NP+M1 simultaneously achieves potent humoral and cell-mediated responses. *Mol Ther* (2014) 22(1):233–8. doi:10.1038/mt.2013.162
66. Pizzolla A, Nguyen TH, Sant S, Jaffar J, Loudovaris T, Mannering SI, et al. Influenza-specific lung-resident memory T cells are proliferative and polyfunctional and maintain diverse TCR profiles. *J Clin Invest* (2018) 128(2): 721–33. doi:10.1172/JCI96957
67. Shin H, Iwasaki A. A vaccine strategy that protects against genital herpes by establishing local memory T cells. *Nature* (2012) 491(7424):463–7. doi:10.1038/nature11522
68. Gilchuk P, Hill TM, Guy C, McMaster SR, Boyd KL, Rabacal WA, et al. A distinct lung-interstitium-resident memory CD8(+) T cell subset confers enhanced protection to lower respiratory tract infection. *Cell Rep* (2016) 16(7):1800–9. doi:10.1016/j.celrep.2016.07.037
69. Wu T, Hu Y, Lee YT, Bouchard KR, Benechet A, Khanna K, et al. Lung-resident memory CD8 T cells (TRM) are indispensable for optimal cross-protection against pulmonary virus infection. *J Leukoc Biol* (2014) 95(2):215–24. doi:10.1189/jlb.0313180
70. Akondy RS, Fitch M, Edupuganti S, Yang S, Kissick HT, Li KW, et al. Origin and differentiation of human memory CD8 T cells after vaccination. *Nature* (2017) 552(7685):362–7. doi:10.1038/nature24633
71. Corti D, Lanzavecchia A. Broadly neutralizing antiviral antibodies. *Annu Rev Immunol* (2013) 31:705–42. doi:10.1146/annurev-immunol-032712-095916
72. Sparrow E, Friede M, Sheikh M, Torvaldsen S, Newall AT. Passive immunization for influenza through antibody therapies, a review of the pipeline, challenges and potential applications. *Vaccine* (2016) 34(45):5442–8. doi:10.1016/j.vaccine.2016.08.057
73. Sui J, Sheehan J, Hwang WC, Bankston LA, Burchett SK, Huang CY, et al. Wide prevalence of heterosubtypic broadly neutralizing human anti-influenza A antibodies. *Clin Infect Dis* (2011) 52(8):1003–9. doi:10.1093/cid/cir121
74. Clemens EB, van de Sandt C, Wong SS, Wakim LM, Valkenburg SA. Harnessing the power of T cells: the promising hope for a universal influenza vaccine. *Vaccines (Basel)* (2018) 6(2). doi:10.3390/vaccines6020018
75. Kumar A, Meldgaard TS, Bertholet S. Novel platforms for the development of a universal influenza Vaccine. *Front Immunol* (2018) 9:600. doi:10.3389/fimmu.2018.00600
76. Lambert LC, Fauci AS. Influenza vaccines for the future. *N Engl J Med* (2010) 363(21):2036–44. doi:10.1056/NEJMra1002842
77. Russell SM, McCahon D, Beare AS. A single radial haemolysis technique for the measurement of influenza antibody. *J Gen Virol* (1975) 27(1):1–10. doi:10.1099/0022-1317-27-1-1
78. Trombetta CM, Montomoli E. Influenza immunology evaluation and correlates of protection: a focus on vaccines. *Expert Rev Vaccines* (2016) 15(8):967–76. doi:10.1586/14760584.2016.1164046
79. Weir JP, Gruber MF. An overview of the regulation of influenza vaccines in the United States. *Influenza Other Respir Viruses* (2016) 10(5):354–60. doi:10.1111/irv.12383
80. Ramilo O, Mejias A. It is time for a comprehensive analytical approach in clinical studies. Virus-versus-host interaction and influenza disease severity. *Am J Respir Crit Care Med* (2014) 189(4):385–6. doi:10.1164/rccm.201401-0008ED
81. de Vries RD, Nieuwkoop NJ, Pronk M, de Bruin E, Leroux-Roels G, Huijskens EGW, et al. Influenza virus-specific antibody dependent cellular cytoxicity induced by vaccination or natural infection. *Vaccine* (2017) 35(2):238–47. doi:10.1016/j.vaccine.2016.11.082
82. Terajima M, Co MD, Cruz J, Ennis FA. High antibody-dependent cellular cytotoxicity antibody titers to H5N1 and H7N9 Avian influenza A viruses in healthy US adults and older children. *J Infect Dis* (2015) 212(7):1052–60. doi:10.1093/infdis/jiv181
83. Valkenburg SA, Zhang Y, Chan KY, Leung K, Wu JT, Poon LL. Preexisting antibody-dependent cellular cytotoxicity-activating antibody responses are stable longitudinally and cross-reactive responses are not boosted by recent influenza exposure. *J Infect Dis* (2016) 214(8):1159–63. doi:10.1093/infdis/jiw346
84. Hobson D, Curry RL, Beare AS, Ward-Gardner A. The role of serum haemagglutination-inhibiting antibody in protection against challenge infection with influenza A2 and B viruses. *J Hyg (Lond)* (1972) 70(4):767–77. doi:10.1017/S0022172400022610
85. Koutsakos M, Wheatley AK, Loh L, Clemens EB, Sant S, Nussing S, et al. Circulating TFH cells, serological memory, and tissue compartmentalization shape human influenza-specific B cell immunity. *Sci Transl Med* (2018) 10(428):eaan8405. doi:10.1126/scitranslmed.aan8405
86. Bentebibel SE, Lopez S, Obermoser G, Schmitt N, Mueller C, Harrod C, et al. Induction of ICOS+CXCR3+CXCR5+ TH cells correlates with antibody

responses to influenza vaccination. *Sci Transl Med* (2013) 5(176):176ra132. doi:10.1126/scitranslmed.3005191

87. Bodewes R, Fraaij PL, Geelhoed-Mieras MM, van Baalen CA, Tiddens HA, van Rossum AM, et al. Annual vaccination against influenza virus hampers development of virus-specific CD8(+) T cell immunity in children. *J Virol* (2011) 85(22):11995–2000. doi:10.1128/JVI.05213-11
88. Nayak JL, Richards KA, Yang H, Treanor JJ, Sant AJ. Effect of influenza A(H5N1) vaccine prepandemic priming on CD4+ T-cell responses. *J Infect Dis* (2015) 211(9):1408–17. doi:10.1093/infdis/jiu616
89. Gostic KM, Ambrose M, Worobey M, Lloyd-Smith JO. Potent protection against H5N1 and H7N9 influenza via childhood hemagglutinin imprinting. *Science* (2016) 354(6313):722–6. doi:10.1126/science.aag1322
90. Bolton KJ, McCaw JM, Brown L, Jackson D, Kedzierska K, McVernon J. Prior population immunity reduces the expected impact of CTL-inducing vaccines for pandemic influenza control. *PLoS One* (2015) 10(3):e0120138. doi:10.1371/journal.pone.0120138
91. Cobey S, Hensley SE. Immune history and influenza virus susceptibility. *Curr Opin Virol* (2017) 22:105–11. doi:10.1016/j.coviro.2016.12.004
92. Cobey S, Gouma S, Parkhouse K, Chambers BS, Ertl HC, Schmader KE, et al. Poor immunogenicity, not vaccine strain egg adaptation, may explain the low H3N2 influenza vaccine effectiveness in 2012-13. *Clin Infect Dis* (2018). doi:10.1093/cid/ciy097
93. Rowell J, Lo CY, Price GE, Misplon JA, Epstein SL, Garcia M. Conventional influenza vaccines influence the performance of a universal influenza vaccine in mice. *Vaccine* (2018) 36(7):1008–15. doi:10.1016/j.vaccine.2017.11.065
94. Monto AS, Malosh RE, Petrie JG, Thompson MG, Ohmit SE. Frequency of acute respiratory illnesses and circulation of respiratory viruses in households with children over 3 surveillance seasons. *J Infect Dis* (2014) 210(11):1792–9. doi:10.1093/infdis/jiu327
95. Nguyen DNT, Mai LQ, Bryant JE, Hang NLK, Hoa LNM, Nadjm B, et al. Epidemiology and etiology of influenza-like-illness in households in Vietnam; it's not all about the kids! *J Clin Virol* (2016) 82:126–32. doi:10.1016/j.jcv.2016.07.014
96. Cowling BJ, Ng S, Ma ES, Cheng CK, Wai W, Fang VJ, et al. Protective efficacy of seasonal influenza vaccination against seasonal and pandemic influenza virus infection during 2009 in Hong Kong. *Clin Infect Dis* (2010) 51(12):1370–9. doi:10.1086/657311
97. Cowling BJ, Perera RA, Fang VJ, Chan KH, Wai W, So HC, et al. Incidence of influenza virus infections in children in Hong Kong in a 3-year randomized placebo-controlled vaccine study, 2009-2012. *Clin Infect Dis* (2014) 59(4):517–24. doi:10.1093/cid/ciu356
98. Cowling BJ, Xu C, Tang F, Zhang J, Shen J, Havers F, et al. Cohort profile: the China Ageing REespiratory infections Study (CARES), a prospective cohort study in older adults in Eastern China. *BMJ Open* (2017) 7(10):e017503. doi:10.1136/bmjopen-2017-017503
99. Gordon A, Kuan G, Aviles W, Sanchez N, Ojeda S, Lopez B, et al. The Nicaraguan pediatric influenza cohort study: design, methods, use of technology, and compliance. *BMC Infect Dis* (2015) 15:504. doi:10.1186/s12879-015-1256-6
100. Thomas S, Rouilly V, Patin E, Alanio C, Dubois A, Delval C, et al. The Milieu Interieur study – an integrative approach for study of human immunological variance. *Clin Immunol* (2015) 157(2):277–93. doi:10.1016/j.clim.2014.12.004
101. Duffy D, Rouilly V, Libri V, Hasan M, Beitz B, David M, et al. Functional analysis via standardized whole-blood stimulation systems defines the boundaries of a healthy immune response to complex stimuli. *Immunity* (2014) 40(3):436–50. doi:10.1016/j.immuni.2014.03.002
102. Duffy D, Rouilly V, Braudeau C, Corbiere V, Djebali R, Ungeheuer MN, et al. Standardized whole blood stimulation improves immunomonitoring of induced immune responses in multi-center study. *Clin Immunol* (2017) 183:325–35. doi:10.1016/j.clim.2017.09.019
103. Pavlova S, D'Alessio F, Houard S, Remarque EJ, Stockhofe N, Engelhardt OG. Workshop report: immunoassay standardisation for "universal" influenza vaccines. *Influenza Other Respir Viruses* (2017) 11(3):194–201. doi:10.1111/irv.12445
104. European Centre for Disease Prevention and Control. *Annual Epidemiological Report for 2015 – Seasonal Influenza [Internet]*. Stockholm: ECDC (2017).
105. CDC. *Influenza Season Vaccination Coverage Report [Online]*. (2014). Available from: https://www.cdc.gov/flu/fluvaxview/reportshtml/reporti1314/reporti/index.html (Accessed: April 24, 2018).
106. CDC. *ACIP Votes Down use of LAIV for 2016-2017 Flu Season.* (2016). Available from: https://www.cdc.gov/media/releases/2016/s0622-laiv-flu.html (Accessed: April 24, 2018).
107. Gorse GJ, Falsey AR, Ozol-Godfrey A, Landolfi V, Tsang PH. Safety and immunogenicity of a quadrivalent intradermal influenza vaccine in adults. *Vaccine* (2015) 33(9):1151–9. doi:10.1016/j.vaccine.2015.01.025
108. Nachbagauer R, Kinzler D, Choi A, Hirsh A, Beaulieu E, Lecrenier N, et al. A chimeric haemagglutinin-based influenza split virion vaccine adjuvanted with AS03 induces protective stalk-reactive antibodies in mice. *NPJ Vaccines* (2016) 1:16015. doi:10.1038/npjvaccines.2016.15
109. Widdice LE, Bernstein DI, Leonard AC, Marsolo KA, Kahn JA. Adherence to the HPV vaccine dosing intervals and factors associated with completion of 3 doses. *Pediatrics* (2011) 127(1):77–84. doi:10.1542/peds.2010-0812
110. Trantham L, Kurosky S, Zhang D, Johnson K. Adherence to multi-dose hepatitis A and hepatitis B vaccine schedules in the United States. *Open Forum Infect Dis* (2017) 4(Suppl_1):S518. doi:10.1093/ofid/ofx163.1347
111. MacDonald NE; SAGE Working Group on Vaccine Hesitancy. Vaccine hesitancy: definition, scope and determinants. *Vaccine* (2015) 33(34):4161–4. doi:10.1016/j.vaccine.2015.04.036
112. Zhou L, Su Q, Xu Z, Feng A, Jin H, Wang S, et al. Seasonal influenza vaccination coverage rate of target groups in selected cities and provinces in China by season (2009/10 to 2011/12). *PLoS One* (2013) 8(9):e73724. doi:10.1371/journal.pone.0073724
113. Black CL, Yue X, Mps, Ball SW, Fink R, de Perio MA, et al. Influenza vaccination coverage among health care personnel – United States, 2016–17 influenza season. *Morb Mortal Wkly Rep* (2017) 66(38):1009–15. doi:10.15585/mmwr.mm6638a1
114. Piedra PA, Gaglani MJ, Kozinetz CA, Herschler G, Riggs M, Griffith M, et al. Herd immunity in adults against influenza-related illnesses with use of the trivalent-live attenuated influenza vaccine (CAIV-T) in children. *Vaccine* (2005) 23(13):1540–8. doi:10.1016/j.vaccine.2004.09.025
115. Cohen SA, Chui KK, Naumova EN. Influenza vaccination in young children reduces influenza-associated hospitalizations in older adults, 2002-2006. *J Am Geriatr Soc* (2011) 59(2):327–32. doi:10.1111/j.1532-5415.2010.03271.x
116. Pebody RG, Green HK, Andrews N, Boddington NL, Zhao H, Yonova I, et al. Uptake and impact of vaccinating school age children against influenza during a season with circulation of drifted influenza A and B strains, England, 2014/15. *Euro Surveill* (2015) 20(39):30029. doi:10.2807/1560-7917.ES.2015.20.39.30029
117. Monto AS, Davenport FM, Napier JA, Francis T Jr. Effect of vaccination of a school-age population upon the course of an A2-Hong Kong influenza epidemic. *Bull World Health Organ* (1969) 41(3):537–42.
118. Medlock J, Galvani AP. Optimizing influenza vaccine distribution. *Science* (2009) 325(5948):1705–8. doi:10.1126/science.1175570
119. Reichert TA, Sugaya N, Fedson DS, Glezen WP, Simonsen L, Tashiro M. The Japanese experience with vaccinating schoolchildren against influenza. *N Engl J Med* (2001) 344(12):889–96. doi:10.1056/NEJM200103223441204
120. Taksler GB, Rothberg MB, Cutler DM. Association of influenza vaccination coverage in younger adults with influenza-related illness in the elderly. *Clin Infect Dis* (2015) 61(10):1495–503. doi:10.1093/cid/civ630
121. Beare AS, Kendal AP, Schild GC. Trials of live influenza A recombinants in man during natural antigenic change in 1971-1976. *Med Microbiol Immunol* (1978) 166(1–4):91–8. doi:10.1007/BF02121138

6

RIG-I-Like Receptors as Novel Targets for Pan-Antivirals and Vaccine Adjuvants Against Emerging and Re-Emerging Viral Infections

Hui Yee Yong[1,2,3] and Dahai Luo [1,2]**

[1] Lee Kong Chian School of Medicine, Nanyang Technological University, Singapore, Singapore, [2] NTU Institute of Structural Biology, Nanyang Technological University, Singapore, [3] School of Biological Sciences, Nanyang Technological University, Singapore

***Correspondence:**
Hui Yee Yong
hyong005@e.ntu.edu.sg;
Dahai Luo
luodahai@ntu.edu.sg

Emerging and re-emerging viruses pose a significant public health challenge around the world, among which RNA viruses are the cause of many major outbreaks of infectious diseases. As one of the early lines of defense in the human immune system, RIG-I-like receptors (RLRs) play an important role as sentinels to thwart the progression of virus infection. The activation of RLRs leads to an antiviral state in the host cells, which triggers the adaptive arm of immunity and ultimately the clearance of viral infections. Hence, RLRs are promising targets for the development of pan-antivirals and vaccine adjuvants. Here, we discuss the opportunities and challenges of developing RLR agonists into antiviral therapeutic agents and vaccine adjuvants against a broad range of viruses.

Keywords: RIG-I-like receptor, pan-antivirals, vaccine adjuvants, interferon, interferon-stimulated genes, RNA therapeutics

INTRODUCTION

RNA viruses account for a third of all emerging and re-emerging infections (1). Due to the changes of abiotic and biotic landscape encountered by RNA viruses and the error-prone nature of viral replication, RNA viruses evolve quickly and contribute to the outbreak of infectious diseases (2). Many recent outbreaks of emerging and re-emerging viruses involve RNA viruses, and thus, there is an urgent need to develop antivirals against these viruses.

The innate immune system confronts viral infection *via* a specialized group of receptors known as pattern recognition receptors (PRRs) (3). Some PRRs recognize RNA viral infections including toll-like receptors 3 and 8 (TLRs), NOD-like receptors NLRP6 and 9 (NLRs), certain DDX/DHX helicases, and RLRs (retinoic acid inducible gene 1 (RIG-I) and melanoma differentiation associated protein 5 (MDA5)) (4–9). These PRRs usually activate interferon production and the secretion of pro-inflammatory cytokines (10). Interferon activates the Janus kinase/signal transducers and activators of transcription (JAK-STAT) signaling pathway in surrounding cells and the expression of interferon-stimulated genes (ISGs). ISGs inhibit virus replication and spread to surrounding cells by degrading viral nucleic acids and inhibiting viral gene expression (11, 12). Here, we focus on RLRs, the major sensors for pathogenic RNA species which trigger antiviral responses and discuss how modulation of RLRs may lead to broad-spectrum antivirals and new vaccine adjuvants.

RIG-I-LIKE RECEPTORS

RIG-I-like receptors are a class of DExD/H box RNA helicases which recognizes double-stranded RNA (dsRNA) (13–17). RLRs consist of RIG-I, MDA5, and laboratory of genetics and physiology 2 (LGP2) (18). RIG-I and MDA5 have similar structural domains with N-terminal caspase activation and recruitment domains (CARDs), central helicase domain, and C-terminal domain, which recognizes viral RNA ligands (19–21). RIG-I recognizes short dsRNA and binds to blunt-ended RNA with 5′ triphosphate moiety (22–27). In contrast, MDA5 binds to the stem region of longer dsRNA in a cooperative manner (28–30). LGP2, on the other hand, only have the helicase and C-terminal domain and are involved in the regulatory function of RIG-I and MDA5 (31, 32).

The CARD domains of RIG-I and MDA5 are involved in the activation of downstream signaling event *via* a protein known as mitochondria antiviral signaling protein (MAVS) (33–36). RIG-I binds to unanchored lysine-63 polyubiquitin chains and promotes efficient interaction with the CARD domain on MAVS (37, 38). MAVS protein polymerizes and forms fibrils when activated and will be polyubiquitinated and phosphorylated (38–42). The MAVS oligomer act as a platform to promote downstream antiviral signaling by recruiting several different proteins, such as tumor necrosis factor receptor type-1-associated death domain (TRADD), receptor interacting serine/threonine-protein kinase 1 (RIP1), Fas-associated protein with death domain (FADD), tumor necrosis factor receptor-associated factors (TRAF6, TRAF2, and TRAF3), as well as caspase 8 and caspase 10 (43, 44). TRAF3 activates TANK binding kinase 1/IκB kinase ε/IκB kinase γ/TANK (TBK1/IKKε/IKKγ/TANK) complex which phosphorylates and dimerizes interferon regulatory factors 3 and 7 (IRF3 and IRF7). The activated IRF3 and IRF7 translocate into the nucleus and activate IFN production (45, 46). TRAF 2 and 6 activate the IKKα/β/γ (also known as NEMO) by ubiquitination and resulting in activation of NFκB and the expression of pro-inflammatory cytokines (**Figure 1**) (41, 47).

PAN-ANTIVIRALS TARGETING RIG-I

Since RLRs are the key component for the antiviral immune response, these sensors are targets for antiviral therapeutics development. Current antiviral interventions focus on the use of direct-acting antivirals (DAAs), which target the essential components in the life cycle of a virus and thus are virus-specific (48). Although DAAs are highly effective, the low fidelity replication of the RNA virus genome could ultimately lead to the emergence of DAA therapies escape mutant (49). To circumvent this problem, broadly targeting antiviral therapeutics need to be used synergistically with DAAs. To this end, RIG-I agonists or RIG-I pathway activators represent a novel group of promising antiviral candidates. Lists of the antiviral candidates are discussed below as three categories based on their chemical nature (**Table 1**).

NUCLEOTIDE-BASED ANTIVIRALS

A dinucleotide-derived small molecule compound, SB9200, has been shown to induce IFN *via* RIG-I and nucleotide-binding oligomerization domain containing protein 2 (NOD2). SB9200 is believed to interact with RIG-I and NOD2 that are associated with pre-genomic RNA thus blocking the HBV viral polymerase from replicating the genomic RNA (60). SB9200 was shown to confer dose-dependent and long-lasting induction of IFNα, IFNβ, and ISGs in liver tissue (50). Treatment of this compound in woodchucks infected with Woodchuck Hepatitis Virus (WHV) showed no sign of toxicity with reduced hepatic WHV antigen and nucleic acid. The sequential treatment of WHV-infected woodchuck with SB9200 followed by entecavir (ETV), a currently used antiviral to treat Hepatitis B (HBV), showed a reduction in viremia and delayed recrudescence of viral replication. The viral reduction from the treatment of SB9200 was comparable with current antivirals, such as Emtricitabine, Tenofovir, and Adefovir, when administered for up to 12 weeks (51). Drugs such as Emtricitabine, Tenofovir, and Adefovir are commonly used for the treatment of HBV. These drugs, however, may cause side effects such as lactic acidosis and possible liver, and kidney failure. SB9200 is effective for HCV patients with relapse after DAA and interferon treatment and could serve as a promising treatment option for patients who are not responding to the current regimen of DAA therapy (52). The phase 1 clinical trial on naïve adult with chronic hepatitis C showed an association between the decline in viral RNA and the peak of SB9200 detection in plasma (Clinical trial no NCT01803308). Currently, SB9200 is being tested in phase 2 clinical trials for treating subjects chronically infected with the HBV.

RNA-BASED ANTIVIRAL CANDIDATES

5′ triphosphorylated and diphosphorylated short dsRNAs are RIG-I specific ligands (22, 26, 61, 62). Goulet et al. showed that 5′pppRNA could activate a broad spectrum of antiviral and inflammatory genes such as IRF3, IRF7, NFkB, and the downstream ISGs. Treatment of lung epithelial cells A549 with 5′pppRNA confers protection against vesicular stomatitis virus (VSV), vaccinia virus, and dengue virus (DENV). The antiviral effect of 5′pppRNA was also detected against HIV in CD4+ T cells and HCV in Huh 7.5 cells (53). Besides that, 5′pppRNA was also an effective antiviral against influenza virus infection *in vitro* and *in vivo*. Treating mice with 5′pppRNA prior to influenza virus challenge also reduces pneumonia related to influenza virus infection (53). In another study, 5′pppRNA was shown to stimulate host antiviral response and reduce the infectivity of DENV and chikungunya virus (CHIKV) in human myeloid, fibroblast, and epithelial cells *via* RIG-I specific activation (54).

Several studies were also carried out to determine factors such as sequence, length, and structure of 5′pppRNA to enhance the antiviral activities of RIG-I (55, 56). Chiang et al. showed that 5′pppRNA with uridine-rich sequence with 99 nucleotides hairpin (M8) triggered higher interferon response when compared to other RIG-I aptamer and poly(I:C). M8 specifically activates RIG-I without triggering MDA5 or TLR3 activation. Prophylactic and therapeutic treatment using M8 protect cells from dengue and influenza viral infections. Furthermore, administration of M8 followed by influenza virus challenge improves the survival rate of mice with low lung virus titer detected at day 3 post-infection (55). In another study carried out by Lee et al., different RNA fold was shown to elicit different antiviral properties *via* RIG-I. Short hairpin RNA with a bent in the stem structure with phosphorothioate backbone was used as antiviral and was more potent than oseltamivir against influenza A H1N1 virus *in vitro* (56). Linehan et al. recently showed that short RNA with stable tetraloop at one

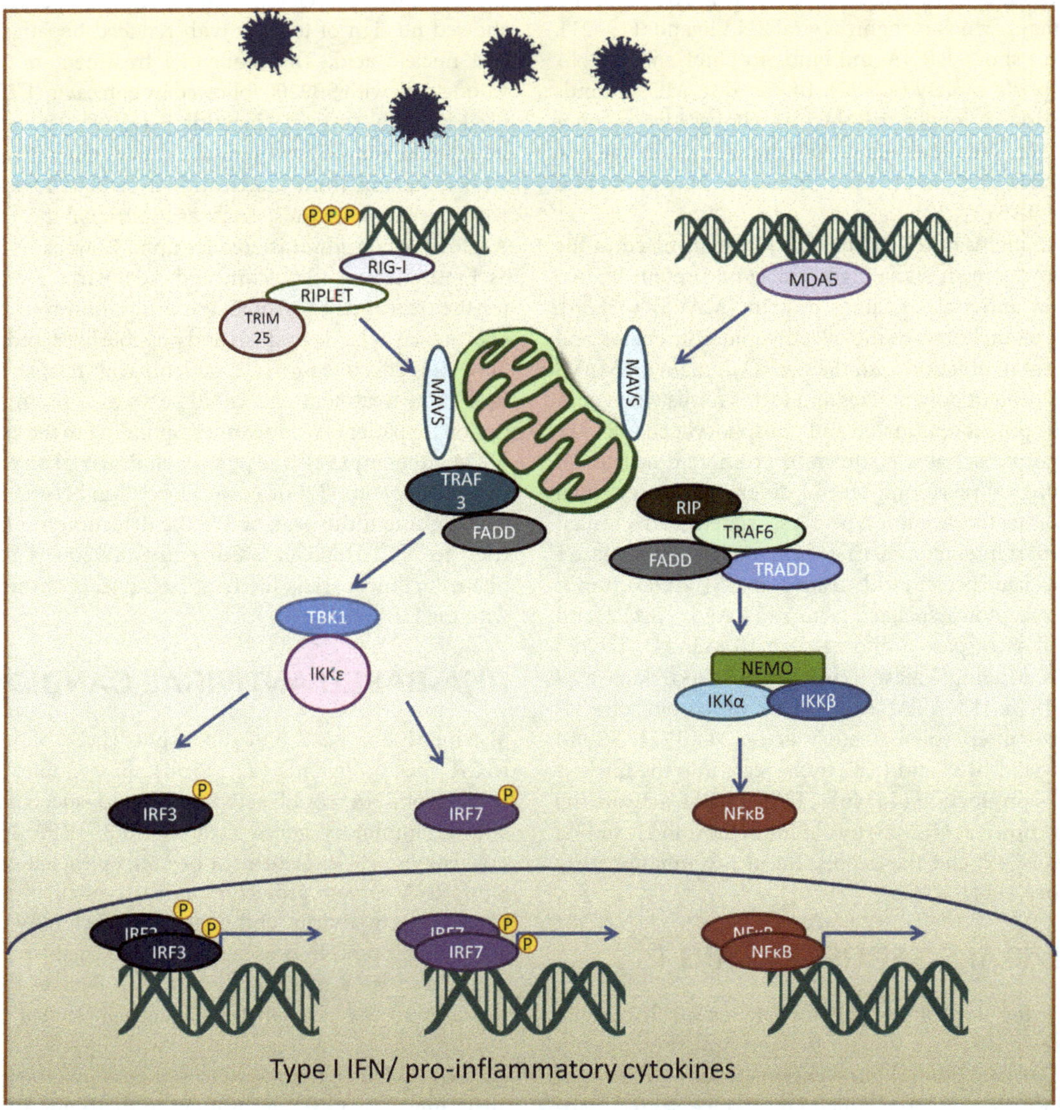

FIGURE 1 | Viral RNA is recognized by RIG-I-like receptors (RLRs), RIG-I, or melanoma differentiation-associated protein 5 (MDA5). Activated RLRs interacts with mitochondria antiviral signaling protein (MAVS) adapter protein *via* CARD–CARD interactions. Activated MAVS then interacts with tumor necrosis factor receptor-associated factors 3 (TRAF3), tumor necrosis factor receptor-associated factors 6 (TRAF6), tumor necrosis factor receptor type-1-associated death domain (TRADD), receptor interacting serine/threonine-protein kinase 1 (RIP1), Fas-associated protein with death domain (FADD), and other signaling molecules. TRAF3 activates TANK binding kinase 1 (TBK1) and IκB kinase ε (IKKε), which phosphorylates interferon regulatory factors 3 and 7 (IRF3 and IRF7). The phosphorylated IRF3 and IRF7 dimerize and translocate into the nucleus to induce type 1 interferon response. On the other hand, MAVS interaction with receptor interacting serine/threonine-protein kinase 1, FADD, TRAF6, and TRADD. TRAF 6 ubiquitinate NF-kappa-B essential modulator (NEMO) which then activates IκB kinase and activates NF-κB. NF-κB transcription factor drives the expression of type 1 interferon and proinflammatory cytokines.

end of duplex RNA triggers a robust IFN 1 response *in vivo*. These short stem-loop RNA (SLR) induces a subset of genes involved in antiviral and effector responses as well as represses gene involved in T cell maturation and could potentially be developed into a highly effective antiviral or vaccine adjuvant (57).

SMALL MOLECULAR COMPOUNDS

High throughput screening (HTS) of small molecule compounds identified a group of novel agonists of the innate immune pathway. The isoflavone-like compound confers protection against HCV and Influenza A virus *in vitro*. These compounds were also shown to activate a narrower subset of genes and thus have potential to be useful antiviral without causing cytokine toxicity (58).

Another class of small molecule compounds, hydroxyquinolines, identified *via* HTS of compound library in cell culture induces the expression of innate immune antiviral genes such as RIG-I, IFIT1, IFIT2, IFITM1, OAS3, and MX1. Remarkably, although these compounds were able to induce high expression of antiviral genes, the expression of type I and III interferon remains low, suggesting the activation of distinct antiviral pathway than that of RIG-I agonists. The specific target(s) of these hydroxyquinoline

TABLE 1 | Pan-antivirals targeting RLRs.

Pan-antivirals	Formula	Target pathway	Reference
Nucleotide-based			
SB9200	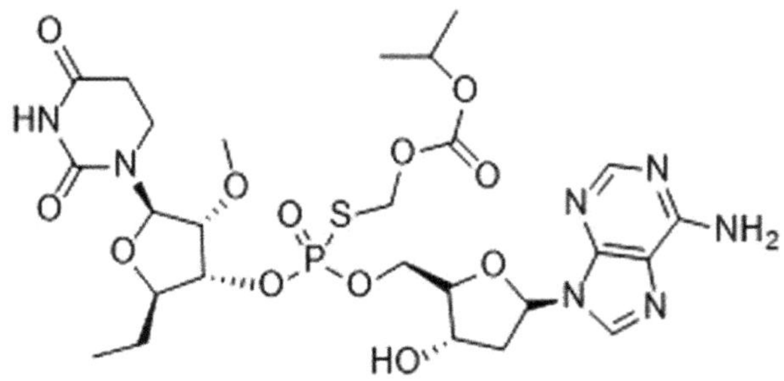	RLR and NLR	(50–52)
RNA-based			
5′ppp RNA derived from the 5′ and 3′ UTRs of the negative-strand RNA virus Vesicular Stomatitis Virus	GACGAAGACC ACAAAACCAG AUAAAAAAUA AAAUUUAAUG AUAAUAAUGG UUUGUUUGUC UUCGUC	RLR	(53, 54)
5′ppp RNA (M8)	GACGAAGACCACAAAACCAGAUAAAAAAAAAAAAAAAAAAAAAAAAAAAAUAAU UUUUUUUUUUUUUUUUUUUUUUUUUUAUCUGGUUUUGUGGUCUUCGUC	RLR	(55)
5′OH RNA with kink (CBS-13-BPS)	GGUAGACGAAACCAGAUAUAAUAUCUGGUUUCGUUUGCC	RIG-I, ISG56	(56)
5′PPP SLR	Stem loop RNA with the length of 10 and 14 base pair (GGACGUACGUUUC GACGUACGUCC) and (GGAUCGAUCGAUCGUUCGCGAUCGAUCGAUCC)	RIG-I	(57)
Small molecular compounds			
KIN 100	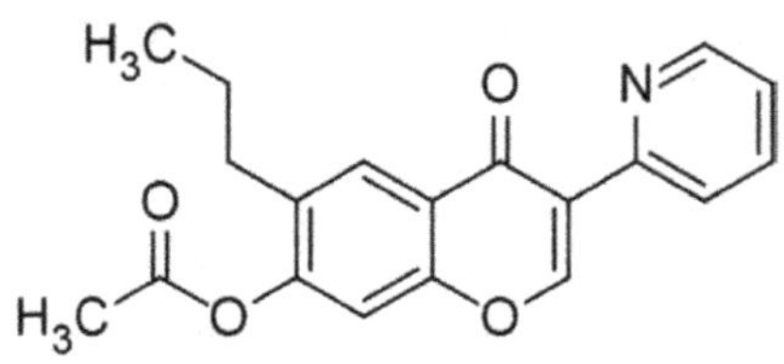	IRF 3	(58)
KIN101	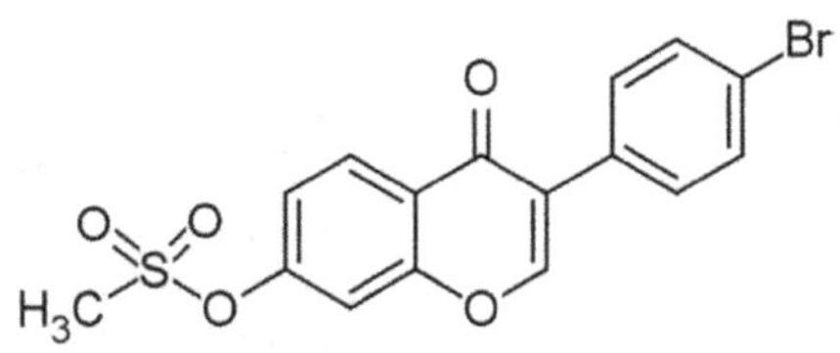	IRF3	(58)
KIN 1000	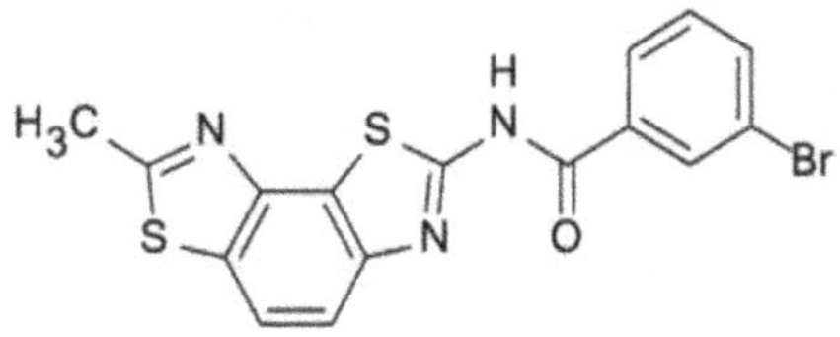	IRF 3	(59)
KIN1400	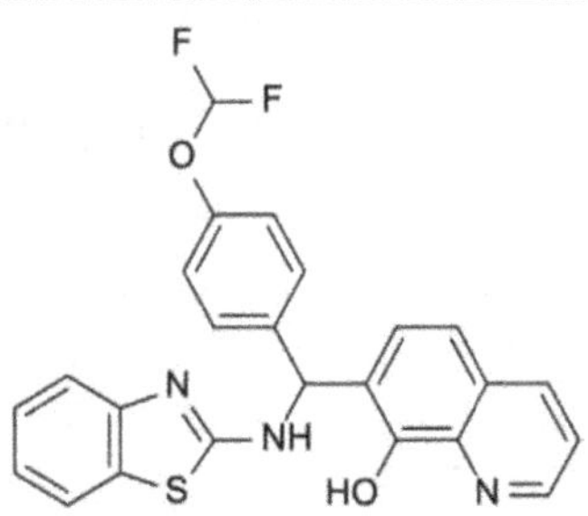	IRF 3	(59)

(Continued)

TABLE 1 | Continued

Pan-antivirals	Formula	Target pathway	Reference
KIN1408	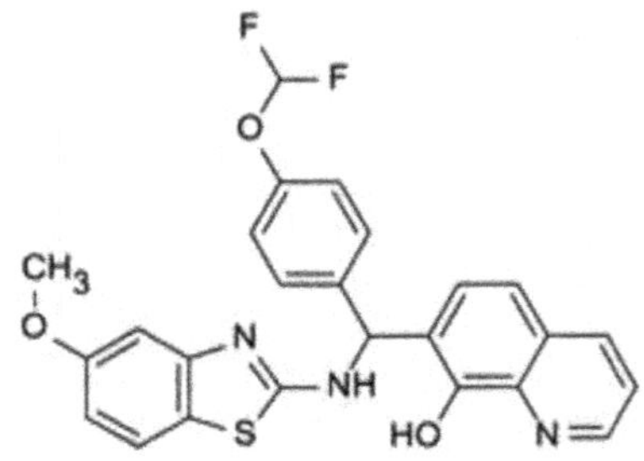	IRF3	(59)
KIN1409	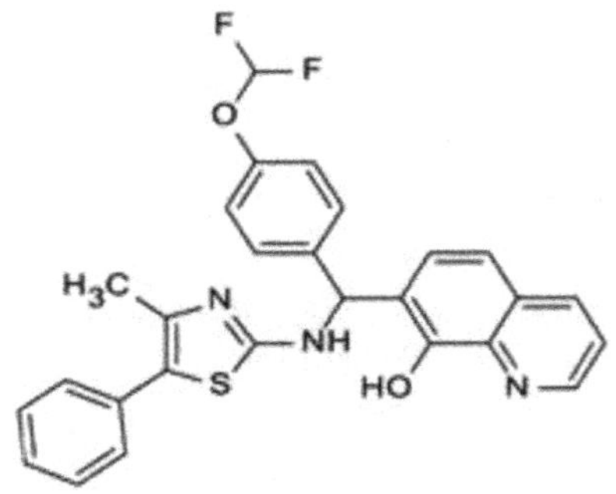	IRF3	(59)

RLRs, RIG-I-like receptors.

compounds are not known. These hydroxyquinoline compounds were effective antivirals against a broad range of RNA viruses from the families Flaviviridae, Filoviridae, Paramyxoviridae, Arenaviridae, and Orthomyxoviridae. Interestingly, these compounds exhibit both prophylactic and therapeutic activity against infection and could be used in combination with other antivirals (59).

INNATE IMMUNE POTENTIATOR AS VACCINE ADJUVANTS

Adjuvants act as an immune enhancer to a vaccine. Several different classes of adjuvant had been approved for use in human vaccines such as alum and oil in emulsion MF59, AS03 (oil in water emulsion), virosomes, and AS04 (aluminum with monophosphoryl lipid A) (63). Alum and MF59 act by increasing antigen uptake at the injection site and activates pro-inflammatory responses (64–66). Alum mainly acts *via* Th2 cellular immune response, which does not confer the best protection for viral infections such as HCV and HIV. Moreover, there are safety concerns with the use of alum as an adjuvant with reported cases of hypersensitivity and erythema (67, 68). Well characterized agonists of innate immunity may serve as a better candidate of targeted vaccine adjuvants (**Figure 2**).

A small molecule compound named KIN 1148, discovered *via* HTS, was shown to activate IRF3 nuclear translocation. When this compound was tested with influenza split virus vaccine H1N1 A/California/07/2009, it confers protection from lethal challenge of influenza virus strain A/California/04/2009. KIN1148 together with the vaccine confers protection *via* IL-10 and Th-2 response to T cells in lung and lung-draining lymph nodes. Immunization with vaccine and KIN 1148 showed a significant increase in IgG antibodies with serum from mice receiving prime-boost immunization conferring protection to naïve mice from influenza challenge. KIN1148 was shown to be able to work alongside the vaccine to boost protective immunity and protect against influenza strain A/California/04/2009 (**Table 2**) (69).

5′triphosphorylated duplex RNA was tested as an adjuvant by Beljanski et al. M8 a potent triphosphorylated RNA was used in conjunction with virus-like particle (VLP) expressing H5N1 influenza hemagglutinin and neuraminidase. The combination of VLP and RNA increases the survival rate of mice infected with H5N1 influenza virus and induces higher antibody titer against influenza virus as compared to other adjuvants such as alum, addavax and poly(I:IC). Furthermore, vaccination with VLP and RNA stimulates TH1-biased CD4 T cells response in mouse sera (70). Another 5′triphosphorylated RNA derived from Sendai virus defective interfering RNA (SeV DI RNA) was also tested as adjuvant together with the H1N1 2009 pandemic vaccine and was shown to enhance production of influenza-specific IgG antibodies and influenza-specific IgA antibodies indicating that this 5′triphosphorylated RNA could potentially be used as influenza vaccine adjuvant (71).

DELIVERY OF RNA-BASED AGENTS REMAINS CHALLENGING

To be effective as therapeutics, functional RNA species must be internalized into targeted cells. The delivery methods commonly used for RNA-based or nucleotide specific antivirals includes the lipid-oligo complexes, nanoparticle-based delivery, and viral-based delivery. The hydrophilic, negatively charge nature of RNA hinders the direct uptake of naked oligos into cells. The administration of RNA *via* inhalation was poorly efficacious in

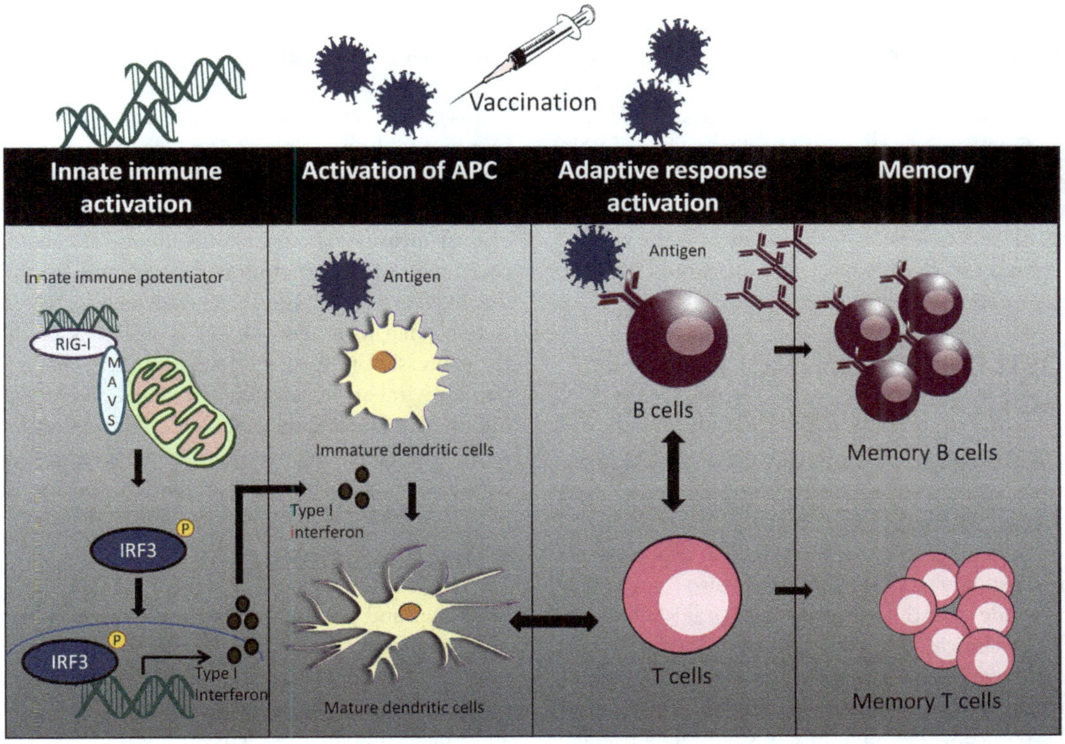

FIGURE 2 | The use of innate immune potentiator as adjuvant triggers the stimulation of adaptive immune responses. Innate immune potentiator stimulates RIG-I-like receptors (RIG-I) and interacts with MAVS adapter. This results in the activation of downstream signaling pathways and release of type I interferon. Type I interferon couple with the presence of antigen trigger DC maturation by enhancing surface marker expression and antigen presentation. The activated DCs interact with CD4+ T cells and thus stimulate Type 1T helper (TH1) cells. TH1 cells in turn interact with B cells to produce antibodies and trigger clonal expansion of B cells and T helper cells.

TABLE 2 | Innate immune potentiator as virus vaccine adjuvants.

Adjuvant	Target	Status	Virus vaccine	Reference
KIN 1148 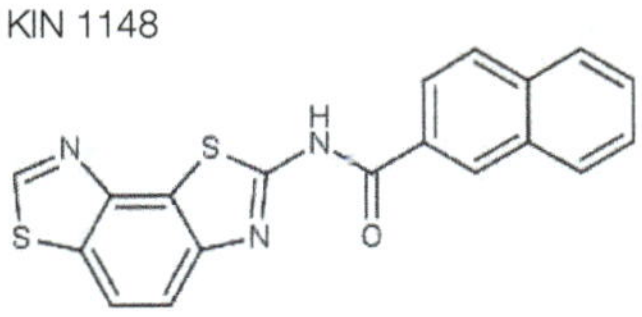	IRF3	Laboratory testing	Influenza H1N1 A/California/07/2009	(69)
M8 5′pppRNA GACGAAGACCACAAAACCAGAUAAA AAAAAAAAAAAAAAAAAAAAAAAUA AUUUUUUUUUUUUUUUUUUUUUUU UUUUUAUCUGGUUUUGUGGUCUUCGUC	RLR	Laboratory testing	H5N1 influenza	(70)
5′pppRNA Derived from SeV DI RNA	RLR	Laboratory testing	H1N1 2009	(71)

RLRs, RIG-I-like receptors.

lung macrophages and only intratracheal administration leads to efficient delivery of RNA into the targeted site (72). Besides suffering from poor uptake, naked RNA is often prone to degradation in plasma (73).

One favored method of delivery for RNA is lipid-oligo complexes. This delivery method is more efficient due to the tendency of lipid to interact with the cell membrane and improve the uptake of RNA (74). A biocompatible lipid-based carrier can further reduce undesired immunogenic activation. However, the cationic nature of lipid is reported to interact with proteins in serum, and these aggregates are cleared by organs such as the spleen, lung and liver (75).

Nanoparticle-based delivery is a versatile method for RNA delivery with many organic or inorganic materials available as nanocarriers. Nanoparticle requires less RNA material with a large surface area for interaction with cells (76). The material used as a carrier could also be tailored for application such as dose, circulation time, as well as passive or active release of RNA (77). To overcome the issue of toxicity or uncontrolled immune activation, multistage delivery of RNA from nanoparticles could be carried put (78). The downside of this strategy is the need to test various materials for RNA delivery and this would drive up the cost of therapeutics or vaccine.

THE DANGER OF UNCONTROLLED IMMUNE ACTIVATION ALWAYS EXISTS

The therapeutic and prophylactic use of pan-antivirals was previously demonstrated in viral infection of influenza and dengue (55, 69, 71). Hotz et al. demonstrated that the pre-exposure of murine APC to synthetic poly(I:C) inhibits RLR activation while augmenting the sensitivity of TLRs. This would also imply a narrow therapeutic window for the use of pan-antiviral RNA targeting RIG-I (79). For clinical usage, the dosage of therapeutics is important to minimize side effects such as exacerbated cytokine storms and toxicity. Prater et al. showed that the injection of pregnant C57BL/6 mice with a high dose of CpG-ODN resulted in high fetal resorptions and craniofacial/limb defects (80). RIG-I agonists face similar concerns.

RIG-I SNPs MAY LEAD TO POOR OR HYPER-RESPONSIVENESS

There are 324 RIG-I SNPs identified from NCBI SNPs database with 8 resulting in amino acid changes or truncation. The S183I mutation on RIG-I weakened the antiviral signaling and produces a low level of IFNβ and NFκB upon IAV and SeV challenges in a cell-based assay. Another SNP of RIG-I at P229 resulted in frameshift mutation at the CARDs domain and triggers constitutive expression of IFNβ suggesting that individual with this mutation could be linked to hyper-responsiveness in the immune system or autoimmune diseases (81). Another commonly found SNP (rs10813831) of RIG-I resulted in the substitution of R7C which could alter RIG-I interaction with MAVS (82). Individuals with these SNPs have a lower rubella-specific IgG titer when immunized with live measles-mumps-rubella (MMR-II) vaccine (83). This SNPs mutation also increased the IFNβ level and RIG-I transcription in human dendritic cells when infected with Newcastle disease virus (NDV) (82). Individuals with these SNPs were also shown to have complications of brainstem encephalitis when infected with enterovirus 71 (84). Several intronic SNPs also alter the cellular and humoral response to the measles vaccine. Genotype of individual carrying the SNP in minor allele of RIG-I (for rs12555727, rs12006123, and rs17289116) also showed less virus-specific IFN-γ secretion against measles. These findings imply that genetic variants are also involved in initial antiviral responses to vaccination (85) The haplotype of RIG-I rs3739674 which is located in the 5′UTR is associated with higher EV71 HFMD risk possibly by altering the expression level of the gene (86). In order to target RIG-I as pan-antiviral or vaccine adjuvant, the different haplotypes affecting the disease outcome should be considered. Dosage concern should be taken into account to enhance the effectiveness of RIG-I as a broadly targeting antiviral or vaccine adjuvant.

CONCLUSION

Emerging and re-emerging viruses present a significant public health concern, and there is an urgent need for novel vaccination and treatment strategies. RIG-I agonists as new adjuvant candidates may work alone or couple to vaccine agents such as VLPs or recombinant proteins to improve the safety and efficacy of conventional vaccines. Antivirals targeting the innate arm of immunity (host-directed therapy) would be useful to confer protection against emerging and re-emerging viruses (87). However, the development of such vaccines and antivirals is still in its infancy and many challenges related to the production and safety evaluation of vaccines and antivirals. Several key issues still need to be addressed including production platform, formulation, delivery, safety, and the ability of such class of the vaccine adjuvant or antivirals to be used in immunocompromised and elderly.

AUTHOR CONTRIBUTIONS

DL and HY discussed, wrote, and revised the manuscript.

ACKNOWLEDGMENTS

This work was supported by (1) a start-up grant from Lee Kong Chian School of Medicine, Nanyang Technological University, (2) MOE2016-T2-2-097 grant, and (3) National Research Foundation grant NRF2016NRF-CRP001-063.

REFERENCES

1. Howard CR, Fletcher NF. Emerging virus diseases: can we ever expect the unexpected? *Emerg Microbes Infect* (2012) 1:e46. doi:10.1038/emi.2012.47
2. Nichol ST, Arikawa J, Kawaoka Y. Emerging viral diseases. *Proc Natl Acad Sci U S A* (2000) 97:12411–2. doi:10.1073/pnas.210382297
3. Yan N, Chen ZJ. Intrinsic antiviral immunity. *Nat Immunol* (2012) 13:214–22. doi:10.1038/ni.2229
4. Creagh EM, O'Neill LA. TLRs, NLRs and RLRs: a trinity of pathogen sensors that co-operate in innate immunity. *Trends Immunol* (2006) 27:352–7. doi:10.1016/j.it.2006.06.003
5. Higgins SC, Mills KH. TLR, NLR agonists, and other immune modulators as infectious disease vaccine adjuvants. *Curr Infect Dis Rep* (2010) 12:4–12. doi:10.1007/s11908-009-0080-9
6. Hornung V. SnapShot: nucleic acid immune sensors, part 1. *Immunity* (2014) 41:868, 868.e1. doi:10.1016/j.immuni.2014.10.005
7. Hornung V. SnapShot: nucleic acid immune sensors, part 2. *Immunity* (2014) 41:1066–1066.e1. doi:10.1016/j.immuni.2014.10.006
8. Kumar H, Kawai T, Akira S. Pathogen recognition in the innate immune response. *Biochem J* (2009) 420:1–16. doi:10.1042/BJ20090272
9. Wu J, Chen ZJ. Innate immune sensing and signaling of cytosolic nucleic acids. *Annu Rev Immunol* (2014) 32:461–88. doi:10.1146/annurev-immunol-032713-120156

10. Iwasaki A, Medzhitov R. Regulation of adaptive immunity by the innate immune system. *Science* (2010) 327:291–5. doi:10.1126/science.1183021
11. Borden EC, Williams BR. Interferon-stimulated genes and their protein products: what and how? *J Interferon Cytokine Res* (2011) 31:1–4. doi:10.1089/jir.2010.0129
12. Schoggins JW, Rice CM. Interferon-stimulated genes and their antiviral effector functions. *Curr Opin Virol* (2011) 1:519–25. doi:10.1016/j.coviro.2011.10.008
13. Bruns AM, Horvath CM. Activation of RIG-I-like receptor signal transduction. *Crit Rev Biochem Mol Biol* (2012) 47:194–206. doi:10.3109/10409238.2011.630974
14. Loo YM, Gale M Jr. Immune signaling by RIG-I-like receptors. *Immunity* (2011) 34:680–92. doi:10.1016/j.immuni.2011.05.003
15. Luo D. Toward a crystal-clear view of the viral RNA sensing and response by RIG-I-like receptors. *RNA Biol* (2014) 11:25–32. doi:10.4161/rna.27717
16. Luo D, Kohlway A, Pyle AM. Duplex RNA activated ATPases (DRAs): platforms for RNA sensing, signaling and processing. *RNA Biol* (2013) 10:111–20. doi:10.4161/rna.22706
17. Schlee M. Master sensors of pathogenic RNA – RIG-I like receptors. *Immunobiology* (2013) 218(11):1322–35. doi:10.1016/j.imbio.2013.06.007
18. Yoneyama M, Kikuchi M, Matsumoto K, Imaizumi T, Miyagishi M, Taira K, et al. Shared and unique functions of the DExD/H-box helicases RIG-I, MDA5, and LGP2 in antiviral innate immunity. *J Immunol* (2005) 175:2851–8. doi:10.4049/jimmunol.175.5.2851
19. Jiang F, Ramanathan A, Miller MT, Tang GQ, Gale M Jr, Patel SS, et al. Structural basis of RNA recognition and activation by innate immune receptor RIG-I. *Nature* (2011) 479:423–7. doi:10.1038/nature10537
20. Kowalinski E, Lunardi T, McCarthy AA, Louber J, Brunel J, Grigorov B, et al. Structural basis for the activation of innate immune pattern-recognition receptor RIG-I by viral RNA. *Cell* (2011) 147:423–35. doi:10.1016/j.cell.2011.09.039
21. Luo D, Ding SC, Vela A, Kohlway A, Lindenbach BD, Pyle AM. Structural insights into RNA recognition by RIG-I. *Cell* (2011) 147:409–22. doi:10.1016/j.cell.2011.09.023
22. Hornung V, Ellegast J, Kim S, Brzozka K, Jung A, Kato H, et al. 5'-Triphosphate RNA is the ligand for RIG-I. *Science* (2006) 314:994–7. doi:10.1126/science.1132505
23. Kohlway A, Luo D, Rawling DC, Ding SC, Pyle AM. Defining the functional determinants for RNA surveillance by RIG-I. *EMBO Rep* (2013) 14:772–9. doi:10.1038/embor.2013.108
24. Pichlmair A, Schulz O, Tan CP, Naslund TI, Liljestrom P, Weber F, et al. RIG-I-mediated antiviral responses to single-stranded RNA bearing 5'-phosphates. *Science* (2006) 314:997–1001. doi:10.1126/science.1132998
25. Schlee M, Roth A, Hornung V, Hagmann CA, Wimmenauer V, Barchet W, et al. Recognition of 5' triphosphate by RIG-I helicase requires short blunt double-stranded RNA as contained in panhandle of negative-strand virus. *Immunity* (2009) 31:25–34. doi:10.1016/j.immuni.2009.05.008
26. Schmidt A, Schwerd T, Hamm W, Hellmuth JC, Cui S, Wenzel M, et al. 5'-triphosphate RNA requires base-paired structures to activate antiviral signaling via RIG-I. *Proc Natl Acad Sci U S A* (2009) 106:12067–72. doi:10.1073/pnas.0900971106
27. Zheng J, Yong HY, Panutdaporn N, Liu C, Tang K, Luo D. High-resolution HDX-MS reveals distinct mechanisms of RNA recognition and activation by RIG-I and MDA5. *Nucleic Acids Res* (2015) 43:1216–30. doi:10.1093/nar/gku1329
28. Peisley A, Jo MH, Lin C, Wu B, Orme-Johnson M, Walz T, et al. Kinetic mechanism for viral dsRNA length discrimination by MDA5 filaments. *Proc Natl Acad Sci U S A* (2012) 109:E3340–9. doi:10.1073/pnas.1208618109
29. Peisley A, Lin C, Wu B, Orme-Johnson M, Liu M, Walz T, et al. Cooperative assembly and dynamic disassembly of MDA5 filaments for viral dsRNA recognition. *Proc Natl Acad Sci U S A* (2011) 108:21010–5. doi:10.1073/pnas.1113651108
30. Wu B, Peisley A, Richards C, Yao H, Zeng X, Lin C, et al. Structural basis for dsRNA recognition, filament formation, and antiviral signal activation by MDA5. *Cell* (2013) 152:276–89. doi:10.1016/j.cell.2012.11.048
31. Bruns AM, Horvath CM. LGP2 synergy with MDA5 in RLR-mediated RNA recognition and antiviral signaling. *Cytokine* (2015) 74:198–206. doi:10.1016/j.cyto.2015.02.010
32. Satoh T, Kato H, Kumagai Y, Yoneyama M, Sato S, Matsushita K, et al. LGP2 is a positive regulator of RIG-I- and MDA5-mediated antiviral responses. *Proc Natl Acad Sci U S A* (2010) 107:1512–7. doi:10.1073/pnas.0912986107
33. Kawai T, Takahashi K, Sato S, Coban C, Kumar H, Kato H, et al. IPS-1, an adaptor triggering RIG-I- and Mda5-mediated type I interferon induction. *Nat Immunol* (2005) 6:981–8. doi:10.1038/ni1243
34. Meylan E, Curran J, Hofmann K, Moradpour D, Binder M, Bartenschlager R, et al. Cardif is an adaptor protein in the RIG-I antiviral pathway and is targeted by hepatitis C virus. *Nature* (2005) 437:1167–72. doi:10.1038/nature04193
35. Seth RB, Sun L, Ea CK, Chen ZJ. Identification and characterization of MAVS, a mitochondrial antiviral signaling protein that activates NF-kappaB and IRF 3. *Cell* (2005) 122:669–82. doi:10.1016/j.cell.2005.08.012
36. Xu LG, Wang YY, Han KJ, Li LY, Zhai Z, Shu HB. VISA is an adapter protein required for virus-triggered IFN-beta signaling. *Mol Cell* (2005) 19:727–40. doi:10.1016/j.molcel.2005.08.014
37. Oshiumi H, Matsumoto M, Seya T. Ubiquitin-mediated modulation of the cytoplasmic viral RNA sensor RIG-I. *J Biochem* (2012) 151:5–11. doi:10.1093/jb/mvr111
38. Wu B, Peisley A, Tetrault D, Li Z, Egelman EH, Magor KE, et al. Molecular imprinting as a signal-activation mechanism of the viral RNA sensor RIG-I. *Mol Cell* (2014) 55:511–23. doi:10.1016/j.molcel.2014.06.010
39. Hou F, Sun L, Zheng H, Skaug B, Jiang QX, Chen ZJ. MAVS forms functional prion-like aggregates to activate and propagate antiviral innate immune response. *Cell* (2011) 146:448–61. doi:10.1016/j.cell.2011.06.041
40. Liu S, Cai X, Wu J, Cong Q, Chen X, Li T, et al. Phosphorylation of innate immune adaptor proteins MAVS, STING, and TRIF induces IRF3 activation. *Science* (2015) 347:aaa2630. doi:10.1126/science.aaa2630
41. Liu S, Chen J, Cai X, Wu J, Chen X, Wu YT, et al. MAVS recruits multiple ubiquitin E3 ligases to activate antiviral signaling cascades. *Elife* (2013) 2:e00785. doi:10.7554/eLife.00785
42. Peisley A, Wu B, Xu H, Chen ZJ, Hur S. Structural basis for ubiquitin-mediated antiviral signal activation by RIG-I. *Nature* (2014) 509:110–4. doi:10.1038/nature13140
43. Shu HB, Takeuchi M, Goeddel DV. The tumor necrosis factor receptor 2 signal transducers TRAF2 and c-IAP1 are components of the tumor necrosis factor receptor 1 signaling complex. *Proc Natl Acad Sci U S A* (1996) 93:13973–8. doi:10.1073/pnas.93.24.13973
44. Zhang D, Lin J, Han J. Receptor-interacting protein (RIP) kinase family. *Cell Mol Immunol* (2010) 7:243–9. doi:10.1038/cmi.2010.10
45. Paz S, Vilasco M, Werden SJ, Arguello M, Joseph-Pillai D, Zhao T, et al. A functional C-terminal TRAF3-binding site in MAVS participates in positive and negative regulation of the IFN antiviral response. *Cell Res* (2011) 21:895–910. doi:10.1038/cr.2011.2
46. Yoneyama M, Suhara W, Fukuhara Y, Fukuda M, Nishida E, Fujita T. Direct triggering of the type I interferon system by virus infection: activation of a transcription factor complex containing IRF-3 and CBP/p300. *EMBO J* (1998) 17:1087–95. doi:10.1093/emboj/17.4.1087
47. Vallabhapurapu S, Karin M. Regulation and function of NF-kappaB transcription factors in the immune system. *Annu Rev Immunol* (2009) 27:693–733. doi:10.1146/annurev.immunol.021908.132641
48. Halfon P, Sarrazin C. Future treatment of chronic hepatitis C with direct acting antivirals: is resistance important? *Liver Int* (2012) 32(Suppl 1):79–87. doi:10.1111/j.1478-3231.2011.02716.x
49. Asselah T, Marcellin P. Interferon free therapy with direct acting antivirals for HCV. *Liver Int* (2013) 33(Suppl 1):93–104. doi:10.1111/liv.12076
50. Korolowicz KE, Iyer RP, Czerwinski S, Suresh M, Yang J, Padmanabhan S, et al. Antiviral efficacy and host innate immunity associated with SB 9200 treatment in the woodchuck model of chronic hepatitis B. *PLoS One* (2016) 11:e0161313. doi:10.1371/journal.pone.0161313
51. Suresh M, Korolowicz KE, Balarezo M, Iyer RP, Padmanabhan S, Cleary D, et al. Antiviral efficacy and host immune response induction during sequential treatment with SB 9200 followed by entecavir in woodchucks. *PLoS One* (2017) 12:e0169631. doi:10.1371/journal.pone.0169631
52. Jones M, Cunningham ME, Wing P, DeSilva S, Challa R, Sheri A, et al. SB 9200, a novel agonist of innate immunity, shows potent antiviral activity against resistant HCV variants. *J Med Virol* (2017) 89:1620–8. doi:10.1002/jmv.24809
53. Goulet ML, Olagnier D, Xu Z, Paz S, Belgnaoui SM, Lafferty EI, et al. Systems analysis of a RIG-I agonist inducing broad spectrum inhibition of virus infectivity. *PLoS Pathog* (2013) 9:e1003298. doi:10.1371/journal.ppat.1003298
54. Olagnier D, Scholte FE, Chiang C, Albulescu IC, Nichols C, He Z, et al. Inhibition of dengue and chikungunya virus infections by RIG-I-mediated

type I interferon-independent stimulation of the innate antiviral response. *J Virol* (2014) 88:4180–94. doi:10.1128/JVI.03114-13

55. Chiang C, Beljanski V, Yin K, Olagnier D, Ben Yebdri F, Steel C, et al. Sequence-specific modifications enhance the broad-spectrum antiviral response activated by RIG-I agonists. *J Virol* (2015) 89:8011–25. doi:10.1128/JVI.00845-15
56. Lee J, Park EB, Min J, Sung SE, Jang Y, Shin JS, et al. Systematic editing of synthetic RIG-I ligands to produce effective antiviral and anti-tumor RNA immunotherapies. *Nucleic Acids Res* (2018) 46(4):1635–47. doi:10.1093/nar/gky039
57. Linehan MM, Dickey TH, Molinari ES, Fitzgerald ME, Potapova O, Iwasaki A, et al. A minimal RNA ligand for potent RIG-I activation in living mice. *Sci Adv* (2018) 4:e1701854. doi:10.1126/sciadv.1701854
58. Bedard KM, Wang ML, Proll SC, Loo YM, Katze MG, Gale M Jr, et al. Isoflavone agonists of IRF-3 dependent signaling have antiviral activity against RNA viruses. *J Virol* (2012) 86:7334–44. doi:10.1128/JVI.06867-11
59. Pattabhi S, Wilkins CR, Dong R, Knoll ML, Posakony J, Kaiser S, et al. Targeting innate immunity for antiviral therapy through small molecule agonists of the RLR pathway. *J Virol* (2015) 90:2372–87. doi:10.1128/JVI.02202-15
60. Sato S, Li K, Kameyama T, Hayashi T, Ishida Y, Murakami S, et al. The RNA sensor RIG-I dually functions as an innate sensor and direct antiviral factor for hepatitis B virus. *Immunity* (2015) 42:123–32. doi:10.1016/j.immuni.2014.12.016
61. Goubau D, Schlee M, Deddouche S, Pruijssers AJ, Zillinger T, Goldeck M, et al. Antiviral immunity via RIG-I-mediated recognition of RNA bearing 5'-diphosphates. *Nature* (2014) 514:372–5. doi:10.1038/nature13590
62. Kato H, Takahasi K, Fujita T. RIG-I-like receptors: cytoplasmic sensors for non-self RNA. *Immunol Rev* (2011) 243:91–8. doi:10.1111/j.1600-065X.2011.01052.x
63. Lee S, Nguyen MT. Recent advances of vaccine adjuvants for infectious diseases. *Immune Netw* (2015) 15:51–7. doi:10.4110/in.2015.15.2.51
64. Dupuis M, Murphy TJ, Higgins D, Ugozzoli M, van Nest G, Ott G, et al. Dendritic cells internalize vaccine adjuvant after intramuscular injection. *Cell Immunol* (1998) 186:18–27. doi:10.1006/cimm.1998.1283
65. Morefield GL, Sokolovska A, Jiang D, HogenEsch H, Robinson JP, Hem SL. Role of aluminum-containing adjuvants in antigen internalization by dendritic cells in vitro. *Vaccine* (2005) 23:1588–95. doi:10.1016/j.vaccine.2004.07.050
66. Mosca F, Tritto E, Muzzi A, Monaci E, Bagnoli F, Iavarone C, et al. Molecular and cellular signatures of human vaccine adjuvants. *Proc Natl Acad Sci U S A* (2008) 105:10501–6. doi:10.1073/pnas.0804699105
67. Clements CJ, Griffiths E. The global impact of vaccines containing aluminium adjuvants. *Vaccine* (2002) 20(Suppl 3):S24–33. doi:10.1016/S0264-410X(02)00168-8
68. Trollfors B, Bergfors E, Inerot A. Vaccine related itching nodules and hypersensitivity to aluminium. *Vaccine* (2005) 23:975–6. doi:10.1016/j.vaccine.2004.08.024
69. Probst P, Grigg JB, Wang M, Munoz E, Loo YM, Ireton RC, et al. A small-molecule IRF3 agonist functions as an influenza vaccine adjuvant by modulating the antiviral immune response. *Vaccine* (2017) 35:1964–71. doi:10.1016/j.vaccine.2017.01.053
70. Beljanski V, Chiang C, Kirchenbaum GA, Olagnier D, Bloom CE, Wong T, et al. Enhanced influenza virus-like particle vaccination with a structurally optimized RIG-I agonist as adjuvant. *J Virol* (2015) 89:10612–24. doi:10.1128/JVI.01526-15
71. Martinez-Gil L, Goff PH, Hai R, Garcia-Sastre A, Shaw ML, Palese P. A Sendai virus-derived RNA agonist of RIG-I as a virus vaccine adjuvant. *J Virol* (2013) 87:1290–300. doi:10.1128/JVI.02338-12
72. Moschos SA, Frick M, Taylor B, Turnpenny P, Graves H, Spink KG, et al. Uptake, efficacy, and systemic distribution of naked, inhaled short interfering RNA (siRNA) and locked nucleic acid (LNA) antisense. *Mol Ther* (2011) 19:2163–8. doi:10.1038/mt.2011.206
73. Deering RP, Kommareddy S, Ulmer JB, Brito LA, Geall AJ. Nucleic acid vaccines: prospects for non-viral delivery of mRNA vaccines. *Expert Opin Drug Deliv* (2014) 11:885–99. doi:10.1517/17425247.2014.901308
74. Xue HY, Guo P, Wen WC, Wong HL. Lipid-based nanocarriers for RNA delivery. *Curr Pharm Des* (2015) 21:3140–7. doi:10.2174/1381612821666150531164540
75. Simoes S, Filipe A, Faneca H, Mano M, Penacho N, Duzgunes N, et al. Cationic liposomes for gene delivery. *Expert Opin Drug Deliv* (2005) 2:237–54. doi:10.1517/17425247.2.2.237
76. Miele E, Spinelli GP, Miele E, Di Fabrizio E, Ferretti E, Tomao S, et al. Nanoparticle-based delivery of small interfering RNA: challenges for cancer therapy. *Int J Nanomedicine* (2012) 7:3637–57. doi:10.2147/IJN.S23696
77. Chan JM, Zhang L, Tong R, Ghosh D, Gao W, Liao G, et al. Spatiotemporal controlled delivery of nanoparticles to injured vasculature. *Proc Natl Acad Sci U S A* (2010) 107:2213–8. doi:10.1073/pnas.0914585107
78. Tasciotti E, Liu XW, Bhavane R, Plant K, Leonard AD, Price BK, et al. Mesoporous silicon particles as a multistage delivery system for imaging and therapeutic applications. *Nat Nanotechnol* (2008) 3:151–7. doi:10.1038/nnano.2008.34
79. Hotz C, Roetzer LC, Huber T, Sailer A, Oberson A, Treinies M, et al. TLR and RLR signaling are reprogrammed in opposite directions after detection of viral infection. *J Immunol* (2015) 195:4387–95. doi:10.4049/jimmunol.1500079
80. Prater MR, Johnson VJ, Germolec DR, Luster MI, Holladay SD. Maternal treatment with a high dose of CpG ODN during gestation alters fetal craniofacial and distal limb development in C57BL/6 mice. *Vaccine* (2006) 24:263–71. doi:10.1016/j.vaccine.2005.07.105
81. Pothlichet J, Burtey A, Kubarenko AV, Caignard G, Solhonne B, Tangy F, et al. Study of human RIG-I polymorphisms identifies two variants with an opposite impact on the antiviral immune response. *PLoS One* (2009) 4:e7582. doi:10.1371/journal.pone.0007582
82. Hu J, Nistal-Villan E, Voho A, Ganee A, Kumar M, Ding Y, et al. A common polymorphism in the caspase recruitment domain of RIG-I modifies the innate immune response of human dendritic cells. *J Immunol* (2010) 185:424–32. doi:10.4049/jimmunol.0903291
83. Ovsyannikova IG, Haralambieva IH, Dhiman N, O'Byrne MM, Pankratz VS, Jacobson RM, et al. Polymorphisms in the vitamin A receptor and innate immunity genes influence the antibody response to rubella vaccination. *J Infect Dis* (2010) 201:207–13. doi:10.1086/649588
84. Pang L, Gong X, Liu N, Xie G, Gao W, Kong G, et al. A polymorphism in melanoma differentiation-associated gene 5 may be a risk factor for enterovirus 71 infection. *Clin Microbiol Infect* (2014) 20:O711–7. doi:10.1111/1469-0691.12618
85. Haralambieva IH, Ovsyannikova IG, Umlauf BJ, Vierkant RA, Shane Pankratz V, Jacobson RM, et al. Genetic polymorphisms in host antiviral genes: associations with humoral and cellular immunity to measles vaccine. *Vaccine* (2011) 29:8988–97. doi:10.1016/j.vaccine.2011.09.043
86. Li YP, Li M, Jia XL, Deng HL, Wang WJ, Wu FP, et al. Association of gene polymorphisms of pattern-recognition receptor signaling pathway with the risk and severity of hand, foot, and mouth disease caused by enterovirus 71 in Chinese Han population. *J Med Virol* (2018) 90:692–8. doi:10.1002/jmv.25000
87. Kaufmann SHE, Dorhoi A, Hotchkiss RS, Bartenschlager R. Host-directed therapies for bacterial and viral infections. *Nat Rev Drug Discov* (2018) 17:35–56. doi:10.1038/nrd.2017.162

7

Advances in Designing and Developing Vaccines, Drugs and Therapies to Counter Ebola Virus

Kuldeep Dhama[1], Kumaragurubaran Karthik[2], Rekha Khandia[3], Sandip Chakraborty[4], Ashok Munjal[3], Shyma K. Latheef[5], Deepak Kumar[6], Muthannan Andavar Ramakrishnan[7], Yashpal Singh Malik[8]*, Rajendra Singh[1], Satya Veer Singh Malik[9], Raj Kumar Singh[10] and Wanpen Chaicumpa[11]*

[1] Division of Pathology, ICAR-Indian Veterinary Research Institute, Bareilly, India, [2] Central University Laboratory, Tamil Nadu Veterinary and Animal Sciences University, Chennai, India, [3] Department of Biochemistry and Genetics, Barkatullah University, Bhopal, India, [4] Department of Veterinary Microbiology, College of Veterinary Sciences and Animal Husbandry, Agartala, India, [5] Immunology Section, ICAR-Indian Veterinary Research Institute, Bareilly, India, [6] Division of Veterinary Biotechnology, ICAR-Indian Veterinary Research Institute, Bareilly, India, [7] Division of Virology, ICAR-Indian Veterinary Research Institute, Nainital, Uttarakhand, India, [8] Division of Biological Standardization, ICAR-Indian Veterinary Research Institute, Bareilly, India, [9] Division of Veterinary Public Health, ICAR-Indian Veterinary Research Institute, Bareilly, India, [10] ICAR-Indian Veterinary Research Institute, Bareilly, Uttar Pradesh, India, [11] Center of Research Excellence on Therapeutic Proteins and Antibody Engineering, Department of Parasitology, Faculty of Medicine Slriraj Hospital, Mahidol University, Bangkok, Thailand

***Correspondence:**
Kuldeep Dhama
kdhama@rediffmail.com;
Yashpal Singh Malik
malikyps@gmail.com

Ebola virus (EBOV), a member of the family *Filoviridae*, is responsible for causing Ebola virus disease (EVD) (formerly named Ebola hemorrhagic fever). This is a severe, often fatal illness with mortality rates varying from 50 to 90% in humans. Although the virus and associated disease has been recognized since 1976, it was only when the recent outbreak of EBOV in 2014–2016 highlighted the danger and global impact of this virus, necessitating the need for coming up with the effective vaccines and drugs to counter its pandemic threat. Albeit no commercial vaccine is available so far against EBOV, a few vaccine candidates are under evaluation and clinical trials to assess their prophylactic efficacy. These include recombinant viral vector (recombinant vesicular stomatitis virus vector, chimpanzee adenovirus type 3-vector, and modified vaccinia Ankara virus), Ebola virus-like particles, virus-like replicon particles, DNA, and plant-based vaccines. Due to improvement in the field of genomics and proteomics, epitope-targeted vaccines have gained top priority. Correspondingly, several therapies have also been developed, including immunoglobulins against specific viral structures small cell-penetrating antibody fragments that target intracellular EBOV proteins. Small interfering RNAs and oligomer-mediated inhibition have also been verified for EVD treatment. Other treatment options include viral entry inhibitors, transfusion of convalescent blood/serum, neutralizing antibodies, and gene expression inhibitors. Repurposed drugs, which have proven safety profiles, can be adapted after high-throughput screening for efficacy and potency for EVD treatment. Herbal and other natural products are also being explored for EVD treatment. Further studies to better understand the pathogenesis and antigenic structures of the virus can help in developing an effective vaccine and identifying appropriate antiviral targets. This review presents the recent advances in designing and developing vaccines, drugs, and therapies to counter the EBOV threat.

Keywords: Ebola virus, Ebola virus disease, vaccines, prophylactics, drugs, therapeutics, treatment

INTRODUCTION

Ebola virus (EBOV; *Zaire ebolavirus*) is the causative agent of a severe hemorrhagic fever disease, Ebola virus disease (EVD; formerly called Ebola hemorrhagic fever). It was first recognized in 1976 in northern Democratic Republic of Congo, at that time Zaire (1–3). Since then, EVD is endemic in Africa. Fruit bats are the best-known reservoirs of EBOV (4). EVD is a well-established zoonotic disease; the initial cases of the EVD outbreaks occur after contact with reservoir or materials contaminated with the virus and followed by human-to-human transmission (5). EBOV is not only a serious public health issue but now also designated as category A pathogen and considered as a potential bioterrorism agent (6, 7). EBOV causes high mortality rates of up to 88% in the infected humans (8); therefore, it is classified as a risk group 4 agent and handled under biosafety level-4 containment. The risk of mortality is relatively greater in the elderly and/or patients with high viral load and poor immune response at the initial stage of the infection (9).

The EBOV belongs to the *Filoviridae* family and has a unique thin filamentous structure that is 80-nm wide and up to 14-µm long. Its envelope is decorated with spikes of trimeric glycoprotein (GP1,2) which are responsible for mediating viral entry into target cells (function of GP1) (10) and release of viral ribonucleoprotein from endosome to cytoplasm for replication (function of GP2) (11, 12). EBOV infects primarily humans, simians, and bats; but other species such as mice, shrew, and duikers may also contact infection (3, 13). Of the five identified EBOV species, four species, *viz.*, EBOV, Sudan virus (SUDV; *Sudan ebolavirus*), Tai Forest virus (TAFV; *Tai Forest ebolavirus*, formerly *Côte d'Ivoire ebolavirus*), and Bundibugyo virus (BDBV; *Bundibugyo ebolavirus*), are known to infect humans and cause disease, whereas Reston virus (RESTV; *Reston ebolavirus)* is non-human primate (NHP) pathogen.

After an initial incubation period of 3–21 days, the disease progresses quickly to fever, intense fatigue, diarrhea, anorexia, abdominal pain, hiccups, myalgia, vomiting, confusion, and conjunctivitis (14) which may lead to the loss of vision (15). EBOV can spread from males to females through semen (16) and from mother to fetus and infant during gestation and lactation, respectively (17). Of the note, in an EBOV-infected patient, higher concentration of Ebola viral RNA in semen was noticed during the recovery period than the viral concentration in the blood during peak time of infection, suggesting male genital organ as virus predilection site for replication (18). Usually the human immune system mounts a response against infectious pathogens by sensing the pathogen-associated molecular patterns *via* a variety of pathogen-recognition receptors. Nevertheless, in the case of EBOV, innate immunity is impaired by the immunosuppressive viral proteins including VP35 and VP24, and lymphocytes are depleted as a result of apoptosis caused by inappropriate dendritic cell (DC)–T-cell interaction (7, 19). A thorough understanding on the pathogenesis of this deadly virus is essential because of its severe health impacts (20).

The increased incidences and fast spread of EBOV paving into a pandemic flight has compelled more focus of research to develop strategies and remedial measures for mitigating the impact and consequential severity of the viral infection. Even before delineating the less studied Ebola viral genome fully, researchers throughout the globe and health industry were pressured to focus on the development of effective and safe Ebola vaccines and therapeutics (21, 22). As of now, no licensed vaccines and direct-acting anti-EBOV agents are available to protect against the lethal viral infection or to treat the disease. To minimize the suffering, EBOV-infected patients are only provided with symptomatic treatment and supportive care. Because of its high pathogenicity and mortality rate, preventive measures, prophylactics, and therapeutics are essential, and researchers worldwide are working to develop effective vaccines, drug, and therapeutics, including passive immunization and antibody-based treatments for EVD (23–26). Prior to the 2014–2016 EBOV outbreak in West Africa, which has been the deadliest EBOV outbreak to date, convalescent blood products from survivors of EVD represented the only recommended treatment option for newly infected persons. Administration of monoclonal antibody (mAb) cocktails (ZMapp, ZMAb, and MB-003) as post-exposure prophylactics have been found to reverse the advanced EVD in NHPs and/or effectively prevented morbidity and mortality in NHPs (27–30).

There is the need for an effective vaccine against EBOV, especially in high-risk areas, to prevent infections in physicians, nurses, and other health-care workers who come into contact with diseased patients (31). Regular monitoring and surveillance of EBOV is essential to control this disease. In the EBOV outbreak, novel surveillance approaches include contact tracing with coordination at the national level and "lockdown" periods, during which household door-to-door reviews are conducted to limit the spread of the virus. Swift identification and confirmation of the Ebola cases and immediate follow-up of appropriate prevention and control measures, including safe burial of dead persons, are crucial practices to counter EBOV (32).

After the onset of EVD, treatment is required, whereas, when EBOV is circulating in population dense areas before infection, prophylactic measures like vaccination are necessary. One of the main challenges in containing EBOV is its presence in remote areas that lack technology and equipment to limit the virus spread. Because of its lethality, EBOV can only be handled in laboratories with biosecurity level-4 containment; thus, only few laboratories in the world can conduct EBOV research and testing of the counter measures against the authentic virus. Recent efforts by several organizations have focused on identifying effective therapies and developing appropriate vaccination strategies (33). Several drugs and vaccines have been developed against EBOV, and the production of low-cost drugs and vaccines against EBOV is essential for everyone, including those in the high-risk areas of the world, to be protected (26, 34). As of the acquisition of better knowledge against the pathogen due to improvement in the field of genomics and proteomics, there has been expansion in the field of vaccine synthesis where epitope-based vaccines are gaining top priority (35–37).

The present review aims to discuss advances in designing and development of EBOV vaccines, drugs, antibody-based treatments, and therapeutics, and their clinical efficacy in limiting EVD, thereby providing protection against the disease and alleviating high public health concerns associated with EBOV.

ADVANCES IN DEVELOPING VACCINES AGAINST EBOV

There is a clear need for an effective vaccine to prevent the rapid spread of EVD. An inactivated EBOV vaccine was first produced in 1980. This vaccine was tested for efficacy in guinea pigs (7). Since that time, several vaccines against EBOV have been developed, but no vaccine is licensed and available in the market (7). After the massive 2014–2016 outbreak of EBOV, several researchers have begun working to develop an effective vaccine (38). For an EBOV vaccine candidate, a long-lasting immune response is essential; as EBOV remains in the seminal fluid of EVD survivors as long as 401 days post-infection (39, 40). Keeping this window of virus persistence, a vaccine conferring immunity at least for 2 years is recommended by the Wellcome Trust-CIDRAP Ebola Vaccine Team B initiative (41). Vaccines like the chimpanzee adenovirus type 3 (ChAd3)-based non-replicating ChAd3-EBO vaccine, prime-boost recombinant adenovirus type 26 vector (Ad26.ZEBOV) followed by the modified vaccinia Ankara vector (MVA-BN-Filoa) vaccine, adenovirus 5-vectored EBOV vaccine, EBOV DNA vaccine, and recombinant vesicular stomatitis virus (rVSV) vector-based vaccine are undergoing clinical trials to evaluate their efficacy against EVD (38). The RNA-dependent RNA polymerase (L) epitope-based vaccine was designed using immunoinformatics. Various software have been used to analyze immunological parameters, and this epitope vaccine was found to be a good candidate for use against EVD (42). Two conserved peptides of EBOV, 79VPSATKRWGFRSGVPP94 from GP1 and 515LHYWTTQDEGAAIGLA530 from GP2, were identified as targets for the development of an epitope-based vaccine (43). Collection of the sequences of EBOV glycoproteins and examination for determining the proteins with greatest immunogenicity have been performed using *in silico* methods. The best corresponding B and T cell epitopes included peptide regions encompassing residues 186–220 and 154HKEGAFFLY162, respectively. Such predicted epitopes can confer the long-lasting immunity against EBOV with better ability of protection (36).

Ebola virus-GP fused with the Fc fragment of a human IgG1 subunit vaccine administrated with alum, QS-21, or polyinosinic-polycytidylic acid-poly-L-lysine carboxymethylcellulose adjuvant induced strong humoral immunity in guinea pigs (44). Effectiveness of a ring vaccine using rVSVΔG/EBOVGP in cases of simulated EBOV disease was studied and even this approach can be employed during an outbreak situation (45). Notably, the neutralizing antibodies play a major role in conferring protection against EBOV infections. Thus, an EBOV vaccine capable of effectively inducing a long-lasting neutralizing antibody response is desirable for developing appropriate prevention strategies in combating the infection. In this line, the mucin-like domain of EBOV envelope glycoprotein GP1 has been identified to be critical in induction of protective humoral immune response (46, 47). Filorab 1 vaccine revealed desirable immunogenicity without the side effects. The main advantage of this vaccine is its higher immune response induction in chimpanzees (captive) when given orally and also with a single dose [instead of multiple doses as is required by virus-like particle (VLP) vaccine] (48). Modified mRNA-based vaccine constructs, formulated with lipid nanoparticles (LNPs) to facilitate delivery, are being tested against EBOV challenge in guinea pigs. These mRNAs induced robust immune responses and conferred up to 100% protection from the infection (49).

It is important to note that compilation of data in relation to immune responses (both induced by vaccines and natural infection) and the records of community members showing IgG seropositivity should be kept systematically. Assimilation of such information will help to handle next outbreaks with more rigidity, thereby helping to check EVD-associated disasters at an early stage (50). *Vis-à-vis* public health workers should also be vaccinated and mass vaccination programs should be undertaken through standardized and coordinated efforts (51).

The following section describes the various types of vaccines and vaccine platforms which are being explored for the development of a successful EBOV vaccine.

Inactivated Vaccines

Even though inactivated vaccines suffer with the problem of reversion to virulence due to inadequate viral inactivation, various strategies have been constantly explored in developing safe and potent non-replicating vaccine candidates for combating the EBOV infection (52). Both heat- and formalin-inactivated EBOV have been found protective against EBOV infection in a guinea pig model. Inclusion of inactivated vaccine with EBOV E-178 along with interferon (IFN) and immune plasma saved the life of a scientist working on EBOV (53). The protective efficacy of liposome-encapsulated irradiated EBOV, tested in a mouse model, was 100%. However, these viral particles failed to protect NHPs (54). This suggests that murine model is excellent for evaluating vaccine efficacy, but the level of protection might be different in different species and, hence, it is essential to test vaccines in NHPs before proceeding to clinical trials in humans. Heat-, formalin-, or gamma irradiation-killed EBOV vaccines have been found ineffective against EBOV disease; thus, the novel effective vaccine is essentially required (55).

DNA Vaccines

In DNA vaccines, plasmids are used to express immunogenic antigens. This is an attractive vaccine approach because of the ease of production and simplicity. In addition, DNA vaccine induces both humoral and cellular immune responses. A three-plasmid DNA vaccine comprising the transmembrane-deleted GP sequences from EBOV species Zaire and SUDV-Gulu as well as nucleoprotein (NP) sequence from EBOV was tested in healthy adults. The vaccine was well tolerated, and both $CD4^+$ and $CD8^+$ T cell responses were elicited (56). An EBOV GP DNA vaccine designed on a consensus alignment of GPs (from strains obtained during 1976–2014), delivered intramuscularly and then electroporated, elicited a strong T cell response, and protected 100% of experimental mice from lethal challenge with EBOV (57). The DNA from three strains of EBOV was used to prime human volunteers and boosted with attenuated adenovirus, which acted as delivery vehicle for EBOV DNA into antigen-presenting cells, induced significant humoral- and cell-mediated immune (CMI) responses (58). Intramuscular inoculation of the DNA vaccine through electroporation with DNA plasmid containing codon-optimized GP genes of EBOV elicited high levels of IgG and a strong CMI response (measured by IFN-γ ELISpot assay) in cynomolgus macaques (59).

Though the preliminary trials using DNA constructs have provided the acceptable safety profiles, the development of low immune titer for a shorter window necessitates repeated vaccinations to overcome this problem. Thus, the use of a potent vaccination regimen based on DNA vaccine platforms does not appear logical for a large population (60, 61).

Virus-Like Particles

Ebola VLPs (EBOV-VLPs or eVLPs) are generated from the expression of viral transmembrane glycoprotein (GP) and structural matrix protein (VP40) in mammalian cells, which undergo self-assembling and budding from host cells and display morphological similarity to infectious EBOV particles (47). Baculovirus-derived eVLPs comprising GP, VP40, and NP of EBOV have been found to induce human myeloid DC maturation, suggesting their immunogenicity. Baculovirus-generated VLPs were able to elicit similar levels of protection as 293T cell-derived VLPs and showed protection against virus challenge in a dose-dependent manner (62). Nano-VLPs, produced by sonication of VLPs and filtering to have a mean diameter of approximately 230 nm, increased their thermostability. Unlike native VLPs where GP protein is denatured in a solution by heating, the nano-VLP maintained the conformational integrity of the GP protein at temperature up to 70°C and could confer protection in a mouse model (63). VLP containing only VP40 was sufficient to protect mice from EBOV infection. VLP injection leads to an enhanced number of natural killer (NK) cells, which play a crucial role in innate immune protection against lethal EBOV. NK cell protection is dependent on perforin, but not recombinant viral vector vaccines on IFN-gamma secretion (64).

Ebola virus VP40 and GP have been demonstrated to interact with the host protein, BST2, and are associated with viral infections by trapping the newly assembled enveloped virions at the plasma membrane in the infected cells, ultimately induce NF-κB activity. The effects of EBOV GP1,2, VP40, and BST2 converge on an intracellular signaling pathway leads to neddylation, resulting in the additive response with respect to the induction of NF-κB activity. Exploring the dynamics of this interaction could provide targets for vaccine developments and therapies that can modulate the inflammatory response during EVD (65).

Quantitation of EBOV antigenic particles using proteomic assays like liquid chromatography high resolution mass spectrometry method can be employed for determining the batch quality of vaccine constructs as well as in optimizing the dosages by assessing the amount of GP1 needed to confer effective protection (47).

It is to be noted that though anti-EBOV antibody can mediate effective protection, VLP-vaccinated murine models were shown to survive the EBOV challenge in the absence of detectable serum anti-EBOV antibodies (66). It could also be revealed that adjuvant signaling may circumvent the necessity for B-cell immunity in conferring protection against EBOV. These studies can be valuable for the future characterization, development, and optimization of effective EBOV vaccine candidates (66).

Virus-Like Replicon Particles (VRPs)

The VRPs are the alternative to live-attenuated vaccines. The use of VRPs eliminates the risk of reversion to the original pathogenic form of live vaccine strains. To generate VRPs, generally filoviruses or alphaviruses are required. Here, while keeping the genes essential for replication, viral structural genes are deleted from full-length genomic cDNA clones. Viral structural genes are replaced with alternative gene(s) coding for an immunogen. Such replicons are able to replicate and transcribe upon transfection in competent cells. The resulting VRPs are able to infect cells only for one cycle. Because of the lack of structural genes, viral progeny are not formed. Viruses such as Venezuelan equine encephalitis virus (VEEV) can be used for production of EBOV antigen instead of structural proteins for the replicon vector. Thus, such vaccines are also quite safe (67). The gene inserted is typically GP, the main target of neutralizing antibodies. VRPs expressing EBOV VP24, VP30, VP35, and VP40 have been evaluated for their protective efficacy in a mouse model, but these were found not to be as protective as EBOV GP and NP antigens. VEEV replicons containing GPs from both EBOV and SUDV showed promising results in cynomolgus macaques after administration of a single dose. Here, two VRPs were constructed that contained the GP of EBOV or SUDV. The animals intramuscularly injected with both of the VRPs, survived viral challenge without exhibiting any clinical signs. The final results indicated that VRP-EBOV GP was able to confer cross-protection against SUDV, whereas VRP-SUDV GP was unable to provide complete protection against EBOV-Zaire challenge (68).

Recently, Ren et al. (69) constructed an alphavirus Semliki forest virus based recombinant replicon vector DREP for efficient and unchecked *ex vivo* co-expression of EBOV GP and VP40. Active immunization with recombinant DREP vectors possessing GP and VP40 induced cellular and humoral immune responses in murine model against EBOV antigens. This path breaking approach may provide key insights and strategies for designing further effective vaccines to contain EBOV permanently.

Reverse Genetics System for EBOV Vaccine

A full-length recombinant EBOV infectious clone was constructed using cDNA. By employing reverse genetics method, viable but replication incompetent virus lacking entire VP30 ORF was constructed. The resultant EbolaΔVP30 is biologically contained and replication deficient, until VP30 is provided extraneously. Virus replication in cell culture was allowed by growing the virus in Vero cell line that stably expresses VP30, designated VeroVP30 (70). The safety of EbolaΔVP30 has been evaluated in mice and guinea pig model and was able to protect from lethal infection (71). The EbolaΔVP30 virus inactivated by using hydrogen peroxide protected NHPs after a single immunization. To avoid any incidence of potential recombination events that might result in regaining the replicative efficiency, the vaccine candidate was inactivated by hydrogen peroxide, that creates nicks and breakages in single- or double-stranded DNA or RNA and the virus is completely inactivated while retaining antigenic determinants unaffected (72).

Recombinant Viral Vector Vaccines

Engineered viruses are gaining popularity because of their ability to efficiently induce CMI responses (a major part of adaptive immunity along with humoral response), as the antigen is expressed and processed in the cytoplasm. Replication-competent rVSV and chimpanzee adenovirus 3 (ChAd-3/cAd3) are the most efficient platforms for designing new vaccines (73). A recombinant vesiculovirus vector containing EBOV GP region (rVSVΔG/EBOVGP) was found to be highly effective after a single injection in NHPs (74, 75). The vaccine evaluated in pigs showed no disease development and no viral shedding. This indicated that the vaccine could be utilized for herd immunization and it also suggested the safety of the live-attenuated rVSVΔG/EBOVGP vaccine (76). Recently, this rVSVΔG/EBOVGP vaccine was evaluated in a randomized double blinded placebo phase III trial in 1,197 humans. There were no adverse effects or death following vaccination, supporting its use as a vaccine (77). The vaccine protected immunocompromised rhesus macaques that had a high number of $CD4^+$ T cells (78). The rVSVΔG/EBOVGP vaccine was also studied for its efficacy as a therapy in rhesus monkeys after exposure to EBOV-Makona. This vaccine showed minimal prophylactic efficacy after exposure (79). Efficacy trials initiated to test the rVSV-vectored EBOV vaccine showed greater efficiency at the time of EVD outbreak, if deployed following the strategy of ring vaccination (80).

Another recombinant vaccine (VSV based), i.e., rVSV-Zaire EBOV has been shown to provide substantial protection. From 10th day of vaccination with this vaccine, no report of any disease was documented, which proved efficacy and effectiveness of rVSV-vectored vaccine in preventing EVD (81). It is interesting to note that seroconversion has been noticed in recipients of recombinant VSV-EBOV (rVSV-EBOV) vaccine by the end of fourth week (i.e., by 28 days) against the Kikwit strain glycoprotein (82). Another recombinant vaccine *viz.*, rVSV-EBOV vaccine was tested as a candidate vaccine. This particular vaccine is under trial in human (phase II/III). It provides protection against only EBOV and is clinically efficient in the clinical set up of ring vaccination format (38, 83, 84). EBOV and SUDV glycoproteins have been assimilated into a cAdVax vector (adenovirus-based vaccine). In mice, this vaccine has provided full protection (85, 86). During recent outbreak in Democratic Republic of the Congo (DRC), rVSVΔG-EBOV-GP is being used for ring vaccination in the affected area. Though the vaccine is yet not approved and still under investigation.

In Russia, clinical trial of a vaccine, GamEvac-Combi, has been performed and has been approved to enter in phase III clinical trial (87). The vaccine GamEvac-Combi contained two heterologous expression systems. One is live-attenuated rVSV and the second is a recombinant replication-defective adenovirus type-5 (Ad5). Both the vectors are expressing the same glycoprotein. The rationale to use a combination of two vectors expressing glycoprotein of EBOV is that widely present preexisting immunity to Ad5 limits the use of Ad5 and also a negative correlation between EBOV glycoprotein-specific immune response and preexisting antibodies to Ad5 has been reported (88). Hence, prime immunization with VSV vectored vaccine and then boosting with AD5 vectored vaccine might contribute in compensating negative impacts of preexisting immune response to Ad5. This heterologous vaccine evoked glycoprotein-specific immune response in 100% volunteers on day 28th. Also, the vaccine is well tolerated and did not significantly altered the body physiological parameters and vital organs. In Liberia, Sierra Leone, and Guinea; the VSV and ChAd3 vectored vaccine are in focus (89).

Another study in mice models has reported that the adoption of a heterologous prime-boost vaccine strategy can result in a durable EBOV-neutralizing antibody response. The chimpanzee serotype 7 adenovirus vectors expressing EBOV GP (AdC7-GP) was used for priming and a truncated version of EBOV GP1 protein (GP1t) was used for boosting. Vaccination response studies showed that AdC7-GP prime/GP1t boost strategy was more potent in generating a sustained and strong immune response as compared to using an individual vaccine construct (90).

Replication-defective recombinant chimpanzee adenovirus type 3-vectored EBOV vaccine (cAd3-EBO) elicited both cell-mediated and humoral immunity in NHPs. A vaccine dose of 2×10^{11} particle units was found sufficient to induce protective immunity in the NHPs and to eliminate the effect of prior immunity to cAd3 (91). Recombinant VSV vaccine expressing EBOV GP and A/Hanoi/30408/2005 H5N1 hemagglutinin (VSVΔG-HA-ZGP) protected mice against challenge with both viruses and also cross-protected against H5N1 viruses (92).

The utility of adenovirus-vectored EBOV vaccines is limited with preexisting anti-adenoviral antibodies, which significantly lower the GP-specific humoral and T cell responses (88). Six mutations in the genome of MVA virus restrict its host specificity and make it unable to replicate in mammalian cells. A randomized study of a multivalent MVA vaccine encoding GPs from EBOV, SUDV, Marburg virus (MARV), and TAFV NP (MVA-BN-Filo) conducted in 87 participants resulted in no fever. The quadrivalent vaccine formulation has demonstrated the boosting up of both cellular and humoral immune responses against EBOV to several folds (93). Twenty-eight days after immunization, GP-specific IgG was detected with EBOV-specific T cell responses (94). EBOV GP and TAFV NP expressed in an MVA platform assembles into VLPs. Heterologous NPs enhanced VLP formation and offered GP-specific IgG1/IgG2a ratios comparable to those of MVA-BN-Filo (95).

Recombinant cytomegalovirus expressing EBOV GP was found to evoke protective immunity in rhesus monkeys challenged with EBOV (79). Baculovirus-expressed EBOV-Makona strain GP administered with Matrix-M (saponin adjuvant) showed better immunogenicity. Administration of Matrix M-adjuvanted vaccine resulted in increased IgG production and $CD4^+$ and $CD8^+$ T cell production (96). A human parainfluenza virus type 3-vectored vaccine expressing the GP of EBOV (HPIV3/EboGP) was developed as an aerosolized vaccine, and studies in Rhesus macaques showed 100% protection against challenge with EBOV (97).

Adenovirus 26 vectored glycoprotein/MVA-BN vaccine has recently passed the phase I trial (94). In the European countries including United Kingdom and United States, for the purpose of clinical trial, administration of ChAd-3 vectored vaccine has been adopted. This vaccine expresses the EBOV GP and is available in monovalent and divalent forms (91, 98).

Ebola vaccine potency trials employing replication defective adenoviral vectors (rAd) encoding EBOV GP have come up with promising results in NHP models. Based on such studies, multiple mutant glycoproteins were developed (such as glycoprotein with deleted transmembrane domain) which offers reduced *in vitro* cytopathogenicity but possessed reduced vaccine-mediated protection. In contrast to this, a point mutated glycoprotein has been reported to offer minimal cytopathogenicity and appropriate immune protection even with a two logs lower vaccine dose (99).

Plant-Based Vaccines and Antibodies

Viral antigens, including GP, VP40, and NP, elicit protective immune responses. ZMapp, the cocktail of antibodies being used to treat EBOV, is a biopharmaceutical drug. To note, the component antibodies in ZMapp are manufactured in *Nicotiana benthamiana* using a rapid antibody manufacturing platform. Gene transfer is mediated by a viral vector, and the expression is transient. *N. benthamiana*-derived antibodies produced stronger antibody-dependent cellular cytotoxicity than the analogous anti-EBOV mAbs produced in a mammalian Chinese hamster kidney cell line (100). Phoolcharoen (101) expressed a GP1 chimera with the heavy chain of 6D8 mAb, forming an immune complex that was co-expressed with the light chain of the same mAb in leaves of tobacco plant. The ammonium sulfate-precipitated purified antibodies, along with poly(I:C) adjuvant, a synthetic analog of double-stranded RNA capable of interacting with toll-like receptor (TLR)-3, was found to elicit strong neutralizing anti-EBOV IgG. In addition, the immune complex along with poly(I:C) adjuvant was capable of stimulating a Th1/Th2 response. The experiment suggested the potential application of plant-produced Ebola immune complexes as vaccine candidates. EBOV VP40 was expressed in tobacco plants, and a mouse immunization study showed results that suggested this approach can be used to produce an EBOV vaccine (102).

The utility of plants as bioreactors for the bulk production of ZMapp could be considered to meet the required demand. The glycosylation pattern of mAbs may alter their efficiency and bioactivity, including their binding with the antigenic epitope. Several glycoforms of EBOV mAb13F6 have been prepared using a magnICON expression system. These glycoforms have human-like biantennary N-glycans with terminal N-acetylglucosamine, resulting in a structure similar to that of human mAbs. Hence, these are beneficial for humans (103).

Both RNA and DNA viruses have been modified to serve as plant-based vectors for the expression of heterologous proteins. Bean yellow dwarf virus, a single stranded-DNA virus, can replicate inside the nucleus of plant cells using their cellular machinery. A vector containing deletions in the coat-encoding genes and gene for the desired antigen may be inserted to form an expression cassette. The delivery of vectors to plants is *Agrobacterium*-mediated (23). mAbs against EBOV are produced by the process of agroinfiltration. In this context, it is noteworthy that lettuce acts as a very good host for the process of agroinfiltration. In lettuce cells, *Agrobacterium tumefaciens* has been used for delivering viral vectors (104). Neutralizing and protective mAb6D8 against EBOV has been expressed at a concentration of 0.5 mg/g of leaf mass. This quantity is similar to that generated in magnICON expression system (105). The plant-derived approach to vaccine development is attractive because of the large amount of transient proteins that can be expressed, with the potential for use during high demand for therapeutics and prophylactics (106). Advances in the field of vector expression like plant transient expression system and associated host cell engineering and manufacturing processes paved way for developing biopharmaceutical proteins and therapeutics in commercial basis. The great potentials of such novel approaches have been exploited for evolving therapeutics to counter emerging pandemics of EBOV and influenza that is evidenced from the production of experimental ZMapp antibodies (107).

An overview of various types of vaccines for countering EVD is presented in **Table 1** and depicted in **Figure 1**.

ADVANCES IN DEVELOPING DRUGS AND THERAPIES AGAINST EBOV

Momentous leap has been witnessed toward the designing of efficacious EBOV drugs and therapeutics during the short span of only few years, even though the efficacy of several biologicals and vaccines were evaluated during the recent West African outbreak, it remained elusive to ratify a licensed EBOV disease treatment regimen (123).

Management of suspected or confirmed EVD patients includes quarantine, symptomatic, and supportive treatments, including fluid replacement, electrolyte imbalance correction, treating complicated infections, and preventing shock (124). For mitigation of the huge fluid loss and resultant hypovolemia, oral rehydration solutions should be provided adequately and if required anti-diarrheal and anti-emetic drugs need to be administered (125). Brincidofovir, a drug used to treat dsDNA viruses such as adenovirus, herpesviruses, orthopoxviruses, papillomavirus, and polyomaviruses, was approved for emergency treatment of two patients with EBOV infection; however, the clinical efficacy of the drug is unknown (126). Many drugs are being tested to identify specific antiviral drugs to treat EBOV, and new drug candidates are being developed by researchers worldwide (26, 127, 128).

Favipiravir (T-705), an antiviral drug found useful in treating influenza, has been studied and found effective against EBOV (129–131). Insertional mutagenesis, a high-throughput method to identify genes responsible for virus replication, can be used to develop drug candidates (132). Molecular docking experiments with EBOV GPs can be used for drug designing and the development of therapeutics (133, 134). Novel flexible nucleosides called fleximers were found to be effective against recombinant EBOV in Huh7 cells (135). Ribavirin antiviral can be recommended for the treatment of EBOV, since in mouse and monkey models, treatment with ribavirin delayed the death and increased survival rate (136). However, adverse effects associated with its use may limit ribavirin use (137). Lamivudine, an anti-retroviral drug, has been tested by Liberian doctor on 15 EBOV patients with survival of 13 patients (138). However, study by Cong et al. (139) found no survival benefits in Guinea pig model. Similar results were obtained by Hensley et al. (140), with no significant antiviral

TABLE 1 | Vaccines for treating Ebola virus disease.

S. No.	Type of vaccine platform	Vaccine	Adjuvant/mode of delivery	Model	Antigen	Inference	Reference
1	Inactivated vaccine	Rabies virus based on inactivated vaccine (FILORAB1)	Glucopyranosyl lipid A	Cyanomolgus and rhesus monkeys	GP	100% protection against lethal Ebola virus (EBOV) challenge, with no to mild clinical signs of disease	Johnson et al. (108)
		Virulent EBOV	Formalin inactivation/heat inactivation	Guinea pig	Complete virus as antigen	Reduction in mortality	Lupton et al. (53)
2	Attenuated vaccine	Live replication-competent EBOV and rabies virus-based bivalent vaccine	Direct inoculation of live-attenuated vaccine	Rhesus macaques	GP	100% protection from lethal challenge	Blaney et al. (109)
3	DNA vaccine	Multiagent filovirus DNA vaccine containing GP of Zaire, Sudan, and Marburg virus (MARV)	Electrical stimulation at an amplitude of 250 V/cm using TriGrid™ electroporation device	BALB/c mice	GP	100% protection from lethal challenge	Grant-Klein et al. (110)
					Mutant GP		
		Synthetic polyvalent-filovirus DNA vaccine against Zaire, Sudan, and MARV	pVAX1 mammalian expression vectors, injected intradermally with 200 µg DNA	Guinea pigs	Codon-optimized GP	100% protection from lethal challenge	Shedlock et al. (111)
		DNA vaccine against EBOV	Intramuscular electroporation (IM-EP) 500 µg dose	Rhesus macaques	Codon-optimized GP	86% protection	Grant-Klein et al. (59)
		DNA encoding Zaire and Sudan glycoproteins	4 mg dose in 1 ml volume	Human healthy adults	Wild-type GP	Antibody response to the Ebola Zaire glycoprotein generated	Kibuuka et al. (60)
4	mRNA vaccine	mRNA molecule encapsulated in a lipid nanoparticle (LNP) formulation	0.2 mg/ml	Guinea pigs	A human Igκ signal peptide or the wild-type signal peptide sequence of GP attached to GP	Potency of mRNA vaccines is enhanced by LNP	Meyer et al. (49)
5	Ebola virus-like particles (VLPs)	pWRG7077 plasmid vectors encoding for Ebola VP40 and GP	10 µg of eVLPs	Balb/c mice	GP and matrix protein (VP40) in mammalian cells	Dose-dependent protection against lethal challenge	Warfield et al. (112)
		MARV GP and EBOV VP40 or vice-versa	Intramuscular vaccination with 100 µg of VLPs + 200 µl RIBI adjuvant	Strain 13 guinea pigs	GP and VP40	Homologous GP is essential and sufficient for protection against lethal challenge with homologous virus	Swenson et al. (113)
		pWRG7077 plasmid vectors encoding for GP, NP, and VP40	3 intramuscular injections of 250 µg of eVLPs + 0.5 ml of RIBI adjuvant	Cynomolgus macaques	GP, NP, and VP40	All animals were protected without showing signs of clinical illness	Warfield et al. (114)
		293T cells transfected with	VLP containing 10 µg GP	C57BL/6 mice	GP + VP40	VLP-mediated anti-EBOV immunity in B cell-deficient mice	Cooper et al. (66)
6	Vaccinia virus-based vaccine	Modified vaccinia virus Ankara-Bavarian Nordic® (MVA-BN) co-expressing VP40 and glycoprotein (GP) of EBOV Mayinga and NP of Taï Forest virus	Intramuscular or intravenous application of 10^8 $TCID_{50}$ of MVA-BN-EBOV-GP or MVA-BN-EBOV-VLP	CBA/J mice	GP + VP40	Production of non-infectious EBOV-VLPs	Schweneker et al. (95)
		Modified vaccinia Ankara (MVA)-based vaccine expressing the EBOV-Makona GP and VP40	1×10^8 $TCID_{50}$	Rhesus macaques	GP + VP40	100% protection with single or prime/boost vaccination	Domi et al. (115)

(*Continued*)

TABLE 1 | Continued

S. No.	Type of vaccine platform	Vaccine	Adjuvant/mode of delivery	Model	Antigen	Inference	Reference
7	Venezuelan equine encephalitis virus (VEEV)-based vaccine	VEEV-like replicon particles (VRP)	10^7 IU VRP	Strain 2 or strain 13 guinea pigs	NP or GP	NP-VRP and GP-VRP immunized animals completely protected against lethal challenge	Pushko et al. (116)
		VRP expressing SUDV GP + EBOV GP	10^{10} focus-forming units	Cynomolgus macaques	GP (EBOV + SUDV)	100% protection against intramuscular challenge with either SUDV or EBOV	Herbert et al. (68)
8	Cytomegalovirus (CMV)-based vaccines	$CD8^+$ T cell epitope from EBOV NP (VYQVNNLEEIC) cloned in mouse CMV vector	5×10^5 plaque forming units	C57BL/6 mice	NP	High levels of long-lasting (>8 months) $CD8^+$ T cells are produced	Tsuda et al. (117)
9	Kunjin virus-based vaccine	Kunjin virus VLPs expressing GP	5×10^6 VLPs	Dunkin–Hartley guinea pigs	GP	More than 75% survival of animals post challenge	Reynard et al. (118)
10	Paramyxovirus-based vaccines	Human parainfluenza virus type 3 (HPIV3) clone containing GP	10^7 plaque-forming units	Rhesus monkeys	GP	Double immunization protected animals	Bukreyev et al. (119)
		Newcastle disease virus clone containing GP	10^7 plaque-forming units	Rhesus monkeys	GP	NDV/GP is highly attenuated for replication in the respiratory tract of immunized animals and developed GP-specific mucosal IgA antibodies	DiNapoli et al. (120)
11	Adenovirus-based vaccines	Adenovirus (rAd5) vaccine GP	2×10^9 virus particle	Phase I human study	GP	Antigen specific humoral and cellular immune responses were generated	Ledgerwood et al. (121)
		Adenovirus (ChAd3) vaccine boosted with MVA	Priming dose 2.5×10^{10} PFU of ChAd3 and a boosting dose of 1.5×10^8 PFU of MVA	Healthy adult volunteers	GP	Elicited B-cell and T-cell immune responses	Ledgerwood et al. (91)
		Chimpanzee serotype 7 adenovirus vaccine expressing GP (AdC7-GP)	Prime boosting with AdC7-GP (1×10^{10}) and boosting with 20 mg *Drosophila* S2 cells expressed truncated GP	BALB/c mice	GP	Long-lasting high-titer neutralizing antibodies production in mice and efficiently prevented luciferase-containing reporter EBOV-like particle entry even at 18 weeks post-immunization	Chen et al. (90)
12	Vesicular stomatitis virus (VSV)-based vaccines	VSV GP replaced with EBOV GP	2×10^7 PFU	Healthy adult volunteers	GP	Anti-Ebola immune responses were documented	Regules et al. (82)
		VSV GP replaced with EBOV GP	3×10^5 PFU	Healthy adult volunteers	GP	Lowered antibody responses observed with vaccine associated side effects like vaccine-induced arthritis and dermatitis	Agnandji et al. (122)
13	Semliki forest virus based vaccines	From DNA-launched replicons (DREP)-eGFP vector, eGFP replaced with GP and NP to make DREP-GP and DREP-VP40 vectors, respectively	10 μg plasmid DNA	Balb/c mice	GP + VP40	EBOV filamentous VLPs were observed in the supernatant of cells resulting from co-expression of GP and VP40 and post immunization, specific humoral accompanied with a mixed Th1/Th2 cellular immune response was obtained	Ren et al. (69)
14	Liposome-encapsulated vaccine	Liposome-encapsulated irradiated EBOV-Zaire (6×10^6 rads of γ-irradiation from a ^{60}Co source)	Intravenous inoculation of 1.0 ml dose containing 194 μg of irradiated EBOV Zaire + 100 μg of lipid A	BALB/c mice and Cynomolgus monkeys	All native EBOV antigens	All mice protected, however the immunization failed to protect Cynomolgus monkeys	Rao et al. (54)

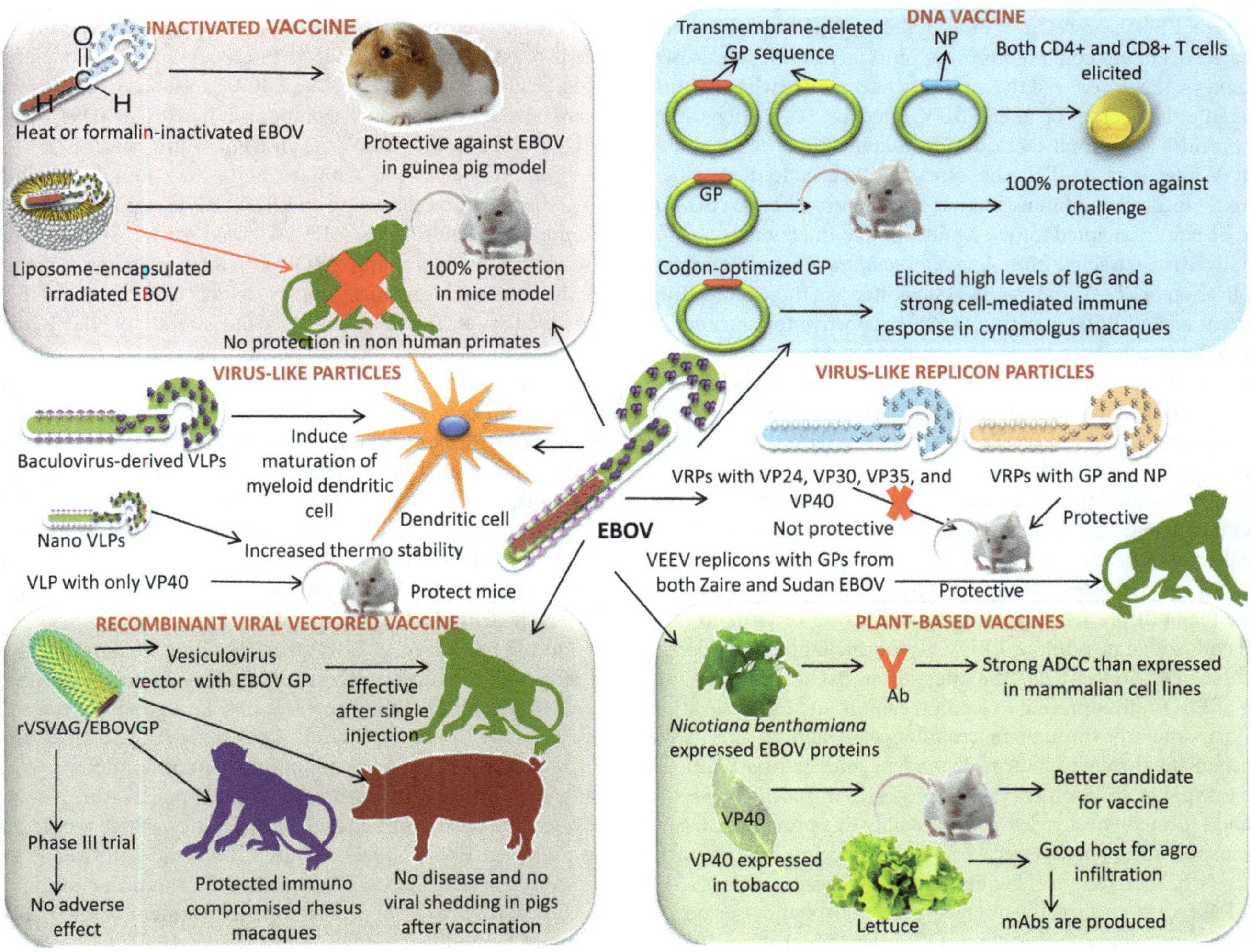

FIGURE 1 | Various vaccine platforms under progress for the development of a successful Ebola virus (EBOV) vaccine. Platforms like inactivated vaccine, DNA vaccine, virus-like particles, virus-like replicon particles (VRPs), plant-based vaccine, and recombinant viral-vectored vaccines are available.

activity of lamivudine against EBOV in Vero E6 cells. Hence, the use of lamivudine may not be advocated.

The docking of VP40, VP35, VP30, and VP24 has been achieved using small molecules belonging to the class of flavonoids and derivatives. Gossypetin and Taxifolin (the two flavonoids of top ranks) showed higher docking scores for every EBOV receptor (141). A virtual analysis of more phytochemicals could help to identify plant-derived products with comparatively higher efficacy and lower toxicity. Adenosine nucleoside analogs such as BCX4430 have been found effective against EBOV in a mouse model. GS-5734, also a nucleoside analog, was found effective against EBOV in a NHP model (142). Using molecular dynamics simulations, graphene sheets are found to associate strongly with VP40 (matrix) protein of EBOV and disrupt VP40 hexamer–hexamer association, crucial to form virus matrix, thereby graphene and similar nanopolymers may be used as therapy or at least disinfectant to reduce the risk of transmission at time of epidemic (143).

The potential of retro-type drugs (molecules that block the retrograde trafficking of bacterial and plant toxins within mammalian cells) must be explored for designing novel therapy against filovirus (144). Retro-2 along with its other two derivatives, Retro-2.1 and compound 25 could effectively block EBOV and MARV progression *in vitro*. The derivatives were shown to be more potent inhibitors of filoviral penetration, replication, and progression when compared with their parent compound, as evidenced by pseudo-typed virus assays (144).

EBOV Entry and Inhibitors

The cell entry of EBOV involves virus binding to the cell surface receptors followed by internalization through macropinocytosis, processing by endosomal proteases, and transport to Niemann–Pick C1 (NPC1; an internal receptor for EBOV) containing endolysosomes. Phosphatidylinositol-3-phosphate 5-kinase is essential for maturation of endosome, a critical step to the EBOV infection (145). *In vitro* studies using apilimod, an antagonist of phosphatidylinositol-3-phosphate 5-kinase, showed inhibition of EBOV by blocking the viral particle trafficking to NPC1 containing endolysosomes (146). IFNs are natural antivirals, and type I (IFN-α/β), particularly, is being widely used for the treatment of viral diseases. Type I IFN-α2b has been evaluated for the treatment of EBOV; however, IFN-α2b was not successful, as only delayed death but could not prevent mortality in EBOV-exposed monkeys. IFN-γ reduced the mortality rate in mice when administered either before or after EBOV infection (147), suggesting its promise as a prophylactic and/or therapeutic drug for use in EBOV infections. As IFN-γ has already been used to treat certain chronic medical conditions and has been approved by the FDA, it can be readily adapted for use against EBOV infections.

Silvestrol extracted from *Aglaia foveolata* was found to inhibit replication of EBOV and has been suggested as a therapeutic drug to treat acute EBOV infection (148). Supportive treatments like oral rehydration therapy are recommended for children under 5 years of age (149). Web-based identification of therapeutic agents indicated that a single siRNA can inhibit mRNA transcription of three species of EBOV, whereas 75 siRNAs can inhibit at least two species of EBOV. The web server Ebola VCR has been developed, with details available for the development of suitable therapeutic agents (150). Numerous treatment options for EVD are discussed below.

Ebola virus possesses only one surface protein and is responsible for both the receptor binding and fusion of virus-to-host cell endosomal membrane. EBOV glycoprotein binds with lectin receptor DC-SIGN (151). The infection initiated with the binding of EBOV glycoprotein to lectin receptors and internalization of virus majorly through macropinocytosis and as alternative mechanism through clathrin-dependent endocytosis (152). In the low pH of endosome, cysteine proteases including cathepsin B and L proteolytically cleave GP. Possibly this proteolytic cleavage exposes the putative receptor-binding region that interacts with NPC1, a receptor facilitating the filovirus entry (153). TIM-1 receptors directly interact with phosphatidylserine on the viral envelope, suggestive of GP independent virus attachment onto the cells. In poorly permissive cells, EBOV infection enhanced by exogenously expressed TIM-1 by 10- to 30-folds (154). Other phosphatidylserine interacting proteins like TIM-4 and Axl (a receptor tyrosine kinase) also have been demonstrated to enhance the infection of several enveloped virus. A benzylpiperazine adamantane diamide-derived compound obtained after screening of a library of small molecules, targets endosomal NPC1, and inhibit infection by VSV particles (VSV) pseudotyped with EBOV GP (155).

Tetrandrin is a potent drug that inhibits the EBOV entry into the cells (156). Two estrogen receptor drugs, clomiphene and toremifene, have been reported to hinder EBOV infection in mice by blocking cell entry and fusion with host cells (157). Amiodarone, an ion channel blocker, has been found to inhibit EBOV entry into cells (158, 159). Dendrimers and fullerene C_{60} have unique symmetrical properties and were recently found effective in inhibiting EBOV entry *in vitro* (160). Clarithromycin, an antibiotic, inhibits the release of calcium (stimulated by nicotinic acid adenine dinucleotide phosphate) from lysosome and exhibit anti-EBOV activity. Alike clarithromycin, posaconazole, an anti-fungal agent also shows similar anti-EBOV activity. In addition, it also inhibits the functions of NPC1 protein and acid sphingomyelinase activity. Both drugs, i.e., clarithromycin and posaconazole, ultimately inhibit the entry of EBOV into the host cell (161). The drug 5-(*N*-ethyl-*N*-isopropyl) amiloride inhibits the process of macropinocytosis (a process required for uptake of large filamentous virions, like EBOV) and thus interferes with the viral entry into the cell. Compounds like MLS000394177 and MLS000733230 also inhibit the viral entry into cells (162).

Prunella vulgaris, a Chinese herb, was found to inhibit EBOV entry into cells, using an EBOV-GP-pseudotyped-human immunodeficiency virus (HIV)-1-based vector system (163). Pseudovirions containing EBOV-GP were used for screening of the Prestwick chemical library, which contains 1,200 FDA approved drugs. The assay was based on cell entry of HIV-1-based surrogate in 384-well format. Twenty chemicals were found to inhibit more than 80% entry and 16 out of them were identified as G protein-coupled receptor (GPCR) antagonists, which target a range of GPCRs including adrenergic receptors, 5-HT (serotonin) receptors, histamine receptors, muscarinic and acetylcholine receptors. The time-of-addition studies suggested that EBOV entry is stopped at level of initial attachment prior to fusion of virus and cell membrane (164). Quercetin 3-β-*O*-D-glucoside (Q3G), a flavonoid derivate, was found to protect mice against EBOV challenge by targeting viral entry (165).

During replication of EBOV, surface GPs undergo proteolytic cleavage in the endosome by several proteases, including cathepsin B (CatB) (166). Thus, proteases may be a good target for the inhibition of EBOV replication. One study showed that, using a synthetic serine protease inhibitor, nafamostat mesilate (NM), caused a reduction in CatB release in rat pancreases. NM was also found to have anti-coagulant properties, which would also be useful in EBOV infections, as EBOV causes disseminated intravascular coagulation. Thus, this drug should be examined in clinical trials to be approved for the treatment of EVD (167). Chemically modified human serum albumin with 3-hydroxyphthalic anhydride (HP-HSA) has been demonstrated with the potential of a therapeutic candidate in resisting the EBOV infection (168).

Transfusion of Convalescent Blood/Serum

Convalescent serum by definition contains immunoglobulins IgM and IgG but is devoid of red blood cells and clotting factors. Transfusing convalescent whole blood and convalescent plasma from disease survivors has been found to neutralize EBOV and reduce its load; thereafter, the immune response of the patient can provide protection against EBOV (169, 170). The use of whole blood and convalescent serum was approved by the World Health Organization (WHO) during critical EBOV conditions (171, 172). Screening of plasma is needed to rule out the presence of residual EBOV RNA and other blood-transmitted pathogens such as HIV, hepatitis B virus, and hepatitis C virus. Protection is conferred in NHPs through antibody therapy (post-exposure). In humans, this has ultimately paved the way for filovirus therapy by the use of polyclonal/mAb (approved by Food and Drug Administration) (173).

Valuable emergency therapeutics for the treatment of EBOV-infected persons include passive immunization with neutralizing antibodies by the transfer of sera from individuals recovering from EVD (174, 175), although it is not considered to render 100% protection especially after exposure (3 days post-exposure) to EBOV (e.g., Zaire Ebolavirus Makona) (176). Precise immunoglobulins retrieved from equine serum against EBOV were found safe and effective as prophylactic therapy in non-allergic patients (177). Recently developed mAb-based treatments for EVD include mAb114 and MB-003, ZMAb, ZMapp, and MIL-77E cocktails (25). ZMAb, consisting of three murine mAbs (1H3, 2G4, and 4G7), administered at a dose of 25 mg/kg three times, completely protected cynomolgus macaques against EVD. Administration of ZMAb with adenovirus-vectored IFN-α resulted in 75 and 100% survival of cynomolgus and rhesus macaques, respectively (29). mAbs that bind to the base of GP (4G7 and 2G4) are neutralizing antibodies, whereas mAbs that bind to the glycan cap (mAb114, 1H3, and 13C6) are non-neutralizing antibodies. The chimeric human mAbs 13C6, 6D8, and 13F6 possess the variable region from mice and Fc region of human; mAbs 13C6 and 6D8 neutralize EBOV in the presence of complement proteins (24). By repeated immunization of mice with glycoproteins of filovirus, generation of pan-EBOV-specific (as well as pan-filovirus) mAbs have been obtained. These pan-EBOV mAbs have shown reaction with RESTV, SUDV, and other viruses (178).

The components of ZMapp are mAbs (chimeric), *viz.*, c13C6 from MB-003 (already known cocktail of antibody) and c2G4 as well as c4G7 from ZMab (different cocktail of antibody). This drug reversed clinical signs in 100% of rhesus macaques, even when administered as late as 5 days after EBOV exposure (30). Use of ZMapp, humanized-mouse antibodies, as a therapeutic agent has shown promise in NHPs (30, 84, 179) and it is a WHO-approved treatment regimen for EVD. Recently, a baby born to an EBOV-infected mother was found positive for EBOV on the first day of life. The baby was treated with ZMapp and the broad spectrum antiviral GS-5734, and, on day 20, the baby was found negative for EBOV (180). MB-003 is another mAb cocktail which is found to be effective in NHPs against variants of EBOV that are resistant to ZMapp (181).

The mechanism of action of mAbs is that they identify the inter-protomer epitope of the GP fusion loop, which is essential for viral membrane fusion, and also neutralize the entry of virus (182). Although several mAbs are available that can neutralize EBOV, there are few mAbs that can neutralize GPs from different EBOV species. In a study by Duehr et al. (183), a panel of eight murine mAbs derived from animals immunized with *Zaire ebolavirus* was evaluated. The mAbs were tested for binding breadth using a set of recombinant surface GPs from RESTV, TAFV, BDBV, EBOV, SUDV, and MARV. Of the eight, two mAbs (KL-2E5 and KL-2H7) showed binding ability. These two mAbs did not neutralize EBOV; however, they protected mice from infection with a VSV expressing the *Zaire ebolavirus* GP. Duehr et al. (183) also suggested that Fc-FcR interactions are responsible for the protection of mice in the absence of neutralization. Although ZMapp was found to be effective against Zaire EBOV, it has not shown cross-protection against other species of EBOV. FVM04 (a mAb) has shown cross neutralizing activity against SUDV. So, it can be used to replace one of the components of ZMapp, thereby increasing the range of protection against SUDV, ultimately leading to generation of cross-protective mAbs cocktail (184).

One Fab, KZ52, obtained by panning of phage display library, was derived from the bone marrow of an EVD survivor. Fab KZ52 exhibited 50% neutralization at a concentration of 8 nM (185). The mAb KZ52 protected guinea pigs from lethal *Zaire ebolavirus* challenge; however, when an experiment was carried out in rhesus macaques, the antibody failed to protect animals prophylactically and did not inhibit viremia (186). EBOV GP is processed by cathepsins, and the cleaved GP fuses with host cells to form a fusion pore, a passage for the EBOV genome to enter the cytosol for replication. Human mAb KZ52 and monkey mAb JP3K11 bind to conformation-dependent epitopes of GP. KZ52 is directed to bind a conformational non-glycosylated epitope at base of GP and a total 23 residues of GP residues remain in contact with antibody. Out of 23, 15 are contacted through van der Waals interactions and remaining 8 through direct hydrogen bonds (187). At 0.4 μg/ml dose, KZ52 lead to 50% neutralization. KZ52 protective efficacy is due to inhibition of cathepsin mediated cleavage of GP (23).

Exploring the synergistic effect of different pairs of neutralizing and non-neutralizing anti-EBOV mAbs could provide 100% protection in mice, revealing the scope of this approach in designing and developing immunotherapeutics and vaccines (188).

Bispecific Trojan-horse antibodies neutralizing other filoviruses have been found to provide protection in mice from multiple EBOV infection (189). Cell-penetrable human scFvs (HuscFvs) (transbodies) that bind to EBOV VP40, a matrix protein pivotal for viral assembly and budding, produced by phage display technology, revealed inhibition of the EBOV-like particles (VLPs) egress from hepatic cells (190). These transbodies were effective in blocking viral assembly and budding within the cells as they bind to several cationic patches in the VP40 C-terminal domain. The transbodies inhibit the function of VP40 by additional mechanisms also; such as binding to N-terminal domain and L-domain peptide WW binding motifs, suggesting the potential of these transbodies as direct acting anti-EBOV agents in future (190). Cell-penetrable HuscFvs specific to a highly conserved interferon-inhibitory domain (IID) of VP35 of EBOV inhibited the VP35 biofunctions in the EBOV replication cycle including polymerase cofactor activity and host IFN–antagonism by forming interface contact with residues of the first basic patch, the central basic patch, end-cap, and residues important for IID multimeric formation for dsRNA binding (191). The cell-penetrable small antibody fragments (HuscFvs) or superantibodies [the term coined by Kohler and Paul (192)] can cross the membrane of all cells but get accumulated intracellularly only where the target antigen is present. Thus, disappearance of the superantibodies from the blood circulation does not imply that they are eliminated from the body. The transbodies to the highly conserved EBOV VP40 and VP35 should be evaluated further using authentic EBOV in animal models of EVD and clinical trials before they can be considered a broadly effective and promising alternative to existing treatment approaches for EVD.

Recently, three mAbs produced in tobacco plants that target the EBOV GP were tested and showed good results in humans (193). Human mAbs against BDBV GP were isolated from patients who survived during the 2007 Uganda outbreak. These mAbs were found to have a neutralizing effect against multiple EBOV species, suggesting the possibility of the use of single mAbs as cross-protecting antibodies (194). Another investigation showed that EBOV GPs were conserved across different EBOV species. ELISA revealed that four mAbs namely S3, S12, S17, and S33 were found to show cross-reaction with GPs of five different species of EBOV (195). The discovery of cross-protective antibodies can aid in the development of therapeutic strategies for treatment of EBOV disease (196). In another study, 349 EBOV GP mAbs were isolated from survivors of EVD in an outbreak in Zaire, and 77% of the mAbs were found to neutralize EBOV (197). Three mAbs of EBOV-GP (Q206, Q314, and Q411) were isolated during the West African EVD outbreak in 2014. Recognition of the novel epitopes has been performed for Q206 and Q411, wherein these mAbs were found protecting mice against EBOV (198). A therapeutic vaccine based on mAbs has been proposed to sufficiently resolve replication of invasive EBOV, even if administered as a single dose 4 days post-infection (199). Non-neutralizing mAb 5D2 or 7C9 expressing adeno-associated virus (AAV), consistently released mAb in body and was found 100% protective against mice adapted EBOV strain. Neutralizing mAb 2G4 conferred 83% protection and a cocktail of these two mAbs provided 100% protection when given 7 days prior to infection and sustained protection when immunized animals were challenged 5 months post AAV-mAb immunization (200).

Potential limitations of mAb-based therapies include the requirement for high doses and mAb mixtures that are outbreak-specific owing to constant viral evolution. Furthermore, epitope mutations could reduce efficacy of the therapeutic mAbs used. Hence, these limiting factors need to be taken care of accordingly with mAbs usages.

EBOV Gene Expression Inhibitors

Viral gene expression is dependent on host cell machinery and is critical for virus replication. A conserved guanine-rich sequence in the EBOV L gene has been reported to assemble into quadruplex RNA, targeted by cationic porphyrin TmPyP4 that directs inhibition of the expression of L gene at the RNA level (86, 201). BCX4430 (a nucleoside analog) is a viral RNA polymerase inhibitor, and it has been found effective in protecting mice against lethal challenge of EBOV (202–204). In addition, double-stranded RNA binding protein 76 has been reported to inhibit EBOV polymerase activity (205).

Small molecular inhibitors needed for the synthesis of polyamine have been found to block the expression of EBOV gene. The eukaryotic initiation factor 5A (eIF5A) hypusination and spermidine (a polyamine) are essentially required for the replication of EBOV. However, if eIF5A hypusination is blocked, the gene expression of EBOV is inhibited which subsequently blocks the replication of the virus. Therefore, in-depth understanding of this mechanism at molecular level is essential for developing anti-EBOV drugs (205).

Repurposed Drugs

It is time taking task to develop a new therapeutic against an infectious agent and till that time new therapy divulged; drug repurposing, *i.e.*, already existing drugs may be screened for their efficacy against pathogen. Owing to the lack of approved EBOV therapies, the screening of potentially efficacious drugs revealed that few of the drugs could be repurposed for EBOV treatment (206) (**Table 2**). Amiodarone, dronedarone, and verapamil, which are used for tachycardia, arrhythmias, and high blood pressure or angina, respectively, have been screened for their ability to inhibit the entry of filoviruses into cells and found efficacious in *in vitro* models (158). The use of statins, angiotensin-converting enzyme inhibitors, and angiotensin receptor blockers has also been suggested to attenuate EBOV infection (126). Phosphoinositide 3-kinases inhibitor LY294002 and calcium/calmodulin kinase (CAMK2) inhibitor KN-93 have been reported to reduce EBOV infection in Vero E6 cells. The p38 mitogen-activated protein kinase inhibitor SB202190 was shown to check virus-mediated cytokine storm, as studied in monocyte-derived DC of humans (207). Estrogen re-uptake modulators, *viz.*, toremiphene and clomiphene, although cause *in vitro* inhibition of the virus entry, but are not free from unwanted side effects like ocular adverse reaction (in case of clomiphene) and serious derangements of electrolytes (in case of toremiphene) at the higher doses. To overcome this, combination therapy is suggested while using such drugs (206). Brincidofovir, a cidofovir analog conjugated with a lipid, can prevent EBOV replication; however, its exact efficacy in an *in vivo* model needs to be determined (208). Because cyclophilin A (CypA) is not essential for EBOV replication, alisporivir, which inhibits the host protein CypA, has shown limited antiviral effects against EBOV strains (Makona, Mayinga) (209). Emetine, an anti-protozoal agent, and its desmethyl analog cephaeline have potently inhibited EBOV replication and cephaeline is well tolerated in patients than emetine (210).

Rosuvastatin, atorvastatin, and pravastatin have been reported to alleviate inflammation, reduce C-reactive protein and TNFα levels, and impede cholesterol-supported EBOV membrane biosynthesis (232). In EBOV infection, overexpression of the procoagulant tissue factor in monocytes and macrophages and participation of endothelial cells leads to an imbalance in coagulation. The use of recombinant nematode anticoagulant protein c2, an inhibitor of tissue factor-mediated blood coagulation, was found to improve survival of macaques from Ebola hemorrhagic fever, and hence suggested to act as a good treatment module targeting the disease development (228). Anti-malarial drugs such as chloroquine and its structural analogs (hydroxychloroquine, pamaquine, primaquine, and plasmaquine) also act as lysosomotropic agents, preventing endosomal/lysosomal acidification, and thus limiting certain viral infections (233). There are conflicting reports on the therapeutic effects of chloroquine in mouse, hamster, and guinea pig models of EVD. Chloroquine was found to inhibit virus replication in *in vitro* studies but failed to protect against EBOV infection and disease development in mice, hamsters, and guinea pigs (234, 235). Esomeprazole and omeprazole were also found to inhibit viral entry during *in vitro* studies but higher concentrations of these drugs may be required when to be used *in vivo* (236). During the EBOV outbreak in Liberia in 2014, a reduction in fever cases was observed following mass administration of malaria chemoprevention drugs (237).

Because of its competitive anti-heparin potential and interference with viral replication and entry into the cell, the anti-trypanosomal agent, Suramin (Germanin or Bayer-205) has been proposed to treat EVD (229). A pyrazine carboxamide derivative namely Favipiravir (an anti-flu medicine), which was used earlier as an inhibitor of influenza virus replication, has been found useful in both therapy and prophylaxis during EBOV epidemic in West Africa (238–240). Favipiravir and the pyrazine carboxamide derivative T-705 showed positive results in treating patients with medium to high viremias, although these drugs were not found to be effective with very high viremias, but revealed acceptable results during EBOV infection in mouse (219, 221, 241).

The microtubule inhibitor drugs (vinblastine, vinorelbine/navelbine, and vincristine), commonly used as anticancer agents,

TABLE 2 | Repurposed drugs used in Ebola virus disease therapy.

S. No.	Method of screening	Repurposed drug	Function of drug	Reference
1	*In vitro* antiviral activities	Verapamil	Hypertension, angina and arrhythmia	Gehring et al. (158)
		Teicoplanin (block a late stage of viral entry)	Glycopeptide antibiotic	Wang et al. (211)
		Nocodazole Cytochalasin B Cytochalasin D Latrunculin A Jasplakinolide	Cell arrest in G2- or M-phase A mycotoxin, inhibits network formation by actin filaments Induces depolymerization of actin filaments Microtubule inhibitor Stabilization of filamentous actin	Yonezawa et al. (212)
		FGI-104	Anti-malarial	Kinch et al. (213)
		Amodiaquine	Anti-malarial	Ekins et al. (214)
		Chloroquine (CQ) Amiodarone Prochlorperazine Benztropine Azithromycin Chlortetracycline Clomiphene	Anti-malarial Anti-arrhythmic Dopamine (D2) receptor antagonist; an antipsychotic agent For treating Parkinson's disease symptoms including muscle spasms, stiffness, tremors, sweating, drooling, and poor muscle control Macrolide antibiotics Antibiotics Induce ovaries to produce two or three eggs per cycle	Madrid et al. (215); Salata et al. (216)
2	A high-throughput assay for Zaire Ebola virus (EBOV) has been developed using the recombinant EBOV engineered to express the enhanced green fluorescent protein (eGFP) (interfere with viral fusion-worked in *in vitro* and *in vivo*)	Clomiphene Toremifene	 For treating gynecomastia	Johansen et al. (157)
3	Mice model (50–90% survival)			Yuan (217)
4	*In vivo* murine EBOV infection model	Bepridil	Calcium channel blocker	Johansen et al. (218)
		Sertraline (block a late stage of viral entry)	Antidepressant	Johansen et al. (218)
5	Recombinant vesicular stomatitis virus containing Ebola GP protein	Tunicamycin	A nucleoside antibiotic	Takada et al. (219)
6	In human—single-arm proof-of-concept trial in Guinea pigs Mouse model (100% protection)	Favipiravir	Broad-spectrum antiviral activity against RNA viruses	Sissoko et al. (220) Oestereich et al. (221)
7	Vero E6 cells infected with infectious Mayinga strain of EBOV	Amiodarone Dronedarone Verapamil	Anti-arrhythmic therapy and multiple ion channel blocker Anti-arrhythmic therapy Ca^{+2} channel blocker	Gehring et al. (158)
8	Primary human monocyte culture	17-allylamino-17-demethoxygeldanamycin (17-AAG)	Inhibitor of heat-shock protein 90	Smith et al. (222)
9	Recombinant EBOV variant Mayinga expressing enhanced GFP	Retro-2, Retro-2.1, and compound 25	Inhibit EBOV cell entry	Shtanko et al. (144)
10	In 293T cells release of Ebola virus-like particles (VLPs) assay	Nilotinib	Treatment for chronic myeloid leukemia in chronic phase	García et al. (223)
11	Mouse infection model and Ebola VLP entry assay	Clomiphene	Induce ovaries to produce two or three eggs per cycle	Nelson et al. (224)

(Continued)

TABLE 2 | Continued

S. No.	Method of screening	Repurposed drug	Function of drug	Reference
12	Ebola VLP entry assay	Vinblastine Vinorelbine Vincristine Colchicine Nocodazole Mebendazole Albendazole Tamoxifen Raloxifene Clemastine Maprotiline Benztropine Clomipramine Thiothixene Trifluoperazine Dronedarone Digoxin Dronedarone Propafenone Sunitinib Daunomycin Clarithromycin	Microtubule inhibitors Estrogen receptor modulators Antihistamine and anticholinergic activities Antipsychotic/antidepressant Pump/channel blocker Anti-arrhythmic drug Receptor tyrosine kinase (RTK) inhibitor Cancer treatment Macrolide antibiotic	Kouznetsova et al. (225)
13	Ebola live virus assays	Posaconazole	Invasive aspergillosis and candidiasis treatment	Sun et al. (161)
14	Laboratory animal model C57BL/6 and BALB/c mice	Chloroquine and amodiaquine	Anti-malarial and anti-inflammatory	Madrid et al. (226)
15	Small molecule chemical screening	NSC 62914	Scavenger of reactive oxygen species	Panchal et al. (227)
16	Rhesus macaque model of Ebola hemorrhagic fever	Recombinant nematode anti-coagulant protein c2	Inhibitor of blood coagulation, attenuates the proinflammatory response	Geisbert et al. (228)
17	Vero E6 cells infected with Mayinga strain of Zaire EBOV	Suramin	Trypanosome-caused river blindness treatment	Henß et al. (229)
18	Computational analysis using Surflex, PLANTS, AutoDock, and AutoDock Vina	Indinavir Sinefungin Maraviroc Abacavir Telbivudine Cidofovir	Human immunodeficiency virus protease inhibitor Anti-fungal Antiviral drug	Zhao et al. (230)
19	Computational analysis of novel drug using CANDOCK (have shown anti-EBOV potential in other modalities also)	Raloxifene Tamoxifen Clemastine Deslanoside Digoxin Mebendazole Sertraline Niclosamide Sertraline	As described above in the table	Chopra et al. (231)

have been found effective in inhibiting EBOV VLP entry into HeLa cells even at low concentrations (48–140 nM). Colchicine, a microtubule modulator primarily used for gout, has also been found to show anti-EBOV activity (225, 242).

Screening of 1766 FDA approved drugs and 259 experimental drugs revealed that Indinavir, an HIV protease inhibitor, may be effective in reducing the severity of EVD (230). The antiviral drugs including Maraviroc, Abacavir, Telbivudine, and Cidofovir could target the MTase domain of EBOV and inhibit the viral RNA-directed RNA polymerase (230). The Computational Analysis of Novel Drug Opportunities platform was recently developed to screen drugs approved by the FDA. Drugs like enfuvirtide, vancomycin, bleomycin, octreotide, lanreotide, somatostatin, and ubidecarenone (CoQ10) have shown higher activity against EBOV (231). Recently, virtual screening of several thousands of repurposing drugs from Drug Bank has been performed and ibuprofen was selected by realizing its possible inhibitory effect on EBOV infection. The drug has been found to show detectable antiviral effect in cell culture and can thus be used as a very useful molecular template for anti-Ebola viral drug development (243).

Nucleotide Analog Prodrug

GS-5734 developed by Gilead Sciences falls under this category. Interestingly, clinical trials have been conducted and it has been found that the drug is effective in clearing virus from semen (181, 244). Administration of GS-5734 in rhesus monkey through intravenous route resulted in suppression of replication of EBOV. It is also important to note that in NHPs, this compound can provide protection post-exposure (245).

Interferons

Interferons act as potent inhibitors of EBOV as has been proved through *in vitro* studies conducted involving various types of cells. IFN-β-1a treatment protected mice against a lethal challenge of EBOV (206). The virus clearance from the blood stream is enhanced by IFN β-1a leading to resolution of the symptoms of the disease at an early stage (246). Even though there is increased therapeutic usage of IFNs, but certain side effects are also associated with such treatment, *viz.*, fever and myalgia, which must be kept in mind while opting for their use. Moreover, the occurrence of malaria additionally should be ruled out before initiating IFN therapy (206). Tilorone hydrochloride induces IFN response in mice and has been found effective against EBOV due to its action mainly mediated through pathway of innate immunity (IFN related) (247).

Oligomer-Mediated Inhibition

RNAi and advanced antisense therapies have been reported to provide post-exposure protection against lethal filovirus infections (248). Small interfering (si)RNA targeting RNA polymerase L protein has shown inhibition of EBOV replication and promising results for its use as a post-exposure therapeutic option (249). siRNAs and phosphorodiamidate morpholino oligomers (PMOs) targeting the EBOV RNA polymerase (L) protein protected NHPs against EVD (248, 249). PMOs target co-polymerase protein VP35 and membrane-associated protein VP24 for this protection (250). Antisense PMO-based drugs like AVI 6002, AVI-6003, and LNPs/siRNA (TKM-Ebola) are in clinical trials. TKM-Ebola is a mixture of three siRNAs that target the L, VP24, and VP35 proteins of Zaire EBOV. In NHPs, it efficiently provided post-exposure protection (249, 251). Although the results were promising, clinicians did not use much TKM-Ebola as it could lead to lethal overproduction of cytokines (a dangerous EBOV-induced inflammatory response) (232). A siRNA LNP product named TKM-130803 has been developed for EVD therapy. Although, the infusion of TKM-130803 at a dosage of 0.3 mg/kg/day through intravenous route to adult patients with severe clinical signs of EVD was comparable, it did not show an improved protection to the existing and classical controls (252). LNP-encapsulated short siRNAs protected 100% of rhesus monkeys exhibiting viremia and clinical illness (253). LNP encapsulation is also an effective drug delivery system (127, 253).

The inhibitors of hsa-miR-1246, hsa-miR-320a, and hsa-miR-196b-5p have been found to decrease EBOV GP cytotoxicity during *in vitro* studies; hence, miRNA technology can be used to develop useful therapeutics (254). Antiviral drug AVI-7537, targeting the VP24 gene of EBOV, has been shown to be efficacious in mice and monkeys (255). The EBOV-GP (cleaved) molecule acts as a ligand for NPC1, a transmembrane transfer protein. For entry of the virus into the target cell, an interaction between EBOV-GP and NPC1 domain C is necessary. Two small molecules, a sulfonamide (MBX2254) and a triazole thioether (MBX2270), have been identified as novel EBOV inhibitors suppressing EBOV infection in an *in vitro* model by blocking the entry of virus into target cell *via* inhibiting GP–NPC1 protein interaction (256). This strategy of targeting viral entry could pave way for the development of an anti-EBOV therapeutic agent.

A brief summary of investigated drugs/biomolecules and therapeutics to treat EBOV infection is presented in **Table 3** and depicted in **Figure 2**.

Of the note, a luciferase reporter system (EBOV-like particle/EBOVLP) has been developed. It helps in evaluating the *in vivo* anti-EBOV agents, *viz.*, vaccines and drugs without the necessity of biosafety level-4 facilities. The system appears suitable in studying the process of viral entry also (259). The molecular tweezer CLR01 has been recently reported to inhibit EBOV and Zika virus infection. CLR01 interacts with the lipids in the viral envelop but not with the cellular membrane, thereby it is having very less effect on viability of cells (270). This small molecule has earlier been shown to possess antiviral activity against HIV-1 and herpes viruses. Such broad-spectrum antiviral agents need to be further explored to develop an effective drug against EBOV.

Currently, priority is being given toward investigating various proteins in the host system and viral targets (druggable) (271). Further research works need to be strengthened to identify potent viral or host targets that can be exploited to treat EVD or inhibit EBOV. With advances in bioinformatics tools, it is now possible to identify the active sites of the viral targets which can be utilized as a critical step toward designing and discovering anti-EBOV drugs (272). The involvement of computational tools has widened our approach toward designing drugs (target based) widely. Computational approaches can also countervail the endemic burdens in development of drugs traditionally (271, 273). Large libraries can now be effectively screened, ultimately stimulating research activities toward identifying potent anti-EBOV drugs. Therapeutic applications of cytokines, recombinant proteins, RNAi technology/RNA interference, TLRs, avian egg yolk antibodies, plant-based pharmaceuticals, nanomedicines, immunomodulatory agents, probiotics, herbs/plant extracts, and others may be explored appropriately to combat EBOV, as these have been found promising against other viral pathogens (2, 249, 274–282).

CONCLUSION AND FUTURE PERSPECTIVES

The 2014 EBOV outbreak has been marked as the most widespread lethal viral hemorrhagic attack and prompted a hasty leap in the researches for developing effective vaccines and therapies to counter it. In the case of Ebola, deviations in the touchstone drug/vaccine research approaches may be permitted by authorities to an appropriate extent, considering the devastating and alarming pandemic threat from the disease. In recent years, several therapies have emerged to tackle lethal EBOV infections. A plant-derived formulation of humanized mAbs: "ZMapp" has been used to treat some patients. However, the shortage of ZMapp supply warrants the evaluation and development of new mAbs.

TABLE 3 | Investigated drugs/biomolecules to treat Ebola virus (EBOV) infection.

S. No.	Name of the therapy	Name of treatment/ biomolecule	Concentration used in experiment	Platform	Experimental model	Inference/notes	Reference
1.	Convalescent blood products therapy	Convalescent whole blood	Transfusion of 150–400 ml blood	–	Human patients	12.5% mortality in treated patients in comparison to 80% in untreated patients	Mupapa et al. (257)
		Polyclonal IgG	Intraperitoneal administration of the purified anti-EBOV IgG (100 mg/kg)	Polyclonal IgG production through trans-chromosomic (Tc) bovine platform technology	Mice	24 h post challenge treatment with SAB-139-V2 antibodies, significant protection was obtained	Dye et al. (258)
2.	Viral entry inhibitors	MBX2254 and MBX2270	MBX2254 (10 μmol/l) and MBX2270 (30 μmol/l) at −1, 0, 2, or 12 h	–	A549 cells	Late stage of EBOV entry is inhibited	Basu et al. (256)
		Tetrandrine	IC_{50} = 55 nM	–	HeLa cells	Inhibits infection of human macrophages, the primary target of EBOV	Sakurai et al. (156)
		MLS000078751 and MLS000534476 MLS000394177, MLS000730532, MLS000733230 MLS000555232 MLS000554255, MLS001101371	8 doses ranging from 0.39 up to 50 μM	Quantitative high-throughput screening (qHTS) approach to screen inhibitor molecules	HeLa cells	Inhibits infection of human macrophages Inhibits early uptake of virus Inhibits early endocytic trafficking Inhibits late endosome trafficking	Anantpadma et al. (162)
		3-hydroxyphthalic anhydride (HP)-modified human serum albumin	EC_{50}s for 0.068 and 0.124, respectively, for Zaire and Sudan pseudoviruses	Lentivirus-based pseudotypes	Huh-7 cell	Blocked pseudovirus entry by inhibiting cell surface attachment	Li et al. (168)
		Benztropine mesylate	IC_{50} ranging from 1.7 to 4.9 μM for different strains of EBOV	Pseudo-virions platform for high-throughput sequencing	A549 and vero cells	Screening of Prestwick Chemical Library containing 1,200 FDA approved drugs	Cheng et al. (164)
		Prunella vulgaris extract	2.5 μg/ml concentration	EBOV-GP pseudo-typed virus (EBOV-GP-V)-mediated infection model	HEK293T cells	Enhance anti-EBOV activity of the monoclonal antibody mAb 2G4 against EBOV-GP	Zhang et al. (163)
		Quercetin 3-β-*O*-D-glucoside (Q3G)	50 mg/kg of body weight	VSV-EBOV inhibition	BALB/c or C57BL/6 mice (Charles River)	Inhibits glycoprotein-mediated virus entry	Qiu et al. (165)
3.	EBOV gene expression inhibitors	Double-stranded RNA binding protein 76 (DRBP76)	shRNA targeting the 3′ UTR of DRBP76 used[a]	Zaire ebolavirus expressing GFP	293T cells	Inhibits EBOV polymerase activity	Shabman et al. (260)
		Silvestrol	IC_{50} = 96 nM	EBOV-infected human primary macrophages	Huh-7 cells and primary human macrophages	Strong reduction of VP40 levels	Biedenkopf et al. (148)

(*Continued*)

TABLE 3 | Continued

S. No.	Name of the therapy	Name of treatment/ biomolecule	Concentration used in experiment	Platform	Experimental model	Inference/notes	Reference
4.	Interferon (IFN)	IFN-α IFN-β	IC_{50} = 0.038 μM IC_{50} = 0.016 μM	*In vitro* model of Ebola Zaire replication with transcription-competent virus-like particles (trVLPs)	HEK 293T cells	Inhibits viral replication 24 h post-infection	McCarthy et al. (261)
		IFN β-1a	30 μg/day	Clinical trial	Human patients	Untreated patients had ~1.5- to 1.9-fold more likeliness to die than those treated	Konde et al. (246)
5.	mAb	ZMAb (combination of 1H3, 2G4, and 4G7)	0.1–100 μg/ml	Pseudo-typed VSV platform	VeroE6 cells	Antibodies target the GP1-GP2 interface and the glycan cap	Audet et al. (262)
		ZMapp (cocktail of humanized-mouse antibodies c2G4 and c4G7 and c13C6)	Totaling dose of 5 mg/animal at 1-day post-infection	–	2 patients evacuated from Liberia to Atlanta	Showed promise in non-human primates and clinical improvements in human subjects	Qiu et al. (30)
		KL-2E5 and KL-2H7	10 mg/kg	Pseudo-typed VSV platform	Stat2$^{-/-}$ mice	Non-neutralizing but protective action of mAb due to Fc-FcR interactions	Duehr et al. (183)
		FVM04	Single intraperitoneal (IP) injection of 10 mg/kg	Mouse-adapted EBOV	Mice	At 1 dpi post infection single dosing led to full protection from lethal challenge	Howell et al. (184)
		KZ52	50 mg/kg	Guinea pig-adapted Ebola Zaire virus	Guinea pigs	Dose-dependent protection of guinea pigs and proven record of efficacy in post-exposure prophylaxis of EBOV infection	Parren et al. (186)
		Q206, Q314, and Q411	100 μg of each mAb	Mouse-adapted EBOV	BALB/c mice	Administration of mAbs cocktail at 1 or 2 days post infection, potently neutralized live EBOV	Zhang et al. (163)
		Cell-penetrable human VP40 binding scFvs (HuscFvs)	40 μg/well	Pseudo-typed lentivirus particles carrying EBOV VP40 and GP genes	Huh7 cells transduced with	Human transbodies effectively inhibit egress of Ebola virus-like particles from mammalian cells	Teimoori et al. (190)
		Cell-penetrable human scFvs to IFN-inhibitory domain of VP35	25 μg/well	EBOV minigenome and VP35 expression cassette	HepG2 cells transduced with EBOV minigenome and VP35 expression cassette	Human transbodies effectively inhibit VP35 co-polymerase activity and antagonize VP35-mediated IFN suppression	Seesuay et al. (191)
		Bispecific antibody (FVM09~548 and FVM09~MR72 dual-variable domain immunoglobulin)	20 mg/kg	Pseudo-typed VSV platform	Female BALB/c mice	Specifically and potently neutralize recombinant VSV-EBOV GP in comparison to the parental mAbs FVM09, mAb-548, and MR72 which has poor neutralizing capacity	Wec et al. (189)
6.	Virus replication inhibitors	Okadaic acid (toxin produced by shell fish)	IC_{50} = 130 nM	–	BSR T7/5 cells	Inhibition of protein phosphatases PP1A and PP2A by okadaic acid blocks multiplication of EBOV in target cells	Modrof et al. (263)
		Pyrazinecarboxamide derivative T-705 (favipiravir)	Treatment (300 mg/kg/day) IC_{90} of 110 μM	Used for treating influenza and other segmented viruses	In IFNAR$^{-/-}$ C57BL/6 mice Vero E6 cells	When treatment initiated 6 days pre-infection or post-infection, it prevented mortality of 100% mice and reduced biochemical correlates of disease Suppression of EBOV replication by 4 log_{10} units	Oestereich et al. (221)

(*Continued*)

TABLE 3 | Continued

S. No.	Name of the therapy	Name of treatment/ biomolecule	Concentration used in experiment	Platform	Experimental model	Inference/notes	Reference
7.	Nucleotide analog	Adenosine nucleoside analog BCX4430 (interrupt viral RNA synthesis)	16 mg/kg BID dose group	–	Cynomolgus macaque	Significantly prolonged mean time to death	Taylor et al. (203)
			25 mg/kg IM BID (treatment started 30–60 min after inoculation)	–	Rhesus macaque	All animals survived	
		FGI-106	3 mg/kg	Cell-based assays also identified inhibitory activity against divergent virus families	C57BL/6 or BALB/c mice	Single dose of FGI-106, administered 24 h post-infection	Aman et al. (264)
8.	Antivirals	Genistein and tyrphostin AG1478 cocktail	Up to 100 μM	–	HEK 293 cells	Higher concentrations of genistein and lower concentrations of tyrphostin AG1478 has higher inhibition of EBOV	Kolokoltsov et al. (265)
		Carbocyclic 3-deazaadenosine (*S*-Adenosylhomocysteine Hydrolase Inhibitors)	Doses ≥0.7 mg/kg every 8 h	–	Adult BALB/c mice	When treatment initiated at 0 or day 1 post infection, it completely protected animals	Huggins et al. (266)
9.	Oligomer-mediated inhibition	siRNAs targeting the Zaire EBOV RNA polymerase L + VP24 + VP35 in stable nucleic acid-lipid particles (SNALPs)	2 mg/kg total siRNA/ dose	–	Chinese rhesus macaques	Macaques given seven treatments with SNALPs were protected after lethal EBOV challenge	Geisbert et al. (249)
		L gene-specific pool of four siRNAs complexed in SNALPs	A single bolus of 0.75 mg/kg siRNA per kilogram of body weight	–	Hartley guinea pigs	One of the 4 siRNAs alone is able to completely protect guinea pigs from a lethal EBOV challenge	Geisbert et al. (267)
		Cell-penetrating peptide conjugated with phosphorodiamidate morpholino oligomers, an uncharged single-stranded DNA analoge; designed to base pair with the translation start site region of VP35	500 μg dose	–	C57Bl/6 mice	Oligomer provided protection to mice when administered before or after an otherwise lethal infection	Enterlein et al. (268)
		TKM-130803	2.24 × 10^9 RNA copies/ ml plasma (0.3 mg/kg)	Single-arm phase II trial, adults with laboratory-confirmed Ebola virus disease (EVD) patients	Human patients	In patients with severe EVD no improvement with treatment	Thi et al. (253)
		miR-607	–	*In silico*	–	Selected mRNA completely blocked all major 4 EBOVs	Golkar et al. (269)

[a]*Dose not mentioned.*

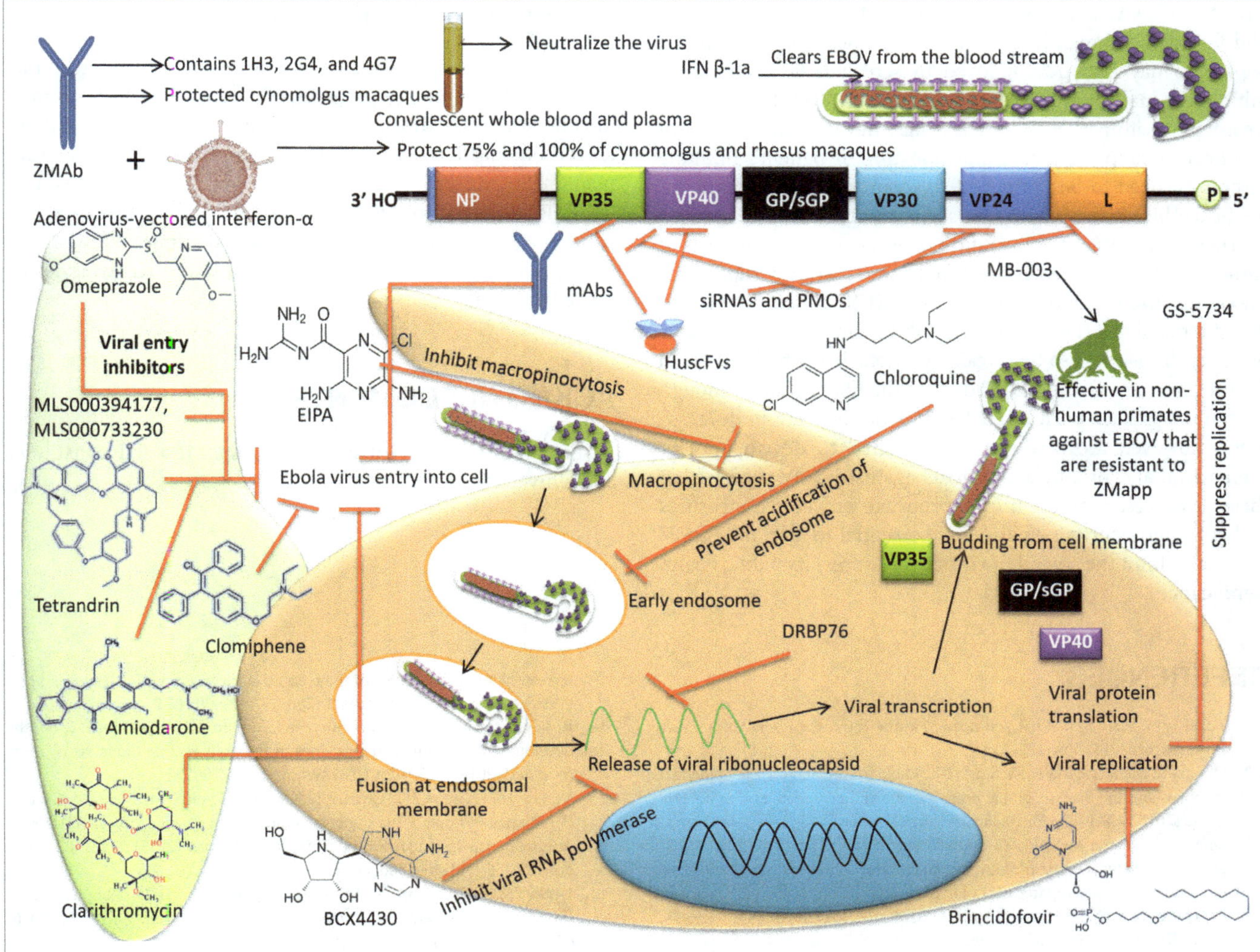

FIGURE 2 | Different therapeutic agents and drugs available for the treatment of Ebola virus disease (EVD). Some agents block the viral entry, some block the RNA polymerase, while some inhibit gene expression. Neutralizing antibodies and mAbs have shown the potential to effectively inhibit Ebola virus (EBOV).

Various drugs have been repurposed to treat potentially lethal disease like EVD. There is a long list of repurposed compounds that have been evaluated as inhibitors of EBOV, including microtubule inhibitors, estrogen receptor and reuptake modulators, kinase inhibitors, histamine antagonists, and ion channel blockers. In-depth studies are still required to understand the pathogenesis and the role of different EBOV peptides, proteins, and antigens and host–virus interactions in EVD. There is also a need to develop economic and effective antivirals and vaccines against EBOV having approach/utility to any part of the world including resource poor countries.

Although the development of vaccines against EBOV began in 1980, there is still no effective vaccine available to prevent this deadly disease. Hence, the hunt for an effective vaccine is still on. Ebola VLPs play an imperative role in high-throughput screening of anti-EBOV compounds. Because five EBOV species have been reported, a polyvalent vaccine having immunogenic determinants such as GP from each of species would provide broader immunity; indeed, in nonhuman primate experimental studies with a DNA vaccine, this is commonly true. The best first-generation vaccine candidates for EBOV are rVSV and ChAd3, as reflected by their application in providing long duration protection during sporadic outbreaks. Various combinations of antigens from different species of EBOV may be explored to achieve higher protective immune response. The rVSV-based vaccine is being used in Democratic Republic of the Congo. Due to absence of preexisting immunity to VSV, it eliminates several drawbacks and safety concerns associated Ad5-based vaccine. Also, it has show long-term protection in several NHP models, it is an ideal vaccine platform to be used at time of outbreak. Together, the GamEvac-Combi vaccine also seems to be equally promising as it generated immune response in 100% volunteers.

In addition, mAbs with broad cross-reactivity that will neutralize all five species of EBOV are required to be developed and evaluated for prophylactic and therapeutic uses. Furthermore, effective antibodies may be engineered for homogeneity with human antibodies. Many nucleic acid-based modalities like siRNA, miRNA, and PMOs have been tested against EBOV and found functional. In the era of genomics, a computational approach may also be employed to screen large numbers of inhibitory molecules to safeguard human health. Available treatments within the disaster settings; mostly combination of appropriate supportive care and boosting of patient's immune responses, need to be optimized to ensure minimum research/medical ethics being followed in such settings.

There is always scope for future investigations on the basis of clinical studies that are designed well and statistically supported. Maximum use of supportive therapy (MUST) should be introduced for studying the effects of new therapeutics. The side effects of newer drugs can also be revealed very efficiently by MUST and for this more resources are needed for the Ebola clinics. Though several drugs have been evaluated and vaccines are in development; however, more research is required to develop potent therapeutic and prophylactic agents against EBOV. Apart from these advances, adaptation of appropriate preventive measures and strict biosecurity principles are essential to stop the EBOV outbreaks, limit the spread of virus, and address its public health significance.

AUTHOR CONTRIBUTIONS

All the authors substantially contributed to the conception, design, analysis and interpretation of data, checking and approving final version of the manuscript, and agreed to be accountable for its contents. KD, RK, AM, and KK initiated this review compilation. SC, SL, and RK updated various sections. RKS, YM, DK, and MR reviewed virology and biotechnology aspects. RKS, SM, RS, and WC reviewed recent vaccines and therapies. RK designed tables. KK designed the figures. WC, AM, and KD overviewed and edited final.

ACKNOWLEDGMENTS

All the authors acknowledge and thank their respective Institutes and Universities.

REFERENCES

1. Vogel WH, Viale PH. What you need to know about the Ebola virus. *J Adv Pract Oncol* (2014) 5(6):471–3.
2. Dhama K, Malik YS, Malik SV, Singh RK. Ebola from emergence to epidemic: the virus and the disease, global preparedness and perspectives. *J Infect Dev Ctries* (2015) 9:441–55. doi:10.3855/jidc.6197
3. Singh RK, Dhama K, Malik YS, Ramakrishnan MA, Karthik K, Khandia R, et al. Ebola virus – epidemiology, diagnosis, and control: threat to humans, lessons learnt, and preparedness plans – an update on its 40 year's journey. *Vet Q* (2017) 37(1):98–135. doi:10.1080/01652176.2017.1309474
4. Leroy EM, Epelboin A, Mondonge V, Pourrut X, Gonzalez J-P, Muyembe-Tamfum J-J, et al. Human Ebola outbreak resulting from direct exposure to fruit bats in Luebo, Democratic Republic of Congo. *Vector Borne Zoonotic Dis* (2007) 9:6. doi:10.1089/vbz.2008.0167
5. Judson SD, Fischer R, Judson A, Munster VJ. Ecological contexts of index cases and spill over events of different ebolaviruses. *PLoS Pathog* (2016) 12(8):e1005780. doi:10.1371/journal.ppat.1005780
6. Kosal ME. A new role for public health in bioterrorism deterrence. *Front Public Health* (2014) 2:278. doi:10.3389/fpubh.2014.00278
7. Wu XX, Yao HP, Wu NP, Gao HN, Wu HB, Jin CZ, et al. Ebolavirus vaccines: progress in the fight against Ebola virus disease. *Cell Physiol Biochem* (2015) 37(5):1641–58. doi:10.1159/000438531
8. Johnson KM, Lange JV, Webb PA, Murphy FA. Isolation and partial characterisation of a new virus causing acute haemorrhagic fever in Zaire. *Lancet* (1977) 1(8011):569–71. doi:10.1016/S0140-6736(77)92000-1
9. Skrable K, Roshania R, Mallow M, Wolfman V, Siakor M, Levine AC. The natural history of acute Ebola virus disease among patients managed in five Ebola treatment units in West Africa: a retrospective cohort study. *PLoS Negl Trop Dis* (2017) 11(7):e0005700. doi:10.1371/journal.pntd.0005700
10. Elliott LH, Kiley MP, McCormick JB. Descriptive analysis of Ebola virus proteins. *Virology* (1985) 147:169–76. doi:10.1016/0042-6822(85)90236-3
11. Adam B, Lins L, Stroobant V, Thomas A, Brasseur R. Distribution of hydrophobic, residues is crucial for the fusogenic properties of the Ebola virus GP2 fusion peptide. *J Virol* (2004) 78:2131–6. doi:10.1128/JVI.78.4.2131-2136.2004
12. Kuhn JH, Andersen KG, Bào Y, Bavari S, Becker S, Bennett RS, et al. Filovirus RefSeq entries: evaluation and selection of filovirus type variants, type sequences, and names. *Viruses* (2014) 6(9):3663–82. doi:10.3390/v6093663
13. Morvan JM, Deubel V, Gounon P, Nakouné E, Barrière P, Murri S, et al. Identification of Ebola virus sequences present as RNA or DNA in organs of terrestrial small mammals of the Central African Republic. *Microbes Infect* (1999) 1:1193–201. doi:10.1016/S1286-4579(99)00242-7
14. Rosales-Mendoza S, Nieto-Gómez R, Angulo C. A perspective on the development of plant-made vaccines in the fight against Ebola virus. *Front Immunol* (2017) 8:252. doi:10.3389/fimmu.2017.00252
15. Varkey JB, Shantha JG, Crozier I, Kraft CS, Lyon GM, Mehta AK, et al. Persistence of Ebola virus in ocular fluid during convalescence. Persistence of Ebola virus in ocular fluid during. *N Engl J Med* (2015) 372(25):2423–7. doi:10.1056/NEJMoa1500306
16. Uyeki TM, Erickson BR, Brown S, McElroy AK, Cannon D, Gibbons A, et al. Ebola virus persistence in semen of male survivors. *Clin Infect Dis* (2016) 62(12):1552–5. doi:10.1093/cid/ciw202
17. Black BO, Caluwaerts S, Achar J. Ebola viral disease and pregnancy. *Obstet Med* (2015) 8(3):108–13. doi:10.1177/1753495X15597354
18. Barnes KG, Kindrachuk J, Lin AE, Wohl S, Qu J, Tostenson SD, et al. Evidence of Ebola virus replication and high concentration in semen of a patient during recovery. *Clin Infect Dis* (2017) 65(8):1400–3. doi:10.1093/cid/cix518
19. Falasca L, Agrati C, Petrosillo N, Di Caro A, Capobianchi MR, Ippolito G, et al. Molecular mechanisms of Ebola virus pathogenesis: focus on cell death. *Cell Death Differ* (2015) 22:1250–9. doi:10.1038/cdd.2015.67
20. He F, Melén K, Maljanen S, Lundberg R, Jiang M, Österlund P, et al. Ebolavirus protein VP24 interferes with innate immune responses by inhibiting interferon-λ1 gene expression. *Virology* (2017) 509:23–34. doi:10.1016/j.virol.2017.06.002
21. Babalola MO. The strengths, weaknesses, opportunities, and threats (SWOTS) analyses of the Ebola virus – paper retracted. *Afr J Infect Dis* (2016) 10(2): 69–88. doi:10.21010/ajid.v10i2.2
22. Banadyga L, Wong G, Qiu X. Small animal models for evaluating filovirus countermeasures. *ACS Infect Dis* (2018). doi:10.1021/acsinfecdis.7b00266
23. Hiatt A, Pauly M, Whaley K, Qiu X, Kobinger G, Zeitlin L. The emergence of antibody therapies for Ebola. *Hum Antibodies* (2015) 23(3–4):49–56. doi:10.3233/HAB-150284
24. Moekotte AL, Huson MA, van der Ende AJ, Agnandji ST, Huizenga E, Goorhuis A, et al. Monoclonal antibodies for the treatment of Ebola virus disease. *Expert Opin Investig Drugs* (2016) 25(11):1325–35. doi:10.1080/13543784.2016.1240785
25. Mendoza EJ, Racine T, Kobinger GP. The ongoing evolution of antibody-based treatments for Ebola virus infection. *Immunotherapy* (2017) 9(5):435–50. doi:10.2217/imt-2017-0010

26. Wu W, Liu S. The drug targets and antiviral molecules for treatment of Ebola virus infection. *Curr Top Med Chem* (2017) 17(3):361–70. doi:10.2174/1568026616666160829161318
27. Marzi A, Yoshida R, Miyamoto H, Ishijima M, Suzuki Y, Higuchi M, et al. Protective efficacy of neutralizing monoclonal antibodies in a nonhuman primate model of Ebola hemorrhagic fever. *PLoS One* (2012) 7:e36192. doi:10.1371/journal.pone.0036192
28. Olinger GG Jr, Pettitt J, Kim D, Working C, Bohorov O, Bratcher B, et al. Delayed treatment of Ebola virus infection with plant-derived monoclonal antibodies provides protection in rhesus macaques. *Proc Natl Acad Sci U S A* (2012) 109:18030–5. doi:10.1073/pnas.1213709109
29. Qiu X, Audet J, Wong G, Pillet S, Bello A, Cabral T, et al. Successful treatment of Ebola virus-infected cynomolgus macaques with monoclonal antibodies. *Sci Transl Med* (2012) 4(138):138ra81. doi:10.1126/scitranslmed.3003876
30. Qiu X, Wong G, Audet J, Bello A, Fernando L, Alimonti JB, et al. Reversion of advanced Ebola virus disease in nonhuman primates with ZMapp. *Nature* (2014) 514(7520):47–53. doi:10.1038/nature13777
31. Kanapathipillai R, Henao Restrepo AM, Fast P, Wood D, Dye C, Kieny M-P, et al. Ebola vaccine — an urgent international priority. *New Engl J Med* (2014) 371:2249–51. doi:10.1056/NEJMp1412166
32. Houlihan CF, Youkee D, Brown CS. Novel surveillance methods for the control of Ebola virus disease. *Int Health* (2017) 9(3):139–41. doi:10.1093/inthealth/ihx010
33. Joffe S. Evaluating novel therapies during the Ebola epidemic. *JAMA* (2014) 312:1299–300. doi:10.1001/jama.2014.12867
34. Rios-Huerta R, Monreal-Escalante E, Govea-Alonso DO, Angulo C, Rosales-Mendoza S. Expression of an immunogenic LTB-based chimeric protein targeting Zaire ebolavirus epitopes from GP1 in plant cells. *Plant Cell Rep* (2017) 36(2):355–65. doi:10.1007/s00299-016-2088-6
35. Sharmin R, Islam AB. A highly conserved WDYPKCDRA epitope in the RNA directed RNA polymerase of human coronaviruses can be used as epitope-based universal vaccine design. *BMC Bioinformatics* (2014) 15(161):1471–2105. doi:10.1186/1471-2105-15-161
36. Dash R, Das R, Junaid M, Akash MFC, Islam A, Hosen SMZ. *In-silico* based vaccine design against Ebola virus glycoprotein. *Adv Appl Bioinform Chem* (2017) 10:11–28. doi:10.2147/AABC.S115859
37. Gera P, Gupta A, Verma P, Singh J, Gupta J. Recent advances in vaccine development against Ebola threat as bioweapon. *Virus disease* (2017) 28(3):242–6. doi:10.1007/s13337-017-0398-0
38. Medaglini D, Siegrist CA. Immunomonitoring of human responses to the rVSV-ZEBOV Ebola vaccine. *Curr Opin Virol* (2017) 23:88–94. doi:10.1016/j.coviro.2017.03.008
39. Mate SE, Kugelman JR, Nyenswah TG, Ladner JT, Wiley MR, Cordier-Lassalle T, et al. Molecular evidence of sexual transmission of Ebola virus. *N Engl J Med* (2015) 373(25):2448–54. doi:10.1056/NEJMoa1509773
40. Sissoko D, Duraffour S, Kerber R, Kolie JS, Beavogui AH, Camara AM, et al. Persistence and clearance of Ebola virus RNA from seminal fluid of Ebola virus disease survivors: a longitudinal analysis and modelling study. *Lancet Glob Health* (2017) 5(1):e80–8. doi:10.1016/S2214-109X(16)30243-1
41. Osterholm M, Moore K, Ostrowsky J, Kimball-Baker K, Farrar J, Wellcome Trust CEVTB. The Ebola Vaccine Team B: a model for promoting the rapid development of medical countermeasures for emerging infectious disease threats. *Lancet Infect Dis* (2016) 16:e1–9. doi:10.1016/S1473-3099(15)00416-8
42. Oany AR, Sharmin T, Chowdhury AS, Jyoti TP, Hasan MA. Highly conserved regions in Ebola virus RNA dependent RNA polymerase may be act as a universal novel peptide vaccine target: a computational approach. *In silico Pharmacol* (2015) 3(1):7. doi:10.1186/s40203-015-0011-4
43. Yasmin T, Nabi AH. B and T cell epitope-based peptides predicted from evolutionarily conserved and whole protein sequences of Ebola virus as vaccine targets. *Scand J Immunol* (2016) 83(5):321–37. doi:10.1111/sji.12425
44. Konduru K, Shurtleff AC, Bradfute SB, Nakamura S, Bavari S, Kaplan G. Ebolavirus glycoprotein Fc fusion protein protects guinea pigs against lethal challenge. *PLoS One* (2016) 11(9):e0162446. doi:10.1371/journal.pone.0162446
45. Merler S, Ajelli M, Fumanelli L, Parlamento S, Pastore Y, Piontti A, et al. Containing Ebola at the source with ring vaccination. *PLoS Negl Trop Dis* (2016) 10(11):e0005093. doi:10.1371/journal.pntd.0005093
46. Cook JD, Lee JE. The secret life of viral entry glycoproteins: moonlighting in immune evasion. *PLoS Pathog* (2013) 9(5):e1003258. doi:10.1371/journal.ppat.1003258
47. Cazares LH, Ward MD, Brueggemann EE, Kenny T, Demond P, Mahone CR, et al. Development of a liquid chromatography high resolution mass spectrometry method for the quantitation of viral envelope glycoprotein in Ebola virus-like particle vaccine preparations. *Clin Proteomics* (2016) 13(1):18. doi:10.1186/s12014-016-9119-8
48. Walsh PD, Kurup D, Hasselschwert DL, Wirblich C, Goetzmann JE, Schnell MJ. The final (oral Ebola) vaccine trial on captive Chimpanzees. *Sci Rep* (2017) 7:43339. doi:10.1038/srep43339
49. Meyer M, Huang E, Yuzhakov O, Ramanathan P, Ciaramella G, Bukreyev A. Modified mRNA-based vaccines elicit robust immune responses and protect guinea pigs from Ebola virus disease. *J Infect Dis* (2018) 217(3):451–5. doi:10.1093/infdis/jix592
50. Lambe T, Bowyer G, Ewer KJ. A review of phase I trials of Ebola virus vaccines: what can we learn from the race to develop novel vaccines? *Phil Trans R Soc B* (2016) 372:20160295. doi:10.1098/rstb.2016.0295
51. Walldorf JA, Cloessner EA, Hyde TB, MacNeil A; CDC Emergency Ebola Vaccine Taskforce. Considerations for use of Ebola vaccine during an emergency response. *Vaccine* (2017). doi:10.1016/j.vaccine.2017.08.058
52. Blaney JE, Wirblich C, Papaneri AB, Johnson RF, Myers CJ, Juelich TL, et al. Inactivated or live-attenuated bivalent vaccines that confer protection against rabies and Ebola viruses. *J Virol* (2011) 85(20):10605–16. doi:10.1128/JVI.00558-11
53. Lupton HW, Lambert RD, Bumgardner DL, Moe JB, Eddy GA. Inactivated vaccine for Ebola virus efficacious in guineapig model. *Lancet* (1980) 2(8207):1294–5. doi:10.1016/S0140-6736(80)92352-1
54. Rao M, Bray M, Alving CR, Jahrling P, Matyas GR. Induction of immune responses in mice and monkeys to Ebola virus after immunization with liposome-encapsulated irradiated Ebola virus: protection in mice requires CD4(+) T cells. *J Virol* (2002) 76(18):9176–85. doi:10.1128/JVI.76.18.9176-9185.2002
55. Ohimain EI. Recent advances in the development of vaccines for Ebola virus disease. *Virus Res* (2016) 211:174–85. doi:10.1016/j.virusres.2015.10.021
56. Martin JE, Sullivan NJ, Enama ME, Gordon IJ, Roederer M, Koup RA, et al. A DNA vaccine for Ebola virus is safe and immunogenic in a phase I clinical trial. *Clin Vaccine Immunol* (2006) 13(11):1267–77. doi:10.1128/CVI.00162-06
57. Patel A, Scott V, Wong G, Reuschel E, Villarreal D, Muthumani K, et al. A single immunization with optimized DNA vaccines protects against lethal Ebola virus challenge in mice (VAC8P.1057). *J Immunol* (2015) 194(1 Suppl):144.13.
58. Vastag B. Ebola vaccines tested in humans, monkeys. *JAMA* (2004) 291:549–50. doi:10.1001/jama.291.5.549
59. Grant-Klein RJ, Altamura LA, Badger CV, Bounds CE, Van Deusen NM, Kwilas SA, et al. Codon-optimized filovirus DNA vaccines delivered by intramuscular electroporation protect cynomolgus macaques from lethal Ebola and Marburg virus challenges. *Hum Vaccin Immunother* (2015) 11(8):1991–2004. doi:10.1080/21645515.2015.1039757
60. Kibuuka H, Berkowitz NM, Millard M, Enama ME, Tindikahwa A, Sekiziyivu AB, et al. Safety and immunogenicity of Ebola virus and Marburg virus glycoprotein DNA vaccines assessed separately and concomitantly in healthy Ugandan adults: a phase 1b, randomised, double-blind, placebo-controlled clinical trial. *Lancet* (2015) 385(9977):1545–54. doi:10.1016/S0140-6736(14)62385-0
61. Sarwar UN, Costner P, Enama ME, Berkowitz N, Hu Z, Hendel CS, et al. Safety and immunogenicity of DNA vaccines encoding Ebola virus and Marburg virus wild-type glycoproteins in a phase I clinical trial. *J Infect Dis* (2015) 211(4):549–57. doi:10.1093/infdis/jiu511
62. Warfield KL, Posten NA, Swenson DL, Olinger GG, Esposito D, Gillette WK, et al. Filovirus-like particles produced in insect cells: immunogenicity and protection in rodents. *J Infect Dis* (2007) 196(Suppl 2):S421–9. doi:10.1086/520612
63. Carra JH, Martins KAO, Schokman RD, Robinson CG, Steffens JT, Bavari S. A thermostable, chromatographically purified Ebola nano-VLP vaccine. *J Transl Med* (2015) 13:228. doi:10.1186/s12967-015-0593-y

64. Warfield KL, Perkins JG, Swenson DL, Deal EM, Bosio CM, Aman MJ, et al. Role of natural killer cells in innate protection against lethal Ebola virus infection. *J Exp Med* (2004) 200(2):169–79. doi:10.1084/jem.20032141
65. Rizk MG, Basler CF, Guatelli J. Cooperation of the Ebola virus proteins VP40 and GP1,2 with BST2 to activate NF-κB independently of virus-like particle trapping. *J Virol* (2017) 91(22):e1308–17. doi:10.1128/JVI.01308-17
66. Cooper CL, Martins KA, Stronsky SM, Langan DP, Steffens J, Van Tongeren S, et al. T-cell-dependent mechanisms promote Ebola VLP-induced antibody responses, but are dispensable for vaccine-mediated protection. *Emerg Microbes Infect* (2017) 6(6):e46. doi:10.1038/emi.2017.31
67. Reynolds P, Marzi A. Ebola and Marburg virus vaccines. *Virus Genes* (2017) 53(4):501–15. doi:10.1007/s11262-017-1455-x
68. Herbert AS, Kuehne AI, Barth JF, Ortiz RA, Nichols DK, Zak SE, et al. Venezuelan equine encephalitis virus replicon particle vaccine protects nonhuman primates from intramuscular and aerosol challenge with ebolavirus. *J Virol* (2013) 87(9):4952–64. doi:10.1128/JVI.03361-12
69. Ren S, Wei Q, Cai L, Yang X, Xing C, Tan F, et al. Alphavirus replicon DNA vectors expressing Ebola GP and VP40 antigens induce humoral and cellular immune responses in mice. *Front Microbiol* (2018) 8:2662. doi:10.3389/fmicb.2017.02662
70. Halfmann P, Kim JH, Ebihara H, Noda T, Neumann G, Feldmann H, et al. Generation of biologically contained Ebola viruses. *Proc Natl Acad Sci U S A* (2008) 105(4):1129–33. doi:10.1073/pnas.0708057105
71. Halfmann P, Ebihara H, Marzi A, Hatta Y, Watanabe S, Suresh M, et al. Replication-deficient ebolavirus as a vaccine candidate. *J Virol* (2009) 83(8):3810–5. doi:10.1128/JVI.00074-09
72. Marzi A, Halfmann P, Hill-Batorski L, Feldmann F, Shupert WL, Neumann G, et al. An Ebola whole-virus vaccine is protective in nonhuman primates. *Science* (2015) 348(6233):439–42. doi:10.1126/science.aaa4919
73. Sameem R, Dias S. Ebola virus: promising vaccine candidates. *Vaccination Res* (2017) 1(1):33–8. doi:10.1080/21645515.2016.1225637
74. Geisbert TW, Feldmann H. Recombinant vesicular stomatitis virus-based vaccines against Ebola and Marburg virus infections. *J Infect Dis* (2011) 204(Suppl 3):S1075–81. doi:10.1093/infdis/jir349
75. Wong G, Qiu X. Designing efficacious vesicular stomatitis virus-vectored vaccines against Ebola virus. *Methods Mol Biol* (2016) 1403:245–57. doi:10.1007/978-1-4939-3387-7_12
76. Wit ED, Marzi A, Bushmaker T, Brining D, Scott D, Richt JA, et al. Safety of recombinant VSV–Ebola virus vaccine vector in pigs. *Emerg Infect Dis* (2015) 21(4):702–4. doi:10.3201/eid2104.142012
77. Halperin SA, Arribas JR, Rupp R, Andrews CP, Chu L, Das R, et al. Six-month safety data of recombinant vesicular stomatitis virus-Zaire Ebola virus envelope glycoprotein vaccine in a phase 3 double-blind, placebo-controlled randomized study in healthy adults. *J Infect Dis* (2017) 215(12):1789–98. doi:10.1093/infdis/jix189
78. Geisbert TW, Daddario-Dicaprio KM, Lewis MG, Geisbert JB, Grolla A, Leung A, et al. Vesicular stomatitis virus-based Ebola vaccine is well-tolerated and protects immunocompromised nonhuman primates. *PLoS Pathog* (2008) 4(11):e1000225. doi:10.1371/journal.ppat.1000225
79. Marzi A, Murphy AA, Feldmann F, Parkins CJ, Haddock E, Hanley PW, et al. Cytomegalovirus-based vaccine expressing Ebola virus glycoprotein protects nonhuman primates from Ebola virus infection. *Sci Rep* (2016) 6:21674. doi:10.1038/srep21674
80. Venkatraman N, Silman D, Folegatti PM, Hill AVS. Vaccines against Ebola virus. *Vaccine* (2017). doi:10.1016/j.vaccine.2017.07.054
81. Henao-Restrepo A, Camacho A, Longini IM, Watson CH, Edmunds WJ, Egger M, et al. Efficacy and effectiveness of an rVSV-vectored vaccine in preventing Ebola virus disease: final results from the Guinea ring vaccination, open-label, cluster-randomized trial (Ebola Ca Suffit!). *Lancet* (2017) 389(10068):505–18. doi:10.1016/S0140-6736(16)32621-6
82. Regules JA, Beigel JH, Paolino KM, Voell J, Castellano AR, Hu Z, et al. A recombinant vesicular stomatitis virus Ebola vaccine. *N Engl J Med* (2017) 376:330–41. doi:10.1056/NEJMoa1414216
83. Folayan MO, Yakubu A, Haire B, Peterson K. Ebola vaccine development plan: ethics, concerns and proposed measures. *BMC Med Ethics* (2016) 17:10. doi:10.1186/s12910-016-0094-4
84. Trad MA, Naughton W, Yeung A, Mazlin L, O'sullivan M, Gilroy N, et al. Ebola virus disease: an update on current prevention and management strategies. *J Clin Virol* (2017) 86:5–13. doi:10.1016/j.jcv.2016.11.005
85. Wang D, Raja NU, Trubey CM, Juompan LY, Luo M, Woraratanadharm J, et al. Development of a cAdVax-based bivalent Ebola virus vaccine that induces immune responses against both the Sudan and Zaire species of Ebola virus. *J Virol* (2006) 80(6):2738–46. doi:10.1128/JVI.80.6.2738-2746.2006
86. Wang SR, Zhang QY, Wang JQ, Ge XY, Song YY, Wang YF, et al. Chemical targeting of a G-quadruplex RNA in the Ebola virus L gene. *Cell Chem Biol* (2016) 23(9):1113–22. doi:10.1016/j.chembiol.2016.07.019
87. Dolzhikova IV, Zubkova OV, Tukhvatulin AI, Dzharullaeva AS, Tukhvatulina NM, Shcheblyakov DV, et al. Safety and immunogenicity of GamEvac-Combi, a heterologous VSV- and Ad5-vectored Ebola vaccine: an open phase I/II trial in healthy adults in Russia. *Hum Vaccin Immunother* (2017) 13(3):613–20. doi:10.1080/21645515.2016.1238535
88. Zhu FC, Hou LH, Li JX, Wu SP, Liu P, Zhang GR, et al. Safety and immunogenicity of a novel recombinant adenovirus type-5 vector-based Ebola vaccine in healthy adults in China: preliminary report of a randomised, double-blind, placebo-controlled, phase 1 trial. *Lancet* (2015) 385(9984): 2272–9. doi:10.1016/S0140-6736(15)60553-0
89. Wong G, Mendoza EJ, Plummer FA, Gao GF, Kobinger GP, Qiu X. From bench to almost bedside: the long road to a licensed Ebola virus vaccine. *Expert Opin Biol Ther* (2018) 18(2):159–73. doi:10.1080/14712598.2018.1404572
90. Chen T, Li D, Song Y, Yang X, Liu Q, Jin X, et al. A heterologous prime-boost Ebola virus vaccine regimen induces durable neutralizing antibody response and prevents Ebola virus-like particle entry in mice. *Antiviral Res* (2017) 145:54–9. doi:10.1016/j.antiviral.2017.07.009
91. Ledgerwood JE, DeZure AD, Stanley DA, Coates EE, Novik L, Enama ME, et al. Chimpanzee adenovirus vector Ebola vaccine. *N Engl J Med* (2017) 376(10):928–38. doi:10.1056/NEJMoa1410863
92. Wong G, Qiu X, Ebihara H, Feldmann H, Kobinger GP. Characterization of a bivalent vaccine capable of inducing protection against both Ebola and cross-clade H5N1 influenza in mice. *J Infect Dis* (2015) 212(Suppl 2): S435–42. doi:10.1093/infdis/jiv257
93. Ewer K, Rampling T, Venkatraman N, Bowyer G, Wright D, Lambe T, et al. A monovalent chimpanzee adenovirus Ebola vaccine boosted with MVA. *New Engl J Med* (2016) 374(17):1635–46. doi:10.1056/NEJMoa1411627
94. Milligan ID, Gibani MM, Sewell R, Clutterbuck EA, Campbell D, Plested E, et al. Safety and immunogenicity of novel adenovirus type 26- and modified vaccinia Ankara-vectored Ebola vaccines: a randomized clinical trial. *JAMA* (2016) 315(15):1610–23. doi:10.1001/jama.2016.4218
95. Schweneker M, Laimbacher AS, Zimmer G, Wagner S, Schraner EM, Wolferstätter M, et al. Recombinant modified vaccinia virus Ankara generating Ebola virus-like particles. *J Virol* (2017) 91(12). doi:10.1128/JVI.00343-17
96. Bengtsson KL, Song H, Stertman L, Liu Y, Flyer DC, Massare MJ, et al. Matrix-M adjuvant enhances antibody, cellular and protective immune responses of a Zaire Ebola/Makona virus glycoprotein (GP) nanoparticle vaccine in mice. *Vaccine* (2016) 34(16):1927–35. doi:10.1016/j.vaccine.2016.02.033
97. Meyer M, Garron T, Lubaki NM, Mire CE, Fenton KA, Klages C, et al. Aerosolized Ebola vaccine protects primates and elicits lung-resident T cell responses. *J Clin Invest* (2015) 125(8):3241–55. doi:10.1172/JCI81532
98. De Santis O, Audran R, Pothin E, Warpelin-Decrausaz L, Vallotton L, Wuerzner G, et al. Safety and immunogenicity of a chimpanzee adenovirus-vectored Ebola vaccine in healthy adults: a randomised, double-blind, placebo controlled, dose-finding, phase 1/2a study. *Lancet Infect Dis* (2016) 16(3):311–20. doi:10.1016/S1473-3099(15)00486-7
99. Sullivan NJ, Geisbert TW, Geisbert JB, Shedlock DJ, Xu L, Lamoreaux L, et al. Immune protection of nonhuman primates against Ebola virus with single low-dose adenovirus vectors encoding modified GPs. *PLoS Med* (2006) 3(6):e177. doi:10.1371/journal.pmed.0030177
100. Budzianowski J. Tobacco against Ebola virus disease. *Przegl Lek* (2015) 72(10):567–71.
101. Phoolcharoen W. *Plant-Produced Ebola Immune Complex as an Ebola Vaccine Candidate*. Ph.D. thesis. Arizona State University (2010).
102. Monreal-Escalante E, Ramos-Vega AA, Salazar-González JA, Bañuelos-Hernández B, Angulo C, Rosales-Mendoza S. Expression of the VP40 antigen from the Zaire ebolavirus in tobacco plants. *Planta* (2017) 246(1):123–32. doi:10.1007/s00425-017-2689-5
103. Zeitlin L, Pettitt J, Scully C, Bohorova N, Kim D, Pauly M, et al. Enhanced potency of a fucose-free monoclonal antibody being developed as an Ebola

virus immunoprotectant. *Proc Natl Acad Sci U S A* (2011) 108(51):20690–4. doi:10.1073/pnas.1108360108

104. Laere E, Ling APK, Wong YP, Koh RY, Lila MAM, Hussein S. Plant-based vaccines: production and challenges. *J Botany* (2016) 2016:1–11. doi:10.1155/2016/4928637
105. Huang Z, Phoolcharoen W, Lai H, Piensook K, Cardineau G, Zeitlin L, et al. High-level rapid production of full-size monoclonal antibodies in plants by a single-vector DNA replicon system. *Biotechnol Bioeng* (2010) 106:9–17. doi:10.1002/bit.22652
106. Dhama K, Wani MY, Deb R, Karthik K, Tiwari R, Barathidasan R, et al. Plant based oral vaccines for human and animal pathogens – a new era of prophylaxis: current and future perspectives. *J Exp Biol Agric Sci* (2013) 1(1): 1–12. doi:10.1177/2051013615613272
107. Kopertekh L, Schiemann J. Transient production of recombinant pharmaceutical proteins in plants: evolution and perspectives. *Curr Med Chem* (2017). doi:10.2174/0929867324666170718114724
108. Johnson RF, Kurup D, Hagen KR, Fisher C, Keshwara R, Papaneri A, et al. An inactivated rabies virus-based Ebola vaccine, filorab1, adjuvanted with glucopyranosyl lipid A in stable emulsion confers complete protection in nonhuman primate challenge models. *J Infect Dis* (2016) 214(Suppl 3):S342–54. doi:10.1093/infdis/jiw231
109. Blaney JE, Marzi A, Willet M, Papaneri AB, Wirblich C, Feldmann F, et al. Antibody quality and protection from lethal Ebola virus challenge in nonhuman primates immunized with rabies virus based bivalent vaccine. *PLoS Pathog* (2013) 9(5):e1003389. doi:10.1371/journal.ppat.1003389
110. Grant-Klein RJ, Van Deusen NM, Badger CV, Hannaman D, Dupuy LC, Schmaljohn CS. A multiagent filovirus DNA vaccine delivered by intramuscular electroporation completely protects mice from Ebola and Marburg virus challenge. *Hum Vaccin Immunother* (2012) 8(11):1703–6. doi:10.4161/hv.21873
111. Shedlock DJ, Aviles J, Talbott KT, Wong G, Wu SJ, Villarreal DO, et al. Induction of broad cytotoxic T cells by protective DNA vaccination against Marburg and Ebola. *Mol Ther* (2013) 21(7):1432–44. doi:10.1038/mt.2013.61
112. Warfield KL, Bosio CM, Welcher BC, Deal EM, Mohamadzadeh M, Schmaljohn A, et al. Ebola virus-like particles protect from lethal Ebola virus infection. *Proc Natl Acad Sci U S A* (2003) 100(26):15889–94. doi:10.1073/pnas.2237038100
113. Swenson DL, Warfield KL, Negley DL, Schmaljohn A, Aman MJ, Bavari S. Virus-like particles exhibit potential as a pan-filovirus vaccine for both Ebola and Marburg viral infections. *Vaccine* (2005) 23(23):3033–42. doi:10.1016/j.vaccine.2004.11.070
114. Warfield KL, Swenson DL, Olinger GG, Kalina WV, Aman MJ, Bavari S. Ebola virus-like particle-based vaccine protects nonhuman primates against lethal Ebola virus challenge. *J Infect Dis* (2007) 196(Suppl 2):S430–7. doi:10.1086/520583
115. Domi A, Feldmann F, Basu R, McCurley N, Shifflett K, Emanuel J, et al. A single dose of modified vaccinia Ankara expressing Ebola virus like particles protects nonhuman primates from lethal Ebola virus challenge. *Sci Rep* (2018) 8:864. doi:10.1038/s41598-017-19041-y
116. Pushko P, Bray M, Ludwig GV, Parker M, Schmaljohn A, Sanchez A, et al. Recombinant RNA replicons derived from attenuated Venezuelan equine encephalitis virus protect guinea pigs and mice from Ebola hemorrhagic fever virus. *Vaccine* (2000) 19(1):142–53. doi:10.1016/S0264-410X(00)00113-4
117. Tsuda Y, Caposio P, Parkins CJ, Botto S, Messaoudi I, Cicin-Sain L, et al. A replicating cytomegalovirus-based vaccine encoding a single Ebola virus nucleoprotein CTL epitope confers protection against Ebola virus. *PLoS Negl Trop Dis* (2011) 5(8):e1275. doi:10.1371/journal.pntd.0001275
118. Reynard O, Mokhonov V, Mokhonova E, Leung J, Page A, Mateo M, et al. Kunjin virus replicon-based vaccines expressing Ebola virus glycoprotein GP protect the guinea pig against lethal Ebola virus infection. *J Infect Dis* (2011) 204(Suppl 3):S1060–5. doi:10.1093/infdis/jir347
119. Bukreyev AA, Dinapoli JM, Yang L, Murphy BR, Collins PL. Mucosal parainfluenza virus-vectored vaccine against Ebola virus replicates in the respiratory tract of vector-immune monkeys and is immunogenic. *Virology* (2010) 399(2):290–8. doi:10.1016/j.virol.2010.01.015
120. DiNapoli JM, Yang L, Samal SK, Murphy BR, Collins PL, Bukreyev A. Respiratory tract immunization of non-human primates with a Newcastle disease virus-vectored vaccine candidate against Ebola virus elicits a neutralizing antibody response. *Vaccine* (2010) 29(1):17–25. doi:10.1016/j.vaccine.2010.10.024
121. Ledgerwood JE, Costner P, Desai N, Holman L, Enama ME, Yamshchikov G, et al. A replication defective recombinant Ad5 vaccine expressing Ebola virus GP is safe and immunogenic in healthy adults. *Vaccine* (2010) 29(2):304–13. doi:10.1016/j.vaccine.2010.10.037
122. Agnandji ST, Huttner A, Zinser ME, Njuguna P, Dahlke C, Fernandes JF, et al. Phase 1 trials of rVSV Ebola vaccine in Africa and Europe. *N Engl J Med* (2016) 374:1647–60. doi:10.1056/NEJMoa1502924
123. Cardile AP, Downey LG, Wiseman PD, Warren TK, Bavari S. Antiviral therapeutics for the treatment of Ebola virus infection. *Curr Opin Pharmacol* (2016) 30:138–43. doi:10.1016/j.coph.2016.08.016
124. Bishop BM. Potential and emerging treatment options for Ebola virus disease. *Ann Pharmacother* (2015) 49(2):196–206. doi:10.1177/1060028014561227
125. Shao X, Ren W, Zhou F. Clinical presentation and care for patients with Ebola virus disease in China Ebola treatment unit, Liberia. *Jpn J Infect Dis* (2016) 70(1):32–7. doi:10.7883/yoken.JJID.2015.597
126. Madariaga MG. Ebola virus disease: a perspective for the United States. *Am J Med* (2015) 128(7):682–91. doi:10.1016/j.amjmed.2015.01.035
127. Choi JH, Croyle MA. Emerging targets and novel approaches to Ebola virus prophylaxis and treatment. *Bio Drugs* (2013) 27(6):565–83. doi:10.1007/s40259-013-0046-1
128. Kilgore PE, Grabenstein JD, Salim AM, Rybak M. Treatment of Ebola virus disease. *Pharmacotherapy* (2015) 35:43–53. doi:10.1002/phar.1545
129. Smither SJ, Eastaugh LS, Steward JA, Nelson M, Lenk RP, Lever MS. Post-exposure efficacy of oral T-705 (Favipiravir) against inhalational Ebola virus infection in a mouse model. *Antiviral Res* (2014) 104:153–5. doi:10.1016/j.antiviral.2014.01.012
130. Duraffour S, Malvy D, Sissoko D. How to treat Ebola virus infections? A lesson from the field. *Curr Opin Virol* (2017) 24:9–15. doi:10.1016/j.coviro.2017.03.003
131. Zhang T, Zhai M, Ji J, Zhang J, Tian Y, Liu X. Recent progress on the treatment of Ebola virus disease with Favipiravir and other related strategies. *Bioorg Med Chem Lett* (2017) 27(11):2364–8. doi:10.1016/j.bmcl.2017.04.028
132. Cheng F, Murray JL, Zhao J, Sheng J, Zhao Z, Rubin DH. Systems biology-based investigation of cellular antiviral drug targets identified by gene-trap insertional mutagenesis. *PLoS Comput Biol* (2016) 12:e1005074. doi:10.1371/journal.pcbi.1005074
133. Ahmad N, Farman A, Badshah SL, Ur Rahman A, Ur Rashid H, Khan K. Molecular modeling, simulation and docking study of Ebola virus glycoprotein. *J Mol Graph Model* (2016) 72:266–71. doi:10.1016/j.jmgm.2016.12.010
134. Alam El-Din HM, Loutfy SA, Fathy N, Elberry MH, Mayla AM, Kassem S, et al. Molecular docking based screening of compounds against VP40 from Ebola virus. *Bioinformation* (2016) 12:192–6. doi:10.6026/97320630012192
135. Yates MK, Raje MR, Chatterjee P, Spiropoulou CF, Bavari S, Flint M, et al. Flex-nucleoside analogues – novel therapeutics against filoviruses. *Bioorg Med Chem Lett* (2017) 27(12):2800–2. doi:10.1016/j.bmcl.2017.04.069
136. Alfson KJ, Worwa G, Carrion R Jr, Griffiths A. Determination and therapeutic exploitation of Ebola virus spontaneous mutation frequency. *J Virol* (2015) 90(5):2345–55. doi:10.1128/JVI.02701-15
137. Tseng CP, Chan YJ. Overview of Ebola virus disease in 2014. *J Chin Med Assoc* (2015) 78:51–5. doi:10.1016/j.jcma.2014.11.007
138. AllAfrica. (2014). Available from: http://allafrica.com/stories/201409292050.html (Accessed: March, 2018).
139. Cong Y, Dyall J, Hart BJ, DeWald LE, Johnson JC, Postnikova E, et al. Evaluation of the activity of lamivudine and zidovudine against Ebola virus. *PLoS One* (2016) 11(11):e0166318. doi:10.1371/journal.pone.0166318
140. Hensley LE, Dyall J, Olinger GG, Jahrling PB. Lack of effect of lamivudine on Ebola virus replication. *Emerg Infect Dis* (2015) 21(3):550–2. doi:10.3201/eid2103.141862
141. Raj U, Varadwaj PK. Flavonoids as multi-target inhibitors for proteins associated with Ebola virus: *in silico* discovery using virtual screening and molecular docking studies. *Interdiscip Sci* (2016) 8(2):142. doi:10.1007/s12539-015-0125-8
142. Bradfute SB. The early clinical development of Ebola virus treatments. *Expert Opin Investig Drugs* (2017) 26(1):1–4. doi:10.1080/13543784.2017.1260545

143. Pokhrel R, Jeevan GC, Bhattarai N, Chapagain P, Gerstman B. Potential disruption of Ebola virus matrix by graphene nano-sheets. *Biophysical J* (2018) 114(3):218a. doi:10.1016/j.bpj.2017.11.1217
144. Shtanko O, Sakurai Y, Reyes AN, Noel R, Cintrat JC, Gillet D, et al. Retro-2 and its dihydroquinazolinone derivatives inhibit filovirus infection. *Antiviral Res* (2018) 149:154–63. doi:10.1016/j.antiviral.2017.11.016
145. Qiu S, Leung A, Bo Y, Kozak RA, Anand SP, Warkentin C, et al. Ebola virus requires phosphatidylinositol (3,5) bisphosphate production for efficient viral entry. *Virology* (2018) 513:17–28. doi:10.1016/j.virol.2017.09.028
146. Nelson EA, Dyall J, Hoenen T, Barnes AB, Zhou H, Liang JY, et al. The phosphatidylinositol-3-phosphate 5-kinase inhibitor apilimod blocks filoviral entry and infection. *PLoS Negl Trop Dis* (2017) 11(4):e0005540. doi:10.1371/journal.pntd.0005540
147. Jerebtsova M, Nekhai S. Therapeutics for postexposure treatment of Ebola virus infection. *Future Virol* (2015) 10(3):221–32. doi:10.2217/fvl.14.109
148. Biedenkopf N, Lange-Grunweller K, Schulte FW, Weißer A, Müller C, Becker D, et al. The natural compound silvestrol is a potent inhibitor of Ebola virus replication. *Antiviral Res* (2017) 137:76–81. doi:10.1016/j.antiviral.2016.11.011
149. Yuan S, Zhang ZW, Li ZL. Improvements in treatment of children younger than age 5 years infected with Ebola virus. *J Pediatr* (2017) 185:251–2. doi:10.1016/j.jpeds.2017.02.025
150. Dhanda SK, Chaudhary K, Gupta S, Brahmachari SK, Raghava GP. A web-based resource for designing therapeutics against Ebola virus. *Sci Rep* (2016) 6:24782. doi:10.1038/srep24782
151. Matsuno K, Kishida N, Usami K, Igarashi M, Yoshida R, Nakayama E, et al. Different potential of C-type lectin-mediated entry between Marburg virus strains. *J Virol* (2010) 84:5140–7. doi:10.1128/JVI.02021-09
152. Aleksandrowicz P, Marzi A, Biedenkopf N, Beimforde N, Becker S, Hoenen T, et al. Ebola virus enters host cells by macropinocytosis and clathrin-mediated endocytosis. *J Infect Dis* (2011) 204(Suppl 3):S957–67. doi:10.1093/infdis/jir326
153. Miller EH, Obernosterer G, Raaben M, Herbert AS, Deffieu MS, Krishnan A, et al. Ebola virus entry requires the host-programmed recognition of an intracellular receptor. *EMBO J* (2012) 31:1947–60. doi:10.1038/emboj.2012.53
154. Kondratowicz AS, Lennemann NJ, Sinn PL, Davey RA, Hunt CL, Moller-Tank S, et al. T-cell immunoglobulin and mucin domain 1 (TIM-1) is a receptor for Zaire Ebolavirus and Lake Victoria Marburgvirus. *Proc Natl Acad Sci U S A* (2011) 108(20):8426–31. doi:10.1073/pnas.1019030108
155. Côté M, Misasi J, Ren T, Bruchez A, Lee K, Filone CM. Small molecule inhibitors reveal Niemann-Pick C1 is essential for Ebola virus infection. *Nature* (2011) 477(7364):344–8. doi:10.1038/nature10380
156. Sakurai Y, Kolokoltsov AA, Chen CC, Tidwell MW, Bauta WE, Klugbauer N, et al. Two-pore channels control Ebola virus host cell entry and are drug targets for disease treatment. *Science* (2015) 347:995–8. doi:10.1126/science.1258758
157. Johansen LM, Brannan JM, Delos SE, Shoemaker CJ, Stossel A, Lear C, et al. FDA-approved selective estrogen receptor modulators inhibit Ebola virus infection. *Sci Transl Med* (2013) 5:190ra79. doi:10.1126/scitranslmed.3005471
158. Gehring G, Rohrmann K, Atenchong N, Mittler E, Becker S, Dahlmann F, et al. The clinically approved drugs amiodarone, dronedarone and verapamil inhibit filovirus cell entry. *J Antimicrob Chemother* (2014) 69:2123–31. doi:10.1093/jac/dku091
159. Salata C, Munegato D, Martelli F, Parolin C, Calistri A, Baritussio A, et al. Amiodarone affects Ebola virus binding and entry into target cells. *New Microbiol* (2018) 41(2):162–4.
160. Illescas BM, Rojo J, Delgado R, Martín N. Multivalent glycosylated nanostructures to inhibit Ebola virus infection. *J Am Chem Soc* (2017) 139(17):6018–25. doi:10.1021/jacs.7b01683
161. Sun W, He S, Martínez-Romero C, Kouznetsova J, Tawa G, Xu M, et al. Synergistic drug combination effectively blocks Ebola virus infection. *Antiviral Res* (2016) 137:165–72. doi:10.1016/j.antiviral.2016.11.017
162. Anantpadma M, Kouznetsova J, Wang H, Huang R, Kolokoltsov A, Guha R, et al. Large-scale screening and identification of novel Ebola virus and Mardburg virus entry inhibitors. *Antimicrob Agents Chemother* (2016) 60(8):4471–81. doi:10.1128/AAC.00543-16
163. Zhang X, Ao Z, Bello A, Ran X, Liu S, Wigle J, et al. Characterization of the inhibitory effect of an extract of *Prunella vulgaris* on Ebola virus glycoprotein (GP)-mediated virus entry and infection. *Antiviral Res* (2016) 127:20–31. doi:10.1016/j.antiviral.2016.01.001
164. Cheng H, Lear-Rooney CM, Johansen L, Varhegyi E, Chen ZW, Olinger GG, et al. Inhibition of Ebola and Marburg virus entry by G protein-coupled receptor antagonists. *J Virol* (2015) 89(19):9932–8. doi:10.1128/JVI.01337-15
165. Qiu X, Kroeker A, He S, Kozak R, Audet J, Mbikay M, et al. Prophylactic efficacy of quercetin 3-β-O-D-glucoside against Ebola virus infection. *Antimicrob Agents Chemother* (2016) 60(9):5182–8. doi:10.1128/AAC.00307-16
166. Bornholdt ZA, Ndungo E, Fusco ML, Bale S, Flyak AI, Crowe JE Jr, et al. Host-primed Ebola virus GP exposes a hydrophobic NPC1 receptor-binding pocket, revealing a target for broadly neutralizing antibodies. *mBio* (2016) 7(1):e2154–2115. doi:10.1128/mBio.02154-15
167. Nishimura H, Yamaya M. A synthetic serine protease inhibitor, nafamostat mesilate, is a drug potentially applicable to the treatment of Ebola virus disease. *Tohoku J Exp Med* (2015) 237(1):45–50. doi:10.1620/tjem.237.45
168. Li H, Yu F, Xia S, Yu Y, Wang Q, Lv M, et al. Chemically modified human serum albumin potently blocks entry of Ebola pseudoviruses and virus like particles. *Antimicrob Agents Chemother* (2017) 61(4):e2168–2116. doi:10.1128/AAC.02168-16
169. van Griensven J, De Weiggheleire A, Delamou A, Smith PG, Edwards T, Vandekerckhove P, et al. The use of Ebola convalescent plasma to treat Ebola virus disease in resource constrained set-tings: a perspective from the field. *Clin Infect Dis* (2015) 62:69–74. doi:10.1093/cid/civ680
170. Garraud O. Use of convalescent plasma in Ebola virus infection. *Transfus Apher Sci* (2017) 56(1):31–4. doi:10.1016/j.transci.2016.12.014
171. Gulland A. First Ebola treatment is approved by WHO. *British Med J* (2014) 349:g5539. doi:10.1136/bmj.g5539
172. Geisen C, Kann G, Strecker T, Wolf T, Schüttfort G, van Kraaij M, et al. Pathogen-reduced Ebola virus convalescent plasma: first steps towards standardization of manufacturing and quality control including assessment of Ebola-specific neutralizing antibodies. *Vox Sang* (2016) 110(4):329–35. doi:10.1111/vox.12376
173. Dye JM, Herbert AS, Kuehne AI, Barth JF, Muhammad MA, Zak SE, et al. Postexposure antibody prophylaxis protects nonhuman primates from filovirus disease. *Proc Natl Acad Sci U S A* (2012) 109:5034–9. doi:10.1073/pnas.1200409109
174. Saphire EO. An update on the use of antibodies against the filoviruses. *Immunotherapy* (2013) 5:1221–33. doi:10.2217/imt.13.124
175. Corti D, Misasi J, Mulangu S, Stanley DA, Kanekiyo M, Wollen S, et al. Protective monotherapy against lethal Ebola virus infection by a potently neutralizing antibody. *Science* (2016) 351:1339–42. doi:10.1126/science.aad5224
176. Mire CE, Geisbert JB, Agans KN, Thi EP, Lee AC, Fenton KA, et al. Passive immunotherapy: assessment of convalescent serum against Ebola virus Makona infection in nonhuman primates. *J Infect Dis* (2016) 214(S3):S367–74. doi:10.1093/infdis/jiw333
177. Borisevich IV, Chemikova NK, Markov VI, Krasnianskiy VP, Borisevich SV, Rozhdestvenskiy EV. An experience in the clinical use of specific immunoglobulin from horse blood serum for prophylaxis of Ebola haemorrhagic fever. *Vopr Virusol* (2017) 62(1):25–9.
178. Holtsberg FW, Shulenin S, Vu H, Howell KA, Patel SJ, Gunn B, et al. Pan-ebolavirus and pan-filovirus mouse monoclonal antibodies: protection against Ebola and Sudan viruses. *J Virol* (2016) 90(1):266–78. doi:10.1128/JVI.02171-15
179. Zhang Y, Li D, Jin X, Huang Z. Fighting Ebola with ZMapp: spotlight on plant-made antibody. *Sci China Life Sci* (2014) 57:987–8. doi:10.1007/s11427-014-4746-7
180. Dornemann J, Burzio C, Ronsse A, Sprecher A, De Clerck H, Van Herp M, et al. First newborn baby to receive experimental therapies survives Ebola virus disease. *J Infect Dis* (2017) 215(2):171–4. doi:10.1093/infdis/jiw493
181. Hayden FG, Friede M, Bausch DG. Experimental therapies for Ebola virus disease: what have we learned? *J Infect Dis* (2017) 215:167–70. doi:10.1093/infdis/jiw496
182. Wec AZ, Herbert AS, Murin CD, Nyakatura EK, Abelson DM, Fels JM, et al. Antibodies from a human survivor define sites of vulnerability for broad protection against Ebola viruses. *Cell* (2017) 169(5):878.e–90.e. doi:10.1016/j.cell.2017.04.037
183. Duehr J, Wohlbold TJ, Oestereich L, Chromikova V, Amanat F, Rajendran M, et al. Novel cross-reactive monoclonal antibodies against Ebolavirus

glycoproteins show protection in a murine challenge model. *J Virol* (2017) 91(16). doi:10.1128/JVI.00652-17

184. Howell KA, Qiu X, Brannan JM, Bryan C, Davidson E, Holtsberg FW, et al. Antibody treatment of Ebola and Sudan virus infection via a uniquely exposed epitope within the glycoprotein receptor-binding site. *Cell Rep* (2016) 15(7):1514–26. doi:10.1016/j.celrep.2016.04.026
185. Maruyama T, Rodriguez LL, Jahrling PB, Sanchez A, Khan AS, Nichol ST, et al. Ebola virus can be effectively neutralized by antibody produced in natural human infection. *J Virol* (1999) 73(7):6024–30.
186. Parren PWHI, Geisbert TW, Maruyama T, Jahrling PB, Burton DR. Pre- and postexposure prophylaxis of Ebola virus infection in an animal model by passive transfer of a neutralizing human antibody. *J Virol* (2002) 76(12):6408–12 doi:10.1128/JVI.76.12.6408-6412.2002
187. Lee JE, Fusco ML, Hessell AJ, Oswald WB, Burton DR, Saphire EO. Structure of the Ebola virus glycoprotein bound to an antibody from a human survivor. *Nature* (2008) 454(7201):177–82. doi:10.1038/nature07082
188. Howell KA, Brannan JM, Bryan C, McNeal A, Davidson E, Turner HL, et al. Cooperativity enables non-neutralizing antibodies to neutralize Ebolavirus. *Cell Rep* (2017) 19(2):413–24. doi:10.1016/j.celrep.2017.03.049
189. Wec AZ, Nyakatura EK, Herbert AS, Howell KA, Holtsberg FW, Bakken RR, et al. A "Trojan horse" bispecific antibody strategy for broad protection against ebolaviruses. *Science* (2016) 354:350–4. doi:10.1126/science.aag3267
190. Teimoori S, Seesuay W, Jittavisutthikul S, Chaisri U, Sookrung N, Densumite J, et al. Human transbodies to VP40 inhibit cellular egress of Ebola virus-like particles. *Biochem Bioph Res Co* (2016) 479:245–52. doi:10.1016/j.bbrc.2016.09.052
191. Seesuay S, Jittavisutthikul S, Sae-lim N, Sookrung N, Sakolvaree Y, Chaicumpa W. Human transbodies that interfere with the functions of Ebolavirus VP35 protein in genome replication and transcription and innate immune antagonism. *Emerg Microbe Infect* (2018) 7(1):41. doi:10.1038/s41426-018-0031-3
192. Kohler H, Paul S. Superantibody activities: new players in innate and adaptive immune response. *Immunol Today* (1998) 9(5):221–7. doi:10.1016/S0167-5699(97)01234-6
193. González-González E, Alvarez MM, Márquez-Ipiña AR, Trujillo-de Santiago G, Rodríguez-Martínez LM, Annabi N, et al. Anti-Ebola therapies based on monoclonal antibodies: current state and challenges ahead. *Crit Rev Biotechnol* (2017) 37(1):53–68. doi:10.3109/07388551.2015.1114465
194. Flyak AI, Shen X, Murin CD, Turner HL, David JA, Fusco ML, et al. Cross-reactive and potent neutralizing antibody responses in human survivors of natural Ebola virus infection. *Cell* (2016) 164(3):392–405. doi:10.1016/j.cell.2015.12.022
195. Hernandez H, Marceau C, Halliday H, Callison J, Borisevich V, Escaffre O, et al. Development and characterization of broadly cross-reactive monoclonal antibodies against all known Ebolavirus species. *J Infect Dis* (2015) 212(Suppl 2):S410–3. doi:10.1093/infdis/jiv209
196. Furuyama W, Marzi A, Nanbo A, Haddock E, Maruyama J, Miyamoto H, et al. Discovery of an antibody for pan-ebolavirus therapy. *Sci Rep* (2016) 6:20514. doi:10.1038/srep20514
197. Bornholdt ZA, Turner HL, Murin CD, Li W, Sok D, Souders CA, et al. Isolation of potent neutralizing antibodies from a survivor of the 2014 Ebola virus outbreak. *Science* (2016) 351(6277):1078–83. doi:10.1126/science.aad5788
198. Zhang Q, Gui M, Niu X, He S, Wang R, Feng Y, et al. Potent neutralizing monoclonal antibodies against Ebola virus infection. *Sci Rep* (2016) 6:25856. doi:10.1038/srep25856
199. Nguyen VK, Hernandez-Vargas EA. Windows of opportunity for Ebola virus infection treatment and vaccination. *Sci Rep* (2017) 7:8975. doi:10.1038/s41598-017-08884-0
200. van Lieshout LP, Soule G, Sorensen D, Frost KL, He S, Tierney K, et al. Intramuscular adeno-associated virus-mediated expression of monoclonal antibodies provides 100% protection against Ebola virus infection in mice. *J Infect Dis* (2018) 217(6):916–25. doi:10.1093/infdis/jix644
201. Ruggiero E, Richter SN. G-quadruplexes and G-quadruplex ligands: targets and tools in antiviral therapy. *Nucleic Acids Res* (2018) 46(7):3270–83. doi:10.1093/nar/gky187
202. Warren TK, Wells J, Panchal RG, Stuthman KS, Garza NL, Van Tongeren SA, et al. Protection against filovirus diseases by a novel broad-spectrum nucleoside analogue BCX4430. *Nature* (2014) 508:402–5. doi:10.1038/nature13027
203. Taylor R, Kotian P, Warren T, Panchal R, Bavari S, Julander J, et al. BCX4430—a broad-spectrum antiviral adenosine nucleoside analog under development for the treatment of Ebola virus disease. *J Infect Public Health* (2016) 9:220–6. doi:10.1016/j.jiph.2016.04.002
204. Cardile AP, Warren TK, Martins KA, Reisler RB, Bavari S. Will there be a cure for Ebola? *Annu Rev Pharmacol Toxicol* (2017) 57:329–48. doi:10.1146/annurev-pharmtox-010716-105055
205. Olsen ME, Filone CM, Rozelle D, Mire CE, Agans KN, Hensley L, et al. Polyamines and hypusination are required for Ebolavirus gene expression and replication. *mBio* (2016) 7(4):e882–816. doi:10.1128/mBio.00882-16
206. Sweiti H, Ekwunife O, Jaschinski T, Lhachimi SK. Repurposed therapeutic agents targeting the Ebola virus: a systematic review. *Curr Therap Res* (2017) 84:10–21. doi:10.1016/j.curtheres.2017.01.007
207. Johnson JC, Martinez O, Honko AN, Hensley LE, Olinger GG, Basler CF. Pyridinyl imidazole inhibitors of p38 MAP kinase impair viral dendritic cells. *Antiviral Res* (2014) 107:102–9. doi:10.1016/j.antiviral.2014.04.014
208. Dunning J, Kennedy SB, Antierens A, Whitehead J, Ciglenecki I, Carson G, et al. Experimental treatment of Ebola virus disease with brincidofovir. *PLoS One* (2016) 11:e0162199. doi:10.1371/journal.pone.0162199
209. Chiramel AI, Banadyga L, Dougherty JD, Falzarano D, Martellaro C, Brees D, et al. Alisporivir has limited antiviral effects against Ebola virus strains Makona and Mayinga. *J Infect Dis* (2016) 214(S3):S355–9. doi:10.1093/infdis/jiw241
210. Yang S, Xu M, Lee EM, Gorshkov K, Shiryaev SA, He S, et al. Emetine inhibits Zika and Ebola virus infections through two molecular mechanisms: inhibiting viral replication and decreasing viral entry. *Cell Discov* (2018) 4:31. doi:10.1038/s41421-018-0034-1
211. Wang Y, Cui R, Li G, Gao Q, Yuan S, Altmeyer R, et al. Teicoplanin inhibits Ebola pseudovirus infection in cell culture. *Antiviral Res* (2016) 125:1–7. doi:10.1016/j.antiviral.2015.11.003
212. Yonezawa A, Cavrois M, Greene WC. Studies of Ebola virus glycoprotein-mediated entry and fusion by using pseudotyped human immunodeficiency virus type 1 virions: involvement of cytoskeletal proteins and enhancement by tumor necrosis factor alpha. *J Virol* (2005) 79(2):918–26. doi:10.1128/JVI.79.2.918-926.2005
213. Kinch MS, Yunus AS, Lear C, Mao H, Chen H, Fesseha Z, et al. FGI-104: a broad-spectrum small molecule inhibitor of viral infection. *Am J Transl Res* (2009) 1(1):87–98.
214. Ekins S, Freundlich JS, Coffee M. A common feature pharmacophore for FDA-approved drugs inhibiting the Ebola virus. Version 2. *F1000Res* (2014) 3:277. doi:10.12688/f1000research.5741.2
215. Madrid PB, Panchal RG, Warren TK, Shurtleff AC, Endsley AN, Green CE, et al. Evaluation of Ebola virus inhibitors for drug repurposing. *ACS Infect Dis* (2015) 1(7):317–26. doi:10.1021/acsinfecdis.5b00030
216. Salata C, Baritussio A, Munegato D, Calistri A, Ha HR, Bigler L, et al. Amiodarone and metabolite MDEA inhibit Ebola virus infection by interfering with the viral entry process. *Pathog Dis* (2015) 73(5):ftv032. doi:10.1093/femspd/ftv032
217. Yuan S. Possible FDA-approved drugs to treat Ebola virus infection. *Infect Dis Poverty* (2015) 4:23. doi:10.1186/s40249-015-0055-z
218. Johansen LM, DeWald LE, Shoemaker CJ, Hoffstrom BG, Lear-Rooney CM, Stossel A, et al. A screen of approved drugs and molecular probes identifies therapeutics with anti-Ebola virus activity. *Sci Transl Med* (2015) 7(290):290ra89. doi:10.1126/scitranslmed.aaa5597
219. Takada A, Robison C, Goto H, Sanchez A, Murti KG, Whitt MA, et al. A system for functional analysis of Ebola virus glycoprotein. *Proc Natl Acad Sci U S A* (1997) 94(26):14764–9. doi:10.1073/pnas.94.26.14764
220. Sissoko D, Laouenan C, Folkesson E, M'Lebing AB, Beavogui AH, Baize S, et al. Experimental treatment with favipiravir for Ebola virus disease (the JIKI Trial): a historically controlled, single-arm proof-of-concept trial in Guinea. *PLoS Med* (2016) 13:e1001967. doi:10.1371/journal.pmed.1001967
221. Oestereich L, Ludtke A, Wurr S, Rieger T, Muñoz-Fontela C, Gunther S. Successful treatment of advanced Ebola virus infection with T-705 (favipiravir) in a small animal model. *Antiviral Res* (2014) 105:17–21. doi:10.1016/j.antiviral.2014.02.014
222. Smith DR, McCarthy S, Chrovian A, Olinger G, Stossel A, Geisbert TW, et al. Inhibition of heat-shock protein 90 reduces Ebola virus replication. *Antiviral Res* (2010) 87(2):187–94. doi:10.1016/j.antiviral.2010.04.015

223. García M, Cooper A, Shi W, Bornmann W, Carrion R, Kalman D, et al. Productive replication of Ebola virus is regulated by the c-Abl1 tyrosine kinase. *Sci Transl Med* (2012) 4(123):123ra24. doi:10.1126/scitranslmed.3003500
224. Nelson EA, Barnes AB, Wiehle RD, Fontenot GK, Hoenen T, White JM. Clomiphene and its isomers block Ebola virus particle entry and infection with similar potency: potential therapeutic implications. *Viruses* (2016) 8(8): E206. doi:10.3390/v8080206
225. Kouznetsova J, Sun W, Martínez-Romero C, Tawa G, Shinn P, Chen CZ, et al. Identification of 53 compounds that block Ebola virus-like particle entry via a repurposing screen of approved drugs. *Emerg Microbes Infect* (2014) 3:e84. doi:10.1038/emi.2014.88
226. Madrid PB, Chopra S, Manger ID, Gilfillan L, Keepers TR, Shurtleff AC, et al. A systematic screen of FDA-approved drugs for inhibitors of biological threat agents. *PLoS One* (2013) 8(4):e60579. doi:10.1371/journal.pone.0060579
227. Panchal RG, Reid SP, Tran JP, Bergeron AA, Wells J, Kota KP, et al. Identification of an antioxidant small-molecule with broad-spectrum antiviral activity. *Antiviral Res* (2012) 93(1):23–9. doi:10.1016/j.antiviral.2011.10.011
228. Geisbert TW, Hensley LE, Jahrling PB, Larsen T, Geisbert JB, Paragas J, et al. Treatment of Ebola virus infection with a recombinant inhibitor of factor VIIa/tissue factor: a study in rhesus monkeys. *Lancet* (2003) 362:1953–8. doi:10.1016/S0140-6736(03)15012-X
229. Henß L, Beck S, Weidner T, Biedenkopf N, Sliva K, Weber C, et al. Suramin is a potent inhibitor of Chikungunya and Ebola virus cell entry. *Virol J* (2016) 13:149. doi:10.1186/s12985-016-0607-2
230. Zhao Z, Martin C, Fan R, Bourne PE, Xie L. Drug repurposing to target Ebola virus replication and virulence using structural systems pharmacology. *BMC Bioinformatics* (2016) 17:90. doi:10.1186/s12859-016-0941-9
231. Chopra G, Kaushik S, Elkin PL, Samudrala R. Combating Ebola with repurposed therapeutics using the CANDO platform. *Molecules* (2016) 21(12):E1537. doi:10.3390/molecules21121537
232. Haque A, Hober D, Blondiaux J. Addressing therapeutic options for Ebola virus infection in current and future outbreaks. *Antimicrob Agents Chemother* (2015) 59:5892–902. doi:10.1128/AAC.01105-15
233. Olsen NJ, Schleich MA, Karp DR. Multifaceted effects of hydroxychloroquine in human disease. *Semin Arthritis Rheum* (2013) 43:264–72. doi:10.1016/j.semarthrit.2013.01.001
234. Dowall SD, Bosworth A, Watson R, Bewley K, Taylor I, Rayner E, et al. Chloroquine inhibited Ebola virus replication *in vitro* but failed to protect against infection anddisease in the *in vivo* guinea pig model. *J Gen Virol* (2015) 96(12):3484–92. doi:10.1099/jgv.0.000309
235. Falzarano D, Safronetz D, Prescott J, Marzi A, Feldmann F, Feldmann H. Lack of protection against Ebola virus from chloroquine in mice and hamsters. *Emerg Infect Dis* (2015) 21(6):1065–7. doi:10.3201/eid2106.150176
236. Long J, Wright E, Molesti E, Temperton N, Barclay W. Antiviral therapies against Ebola and other emerging viral diseases using existing medicines that block virus entry. Version 2. *F1000Res* (2015) 4:30. doi:10.12688/f1000research.6085.2
237. Kuehne A, Tiffany A, Lasry E, Janssens M, Besse C, Okonta C, et al. Impact and lessons learned from mass drug administrations of malaria chemoprevention during the Ebola outbreak in Monrovia, Liberia, 2014. *PLoS One* (2016) 11:e0161311. doi:10.1371/journal.pone.0161311
238. Furuta Y, Takahashi K, Fukuda Y, Kuno M, Kamiyama T, Kozaki K, et al. In vitro and in vivo activities of anti-influenza virus compound T-705. *Antimicrob Agents Chemother* (2002) 46:977–81. doi:10.1128/AAC.46.4.977-981.2002
239. Van Herp M, Declerck H, Decroo T. Favipiravir–a prophylactic treatment for Ebola contacts? *Lancet* (2015) 385:2350. doi:10.1016/S0140-6736(15)61095-9
240. Chinello P, Petrosillo N, Pittalis S, Biava G, Ippolito G, Nicastri E, et al. QTc interval prolongation during favipiravir therapy in an Ebolavirus-infected patient. *PLoS Negl Trop Dis* (2017) 11(12):e0006034. doi:10.1371/journal.pntd.0006034
241. Nagata T, Lefor AK, Hasegawa M, Ishii M. Favipiravir: a new medication for the Ebola virus disease pandemic. *Disaster Med Public Health Prep* (2015) 9:79–81. doi:10.1017/dmp.2014.151
242. Veljkovic V, Loiseau PM, Figadere B, Glisic S, Veljkovic N, Perovic VR, et al. Virtual screen for repurposing approved and experimental drugs for candidate inhibitors of EBOLA virus infection. *F1000Res* (2015) 4:34. doi:10.12688/f1000research.6110.1
243. Paessler S, Huang C, Sencanski M, Veljkovic N, Perovic V, Glisic S, et al. Ibuprofen as a template molecule for drug design against Ebola virus. *Front Biosci (Landmark Ed)* (2018) 23:947–53. doi:10.2741/4627
244. Siegel D, Hui HC, Doerffler E, Clarke MO, Chun K, Zhang L, et al. Discovery and synthesis of a phosphoramidate prodrug of a Pyrollo[2,*1f*] [triazin-4-amino] Adenine *C*-nucleoside (GS-5734) for the treatment of Ebola and emerging viruses. *J Med Chem* (2017) 60(5):1648–61. doi:10.1021/acs.jmedchem.6b01594
245. Warren TK, Jordan R, Lo MK, Ray AS, Mackman RL, Soloveva V, et al. Therapeutic efficacy of the small molecule GS-5734 against Ebola virus in rhesus monkeys. *Nature* (2016) 531(7594):381–5. doi:10.1038/nature17180
246. Konde MK, Baker DP, Traore FA, Sow MS, Camara A, Barry AA, et al. Interferon β-1a for the treatment of Ebola virus disease: a historically controlled, single-arm proof-of-concept trial. *PLoS One* (2017) 12(2):e0169255. doi:10.1371/journal.pone.0169255
247. Ekins S, Lingerfelt MA, Comer JE, Freiberg AN, Mirsalis JC, O'Loughlin K, et al. Efficacy of tilorone dihydrochloride against Ebola virus infection. *Antimicrob Agents Chemother* (2017) 62:e1711–7. doi:10.1128/AAC.01711-17
248. Warren TK, Warfield KL, Wells J, Swenson DL, Donner KS, Van Tongeren SA, et al. Advanced antisense therapies for postexposure protection against lethal filovirus infections. *Nat Med* (2010) 16:991–4. doi:10.1038/nm.2202
249. Geisbert TW, Lee AC, Robbins M, Geisbert JB, Honko AN, Sood V, et al. Post exposure protection of non-human primates against a lethal Ebola virus challenge with RNA interference: a proof-of-concept study. *Lancet* (2010) 375:1896–905. doi:10.1016/S0140-6736(10)60357-1
250. Warren TK, Whitehouse CA, Wells J, Welch L, Heald AE, Charleston JS, et al. A single phosphorodiamidate morpholino oligomer targeting VP24 protects rhesus monkeys against lethal Ebola virus infection. *mBio* (2015) 6:e2344–2314. doi:10.1128/mBio.02344-14
251. Bixler SL, Duplantier AJ, Bavari S. Discovering drugs for the treatment of Ebola virus. *Curr Treat Options Infect Dis* (2017) 9(3):299–317. doi:10.1007/s40506-017-0130-z
252. Dunning J, Sahr F, Rojek A, Gannon F, Carson G, Idriss B, et al. Experimental treatment of Ebola virus disease with TKM-130803: a single-arm phase 2 clinical trial. *PLoS Med* (2016) 13(4):e1001997. doi:10.1371/journal.pmed.1001997
253. Thi EP, Mire CE, Lee AC, Geisbert JB, Zhou JZ, Agans KN, et al. Lipid nanoparticle siRNA treatment of Ebola-virus-Makona-infected nonhuman primates. *Nature* (2015) 521:362–5. doi:10.1038/nature14442
254. Sheng M, Zhong Y, Chen Y, Du J, Ju X, Zhao C, et al. Hsa-miR-1246, hsamiR-320a and hsa-miR-196b-5p inhibitors can reduce the cytotoxicity of Ebola virus glycoprotein in vitro. *Sci China Life Sci* (2014) 57:959–72. doi:10.1007/s11427-014-4742-y
255. Iversen PL, Warren TK, Wells JB, Garza NL, Mourich DV, Welch LS, et al. Discovery and early development of AVI-7537 and AVI-7288 for the treatment of Ebola virus and Marburg virus infections. *Viruses* (2012) 4:2806–30. doi:10.3390/v4112806
256. Basu A, Mills DM, Mitchell D, Ndungo E, Williams JD, Herbert AS, et al. Novel small molecule entry inhibitors of Ebola virus. *J Infect Dis* (2015) 212(Suppl 2):S425–34. doi:10.1093/infdis/jiv223
257. Mupapa K, Massamba M, Kibadi K, Kuvula K, Bwaka A, Kipasa M, et al. Treatment of Ebola hemorrhagic fever with blood transfusions from convalescent patients. International Scientific and Technical Committee. *J Infect Dis* (1999) 179(Suppl 1):S18–23. doi:10.1086/514298
258. Dye JM, Wu H, Hooper JW, Khurana S, Kuehne AI, Coyle EM, et al. Production of potent fully human polyclonal antibodies against Ebola Zaire virus in transchromosomal cattle. *Sci Rep* (2016) 6:24897. doi:10.1038/srep24897
259. Li D, Chen T, Hu Y, Zhou Y, Liu Q, Zhou D, et al. An Ebola virus-like particle-based reporter system enables evaluation of antiviral drugs *in vitro* under non-biosafety level 4 conditions. *J Virol* (2016) 90(19):8720–8. doi:10.1128/JVI.01239-16
260. Shabman RS, Leung DW, Johnson J, Glennon N, Gulcicek EE, Stone KL, et al. DRBP76 associates with Ebola virus VP35 and suppresses viral polymerase function. *J Infect Dis* (2011) 204:S911–8. doi:10.1093/infdis/jir343
261. McCarthy SD, Majchrzak-Kita B, Racine T, Kozlowski HN, Baker DP, Hoenen T, et al. A rapid screening assay identifies monotherapy with

interferon-ß and combination therapies with nucleoside analogs as effective inhibitors of Ebola virus. *PLoS Negl Trop Dis* (2016) 10(1):e0004364. doi:10.1371/journal.pntd.0004364
262. Audet J, Wong G, Wang H, Lu G, Gao GF, Kobinger G, et al. Molecular characterization of the monoclonal antibodies composing ZMAb: a protective cocktail against Ebola virus. *Sci Rep* (2014) 4:6881. doi:10.1038/srep06881
263. Modrof J, Mühlberger E, Klenk HD, Becker S. Phosphorylation of VP30 impairs Ebola virus transcription. *J Biol Chem* (2002) 277(36):33099–104. doi:10.1074/jbc.M203775200
264. Aman MJ, Kinch MS, Warfield K, Warren T, Yunus A, Enterlein S, et al. Development of a broad-spectrum antiviral with activity against Ebola virus. *Antiviral Res* (2009) 83(3):245–51. doi:10.1016/j.antiviral.2009.06.001
265. Kolokoltsov AA, Adhikary S, Garver J, Johnson L, Davey RA, Vela EM. Inhibition of Lassa virus and Ebola virus infection in host cells treated with the kinase inhibitors genistein and tyrphostin. *Arch Virol* (2012) 157(1):121–7. doi:10.1007/s00705-011-1115-8
266. Huggins J, Zhang ZX, Bray M. Antiviral drug therapy of filovirus infections: S-adenosylhomocysteine hydrolase inhibitors inhibit Ebola virus in vitro and in a lethal mouse model. *J Infect Dis* (1999) 179(Suppl 1):S240–7. doi:10.1086/514316
267. Geisbert TW, Hensley LE, Kagan E, Yu EZ, Geisbert JB, Daddario-DiCaprio K, et al. Postexposure protection of guinea pigs against a lethal Ebola virus challenge is conferred by RNA interference. *J Infect Dis* (2006) 193(12):1650–7. doi:10.1086/504267
268. Enterlein S, Warfield KL, Swenson DL, Stein DA, Smith JL, Gamble CS, et al. VP35 knockdown inhibits Ebola virus amplification and protects against lethal infection in mice. *Antimicrob Agents Chemother* (2006) 50(3):984–93. doi:10.1128/AAC.50.3.984-993.2006
269. Golkar Z, Battaria R, Pace DG, Bagasra O. Inhibition of Ebola virus by anti-Ebola miRNAs *in silico*. *J Infect Dev Ctries* (2016) 10(6):626–34. doi:10.3855/jidc.7127
270. Rocker AE, Müller JA, Dietzel E, Harms M, Krüger F, Heid C, et al. The molecular tweezer CLR01 inhibits Ebola and Zika virus infection. *Antiviral Res* (2018) 152:26–35. doi:10.1016/j.antiviral.2018.02.003
271. Balmith M, Faya M, Soliman ME. Ebola virus: a gap in drug design and discovery – experimental and computational perspective. *Chem Biol Drug Des* (2017) 89(3):297–308. doi:10.1111/cbdd.12870
272. Balmith M, Soliman MES. Potential Ebola drug targets – filling the gap: a critical step forward towards the design and discovery of potential drugs. *Biologia* (2017) 72(1):1–13. doi:10.1515/biolog-2017-0012
273. Schuler J, Hudson ML, Schwartz D, Samudrala R. A systematic review of computational drug discovery, development, and repurposing for Ebola virus disease treatment. *Molecules* (2017) 22(1777):1–27. doi:10.3390/molecules22101777
274. Dhama K, Chakraborty S, Mahima, Wani MY, Verma AK, Deb R, et al. Novel and emerging therapies safeguarding health of humans and their companion animals: a review. *Pak J Biol Sci* (2013) 16:101–11. doi:10.3923/pjbs.2013.101.111
275. Dhama K, Karthik K, Khandia R, Munjal A, Tiwari R, Rana R, et al. Medicinal and therapeutic potential of herbs and plant metabolites/extracts countering viral pathogens – current knowledge and future prospects. *Curr Drug Metab* (2018). doi:10.2174/1389200219666180129145252
276. Malik YS, Sharma K, Jeena LM, Kumar N, Sircar S, Rajak KK, et al. Toll-like receptors: the innate immune receptors with ingenious anti-viral paradigm. *South Asian J Exp Biol* (2013) 3:207–13.
277. Gao J, Yin L. Drug development for controlling Ebola epidemic – a race against time. *Drug Discov Ther* (2014) 8:229–31. doi:10.5582/ddt.2014.01040
278. Arntzen C. Plant-made pharmaceuticals: from "Edible Vaccines" to Ebola therapeutics. *Plant Biotechnol* (2015) 13:1013–6. doi:10.1111/pbi.12460
279. Streatfield SJ, Kushnir N, Yusibov V. Plant-produced candidate countermeasures against emerging and re-emerging infections and bioterror agents. *Plant Biotechnol J* (2015) 13:1136–59. doi:10.1111/pbi.12475
280. Yao J, Weng Y, Dickey A, Wang KY. Plants as factories for human pharmaceuticals: applications and challenges. *Int J Mol Sci* (2015) 16:28549–65. doi:10.3390/ijms161226122
281. Iqbal HM, Villalba A, Khandia R, Munjal A, Dhama K. Recent trends in nanotechnology-based drugs and formulations for targeted therapeutic delivery. *Recent Pat Inflamm Allergy Drug Discov* (2016) 10(2):86–93. doi:10.2174/1872213X10666161213162823
282. Prasad M, Lambe UP, Brar B, Shah I, Manimegalai J, Ranjan K, et al. Nanotherapeutics: an insight into healthcare and multi-dimensional applications in medical sector of the modern world. *Biomed Pharmacother* (2018) 97:1521–37. doi:10.1016/j.biopha.2017.11.026

8

Neutrophil Activation in Acute Hemorrhagic Fever with Renal Syndrome is Mediated by Hantavirus-Infected Microvascular Endothelial Cells

Tomas Strandin [1], Satu Mäkelä [2], Jukka Mustonen [2] and Antti Vaheri [1]*

[1] *Department of Virology, Medicum, Faculty of Medicine, University of Helsinki, Helsinki, Finland,* [2] *Department of Internal Medicine, Faculty of Medicine and Life Sciences, Tampere University Hospital, University of Tampere, Tampere, Finland*

Correspondence:
Tomas Strandin
tomas.strandin@helsinki.fi

Hantaviruses cause hemorrhagic fever with renal syndrome (HFRS) and hantavirus cardiopulmonary syndrome (HCPS) in humans. Both diseases are considered to be immunologically mediated but the exact pathological mechanisms are still poorly understood. Neutrophils are considered the first line of defense against invading microbes but little is still known of their role in virus infections. We wanted to study the role of neutrophils in HFRS using blood and tissue samples obtained from Puumala hantavirus (PUUV)-infected patients. We found that neutrophil activation products myeloperoxidase and neutrophil elastase, together with interleukin-8 (the major neutrophil chemotactic factor in humans), are strongly elevated in blood of acute PUUV-HFRS and positively correlate with kidney dysfunction, the hallmark clinical finding of HFRS. These markers localized mainly in the tubulointerstitial space in the kidneys of PUUV-HFRS patients suggesting neutrophil activation to be a likely component of the general immune response toward hantaviruses. We also observed increased levels of circulating extracellular histones at the acute stage of the disease supporting previous findings of neutrophil extracellular trap formation in PUUV-HFRS. Mechanistically, we did not find evidence for direct PUUV-mediated activation of neutrophils but instead primary blood microvascular endothelial cells acquired a pro-inflammatory phenotype and promoted neutrophil degranulation in response to PUUV infection *in vitro.* These results suggest that neutrophils are activated by hantavirus-infected endothelial cells and may contribute to the kidney pathology which determines the severity of HFRS.

Keywords: hantavirus, HFRS, neutrophils, IL-8, endothelial cells, degranulation, NETs, NETosis

INTRODUCTION

Hantaviruses are the causative agents of two human diseases: hemorrhagic fever with renal syndrome (HFRS) in Eurasia and hantavirus cardiopulmonary syndrome (HCPS) in the Americas. Each hantavirus species is carried by its specific rodent host with no or minimal signs of disease but cause occasional human spillover infections with immune-mediated pathology (1). A hallmark of both hantavirus diseases is increased vascular permeability which mediates kidney and lung failure associated with HFRS and HCPS, respectively (1). Endothelial cells lining the vasculature are also the prime target of viral replication in patients (2, 3). Puumala hantavirus (PUUV) circulates in Northern Europe and Russia causing a relatively mild form of HFRS as compared to Hantaan (HTNV) or Dobrava hantavirus (DOBV)-caused HFRS and especially Andes (ANDV)- or Sin Nombre (SNV)-caused HCPS in which fatality rates can reach 40% (4).

Typical laboratory findings in acute PUUV-caused HFRS are leukocytosis, thrombocytopenia, increased C-reactive protein (CRP) level, and as signs of acute kidney injury (AKI), proteinuria, haematuria and elevated serum creatinine concentration (5). In addition to thrombocytopenia, hematological abnormalities include increased coagulation and fibrinolysis, complement activation, and elevated levels of pro-inflammatory cytokines which all have the potential to contribute to vascular permeability. Vascular permeability, in turn, could be the underlying cause of proteinuria which typically precedes AKI (6). The pathophysiology of PUUV-HFRS associated AKI is usually described as tubulointerstitial nephritis and infiltration of several immune cell types such as lymphocytes, monocytes, and polymorphonuclear leukocytes into kidneys have been observed (7, 8).

Neutrophils are the most abundant circulating leukocytes in humans and play a fundamental role in the innate immune response (9). Circulating neutrophils are the first type of immune cells recruited to sites of inflammation or infection. In humans, one of the most important chemotactic factors for neutrophils is interleukin (IL)-8, released at the site inflammation/infection (10). After receiving chemotactic signals neutrophils interact with endothelial cells lining the vasculature in order to traverse the endothelium and into the inflamed tissues (11). *In vivo*, the interactions between neutrophils and endothelial cells include initial rolling followed by firm adhesion and finally transendothelial migration. Firm adhesion is facilitated, among other factors, by endothelial intercellular adhesion molecule (ICAM)-1 expressed on the surface of endothelial cells and CD11b/CD18 integrin complex (also known as Mac-1, CR3 or $\alpha_M\beta_2$) on neutrophils (12). Once neutrophils reach the site of infection their primary role is to kill invading microbes by production of reactive oxygen species (ROS) and the release of antimicrobial proteins such as myeloperoxidase (MPO) and human neutrophil elastase (HNE) in a process of degranulation (13, 14). In addition to ROS formation and degranulation, neutrophils are also able to release neutrophil extracellular traps (NETs), consisting of extracellular chromatin decorated with histones and granular proteins such as MPO and HNE, and with the potential to entrap and kill pathogens (15, 16).

The activation of neutrophils in several bacterial infections is well-described but their role in virus-mediated diseases has been neglected to a large extent (17). The involvement of neutrophils in the pathogenesis of hantavirus diseases is suggested by acutely increased serum levels of cytokines and chemokines with known functions in neutrophil chemotaxis, differentiation and mobilization (18–20). Increased numbers of circulating histones, cell-fee DNA and histone-DNA complexes have been described in the acute stage of PUUV infection (21–23), suggesting that neutrophils release NETs during HFRS. NETosis could potentially explain capillary leakage in HFRS (24). Interestingly, neutrophils are crucial for increased vascular permeability observed in response to HTNV infection in SCID mice (25). Furthermore, HTNV has also been shown to cause NETosis *in vitro* (21).

In this study we wanted to elucidate the role of neutrophil activation in HFRS by determining markers of neutrophil activation (MPO, HNE, histones, and IL-8) in blood and tissues of patients suffering from acute PUUV-caused HFRS. In addition, to directly determine the role that hantavirus plays in mediating neutrophil responses in PUUV-HFRS, we investigated the potential of purified PUUV or PUUV-infected endothelial cells to activate neutrophils *in vitro*. Taken together, we found that the levels of circulating and tissue-localized MPO, HNE and IL-8 are elevated in acute PUUV-HFRS and correlate with kidney dysfunction, thereby corroborating the role of neutrophils in hantavirus pathogenesis. Mechanistically, our results do not support direct virus-mediated neutrophil activation but rather an indirect mechanism through infected endothelial cells. Finally, the antiviral function of neutrophils was pinpointed strongly to the release of proteases from neutrophils.

MATERIALS AND METHODS

Patient Samples

The study was approved by the Ethics Committee of Tampere University Hospital (Nos. 99256 and R04180). All subjects gave written informed consent in accordance with the Declaration of Helsinki. The study consisted of plasma samples from patients treated for serologically confirmed acute PUUV infection at the Tampere University Hospital, Finland, during September 2000–March 2009. We assessed the extracellular circulating levels of MPO, HNE, histone H3 and IL-8 in plasma samples obtained from patients with acute PUUV-caused HFRS at 1st day of hospitalization (acute stage; median days after onset of fever 4 ± 2), early recovery phase (15–30 days after hospitalization) and healthy controls.

The study included Boiun-fixed, paraffin-embedded kidney biopsies obtained at Tampere University Hospital during 1985–1987. The biopsies among patients with PUUV-HFRS were performed for clinical reasons at the time when there was no reliable serological test for PUUV infection available. All these biopsies were performed during the acute phase of the disease. The highest measured serum creatinine level of the patients ranged from 220 to 1,050 μmol/L. The biopsy findings were acute interstitial in two cases and acute tubulointerstitial nephritis in three, both findings being typical for PUUV-induced AKI (5).

PUUV-negative cases served as controls. Indications for renal biopsies were AKI in one case, microscopic hematuria and/or proteinuria in four cases. The biopsy findings were normal morphology in two cases, acute tubulointerstitial nephritis, mesangial proliferative glomerulonephritis and IgM-glomerulonephritis in one case each. In both groups of biopsy patients a positive (PUUV-HFRS cases) or negative (controls)

PUUV-serology was determined using stored serum samples obtained at the time of renal biopsy.

Primary Antibodies

Primary antibodies used in this study were rabbit polyclonal antibodies to MPO (Thermo scientific, #RB-373-A), Histone H3 (Abcam, #ab18521) or HNE (Abcam, #ab68672) and mouse monoclonal antibodies to IL-8 (RnD Systems; #Mab-208), CD18 (Millipore, #TS1-18) and ICAM-1 (RnD systems, #BBIG-I1) in addition to IgG1 isotype control (Immunotools). Rabbit polyclonal antibodies for PUUV nucleocapsid protein and glycoproteins have been described before (26).

Histone Quantification

Histones were measured by a dot-blot assay where 2 μl of patient or healthy control EDTA-plasma were pipetted on nitrocellulose membrane, air-dried and probed with Histone H3 antibody in blocking buffer [1.5% milk in Tris–EDTA–NaCl–Tween (TENT)]. After washing with TENT, the primary antibody was detected with IR800-conjugated anti-rabbit antibody (Li-cor) in blocking buffer. After additional washing, signal intensity was determined by Odyssey instrumentation (Li-cor). Recombinant Histone H3 (New England Biolabs) was used for standard preparation.

Enzyme-Linked Immunosorbent Assays (ELISAs)

The levels of MPO, HNE, and IL-8 were measured from patient or control plasma using ELISA kits provided by Abcam (for MPO, HNE, and IL-8) or Immunotools (for IL-8).

Immunohistochemistry (IHC)

IHC was performed on kidney sections after heat-mediated antigen retrieval using the protocol provided in Vectastain ABC Elite HRP kit from Vector labs. Avidin/biotin blocking kit, biotinylated goat anti-mouse IgG or anti-rabbit secondary antibodies and DAB substrate were used as suggested by the vendor (Vector labs). The mean percentage of DAB positive area was counted from four images taken (1.5 × 1.5 mm) from each individual section using Fiji Image J software.

Cultures of Primary Blood Microvascular Endothelial Cells (BECs)

BECs were obtained from Lonza and maintained in endothelial basal medium (EBM-2) supplemented with SingleQuots™ Kit containing 5% fetal bovine serum (FBS), human endothelial growth factor, hydrocortisone, vascular endothelial growth factor, human fibroblast growth factor-basic, ascorbic acid, R^3-insulin like growth factor-1, gentamicin and amphotericin-B (Lonza). For experiments the cells were used at passages 7–10.

Virus Propagation and Titration

PUUV Kazan strain was propagated in Vero E6 cells (green monkey kidney epithelial cell line; ATCC no. CRL-1586) grown in Minimum Essential Medium containing 10% FCS, penicillin and streptomycin (cMEM). For experiments, PUUV was purified from Vero E6 cell supernatant through a 30% sucrose cushion by ultracentrifugation. Virus titers were measured by incubating diluted virus stocks on Vero E6 cells for 24 h at 37°C and subsequently staining acetone-fixed cells with a polyclonal antibody specific for PUUV nucleocapsid protein and AlexaFluor488-conjugated secondary antibody. Focus-forming units (FFU)/ml were counted under an UV-microscope.

Infection of BECs

Confluent BECs were infected for 1 h at 37°C using purified PUUV diluted in BEC growth medium at multiplicity of infection (MOI) of 10. For inactivation of PUUV, virus stocks were kept under UV light for 30 min.

Immunofluorescence

Immunofluorescence of either mock-, UV-PUUV or live PUUV-infected BECs was performed on cells grown on black, glass-bottomed cell culture plates. After fixation with 4% formaldehyde, cells were permeabilized (3% BSA, 0.3% TritonX-100) for 10 min and incubated with primary antibodies to MPO, HNE, ICAM-1 or viral nucleocapsid protein followed by appropriate Alexafluor488- or Alexafluor594-conjugated secondary antibodies (Thermo Scientific). To stain the nuclei, cells were incubated with Hoechst 33258. After washing, fluorescence intensity was counted using Hidex sense microplate reader (Hidex) and images taken using Leica TCS SP8 X confocal microscope (Biomedicum Imaging Unit, Biomedicum, University of Helsinki, Helsinki, Finland). Neutrophil activation was quantitated by the percentage of decondensed polymorphonuclear cells with simultaneous MPO relocalization in 4 immunofluorescence images (500 × 500 μm) taken randomly from each well by confocal microscope.

PMN Cultures

Fresh blood from healthy volunteers was drawn into EDTA-tubes and PMNs immediately isolated using Polymorphoprep separation medium (Axis-Shield) according to manufacturer's protocol. PMN purity and viability were assessed by phenotypic polymorphonuclear characterization using Hoechst 33258 fluorescence microscopy and trypan blue exclusion test, respectively (both were routinely found to be over 90%). Isolated PMNs were diluted into BEC growth medium (10^6 cells/ml) and incubated with mock-, UV-PUUV or live PUUV-infected BECs for 1 or 3 h at 37°C (10 times excess PMNs over BECs). Cells were washed and subjected directly to immunofluorescence staining as described above for determination of PMN binding. When PMN-BEC co-cultures were incubated in the presence of 10 μg/ml neutralizing antibodies to IL-8, CD18 or viral glycoproteins, PMNs were pre-treated with FcR blocking reagent (Immunostep) for 10 min.

Neutrophil Activation Assays

Purified virus or virus-containing Vero E6 cell culture supernatants were incubated with freshly isolated PMNs (MOI 1) in cMEM for 3 h at 37°C. The incubation time was chosen based on the optimal time needed to detect adequate levels of PMN activation marker expression with low concurrent spontaneous activation due to culturing. After fixation with

2% formaldehyde, extracellular DNA was quantitated with the fluorescent, cell-impermeable Pico-Green dsDNA binding reagent (Thermo Scientific) using Hidex Sense microplate reader. Peroxidase activity was assessed from supernatants of pelleted PMNs (400 × g 5 min) by the chromogenic peroxidase substrate 3,3′,5,5′-tetramethylbenzidine (TMB).

PUUV Viability Assay

Purified PUUV was incubated for 3 h with freshly isolated PMNs (in a 1:1 ratio) in assay buffer (10 mM Hepes pH 7,4; 150 mM NaCl). Neutrophil activator phorbol myristate acetate (PMA; 1 μg/ml) and one of the following inhibitors NaN_3 (0.01 or 0.002%), PMSF (0.2 or 1 mM), EDTA (2 mM) or DNAse I (10 U/ml) were added where indicated. After incubation, PMNs were pelleted by centrifugation (400 × g 5 min) and one third of the supernatant used for PUUV titer measurement as described above. The rest of the sample was used for immunoblotting by standard procedures for PUUV structural proteins (27) using polyclonal antibodies specific for Gn, Gc or N followed by IRD800-conjugated secondary antibody (Li-Cor) and detection by Odyssey.

Statistics

Significant differences between groups of normally distributed data was assessed by student's T-test and non-normally distributed data by Mann-Whitney U-test or Kruskal-Wallis H-test for multiple populations. The normality of data was estimated by Shapiro-Wilk test. Correlations between parameters were assessed using Spearman's rank correlation test. All analyses were done with SPSS software version 24 (SPSS Inc., Chicago, IL, USA) or GraphPad prism (La Jolla, CA, United States).

RESULTS

Circulating Levels of MPO, HNE, Histones, and IL-8 Are Elevated in Acute PUUV-Caused HFRS

Circulating levels of MPO, HNE, histones, and IL-8 were all significantly higher in the acute stage of the disease as compared to the recovery stage or healthy controls (**Figure 1**). The levels of all the measured markers remained elevated also in the recovery stage as compared to controls but this difference was not statistically significant. Strongly elevated circulating levels of MPO and HNE suggest that neutrophils are activated in acute PUUV-HFRS. Furthermore, increased numbers of extracellular histones imply that neutrophil activation could, at least in part, be due to NETosis (21). Interestingly, in the present study, neutrophil activation was accompanied by elevated levels of IL-8, a chemotactic and priming factor for neutrophils.

To get further insight to the role of neutrophil activation in the pathogenesis of PUUV-HFRS by we correlated the acute plasma levels of MPO, HNE, histone H3, and IL-8 to variables reflecting severity of AKI (maximum plasma creatinine level measured during the hospital stay), and to hematological variables (minimum blood platelet count, maximum blood leukocyte count, and plasma tissue plasminogen activator (tPA) level) (**Table 1**). We found that HNE and histone H3 positively correlated with the severity of AKI. In addition, MPO and HNE correlated with all the tested hematological variables. Not surprisingly, given the likely neutrophil origin of MPO and HNE, they also correlated strongly with each other. The acute IL-8 levels correlated significantly with low platelets and exceptionally strongly with MPO, HNE and histones ($p < 0.005$ for all) suggesting that IL-8 could play a role in neutrophil activation.

Localization of MPO, HNE, and IL-8 in the Kidneys of Acute PUUV-HFRS

In order to investigate whether markers of neutrophil activation could also be detected in tissues of patients suffering from acute PUUV-HFRS, we made use of archival biopsies to detect the expression of MPO, HNE and IL-8 in patient kidneys by immunohistochemistry. We did not include histones in this analysis since we expected that differentiating NET-associated histones from viable cells would be challenging. Elevated expression of MPO, HNE and IL-8 could be detected more readily in acute PUUV-HFRS patients than PUUV-negative control patient samples (**Figure 2A**). By counting the tissue area staining positive for MPO, HNE, or IL-8 we could observe a statistically significant difference in MPO expression between PUUV positive and negative cases ($n = 5$; $p = 0.04$; **Figure 2B**). In the case of HNE and IL-8 higher expression was found in 2 and 3 PUUV cases, respectively, as compared to controls but this was not enough to reach statistical significance ($n = 5$; $p = 0.08$ and $p = 0.15$, respectively). The most prominent localization of MPO, HNE and IL-8 in HFRS patients was the tubulointerstitial space, in line with the diagnosis of tubulointerstitial nephritis. Therein we could observe both cell-associated (arrowheads) and extracellular expression (filled arrows) of MPO and HNE suggesting both neutrophil infiltration and activation, respectively. Interestingly, HNE and IL-8 localized also to in the tubular epithelial cells in two HFRS patients (empty arrows). IL-8 could also occasionally be observed in the tubular cells of PUUV-negative patients albeit with a lower intensity and frequency as compared to HFRS patients (**Figures 2A,B**). Taken together, these results show that MPO is a component of the inflammatory response toward PUUV in the kidneys of acute HFRS, possibly accompanied by HNE and IL-8, and suggest that neutrophils (and their activation products) infiltrate kidneys through the capillary endothelium. In addition, the current findings together with our previous observations of elevated IL-8 levels in urine of acute PUUV-HFRS (28) suggest that IL-8 is produced locally by kidney epithelial cells in PUUV-HFRS and likely acts as a chemotactic factor inviting neutrophil recruitment and extravasation in the kidney.

Live PUUV Does Not Activate Neutrophils *in vitro*

It has been shown that HTNV can directly bind CD18 integrin on neutrophils and induce NETosis (21). We wanted to determine whether PUUV can also induce NETosis which could explain our findings of neutrophil activation in acute PUUV-HFRS. We did this by incubating mock- or PUUV-infected Vero E6 cell culture supernatants or purified PUUV (with the same infectious titer) with freshly isolated PMNs and subsequently quantified the release of extracellular DNA from PMNs. NETosis was

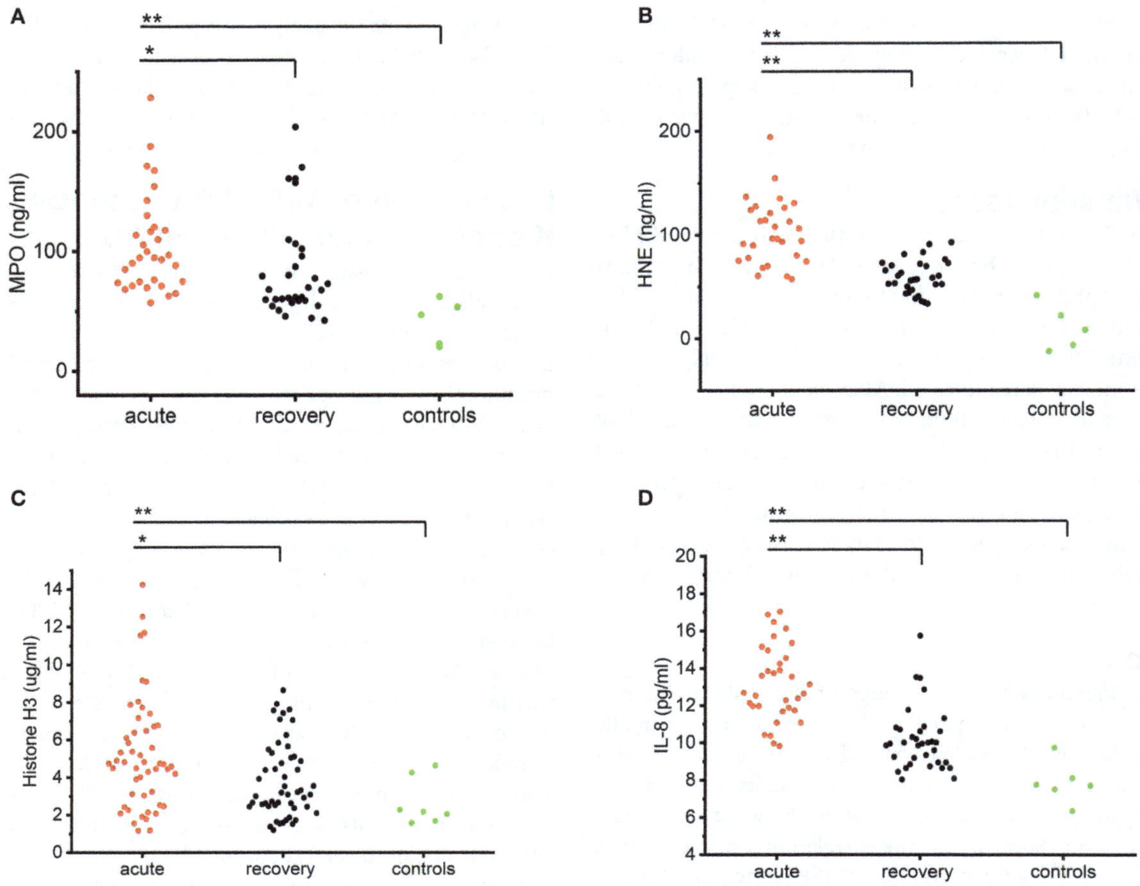

FIGURE 1 | Circulating levels of MPO, HNE, histone H3 and IL-8 in PUUV-HFRS. Plots of the acute (median days after onset of fever 4 ± 2) and recovery stage (15–30 days post onset) levels of MPO **(A)**, HNE **(B)**, histones **(C)** or IL-8 **(D)** in PUUV-infected patient plasma samples (n = 32, 30, 53 and 36, respectively) as compared to healthy controls (n = 5, 5, 5, and 8, respectively) distributions across groups were compared by Kruskal-Wallis H test and statistically significant differences indicated as either $^{*}p < 0.05$ or $^{**}p < 0.01$.

clearly induced above mock control by PUUV-containing Vero E6 supernatant but not with purified PUUV (**Figure 3A**). To elaborate on the finding that live PUUV does not cause NETosis, UV-inactivation of PUUV-infected Vero E6 supernatant did not affect its ability to induce NETosis (**Figure 3B**). These findings indicate that live PUUV alone is not capable of inducing NETosis but instead involves other factor/s released from hantavirus-infected Vero E6 cells supernatants which might act alone or synergistically with the inactivated virus. In order to analyze whether purified hantaviruses could induce PMN degranulation we incubated fresh PMNs with purified PUUV, TULV, HTNV, or PMA (as a positive control) and analyzed peroxidase activity in cell supernatants (**Figure 3B**). MPO activity was induced by PMA but not with any of the hantaviruses tested, suggesting that hantavirus do not induce significant PMN degranulation. These results imply that neutrophil activation in HFRS is not caused by direct contact with hantavirus but instead requires additional factors. Thus, we wanted to analyze whether PUUV-infected endothelial cells could play a role in neutrophil activation during HFRS.

PUUV Induces a Pro-Inflammatory Phenotype in BECs

Endothelial cells are the prime target of hantavirus infection *in vivo* (2, 3). Thus, we hypothesized that PUUV could mediate neutrophil activation through infected endothelial cells. To test this, we either mock-infected or infected primary blood endothelial cells (BECs) with purified live PUUV or UV-inactivated PUUV (UV-PUUV). By visualizing the expression of viral nucleocapsid protein N in the cells by immunofluorescence we observed that BECs were close to 100% infected at 3 days post infection (dpi), followed by significant drop in infectivity levels at 6 dpi (**Figure 4A**). The downregulation of PUUV infection in BECs is type I interferon-mediated, as reported previously (29), and is probably due to MxA protein sequestering the viral N protein (30) We analyzed the supernatants of infected BECs for the presence of IL-8 by ELISA and observed that BECs infected with live PUUV upregulate the secretion of IL-8 at 3 dpi as compared to mock- or UV-PUUV infections (**Figure 4B**). However, longer culturing of mock- or UV-PUUV infected BECs also upregulated IL-8 in the cell supernatants which finally led to

TABLE 1 | Correlation between different clinical variables reflecting HFRS disease severity and markers of neutrophil activation.

		Creatinine (max)	Platelets (min)	Leukocyte count (max)	tPA	MPO	HNE	Histones	IL-8
MPO	*r*	0.215	−0.582**	0.405**	0.571*	1.000	0.363**	0.329*	0.659**
	Sig.	0.123	0.000	0.003	0.021		0.008	0.016	0.000
	n	53	52	52	16	53	53	53	36
HNE	*r*	0.364**	−0.420**	0.296*	0.636**	0.363**	1.000	0.130	0.474**
	Sig.	0.007	0.002	0.033	0.008	0.008		0.352	0.004
	n	53	52	52	16	53	53	53	36
Histones	*r*	0.228*	−0.260	0.273	−0.101	0.329*	0.130	1.000	0.464**
	Sig.	0.036	0.063	0.050	0.632	0.016	0.352		0.004
	n	53	52	52	16	53	53	53	36
IL-8	*r*	0.138	−0.379*	0.292	0.536	0.659**	0.474**	0.464**	1.000
	Sig.	0.423	0.025	0.089	0.089	0.000	0.004	0.004	
	n	36	35	35	11	36	36	36	36

*The clinical variables creatinine, platelet and leukocyte counts are maximum or minimum values from the course of hospital stay whereas tPA and markers of neutrophil activation are from 1st day of hospitalization. r, Spearman's rho correlation coefficient; Sig., Significance of correlation (p); n, number of patients; MPO, Myeloperoxidase; HNE, Neutrophil elastase; IL-8, Interleukin-8; tPA, Tissue plasminogen activator; *p < 0.05, **p < 0.01.*

comparable, high levels of IL-8 irrespective of PUUV infection at 6 dpi. Since IL-8 could act as a general marker of inflammation (10), we wanted to see whether PUUV-infected BECs would upregulate also other inflammatory factors potentially important for neutrophil recruitment. Thus we assessed the expression of ICAM-1, a ligand for neutrophil-expressed CD11b/CD18 integrin complex, on the plasma membrane of BECs by immunofluorescence-based imaging and quantification assays. We found elevated levels ICAM-1 on the surface of PUUV-infected BECs as compared to mock- or UV-PUUV infected BECs at 3 dpi (**Figure 4C**). The elevated ICAM-1 levels remained only slightly lower as compared to TNF-α treated BECs, used as a positive control. At 6 dpi, ICAM-1 expression returned to baseline levels in PUUV-infected BECs concomitantly with the reduction of viral replication. As expected, TNF-α was found to be a robust inducer of ICAM-1 in BECs and thus we hypothesized that TNF-α could induce ICAM-1 also in PUUV-infected BECs. However, we did not find any evidence for TNF-α in PUUV-infected BEC supernatants by ELISA suggesting that the induction of ICAM-1 in PUUV-infected BECs is independent of this cytokine (data not shown).

PMNs Adhere to PUUV-Infected BECs

Next, we wanted to determine whether freshly isolated PMNs (containing mainly neutrophils) could adhere to PUUV-infected BECs which express elevated levels of IL-8 and ICAM-1. Fresh PMNs were incubated with mock-, UV-PUUV or live PUUV-infected BECs for 1 h, non-bound PMNs removed by washing and remaining numbers of BEC-bound PMNs determined by immunofluorescence-based imaging and quantitation of MPO (used as a marker of PMNs). In addition to MPO, bound PMNs were differentiated from BECs based on their segmented nuclear morphology by DNA staining. We found that PMN binding to PUUV-infected BECs was significantly elevated as compared to mock- or UV-PUUV infected BECs at 3 dpi, but not at 6 dpi (**Figures 5A,B**), consistent with the elevated expression of ICAM-1 and higher virus replication in PUUV-infected BECs at 3 dpi. As positive and negative controls, we used TNF-α treated BECs and PUUV infected-BECs without PMN incubation, respectively. Based on these results we consistently allowed PMNs to bind the 3-day BEC cultures for 1 h in the following experiments assessing PMN-BEC interaction as shown in **Figure 5**.

We wanted to analyze further whether the binding of PMNs to PUUV-infected BECs is mediated by chemotactic signals driven by IL-8 and/or is dependent of the neutrophil-expressed CD11b/CD18 binding to ICAM-1 on BECs. We did this by incubating PMNs with either BECs infected with either live PUUV or UV-PUUV as the negative control for infection in the presence of neutralizing antibodies to IL-8 or CD18. We could determine that binding to PUUV-infected BECs was dependent on CD11b/CD18 on neutrophils but not on the presence of IL-8 (**Figures 5A,C**). Not surprisingly, CD11b/CD18 seemed to mediate the adhesion of PMNs also to TNF-α treated BECs, although less dramatically (**Figure 5D**). The fact that CD18 neutralizing antibody was not as efficient in blocking PMN adhesion to TNF-α treated BECs could be due to the excess level of ICAM-1 upregulated by TNF-α as compared to PUUV infection (**Figure 4C**). Given that HTNV has been shown to bind CD18 integrin (21) we also tested the effect of viral glycoprotein (Gn and Gc) neutralizing antibodies (31) on PMN-BEC interaction. However, we could not observe any significant effects (**Figure 5E**) by Gn or Gc neutralizing antibodies suggesting that PMN adhesion to infected BECs is mediated by host-derived inflammatory factors but not viral proteins. Unfortunately, we could not reliably determine the role of ICAM-1 in PMN-BEC interaction since the presence of ICAM-1 specific antibodies resulted in further elevated binding of PMNs to BECs regardless of BECs being infected with PUUV or not (data not shown). We hypothesize that this phenomenon could be due to antibody-mediated cross-linking of neutrophil- and BEC-associated ICAM-1 proteins. In addition, ICAM-1 antibodies are known to activate cross-linking and activation

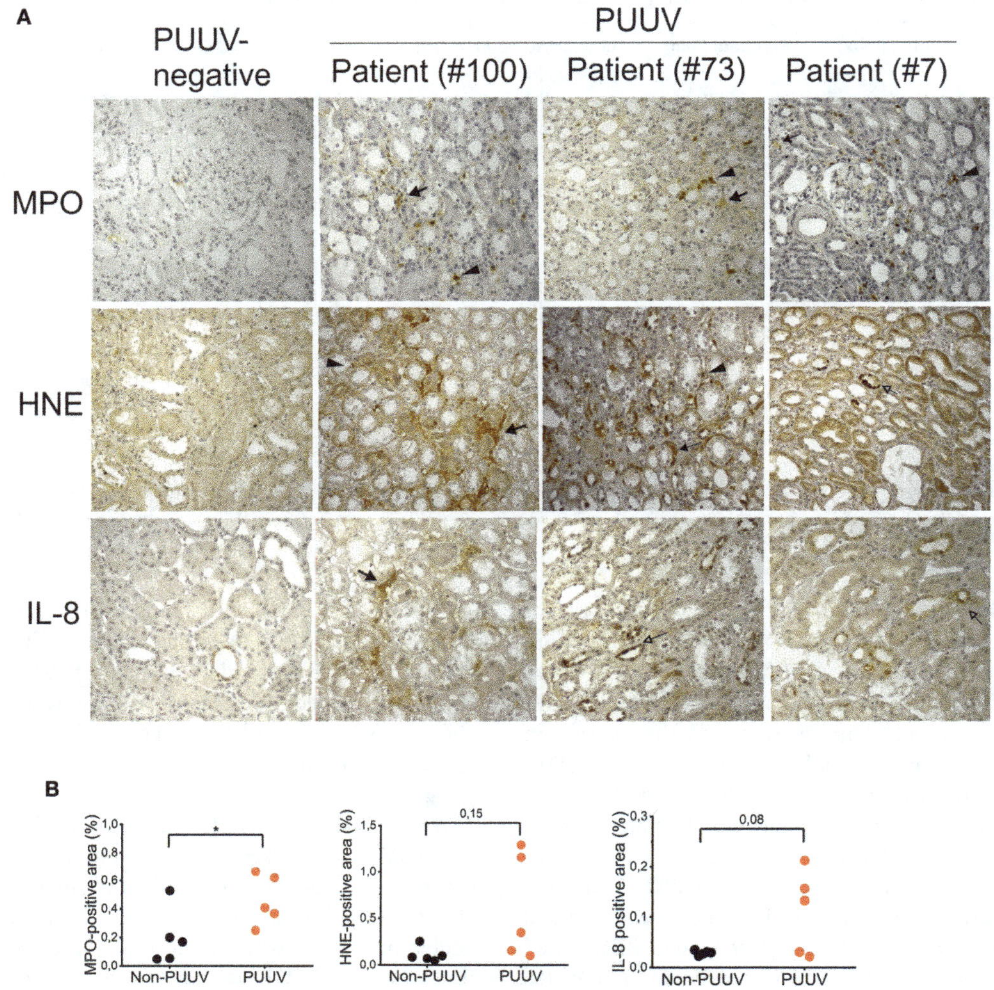

FIGURE 2 | Immunohistochemical analysis of MPO, HNE and IL-8 in kidney sections from patients with acute PUUV-HFRS. Kidney sections from acute PUUV-HFRS or unrelated kidney diseases ($n = 5$ for both) were analyzed for the presence of MPO, HNE or IL-8 by standard immunohistochemical techniques and visualized by DAB staining. **(A)** Images from three cases with acute PUUV-HFRS and one PUUV-negative control section is shown. **(B)** The tissue area positive for MPO, HNE or IL-8 was evaluated as percentages in all sections and mean values ± standard deviation reported for acute PUUV-HFRS and PUUV-negative sections. Significant differences were assessed by student's *T*-test and statistically significant differences indicated as $^*p < 0.05$.

of ECs on cell surfaces in some conditions (32) which could potentially explain this finding.

PUUV-Infected BECs Induce PMN Degranulation

Next, we wanted to determine whether more extensive co-culturing of PMNs and PUUV-infected BECs could result in PMN activation (degranulation or NETosis) which could explain our findings of increased levels of extracellular neutrophil markers in PUUV-HFRS patients (**Figures 1, 2**). We observed a time-dependent morphological change in PMNs bound to PUUV-infected BECs but not in mock- or UV-PUUV infected BECs which was visible after 3 but not 1 h of co-culture (**Figures 6A,B**). This was evident by increased nuclear swelling of PMNs together with altered localization of MPO from diffuse to plasma membrane-associated staining. Furthermore, MPO could be observed also extracellularly, which strongly suggests that PMN degranulation was taking place. The fluorescent phenotype of PMNs bound to PUUV-infected BECs was strikingly similar although less pronounced as observed for PMNs bound to TNF-α treated cells after a 3 h of co-culture. We did not find any evidence for NETosis in PMNs bound either on PUUV-infected or TNF-α treated cells or by PUUV-infected BEC supernatants (data not shown) in these experimental conditions.

Antiviral Effect of PMNs Is Mediated by Protease Release *in vitro*

Finally, we wanted to determine whether neutrophils possess antiviral function and if so, by which mechanism. We incubated purified PUUV with freshly isolated PMNs, which were either non-activated or activated with PMA. Furthermore, incubations

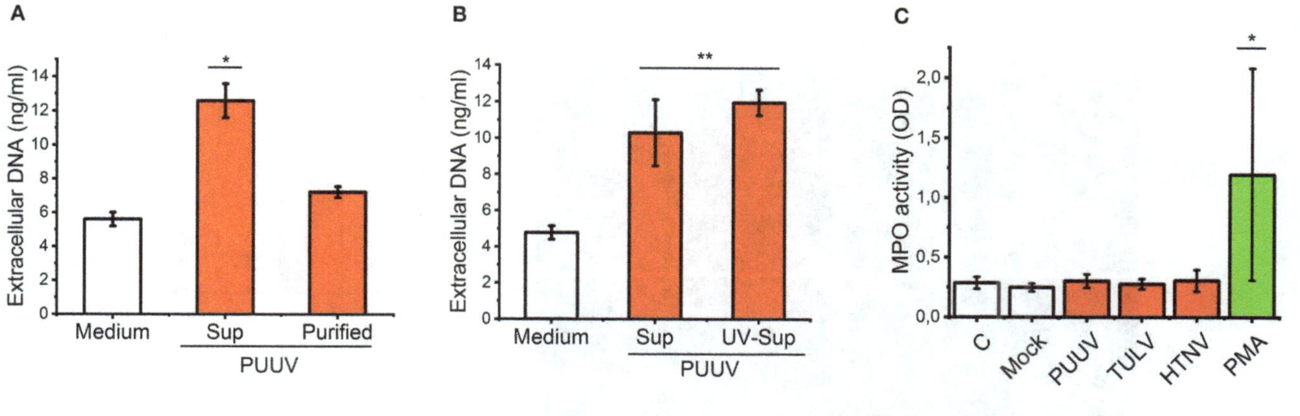

FIGURE 3 | Live PUUV does not induce neutrophil activation. **(A)** Mock- or PUUV-containing Vero E6 supernatants (Sup) or purified PUUV were incubated with freshly isolated PMNs for 3 h (MOI 1) ($n = 2$). The release of extracellular DNA was assessed by an impermeable DNA binding fluorescent dye. **(B)** Mock-, live PUUV- or UV-inactivated PUUV-containing Vero E6 supernatants were incubated with PMNs and assessed for DNA release as in **(A)** ($n = 3$). **(C)** Purified PUUV, TULV or HTNV were incubated with fresh PMNs for 3 h (MOI 1) and peroxidase activity assessed from cell culture supernatants by TMB ($n = 3$). PMA-treated PMNs were used as a positive controls. Difference between groups were assessed by one-way ANOVA + Dunnett's multiple comparisons test and statistically significant differences indicated as either $^{*}p < 0.05$ or $^{**}p < 0.01$.

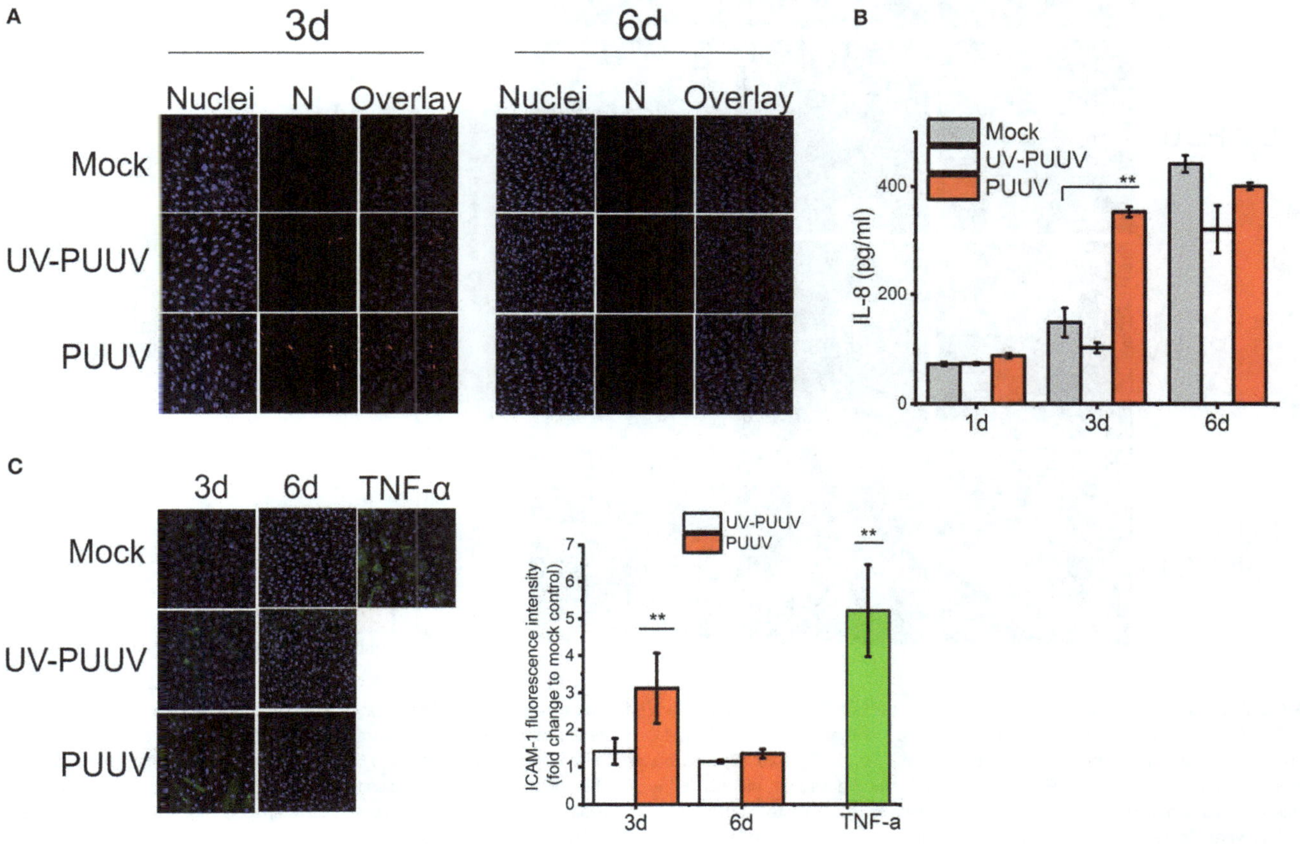

FIGURE 4 | PUUV infection causes pro-inflammatory responses in BECs. **(A)** BECs were either mock-infected or infected with live or UV-inactivated PUUV (UV-PUUV) and assessed for viral nucleocapsid protein expression at 3 and 6 days post infection by immunofluorescence (red). The nuclei of BECs were visualized with Hoechst 33420 (blue). **(B)** IL-8 was measured from the respective supernatants of mock, UV-PUUV or PUUV-infected BECs by ELISA. **(C)** ICAM-1 expression in TNF-α treated or mock-, UV-PUUV or PUUV-infected BECs was visualized by immunofluorescence (green) and shown as an overlay with Hoechst 33258 staining (blue). Fluorescence intensity of ICAM-1 expression on BECs was quantified and reported as fold change to mock-infected cells. Differences between groups were assessed by one-way ANOVA with Dunnett's multiple comparisons test and statistically significant differences indicated as $^{**}p < 0.01$. $n = 2$ in all panels. Results shown are representatives of three independent experiments.

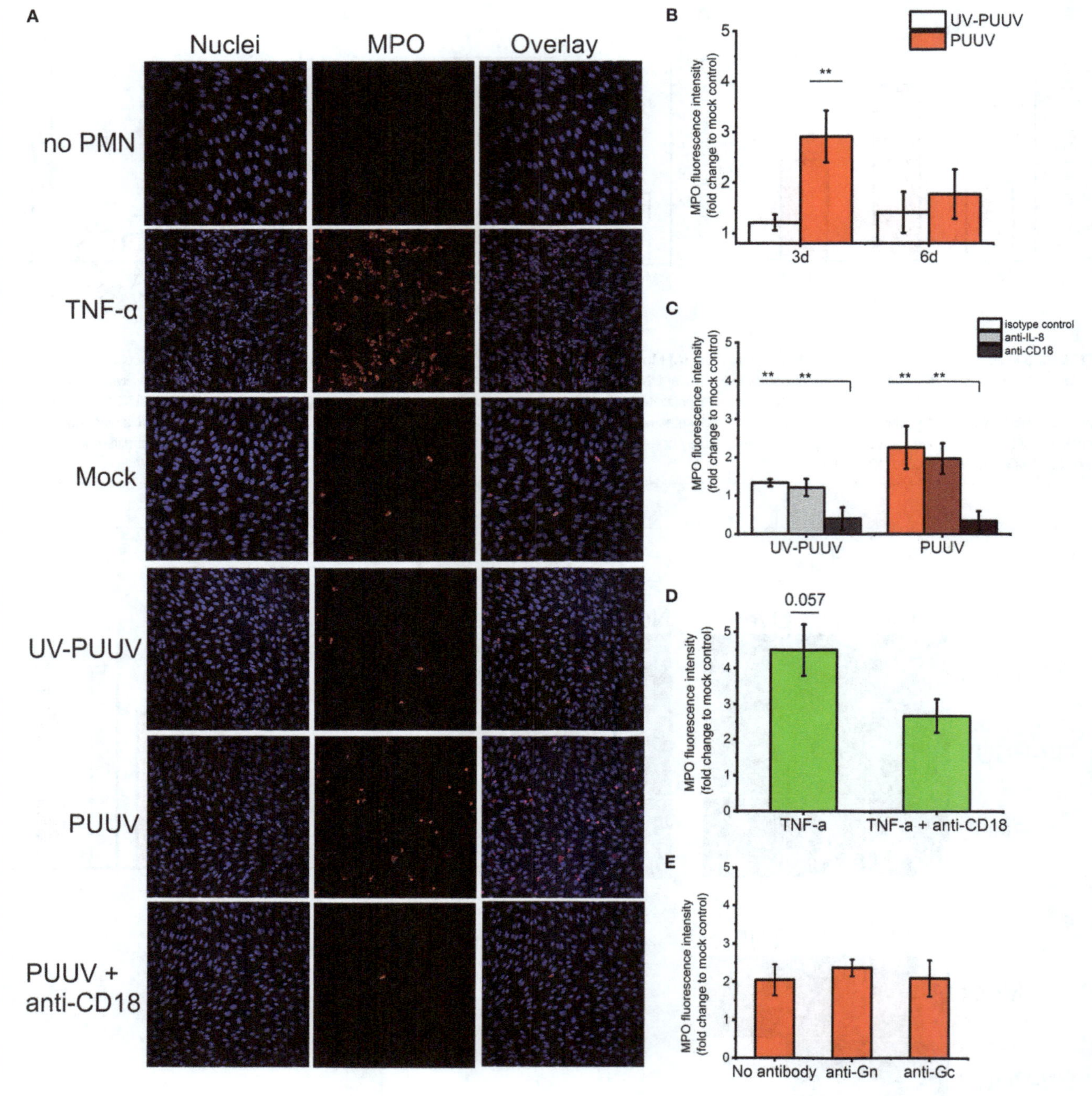

FIGURE 5 | Binding of quiescent PMNs to PUUV-infected BECs. Freshly isolated PMNs were allowed to bind to mock-, UV-PUUV or live PUUV-infected BECs for 1 h at 3 or 6 days post infection (dpi). **(A)** PMNs bound to either TNF-α treated, UV-PUUV or PUUV-infected BECs were visualized at 3 dpi by immunofluorescence using MPO-specific antibody. The nuclei were stained with Hoechst 33420. **(B)** BEC-bound PMNs were quantified at 3 and 6 dpi as fold change to mock-infected cells. **(C)** PMNs were allowed to bind to PUUV-infected BECs at 3 days post infection in the presence of neutralizing antibodies to IL-8, CD18 or an isotype control and quantified as above. **(D)** PMNs were allowed to bind to BECs treated with TNF-α for 3 days in the presence or absence of CD18 antibody and quantified as above. **(E)** PMNs were allowed to bind at 3 days post infection to PUUV-infected BECs treated with Gn- or Gc-specific neutralizing antibodies and quantified as above. Statistically significant differences between groups were assessed either by student's *T*-test **(B,D)** or one-way ANOVA with Dunnett's multiple comparison test **(C,E)** and indicated as $^{**}p < 0.01$. $n = 2$ in all panels. Results shown are representatives of three independent experiments.

of virus with PMA-activated PMNs were performed in the presence of one of the following inhibitors: NaN_3 (an inhibitor of MPO activity), phenylmethylsulfonylfluoride (PMSF; inhibitor of serine proteases), EDTA (inhibitor of metalloproteinases) and DNAse (degradation of NETs). After incubation, samples were subjected to immunoblotting in order to detect degradation of

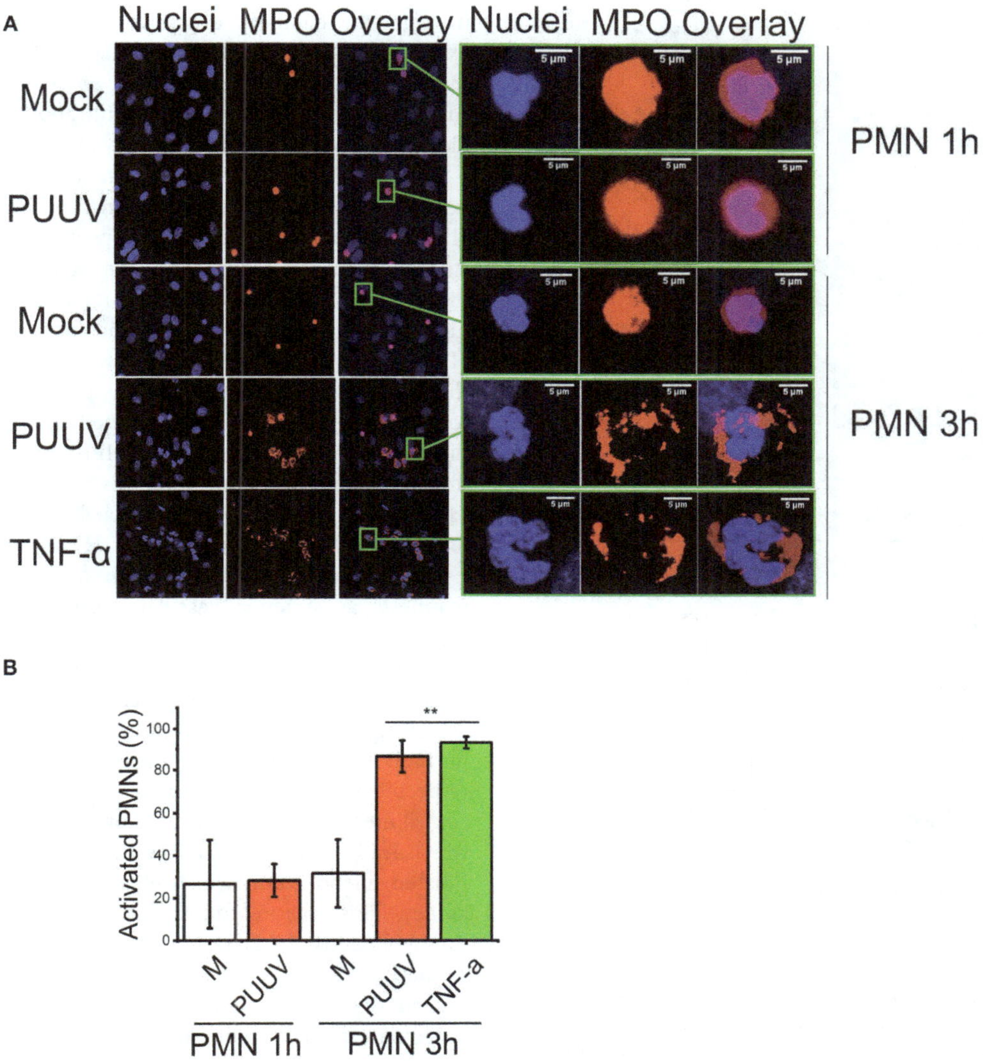

FIGURE 6 | PUUV-infected BECs induce PMN degranulation. **(A)** PMNs were allowed to bind to mock- or PUUV-infected BECs at 3 days post infection for 1 or 3 h. BECs treated with TNF-α for 1 day and exposed to PMNs for 3 h were used positive control for PMN activation. PMN activation was assessed by morphological changes of bound PMNs as observed by immunofluorescence staining for MPO (red) and nuclei (Hoechst 33420, blue). On the right, the fluorescence image of one individual BEC-bound PMN from each treatment group is enlarged for better visualization of PMN activation. **(B)** The percentage of swollen nuclei with concomitant changes in MPO expression from diffuse cytoplasmic to plasma membrane localization were counted in individual wells and mean values ± standard deviation reported. Statistically significant differences between groups is assessed by student's *T*-test and indicated as $^{**}p < 0.01$. $n = 3$. Results shown are representatives of two independent experiments.

viral structural proteins Gn, Gc and N protein (**Figure 7A**) and virus titer determinations in Vero E6 cells (**Figure 7B**). The PUUV Gc and N proteins migrated as expected based on their molecular size of ~54 and 50 kDa, respectively, whereas Gn is known to form SDS-stabile tetramers of ~240 kDa in SDS-PAGE [**Figure 7A**, (27)]. PMA-treated PMNs complete destroyed PUUV infectivity and the surface glycoproteins Gn and Gc while it has almost no effect on N protein, which is retained inside the virus particle, whereas quiescent PMNs decreased PUUV viability only marginally (50%) with the concomitant low-level cleavage of Gc. PMSF totally blocked the cleavage of Gn and Gc while retaining almost 10% of PUUV infectivity indicating strong involvement of serine proteases (such as HNE) in the antiviral effect of activated PMNs. Also, EDTA treatment retained significant levels of infectivity (5%) although not being able to block the degradation of Gn and Gc significantly. However, NaN_3 or DNAse treatments had no effect on the ability of PMA-treated PMNs to kill virus or degrade its glycoproteins, indicating that MPO or the formation of NETs do not play a direct role in the antiviral effects of PMNs in this experimental setup. The fact that the infectivity of PUUV was not significantly reduced after treatment with quiescent PMNs is further proof (see **Figure 3**) that hantaviruses are unable to significantly activate PMNs.

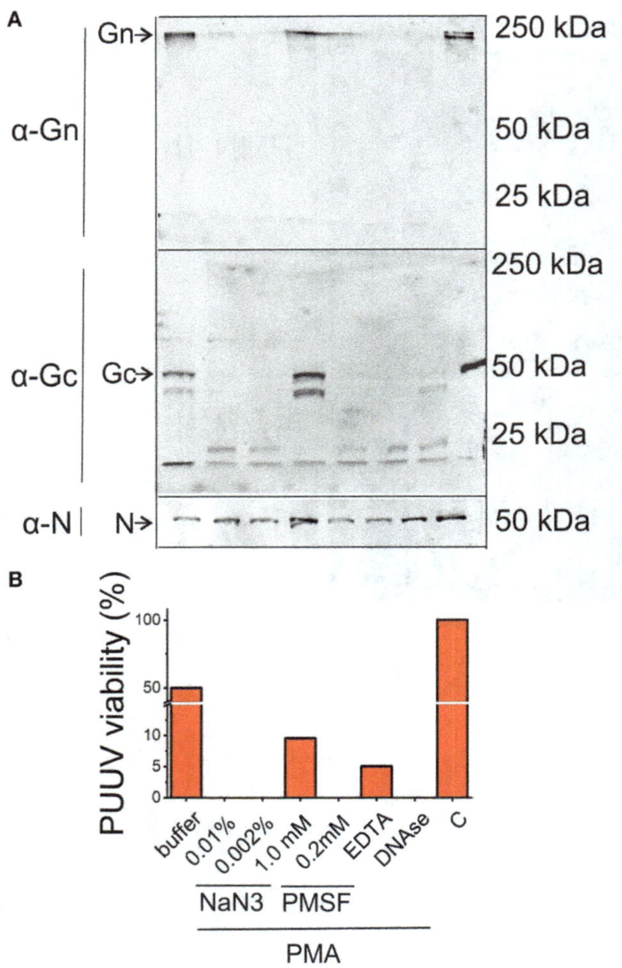

FIGURE 7 | Antiviral activity of activated PMNs. Purified PUUV was incubated with quiescent or PMA-activated freshly isolated PMNs in the presence of inhibitors for MPO (0.01 or 0.002% NaN_3), serine proteases (1 or 0.2 mM PMSF), metalloproteinases (1 mM EDTA) or NETs (10 U/ml DNAse) and **(A)** subjected to immunoblotting for viral proteins Gn, Gc and N protein and infectious titer measurement in Vero E6 cells **(B)**. C, Control without the addition of PMNs.

DISCUSSION

We observed elevated levels of circulating extracellular MPO, HNE and histones in the acute stage of PUUV-caused HFRS as compared to the recovery stage and healthy controls. MPO and HNE are expressed in neutrophil granules and released to the extracellular space through neutrophil degranulation or alternatively as components of NETs. Histones, on the other hand, are essential components of NETs but could be also released from other types of dying cells. The circulating levels of histone H3 correlated with MPO and HNE suggesting that all these factors are released simultaneously from neutrophils during NETosis, which presence in acute PUUV-HFRS has been reported previously (21). Interestingly, we found strong positive correlations between the levels of HNE or histone H3 and variable reflecting the severity of AKI (maximum creatinine); indicating that neutrophils could play a role in mediating kidney damage, the hallmark of HFRS. We could observe elevated expression of MPO in kidneys of acute PUUV-HFRS where it mainly localized to the interstitial space surrounding tubules, supporting earlier findings that infiltration of neutrophils into kidneys is a part of the inflammatory response toward PUUV (7).

In addition, we found that the major chemotactic factor for neutrophils, IL-8, is upregulated in the acute stage of PUUV-HFRS in blood, as previously reported (33), and correlated strongly with neutrophil activation markers (MPO, HNE and histone H3). This was also accompanied by a tendency of higher IL-8 expression also in the kidneys of acute PUUV-HFRS patients. The kidney IL-8 was found to be localized to the tubulointerstitial space, similarly to MPO and HNE, but also to tubular epithelial cells. This suggests IL-8 could be expressed directly by the kidney in PUUV-HFRS and plays a major role in recruiting neutrophils into this tissue. Furthermore, local expression of IL-8 in the kidney probably explains the high levels of IL-8 found in the urine of PUUV-HFRS patients (28).

AKI is the hallmark symptom of HFRS but the disease manifests as systemic vascular dysfunction as indicated by capillary leakage in several organs (1). It is of interest to note that neutrophil activation markers not only correlate with kidney injury, but also with different hematological parameters indicating the extent of thrombocytopenia, leukocytosis and fibrinolysis (low platelets, high leukocytes and high tPA, respectively). This suggests that neutrophil activation either contributes to or is in fact caused by the same underlying factors which lead to capillary leakage in PUUV-HFRS and is not an isolated phenomenon which effect would be restricted to the kidney. This calls for future studies aimed at determining the extent of neutrophil activation also in other forms of hantavirus-mediated diseases such as HCPS which severely affect lungs instead of kidneys. In fact, neutrophils have been shown as the main culprits of pulmonary vascular permeability in mouse model of HTNV infection (25).

A previous report indicates that HTNV binds CD11b/CD18 integrin complex on the surface of neutrophils and, as shown using HTNV-containing Vero E6 cell culture supernatants, activates NETosis in freshly isolated PMNs (21). Given the high degree of similarity between different hantaviruses (1), we hypothesized that also PUUV is be able to activate in NET formation in PMNs. However, we observed that, while PUUV-containing Vero E6 cell culture supernatant was able to activate NETosis, purified PUUV was not (**Figure 3A**), suggesting that NETosis is not mediated by live, intact virus but rather other factor/s present in the cell culture supernatant of infected Vero E6 cells. We therefore sought for an alternative mechanism of neutrophil activation in PUUV-HFRS and turned our attention toward microvascular endothelial cells, the prime target of hantavirus infection *in vivo*. To begin with, we found that PUUV-infected blood microvascular cells (BECs) secreted elevated levels of IL-8 and expressed more ICAM-1 on their surface than non-infected BECs; suggesting that PUUV infection induces a pro-inflammatory phenotype in BECs. Importantly, elevated expression of ICAM-1 has been also detected in kidneys of acute PUUV-HFRS (8). We observed that freshly isolated PMNs adhered to PUUV-infected, pro-inflammatory BECs which was dependent on CD11b/CD18 integrin complex on the surface of neutrophils but not IL-8 or viral glycoproteins. We then asked whether the BEC-adhered PMNs would become activated to explain the observed elevated levels of MPO, HNE and histones in patients. We found that extensive co-culturing of fresh PMNs together with PUUV-infected BECs resulted in morphological changes in PMNs, which suggested degranulation of PMNs. However, we did not find any evidence of increased NETosis in these co-cultures.

These results imply that PUUV infection causes pro-inflammatory changes in endothelial cells to attract and activate neutrophils on the surface of the endothelium by an IL-8 dependent mechanism. It is previously noted that pro-inflammatory endothelial cells can induce NETosis partially through EC-derived IL-8 causing endothelial cell death (34). The interactions of neutrophils with the endothelium in inflammatory conditions is well-documented (9, 12, 35, 36) and typically these events are not associated with clinically significant vascular permeability. In typical inflammatory reactions, however, the chemotactic signals that induce inflammation originate from tissues from where neutrophil diapedesis across the endothelium is locally dictated. This is in contrast to hantavirus infections where the viruses replicate in endothelial cells to cause systemic inflammation of the vasculature. In addition to endothelial cells, hantavirus glycoproteins have been detected in renal tubular cells in acute HTNV-caused HFRS (37), where we observed increased levels of HNE and IL-8 in this study, suggesting that hantavirus-infected tubular cells could behave similarly to infected endothelial cells and recruit and activate neutrophils by an IL-8 dependent mechanism. The fact that depletion of neutrophils suppress lung pathology in a mouse model for HTNV certainly supports the idea of neutrophils as the driving force of HFRS pathogenesis (25). Similar mechanisms could play a role also in other hemorrhagic fevers (38). It is known that for instance that flavi- and filoviruses induce pro-inflammatory changes in endothelial cells (39–41). Of note, ICAM-1 polymorphism is associated with dengue disease severity (42).

Neutrophils are well-known for their antibacterial effects but their ability to counteract viral infections are only beginning to be unraveled (17, 35, 43). Early research indicates that defensins, which are peptides released from neutrophils upon activation, show antiviral activity against enveloped viruses (44). MPO can also cause oxidative damage to viruses upon neutrophil oxidative burst and degranulation (45). Lately, the antiviral effects of NETs have been implicated (46). In the present study we observed that serine proteases (such as HNE) play a major role in the virucidal function of neutrophils against PUUV. However, we did not obtain evidence for a direct role of NETs or MPO-mediated oxidative effects in killing PUUV. Furthermore, the fact that PUUV was not killed by PMNs which were non-activated at the start of the experiment, show that PUUV doesn't directly cause significant protease release by PMNs. The inability of PMNs to produce NETs through direct contact with hantaviruses is not surprising since typically NETs are produced in response to larger microbes (47) but given the known expression of several Toll-like receptors by neutrophils (48), their inability to release proteases (degranulate) in response to PUUV is peculiar. However, some viruses are known to block the activation of neutrophils (49, 50) and whether this is also the case for hantaviruses remain a topic for future studies.

To conclude, we have found that patients suffering from acute PUUV-caused HFRS show elevated levels of circulating MPO, HNE, histone H3 and IL-8 indicating neutrophil activation through degranulation and/or NETosis. The expression levels of these markers positively correlate with parameters reflecting disease severity suggesting that neutrophil activation could play a major role in the pathogenesis of HFRS. Mechanistically, our data indicates that neutrophil activation is more likely to occur indirectly via virus-infected microvascular endothelial cells rather than directly through virus contact with neutrophils. Future studies are still needed to elucidate whether either neutrophil degranulation or NETosis has the stronger impact on hantavirus pathogenesis.

AUTHOR CONTRIBUTIONS

TS and AV conceived and designed the research. TS performed the experiments and analyzed the data. SM and JM contributed to sample collection. TS wrote the paper. All authors reviewed the manuscript.

ACKNOWLEDGMENTS

We thank Ms. Sanna Mäki, Ms. Katriina Ylinikkilä, and Ms. Marja-Leena Koskinen for excellent technical assistance.

REFERENCES

1. Vaheri A, Strandin T, Hepojoki J, Sironen T, Henttonen H, Makela S, et al. Uncovering the mysteries of *Hantavirus* infections. *Nat Rev Microbiol.* (2013) 11:539–50. doi: 10.1038/nrmicro3066
2. Mackow ER, Gorbunova EE, Gavrilovskaya IN. Endothelial cell dysfunction in viral hemorrhage and edema. *Front Microbiol.* (2015) 5:733. doi: 10.3389/fmicb.2014.00733
3. Hepojoki J, Vaheri A, Strandin T. The fundamental role of endothelial cells in *Hantavirus* pathogenesis. *Front Microbiol.* (2014) 5:727. doi: 10.3389/fmicb.2014.00727
4. Jonsson CB, Figueiredo LT, Vapalahti O. A global perspective on *Hantavirus* ecology, epidemiology, and disease. *Clin Microbiol Rev.* (2010) 23:412–41. doi: 10.1128/CMR.00062-09.
5. Mustonen J, Outinen T, Laine O, Porsti I, Vaheri A, Makela S. Kidney disease in Puumala *Hantavirus* infection. *Infect*

Dis (Lond). (2017) 49:321–32. doi: 10.1080/23744235.2016.1274421
6. Bunz H, Weyrich P, Peter A, Baumann D, Tschritter O, Guthoff M, et al. Urinary neutrophil gelatinase-associated lipocalin (NGAL) and proteinuria predict severity of acute kidney injury in *Puumala virus* infection. *BMC Infect Dis.* (2015) 15:464. doi: 10.1186/s12879-015-1180-9
7. Mustonen J, Helin H, Pietila K, Brummer-Korvenkontio M, Hedman K, Vaheri A, et al. Renal biopsy findings and clinicopathologic correlations in nephropathia epidemica. *Clin Nephrol* (1994) 41:121–6.
8. Temonen M, Mustonen J, Helin H, Pasternack A, Vaheri A, Holthofer H. Cytokines, adhesion molecules, and cellular infiltration in nephropathia epidemica kidneys: an immunohistochemical study. *Clin Immunol Immunopathol.* (1996) 78:47–55. doi: 10.1006/clin.1996.0007
9. Summers C, Rankin SM, Condliffe AM, Singh N, Peters AM, Chilvers ER. Neutrophil kinetics in health and disease. *Trends Immunol.* (2010) 31:318–24. doi: 10.1016/j.it.2010.05.006
10. Harada A, Sekido N, Akahoshi T, Wada T, Mukaida N, Matsushima K. Essential involvement of interleukin-8 (IL-8) in acute inflammation. *J Leukoc Biol.* (1994) 56:559–64.
11. Borregaard N. Neutrophils, from marrow to microbes. *Immunity* (2010) 33:657–70. doi: 10.1016/j.immuni.2010.11.011
12. Vestweber D. How leukocytes cross the vascular endothelium. *Nat Rev Immunol.* (2015) 15:692–704. doi: 10.1038/nri3908
13. Pham CT. Neutrophil serine proteases: specific regulators of inflammation. *Nat Rev Immunol.* (2006) 6:541–50. doi: 10.1038/nri1841
14. Odobasic D, Kitching AR, Holdsworth SR. Neutrophil-mediated regulation of innate and adaptive immunity: the role of myeloperoxidase. *J Immunol Res.* (2016) 2016:2349817. doi: 10.1155/2016/2349817
15. Yipp BG, Kubes P. NETosis: how vital is it? *Blood* (2013) 122:2784–94. doi: 10.1182/blood-2013-04-457671
16. Brinkmann V, Reichard U, Goosmann C, Fauler B, Uhlemann Y, Weiss DS, et al. Neutrophil extracellular traps kill bacteria. *Science* (2004) 303:1532–5. doi: 10.1126/science.1092385
17. Gabriel C, Her Z, Ng LF. Neutrophils: neglected players in viral diseases. *DNA Cell Biol.* (2013) 32:665–75. doi: 10.1089/dna.2013.2211
18. Baigildina AA, Khaiboullina SF, Martynova EV, Anokhin VA, Lombardi VC, Rizvanov AA. Inflammatory cytokines kinetics define the severity and phase of nephropathia epidemica. *Biomark Med.* (2015) 9:99–107. doi: 10.2217/bmm.14.88
19. Morzunov SP, Khaiboullina SF, St Jeor S, Rizvanov AA, Lombardi VC. Multiplex analysis of serum cytokines in humans with *Hantavirus* pulmonary syndrome. *Front Immunol.* (2015) 6:432. doi: 10.3389/fimmu.2015.00432
20. Khaiboullina SF, Martynova EV, Khamidullina ZL, Lapteva EV, Nikolaeva IV, Anokhin VV, et al. Upregulation of IFN-gamma and IL-12 is associated with a milder form of *Hantavirus* hemorrhagic fever with renal syndrome. *Eur J Clin Microbiol Infect Dis.* (2014) 33:2149–56. doi: 10.1007/s10096-014-2176-x
21. Raftery MJ, Lalwani P, Krautkrmer E, Peters T, Scharffetter-Kochanek K, Kruger R, et al. Beta2 integrin mediates *Hantavirus*-induced release of neutrophil extracellular traps. *J Exp Med.* (2014) 211:1485–97. doi: 10.1084/jem.20131092
22. Outinen TK, Kuparinen T, Jylhava J, Leppanen S, Mustonen J, Makela S, et al. Plasma cell-free DNA levels are elevated in acute Puumala *Hantavirus* infection. *PLoS ONE* (2012) 7:e31455. doi: 10.1371/journal.pone.0031455
23. Vaheri A, Strandin T, Jaaskelainen AJ, Vapalahti O, Jarva H, Lokki ML, et al. Pathophysiology of a severe case of Puumala *Hantavirus* infection successfully treated with bradykinin receptor antagonist icatibant. *Antiviral Res.* (2014) 111:23–5. doi: 10.1016/j.antiviral.2014.08.007
24. Schonrich G, Kruger DH, Raftery MJ. *Hantavirus*-induced disruption of the endothelial barrier: neutrophils are on the payroll. *Front Microbiol.* (2015) 6:222. doi: 10.3389/fmicb.2015.00222
25. Koma T, Yoshimatsu K, Nagata N, Sato Y, Shimizu K, Yasuda SP, et al. Neutrophil depletion suppresses pulmonary vascular hyperpermeability and occurrence of pulmonary edema caused by *Hantavirus* infection in C.B-17 SCID mice. *J Virol.* (2014) 88:7178–88. doi: 10.1128/JVI.00254-14
26. Vapalahti O, Kallio-Kokko H, Narvanen A, Julkunen I, Lundkvist A, Plyusnin A, et al. Human B-cell epitopes of *Puumala virus* nucleocapsid protein, the major antigen in early serological response. *J Med Virol.* (1995) 46:293–303.
27. Hepojoki J, Strandin T, Vaheri A, Lankinen H. Interactions and oligomerization of *Hantavirus* glycoproteins. *J Virol.* (2010) 84:227–42. doi: 10.1128/JVI.00481-09.
28. Libraty DH, Makela S, Vlk J, Hurme M, Vaheri A, Ennis FA, et al. The degree of leukocytosis and urine GATA-3 mRNA levels are risk factors for severe acute kidney injury in *Puumala virus* nephropathia epidemica. *PLoS ONE* (2012) 7:e35402. doi: 10.1371/journal.pone.0035402
29. Strandin T, Hepojoki J, Laine O, Makela S, Klingstrom J, Lundkvist A, et al. Interferons induce STAT1-dependent expression of tissue plasminogen activator, a pathogenicity factor in Puumala *Hantavirus* disease. *J Infect Dis.* (2016) 213:1632–41. doi: 10.1093/infdis/jiv764
30. Khaiboullina SF, Rizvanov AA, Deyde VM, St Jeor SC. Andes virus stimulates interferon-inducible MxA protein expression in endothelial cells. *J Med Virol.* (2005) 75:267–75. doi: 10.1002/jmv.20266
31. Lundkvist A, Niklasson B. Bank vole monoclonal antibodies against *Puumala virus* envelope glycoproteins: identification of epitopes involved in neutralization. *Arch Virol.* (1992) 126:93–105.
32. Sano H, Nakagawa N, Chiba R, Kurasawa K, Saito Y, Iwamoto I. Cross-linking of intercellular adhesion molecule-1 induces interleukin-8 and RANTES production through the activation of MAP kinases in human vascular endothelial cells. *Biochem Biophys Res Commun.* (1998) 250:694–8.
33. Sadeghi M, Eckerle I, Daniel V, Burkhardt U, Opelz G, Schnitzler P. Cytokine expression during early and late phase of acute Puumala *Hantavirus* infection. *BMC Immunol.* (2011) 12:65. doi: 10.1186/1471-2172-12-65
34. Gupta AK, Joshi MB, Philippova M, Erne P, Hasler P, Hahn S, et al. Activated endothelial cells induce neutrophil extracellular traps and are susceptible to NETosis-mediated cell death. *FEBS Lett.* (2010) 584:3193–7. doi: 10.1016/j.febslet.2010.06.006
35. Camp JV, Jonsson CB. A role for neutrophils in viral respiratory disease. *Front Immunol.* (2017) 8:550. doi: 10.3389/fimmu.2017.00550
36. Jenne CN, Wong CH, Zemp FJ, McDonald B, Rahman MM, Forsyth PA, et al. Neutrophils recruited to sites of infection protect from virus challenge by releasing neutrophil extracellular traps. *Cell Host Microbe.* (2013) 13:169–80. doi: 10.1016/j.chom.2013.01.005
37. Kim S, Kang ET, Kim YG, Han JS, Lee JS, Kim YI, et al. Localization of *Hantaan* viral envelope glycoproteins by monoclonal antibodies in renal tissues from patients with Korean hemorrhagic fever H. *Am J Clin Pathol.* (1993) 100:398–403. doi: 10.1055/s-0037-1613397
38. Schnittler HJ, Feldmann H. Viral hemorrhagic fever–a vascular disease? *Thromb Haemost.* (2003) 89:967–72. doi: 10.4269/ajtmh.2000.63.71
39. Huang YH, Lei HY, Liu HS, Lin YS, Liu CC, Yeh TM. Dengue virus infects human endothelial cells and induces IL-6 and IL-8 production. *Am J Trop Med Hyg.* (2000) 63:71–5.
40. Harcourt BH, Sanchez A, Offermann MK. *Ebola virus* selectively inhibits responses to interferons, but not to interleukin-1beta, in endothelial cells. *J Virol.* (1999) 73:3491–6.
41. Dalrymple NA, Mackow ER. Endothelial cells elicit immune-enhancing responses to dengue virus infection. *J Virol.* (2012) 86:6408–15. doi: 10.1128/JVI.00213-12
42. Sharma S, Singh SK, Kakkar K, Nyari N, Singh D, Dhole TN, et al. Association of ICAM-1 K469E polymorphism with dengue infection in North Indian population. *Microb Pathog.* (2016) 96:80–4. doi: 10.1016/j.micpath.2016.05.006
43. Galani IE, Andreakos E. Neutrophils in viral infections: current concepts and caveats. *J Leukoc Biol.* (2015) 98:557–64. doi: 10.1189/jlb.4VMR1114-555R
44. Daher KA, Selsted ME, Lehrer RI. Direct inactivation of viruses by human granulocyte defensins. *J Virol.* (1986) 60:1068–74.
45. Klebanoff SJ, Coombs RW. Viricidal effect of polymorphonuclear leukocytes on human immunodeficiency virus-1. Role of the myeloperoxidase system. *J Clin Invest.* (1992) 89:2014–7. doi: 10.1172/JCI115810
46. Agraz-Cibrian JM, Giraldo DM, Mary FM, Urcuqui-Inchima S. Understanding the molecular mechanisms of NETs and their role in antiviral innate immunity. *Virus Res.* (2017) 228:124–33. doi: 10.1016/j.virusres.2016.11.033
47. Branzk N, Lubojemska A, Hardison SE, Wang Q, Gutierrez MG, Brown GD, et al. Neutrophils sense microbe size and selectively release neutrophil extracellular traps in response to large pathogens. *Nat Immunol.* (2014) 15:1017–25. doi: 10.1038/ni.2987

48. Thomas CJ, Schroder K. Pattern recognition receptor function in neutrophils. *Trends Immunol.* (2013) 34:317–28. doi: 10.1016/j.it.2013.02.008
49. Saitoh T, Komano J, Saitoh Y, Misawa T, Takahama M, Kozaki T, et al. Neutrophil extracellular traps mediate a host defense response to human immunodeficiency virus-1. *Cell Host Microbe* (2012) 12:109–16. doi: 10.1016/j.chom.2012.05.015
50. Hartshorn KL, Liou LS, White MR, Kazhdan MM, Tauber JL, Tauber AI. Neutrophil deactivation by influenza A virus. Role of hemagglutinin binding to specific sialic acid-bearing cellular proteins. *J Immunol.* (1995) 154:3952–60.

9

Pathogenicity and Viral Shedding of MERS-CoV in Immunocompromised Rhesus Macaques

*Joseph Prescott[1], Darryl Falzarano[1], Emmie de Wit[1], Kath Hardcastle[2], Friederike Feldmann[2], Elaine Haddock[1], Dana Scott[2], Heinz Feldmann[1] and Vincent Jacobus Munster[1]**

[1] Laboratory of Virology, Division of Intramural Research, Rocky Mountain Laboratories, National Institute of Allergy and Infectious Diseases, National Institutes of Health, Hamilton, MT, United States, [2] Rocky Mountain Veterinary Branch, Division of Intramural Research, Rocky Mountain Laboratories, National Institute of Allergy and Infectious Diseases, National Institutes of Health, Hamilton, MT, United States

***Correspondence:**
Vincent Jacobus Munster
munstervj@niaid.nih.gov

Middle East respiratory syndrome coronavirus (MERS-CoV) has recently emerged in the Middle East. Since 2012, there have been approximately 2,100 confirmed cases, with a 35% case fatality rate. Disease severity has been linked to patient health status, as people with chronic diseases or an immunocompromised status fare worse, although the mechanisms of disease have yet to be elucidated. We used the rhesus macaque model of mild MERS to investigate whether the immune response plays a role in the pathogenicity in relation to MERS-CoV shedding. Immunosuppressed macaques were inoculated with MERS-CoV and sampled daily for 6 days to assess their immune statues and to measure viral shedding and replication. Immunosuppressed macaques supported significantly higher levels of MERS-CoV replication in respiratory tissues and shed more virus, and virus disseminated to tissues outside of the respiratory tract, whereas viral RNA was confined to respiratory tissues in non-immunosuppressed animals. Despite increased viral replication, pathology in the lungs was significantly lower in immunosuppressed animals. The observation that the virus was less pathogenic in these animals suggests that disease has an immunopathogenic component and shows that inflammatory responses elicited by the virus contribute to disease.

Keywords: Middle East respiratory syndrome coronavirus, immunosuppression, pathology, shedding, macaque monkey

INTRODUCTION

A novel coronavirus (CoV) emerged in Saudi Arabia in June of 2012 that is the causative agent of a severe respiratory disease called Middle East respiratory syndrome (MERS) (1). Thus far, there have been almost 2,100 diagnosed cases (2). Despite increased surveillance and the identification of many new cases, the case fatality rate has remained high and is currently approximately 35%.

Although there have been a high number of cases, little is known about the mechanisms of pathogenesis and the disease progression in humans is poorly described. Clinical features range from asymptomatic infection, to an acute respiratory distress syndrome, and multi-organ failure (3). The majority of patients that have succumbed to MERS-CoV have had comorbidities (4, 5) and disease is thought to be more severe in immunocompromised patients. However, the actual mechanisms of disease remain to be elucidated. The virus has been shown to replicate in human primary epithelial and *ex vivo* human lung cultures, especially in non-ciliated bronchial epithelial cells and alveolar type II pneumocytes (6–8) and the receptor has been identified as dipeptidyl peptidase 4, which is expressed on these cell types (9). MERS-CoV shedding is higher in patients with more severe disease manifestations compared to milder cases (10).

Our laboratory has recently developed two non-human primate models of MERS, utilizing the rhesus macaque and the common marmoset (11–13). Rhesus macaques develop a mild pneumonia upon intratracheal inoculation with MERS-CoV (12). In this model, virus replicates within the respiratory tract to modest levels, and is detectible in oral and nasal swabs. However, clinical disease is most prominent within the first few days after inoculation and animals show signs of disease resolution soon after. Disease in rhesus likely models the mild form of the human disease, where the infection is self-limiting and clinical signs and symptoms are mild (10, 14, 15). In an effort to examine whether the immune status of an individual influences the disease severity and pathogenicity and replication kinetics of the virus, we downregulated the immune system of rhesus macaques using immunosuppressive drugs. We found that MERS-CoV replicated to significantly higher titers and disseminated outside of the respiratory tract in immunosuppressed animals, yet pathology was markedly reduced in these animals, showing that disease has an immunopathogenic component.

MATERIALS AND METHODS

Ethics Statement

The use of study animals was approved by the Institutional Animal Care and Use Committee of the Rocky Mountain Laboratories and experiments were performed following the guidelines of the Association for Assessment and Accreditation of the Laboratory Animal Care by certified staff in an approved facility. The guidelines and basic principles in the United States Public Health Service Policy on Humane Care and Use of Laboratory Animals and the Guide for the Care and Use of Laboratory Animals were followed. All procedures were carried out under anesthesia using Ketamine by trained personnel under veterinarian supervision and efforts were made to provide for the welfare of animals and to minimize suffering. All animals were humanely euthanized at the endpoint of the study (6 days post-inoculation) by exsanguination under deep anesthesia. All standard operating procedures for MERS-CoV were approved by the Institutional Biosafety committee of the Rock Mountain Laboratories, and sample inactivation was carried out according to approved standard operating procedures prior to removal from high containment.

Virus Propagation

Middle East respiratory syndrome coronavirus (isolate EMC/2012) was propagated in Vero E6 cells in DMEM (Sigma) supplemented with 2% FBS (Logan), 1 mM L-glutamine (Lonza), 50 U/mL penicillin, and 50 μg/mL streptomycin (both from Gibco).

Rhesus Macaque Immunosuppression and Inoculation

Five Rhesus macaques (female, weighing 7–11 kg, 11 years of age) were enrolled in this study. Immunosuppression (animals ISCoV1-3) was achieved by administration of cyclophosphamide (CyP) (Roxane Laboratories) (10 mg/kg dissolved in 30 mL of a meal supplement (Boost) and delivered *via* an orogastric tube under anesthesia every other day starting 16 days prior to virus inoculation and ending 2 days after inoculation), and dexamethasone (Dex, 2 mg/kg daily by subcutaneous injection beginning 16 days prior to virus inoculation and ending 5 days after inoculation). Mock immunosuppression (CoV1-2) was performed following the same schedule, but orogastric feeding did not contain CyP and injections consisted of sterile PBS. Immunosuppression was confirmed by monitoring white blood cell (WBC) populations using a HemaVet (Drew Scientific). For inoculation, 7×10^6 $TCID_{50}$ of MERS-CoV was diluted in 7 mL of DMEM and delivered *via* intratracheal (4 mL) oral (1 mL) nasal (1 mL), and ocular (1 mL) routes as previously described (12). Clinical exams were performed on days −18, −16, −10, −4, −2, 0, and +1 to +6 relative to virus inoculation. Blood was obtained at these times as well as nasal and oral swabbing and chest radiographs starting on day 0. Six days after inoculation, all five animals were euthanized and necropsies performed to obtain samples of the following tissues: lungs (all six lobes), bronchi, oro/nasopharynx, trachea, tonsils, heart, liver, spleen, kidney, adrenal gland, pancreas, inguinal, axillary, mesenteric, and mediastinal lymph nodes.

Virus Quantitation

We used a one-step real-time quantitative RT-PCR to measure viral RNA in the samples. RNA was extracted from swabs using the QiaAmp Viral RNA extraction kit and tissues using the RNeasy kit (both from Qiagen). RNA was then used along with a MERS-CoV-specific primer/probe set using the Rotor-Gene Probe kit (Qiagen). Tissue culture infectious dose 50% (TCID50) equivalents were calculated by comparing cycle threshold values to a standard curve generated from virus stocks of known titer. Primers and probe sequences were described previously (16).

Histopathology

Tissues were fixed in 10% neutral buffered formalin with two changes, for a minimum of 7 days and processed with a Sakura VIP-5 Tissue Tek, on a 12 h automated schedule, using a graded series of ethanol, xylene, and ParaPlast Extra. Embedded tissues were then sectioned at 5 μm and dried overnight at 42°C prior to staining.

For immunohistochemistry (IHC), tissues were processed using the Discovery XT automated processor with a DAPMap kit (both from Ventana). Specific primary antibodies used were: anti-HCoV-EMC polyclonal rabbit antibody (17) against CoV at a 1:1,000 dilution, anti-CD3 (2GV6) rabbit monoclonal primary antibody applied neat, and anti-CD20 (Thermo Scientific) at a 1:100 dilution. For CD3 and CD20, IHC stained sections were scanned with an Aperio ScanScope XT (Aperio Technologies, Inc., Vista, CA, USA) and analyzed using the ImageScope Positive Pixel

Count algorithm (version 9.1). Approximately 25 mm squared were evaluated at 2× magnification. The default parameters of the Positive Pixel Count (hue of 0.1 and width of 0.5) were used.

RESULTS

Rhesus Macaque Immunosuppression

To assess the contribution of the immune response to protection from MERS disease, we immunosuppressed three rhesus macaques using CyP and Dex for 16 days prior to inoculation with 7×10^6 $TCID_{50}$ of MERS-CoV. Two animals were used for mock immunosuppression controls and received the identical inoculum. Throughout immunosuppression, we monitored WBC populations in the blood to determine the efficacy of the immunosuppression regimen. Total WBC counts were decreased by approximately twofold compared to the control animals in response to CyP and Dex administration at the time of MERS-CoV inoculation. This reduction was due to decreases in all measured cell types (lymphocytes, neutrophils, monocytes, eosinophils, and basophils) (**Figure 1**). Following MERS-CoV inoculation, the absolute counts of these cell populations remained low in the immunosuppressed animals, suggesting their inability to respond to infection. Conversely, the two mock immunosuppressed animals had increased numbers of monocytes and eosinophils in response to infection. To quantify immunosuppression at the tissue level, the spleens and mediastinal lymph nodes of all animals were stained immunohistochemically with T cell and B cell markers (CD3 and CD20, respectively) post-mortem. The amount of staining was quantitatively assessed using imaging software. The quantity of CD3 staining was approximately 2-fold lower in the spleen and 2.7-fold in a mediastinal lymph node in the immunosuppressed animals. Likewise, CD20 was 2.4-fold lower in the spleen and 3-fold lower in the lymph nodes, showing a general reduction in lymphocytes in these tissues and confirming that the suppressive drug therapy was effective in reducing immune cell populations (**Figures 2A,B**). Immunosuppression also disrupted the normal architecture of these tissues.

Virus Shedding and Replication

Oral and nasal swab samples were obtained daily throughout the course of MERS-CoV infection to monitor the shedding of viral RNA. While shedding was detected from all animals, detection of viral RNA occurred earlier, persisted longer, and was several logs higher, in the immunosuppressed animals compared to the control animals (**Figures 3A,B**). Viral RNA was detectable at 6 days post-inoculation in nasal swabs from all three immunosuppressed animals and oral swabs from two animals, whereas the control animals were negative by this time point.

To assess virus replication in the tissues, we enlisted three rhesus macaques from a previous study to serve as historic controls, along with the two controls in this study (11). All animals were given the same inoculum (from the same stock of virus) *via* the same route and all were euthanized 6 days post-inoculation. When comparing the viral abundance in the lungs (all six lobes) between the controls from this study and the historic controls,

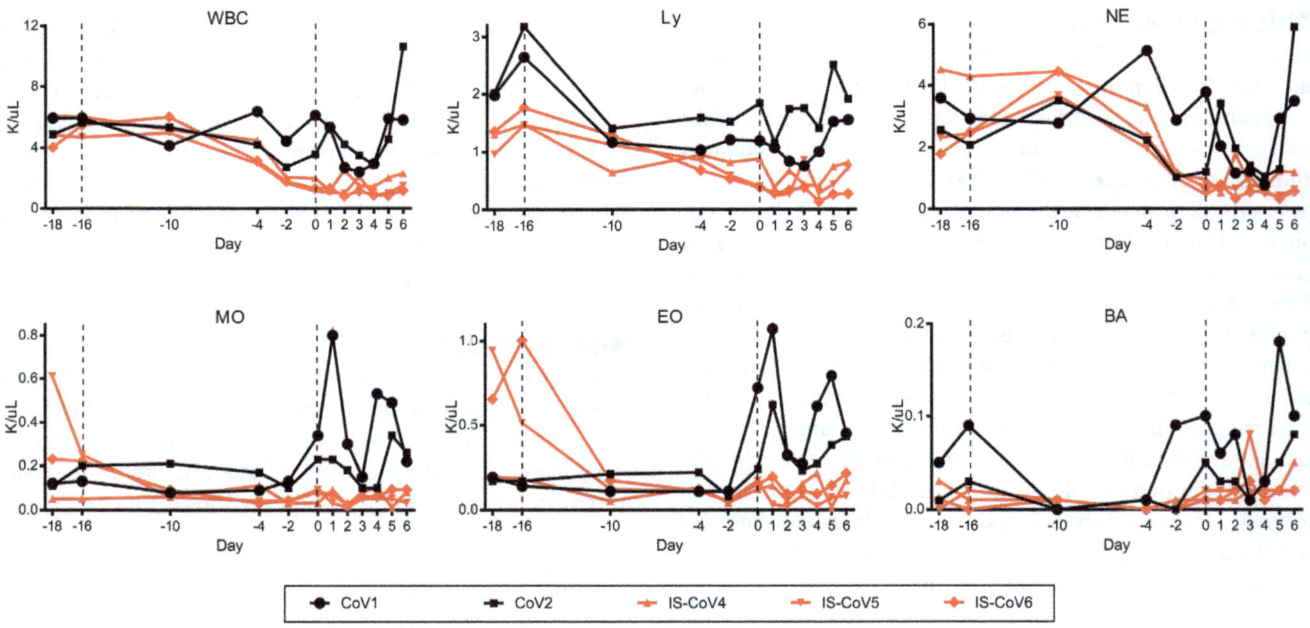

FIGURE 1 | Immunosuppression of rhesus macaques. Three rhesus macaques were immunosuppressed using a combination of cyclophosphamide (10 mg/kg every other day) and dexamethasone (2 mg/kg daily) for 16 days (−16) prior to inoculation with Middle East respiratory syndrome coronavirus, and for 5 days thereafter. Blood samples were collected at the indicated time points, inclusive of a control bleed 2 days prior to the initiation of the study (−18), and blood cells were enumerated. All blood cell types measured were decreased in the immunosuppressed animals (red lines) at the time of inoculation and remained depressed. Control animals given PBS (black lines) had no reduction in cell counts and cell counts increased in response to infection. Total white blood cells (WBC), lymphocytes (Ly), neutrophils (NE), monocytes (MO), eosinophils (EO), and basophils (BA) were measured.

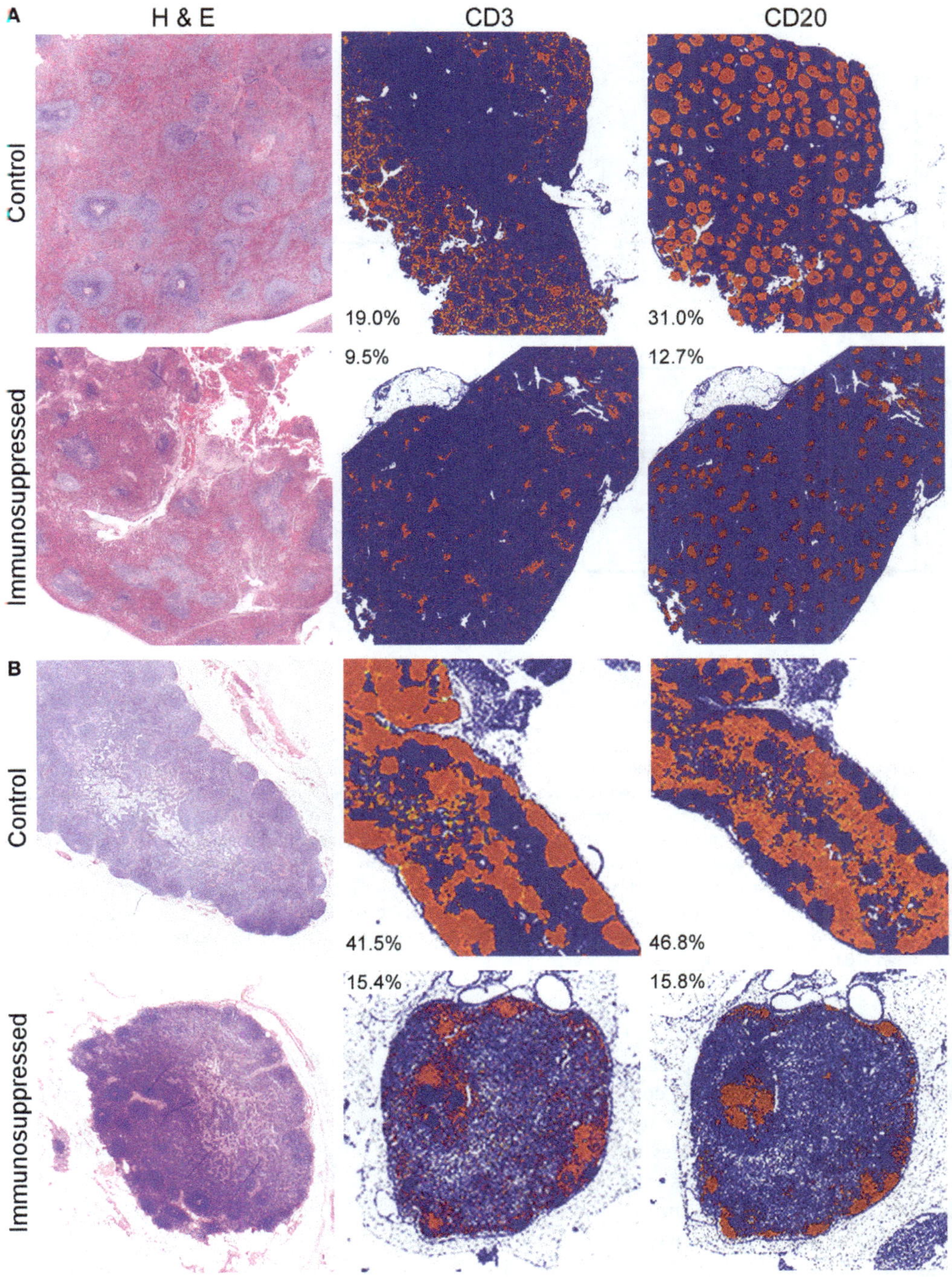

FIGURE 2 | Depletion of immune cells in lymphoid tissues. Tissues collected from control and immunosuppressed animals at the time of euthanasia (6 dpi) were stained with H&E or markers for T cells (CD3) and B cells (CD20). The spleens **(A)** and mediastinal lymph nodes **(B)** of immunosuppressed animals showed disruption of the normal architecture of the white pulp visualized after H&E staining. Quantitation of the amount of specific CD marker staining (red), compared to the absence of staining (blue) showed that the amount of CD3 staining was reduced approximately 2-fold in the spleen **(A)** and 2.7-fold in the lymph node **(B)** in the immunosuppressed animals. Likewise, CD20 staining was reduced by 2.4-fold in the spleen and 3-fold in the lymph nodes, showing a reduction in these cells. Values shown are the percent of positive (red) staining within a tissue and are the average for all animals within each group.

there was no significant difference in the geometric means of viral RNA abundance between these two groups, although the historic controls had slightly more measurable viral RNA (**Figure 3C**). However, the immunosuppressed animals had significantly increased MERS-CoV replication (measured by RNA abundance) in the lungs (Kolmogorov–Smirnov test, $p \leq 0.001$). Similarly, there was significantly more virus detected in several respiratory, or respiratory tract-associated

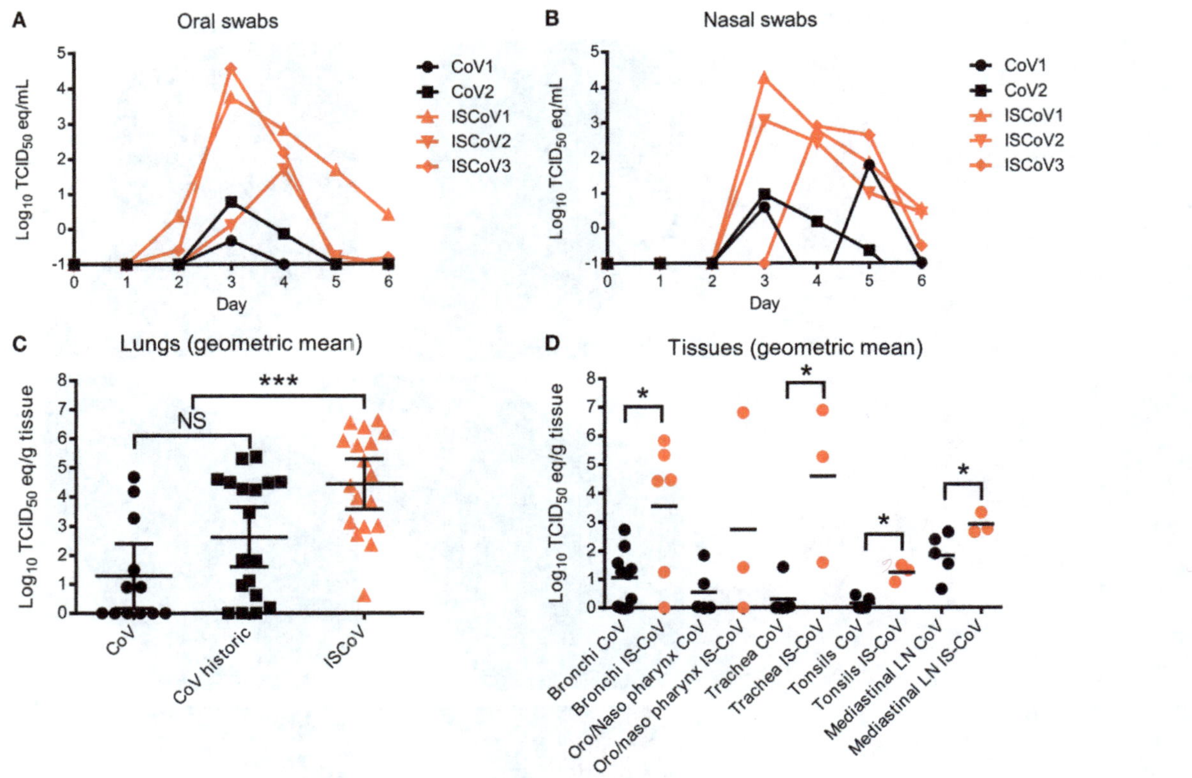

FIGURE 3 | Middle East respiratory syndrome coronavirus shedding and replication. Shedding of virus was monitored by measuring viral RNA in nasal **(A)** and oral **(B)** swabs using MERS-CoV-specific qRT-PCR. Nasal swabs were positive for viral RNA for all but one immunosuppressed animal starting 3 dpi, with immunosuppressed animals (red lines) reaching higher titers and more sustained shedding. Oral swabs **(B)** showed a similar trend. Viral replication was assessed in the lungs **(C)** by performing qRT-PCR using tissue samples from each of the six lobes from each animal. Data are represented as the geometric mean and 95% confidence interval from each group. qRT-PCR was performed on an additional three animals from a previous macaque study (CoV historic) to compare to the immunosuppressed animals. Tissues from the respiratory tracts were also analyzed for RNA levels **(D)** and the samples from the historic control macaques were grouped with the two control animals from this study (black circles). Data are represented as the geometric means of the groups. To compare the data sets within **(C,D)**, a Kolmogorov–Smirnov test was performed to determine statistical differences between the control and immunosuppressed groups. Asterisks (*) indicate significant differences, with $^{*}p \leq 0.05$ and $^{***}p \leq 0.001$.

tissues, including the bronchi, trachea, tonsils, and mediastinal lymph nodes of immunosuppressed animals, compared to the controls (**Figure 3D**) (Kolmogorov–Smirnov test, $p \leq 0.05$). When assessing viral dissemination in tissues outside of the respiratory tract, immunosuppressed animals were positive for low levels of viral RNA in several tissues, including the liver and spleen, as well as several lymph nodes, whereas virus was undetectable outside of the respiratory tract in the control animals, with the exception of one inguinal lymph node sample (**Table 1**).

Lung Histopathology

Samples from all animals were evaluated for the presence of histopathologic changes. Each of the animals, with the exception of IS-CoV3, developed some degree of pulmonary pathology upon examination of tissue following necropsy 6 days after inoculation (**Figure 4A**). Lesions were characterized as multifocal, mild-to-marked, interstitial pneumonia and were frequently centered on terminal bronchioles. The pneumonia was characterized by thickening of alveolar septae by congestion, edema and fibrin, and small to moderate numbers of macrophages and neutrophils. Alveoli contained moderate numbers of pulmonary macrophages and neutrophils. In lungs with marked changes, there was abundant alveolar edema and fibrin with the formation of hyaline membranes. Multifocal type II pneumocyte hyperplasia

TABLE 1 | Middle East respiratory syndrome coronavirus (MERS-CoV) dissemination in rhesus macaque tissues detected by qRT-PCR.

Tissue	CoV1	CoV2	IS-CoV1	IS-CoV2	IS-CoV3
Heart	–	–	–	+	–
Liver	–	–	+	–	+
Spleen	–	–	+	–	+
Kidney	–	–	–	–	+
Adrenal gland	–	–	+	–	–
Pancreas	–	–	+	+	–
Inguinal LN	–	+	+	+	+
Axillary LN	–	–	+	+	+
Mesenteric LN	–	–	+	+	+

(–) indicates that no viral RNA was detected, (+) indicates that viral RNA was detected by qRT-PCR. LN, lymph node.

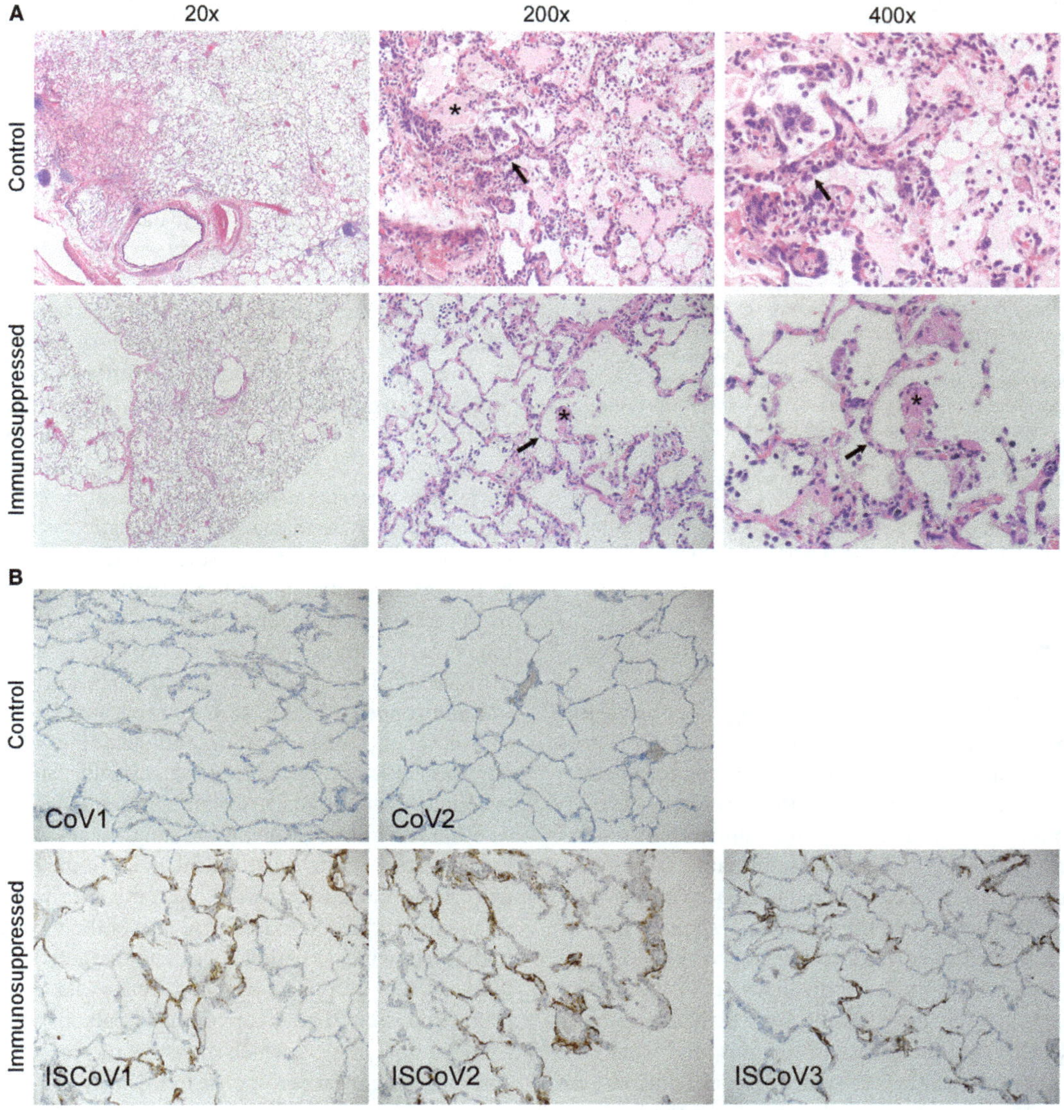

FIGURE 4 | Histopathologic changes induced by Middle East respiratory syndrome coronavirus (MERS-CoV). Lung tissue samples from control and immunosuppressed animals were stained with H&E **(A)** or an antibody specific for MERS-CoV **(B)**. Lung tissue from representative animals from each group were stained with H&E **(A)** and demonstrate that control animals developed multifocal, mild-to-marked, interstitial pneumonia, and thickening of alveolar septae by congestion, edema and fibrin, and formation of hyaline membranes. Multifocal type II pneumocyte hyperplasia was noted. The lungs of immunosuppressed macaques showed few pathologic changes. Asterisks show fibrin deposits and arrows indicate edema. Immunohistochemistry **(B)** of control animals showed little or no viral antigen present. By contrast, immunosuppressed animals showed significant levels of viral antigen, which was multifocal throughout the tissue and predominant within type I pneumocytes.

was noted and there were also perivascular infiltrates of inflammatory cells within, and adjacent to, affected areas of the lung. Samples from each lung lobe for each animal were individually scored for the presence and extent of pathologic changes, with scores ranging from 0 (no pathology) to 4 (multiple coalescing inflammatory foci with fibrin and edema). Animals CoV1 and CoV2 had average histology scores of 1.3 and 1.2, with individual lung lobe scores ranging from 0 to 4 and from 0 to 3, respectively (**Table 2**). Immunosuppressed animals displayed much milder pathology with average scores for IS-CoV1, IS-CoV2, and IS-CoV3 of 0.2, 0.6, and 0, respectively, and no lobe showing a score greater than 1.

The animals that did not undergo immunosuppression developed the most severe pulmonary pathology, but demonstrated little or no viral antigen in the lung tissue examined by IHC (**Figure 4B**), reflecting the qRT-PCR results, where much less viral RNA was detected and viral RNA was undetectable in many of the individual lung lobes. Conversely, macaques that had undergone immunosuppression had very mild lung lesions, but demonstrated MERS-CoV viral antigen multifocally throughout the lung; predominantly within type I pneumocytes. This suggests that pulmonary pathology associated with MERS-CoV in these animals may be tightly associated with the immune response.

TABLE 2 | Histopathologic scoring of lungs from rhesus macaques.

Tissue	CoV1	CoV2	ISCoV1	ISCoV2	ISCoV3
Right upper lobe	0	1	0	1	0
Right middle lobe	2	0	1	1	0
Right lower lobe	0	1	0	0	0
Left upper lobe	2	0	0	0	0
Left middle lobe	0	2	0	1	0
Left lower lobe	4	3	0	1	0
Average score	1.3	1.2	0.2	0.6	0

(0) = no pathology, (1) = few inflammatory foci scattered between multiple lung lobes; alveolar interstitium minimally thickened by congestion and small numbers of neutrophils and macrophages; few neutrophils and macrophages within alveoli, (2) = multiple inflammatory foci in multiple lung lobes; alveolar interstitium is mildly thickened, edema and small numbers of neutrophils and macrophages; small numbers of neutrophils and macrophages within alveoli, (3) = multiple inflammatory foci scattered within single lung lobes; alveolar interstitium is moderately thickened, edema and moderate numbers of neutrophils and macrophages; many neutrophils and macrophages within alveoli; small amounts of fibrin and edema in alveoli, (4) = multiple to coalescing inflammatory foci within a single lung lobe; alveolar interstitium is markedly thickened by congestion, edema, fibrin, and large numbers of neutrophils and macrophages; large numbers of neutrophils, macrophages, cellular debris, fibrin, and edema within alveoli.

DISCUSSION

Little is known regarding how several emerging zoonotic viruses infecting the respiratory tract cause disease, and what risk factors contribute to poor outcome. Some viruses are thought to cause disease by dysregulating the immune response, whereby destruction of infected cells or secretion of pro-inflammatory mediators leads to immunopathology, as in the case of hantaviruses (18). Conversely, pathogenesis caused by some viruses correlates with deficiencies, or inefficiencies of the immune response, such as in the case of pathogenic viruses affecting the very young and elderly, or immune compromised individuals, as in the case of influenza virus (19). The mechanisms by which the recently emerged MERS-CoV causes disease in humans, and what host factors are associated with either resistance or a poor outcome are not known (15). These questions are important for the development of countermeasures that either directly target the virus to inhibit its replication or modulate the immune response to limit immunopathogenesis.

Early epidemiologic studies of MERS suggested that patients with comorbidities fared worse than healthy patients upon infection, and the number of comorbidities correlated with a worse outcome (20). In addition, a few patients with lethal infections were reported to be immunosuppressed (21–23). These reports were from cases where diagnoses were primarily in patients already in hospitals, including a relatively large number of nosocomial infections affecting 23 patients in a hospital outbreak in Al-Hasa (24). Since these initial case reports, more than 2,000 additional cases of MERS-CoV infection have been confirmed (2). Although many of these new cases are reported to be health care related, either stemming from patients or health care workers, it is unclear how many of these cases involve immunocompromised individuals.

Risk factors that have been associated with disease (or infection) include weakened immune systems and chronic diseases, such as diabetes, cancer, and chronic lung disease, as well as co-infections (5, 20, 25). Although these comorbidities clearly affect the status of the immune response, acute immunosuppression using drugs, as we have done here, provides a more controlled deficit in immune responses, whereas immune dysregulation brought on by chronic disease, infection, and aging is a complex phenomenon that involves deficiencies in the immune response, chronic inflammatory responses, and other known and yet to be described complex changes. For instance, the majority of patients had diabetes as a comorbidity and several others were immunosuppressed with HIV/AIDS. Both of these conditions alter the immune response in a way that both inhibits normal T cell functions, as well as inducing an inflammatory response by altering Th17 responses and secretion of inflammatory cytokines (26–30). The immunosuppression in our study mimics some aspects of the human condition in these patients, such as inhibition of $CD4^+$ T cell responses by HIV-infected patients. However, the chemical immunosuppression used herein is unlikely to mimic the chronic inflammatory state in many of these patients. This higher basal level of immune activation associated with these conditions may be important contributions to the manifestation of the clinically overt serious disease following MERS-CoV infection, and would imply that the immune system plays a role in the pathogenesis of MERS-CoV. This agrees with our observation that upon simple immunosuppression, MERS-CoV replicated to higher levels and showed greater dissemination and shedding, while the pathology was actually reduced in these animals. Pathology was likely lessened due to the absence of inflammatory cells and mediators, as observed histologically in the lung tissues. This suggests that the virus itself might cause little damage to the cells that it infects and this would lead toward a mechanism in which the absence of an efficient immune response allows the virus to replicate to high levels, whereas pathology can be attributed to the overactive inflammatory response, which patients with comorbidities are prone to possess. This is supported by data in the resus and marmoset animal models, which show that increased viral replication and the local immune response to this plays an important role in the pulmonary severity of disease (31). Although not performed in this study, a control group treated with immunosuppressive drugs, and not challenged, would be necessary for a comprehensive picture of the immune status of these animals at the time of necropsy.

Recent experiments using human-derived blood cells have shown that infection with MERS-CoV results in a dramatic increase in the production of cytokines and immune cell-recruiting chemokines and the authors hypothesize that these inflammatory responses could lead to severe inflammation and tissue damage (32, 33). This is supported by the observation that bronchoalveolar lavage fluid of humans infected with MERS-CoV contain high numbers of neutrophils and macrophages (1, 22). Furthermore, lymphopenia has been associated with disease and is potentially caused by infiltration of lymphocytes in the lung tissue and egress from the blood (34). Taking these findings into account, we can envision a model in which infection of the lung tissue and resident immune cells, such as alveolar macrophages, leads to the hyper-production of inflammatory cytokines and immune cell recruitment chemokines, which together limit virus replication, but result in an immunopathologic state. Upon immunosuppression of our macaques, the virus was still able to infect and replicate in the lung tissue, and likely induced local cytokine and chemokine expression; however, the depletion of immune cell populations upon chemical immunosuppression inhibited recruitment of inflammatory cells to the lungs (or infected tissues) and, thus, limited pathology. This is the first direct experimental evidence showing that MERS-CoV has an immunopathogenic component. This is in line with the observation in one patient in South Korea, which was taking prolonged high-dose corticosteroid therapy to control lymphoma activity and hemolytic anemia and displayed persistant viral shedding without clinical progression of the disease (23).

The shedding of MERS-CoV was more extensive in the immunosuppressed animals, both in duration as in peak shedding. This suggests that the immune status has direct influence on virus shedding and subsequent potential of transmission. The epidemiological analyses of the 2015 MERS-CoV outbreak in South Korea clearly showed that only the level of MERS-CoV shedding was directly associated with transmission potential. Where spreaders had statistically lower Ct values compared to non-spreaders (25). The persistent MERS-CoV shedding in immunocompromised patients (23) could, therefore, contribute to enhanced nosocomial transmission.

As of yet, no specific treatment options have been identified for MERS-CoV infection. The results presented herein show that inflammatory responses contribute to the pathogenic process. This would suggest that treatment for patients with symptomatic infections would benefit from additional therapy that lessens the inflammatory response, especially in the lung, and not be based solely on therapies that are aimed at controlling virus replication.

ETHICS STATEMENT

The use of study animals was approved by the Institutional Animal Care and Use Committee of the Rocky Mountain Laboratories and experiments were performed following the guidelines of the Association for Assessment and Accreditation of the Laboratory Animal Care by certified staff in an approved facility. The guidelines and basic principles in the United States Public Health Service Policy on Humane Care and Use of Laboratory Animals and the Guide for the Care and Use of Laboratory Animals were followed. All procedures were carried out under anesthesia using Ketamine by trained personnel under veterinarian supervision and efforts were made to provide for the welfare of animals and to minimize suffering. All animals were humanely euthanized at the endpoint of the study (6 days post-inoculation) by exsanguination under deep anesthesia. All standard operating procedures for MERS-CoV were approved by the Institutional Biosafety committee of the Rock Mountain Laboratories, and sample inactivation was carried out according to approved standard operating procedures prior to removal from high containment.

AUTHOR CONTRIBUTIONS

JP, DF, EW, HF, and VM designed the study; JP, DS, HF, and VM analyzed the data; JP, HF, and VM wrote the manuscript; and JP, KH, FF, EH, VM, and DS performed the experiments and assays.

ACKNOWLEDGMENTS

We would like to thank Doug Brining for veterinarian services; Dan Long, Tina Thomas, and Rebecca Rosenke for histology support; and Anita Mora for graphics. We would also like to thank Drs. Bart Haagmans and Ron Fouchier (Erasmus MC, Netherlands) for providing the MERS-CoV isolate.

REFERENCES

1. Zaki AM, van Boheemen S, Bestebroer TM, Osterhaus AD, Fouchier RA. Isolation of a novel coronavirus from a man with pneumonia in Saudi Arabia. *N Engl J Med* (2012) 367:1814–20. doi:10.1056/NEJMoa1211721
2. WHO. *Middle East Respiratory Syndrome Coronavirus (MERS-CoV)*. Geneva: World Health Organisation (2015). Available from: http://www.who.int/mediacentre/factsheets/mers-cov/en/
3. de Wit E, van Doremalen N, Falzarano D, Munster VJ. SARS and MERS: recent insights into emerging coronaviruses. *Nat Rev Microbiol* (2016) 14:523–34. doi:10.1038/nrmicro.2016.81
4. Hui DS, Memish ZA, Zumla A. Severe acute respiratory syndrome vs. The Middle East respiratory syndrome. *Curr Opin Pulm Med* (2014) 20:233–41. doi:10.1097/MCP.0000000000000046
5. Saad M, Omrani AS, Baig K, Bahloul A, Elzein F, Matin MA, et al. Clinical aspects and outcomes of 70 patients with Middle East respiratory syndrome coronavirus infection: a single-center experience in Saudi Arabia. *Int J Infect Dis* (2014) 29:301–6. doi:10.1016/j.ijid.2014.09.003
6. Kindler E, Jónsdóttir H, Muth D, Hamming O, Hartmann R, Rodriguez R, et al. Efficient replication of the novel human betacoronavirus EMC on primary human epithelium highlights its zoonotic potential. *mBio* (2013) 4:12. doi:10.1128/mBio.00611-12
7. Chan RW, Chan MC, Agnihothram S, Chan LL, Kuok DI, Fong JH, et al. Tropism of and innate immune responses to the novel human betacoronavirus lineage C virus in human ex vivo respiratory organ cultures. *J Virol* (2013) 87:6604–14. doi:10.1128/JVI.00009-13
8. Chan RW, Hemida MG, Kayali G, Chu DK, Poon LL, Alnaeem A, et al. Tropism and replication of Middle East respiratory syndrome coronavirus from dromedary camels in the human respiratory tract: an in-vitro and ex-vivo study. *Lancet Respir Med* (2014) 2:813–22. doi:10.1016/S2213-2600(14)70158-4
9. Raj VS, Mou H, Smits SL, Dekkers DH, Muller MA, Dijkman R, et al. Dipeptidyl peptidase 4 is a functional receptor for the emerging human coronavirus-EMC. *Nature* (2013) 495:251–4. doi:10.1038/nature12005
10. Oh MD, Park WB, Choe PG, Choi SJ, Kim JI, Chae J, et al. Viral load kinetics of MERS coronavirus infection. *N Engl J Med* (2016) 375:1303–5. doi:10.1056/NEJMc1511695
11. Munster V, de Wit E, Feldmann H. Pneumonia from human coronavirus in a macaque model. *N Engl J Med* (2013) 368:1560–2. doi:10.1056/NEJMc1215691
12. de Wit E, Rasmussen A, Falzarano D, Bushmaker T, Feldmann F, Brining D, et al. Middle East respiratory syndrome coronavirus (MERS-CoV) causes transient lower respiratory tract infection in Rhesus macaques. *Proc Natl Acad Sci U S A* (2013) 110:16598–603. doi:10.1073/pnas.1310744110
13. Falzarano D, de Wit E, Feldmann F, Rasmussen AL, Okumura A, Peng X, et al. Infection with MERS-CoV causes lethal pneumonia in the common

marmoset. *PLoS Pathog* (2014) 10:e1004250. doi:10.1371/journal.ppat.1004250
14. Memish ZA, Al-Tawfiq JA, Assiri A, AlRabiah FA, Al Hajjar S, Albarrak A, et al. Middle East respiratory syndrome coronavirus disease in children. *Pediatr Infect Dis J* (2014) 33:904–6. doi:10.1097/INF.0000000000000325
15. Al-Tawfiq JA, Memish ZA. Middle East respiratory syndrome coronavirus: epidemiology and disease control measures. *Infect Drug Resist* (2014) 7:281–7. doi:10.2147/IDR.S51283
16. Corman VM, Muller MA, Costabel U, Timm J, Binger T, Meyer B, et al. Assays for laboratory confirmation of novel human coronavirus (hCoV-EMC) infections. *Euro Surveill* (2012) 17. doi:10.2807/ese.17.49.20334-en
17. de Wit E, Prescott J, Baseler L, Bushmaker T, Thomas T, Lackemeyer M, et al. The Middle East respiratory syndrome coronavirus (MERS-CoV) does not replicate in Syrian hamsters. *PLoS One* (2013) 8:e69127. doi:10.1371/journal.pone.0069127
18. Charbonnel N, Pages M, Sironen T, Henttonen H, Vapalahti O, Mustonen J, et al. Immunogenetic factors affecting susceptibility of humans and rodents to hantaviruses and the clinical course of hantaviral disease in humans. *Viruses* (2014) 6:2214–41. doi:10.3390/v6052214
19. Meyer KC. The role of immunity and inflammation in lung senescence and susceptibility to infection in the elderly. *Semin Respir Crit Care Med* (2010) 31:561–74. doi:10.1055/s-0030-1265897
20. Assiri A, Al-Tawfiq J, Al-Rabeeah A, Al-Rabiah F, Al-Hajjar S, Al-Barrak A, et al. Epidemiological, demographic, and clinical characteristics of 47 cases of Middle East respiratory syndrome coronavirus disease from Saudi Arabia: a descriptive study. *Lancet Infect Dis* (2013) 13:752–61. doi:10.1016/S1473-3099(13)70204-4
21. Arabi YM, Arifi AA, Balkhy HH, Najm H, Aldawood AS, Ghabashi A, et al. Clinical course and outcomes of critically ill patients with Middle East respiratory syndrome coronavirus infection. *Ann Intern Med* (2014) 160:389–97. doi:10.7326/M13-2486
22. Guery B, Poissy J, el Mansouf L, Sejourne C, Ettahar N, Lemaire X, et al. Clinical features and viral diagnosis of two cases of infection with Middle East Respiratory Syndrome coronavirus: a report of nosocomial transmission. *Lancet* (2013) 381:2265–72. doi:10.1016/S0140-6736(13)60982-4
23. Kim SH, Ko JH, Park GE, Cho SY, Ha YE, Kang JM, et al. Atypical presentations of MERS-CoV infection in immunocompromised hosts. *J Infect Chemother* (2017) 23:769–73. doi:10.1016/j.jiac.2017.04.004
24. Assiri A, McGeer A, Perl T, Price C, Al Rabeeah A, Cummings D, et al. Hospital outbreak of Middle East respiratory syndrome coronavirus. *N Engl J Med* (2013) 369:407–16. doi:10.1056/NEJMoa1306742
25. Kim SW, Park JW, Jung HD, Yang JS, Park YS, Lee C, et al. Risk factors for transmission of Middle East respiratory syndrome coronavirus infection during the 2015 outbreak in South Korea. *Clin Infect Dis* (2017) 64:551–7. doi:10.1093/cid/ciw768
26. Dandona P, Aljada A, Bandyopadhyay A. Inflammation: the link between insulin resistance, obesity and diabetes. *Trends Immunol* (2004) 25:4–7. doi:10.1016/j.it.2003.10.013
27. Bastard JP, Maachi M, Lagathu C, Kim MJ, Caron M, Vidal H, et al. Recent advances in the relationship between obesity, inflammation, and insulin resistance. *Eur Cytokine Netw* (2006) 17:4–12.
28. DeFuria J, Belkina AC, Jagannathan-Bogdan M, Snyder-Cappione J, Carr JD, Nersesova YR, et al. B cells promote inflammation in obesity and type 2 diabetes through regulation of T-cell function and an inflammatory cytokine profile. *Proc Natl Acad Sci U S A* (2013) 110:5133–8. doi:10.1073/pnas.1215840110
29. Deeks SG, Tracy R, Douek DC. Systemic effects of inflammation on health during chronic HIV infection. *Immunity* (2013) 39:633–45. doi:10.1016/j.immuni.2013.10.001
30. Hunt PW. Th17, gut, and HIV: therapeutic implications. *Curr Opin HIV AIDS* (2010) 5:189–93. doi:10.1097/COH.0b013e32833647d9
31. Baseler LJ, Falzarano D, Scott DP, Rosenke R, Thomas T, Munster VJ, et al. An acute immune response to Middle East respiratory syndrome coronavirus replication contributes to viral pathogenicity. *Am J Pathol* (2016) 186:630–8. doi:10.1016/j.ajpath.2015.10.025
32. Zhou J, Chu H, Li C, Wong B, Cheng Z-S, Poon V, et al. Active MERS-CoV replication and aberrant induction of inflammatory cytokines and chemokines in human macrophages: implications for pathogenesis. *J Infect Dis* (2013) 209(9):1331–42. doi:10.1093/infdis/jit504
33. Scheuplein VA, Seifried J, Malczyk AH, Miller L, Hocker L, Vergara-Alert J, et al. High secretion of interferons by human plasmacytoid dendritic cells upon recognition of Middle East respiratory syndrome coronavirus. *J Virol* (2015) 89:3859–69. doi:10.1128/JVI.03607-14
34. Drosten C, Seilmaier M, Corman V, Hartmann W, Scheible G, Sack S, et al. Clinical features and virological analysis of a case of Middle East respiratory syndrome coronavirus infection. *Lancet Infect Dis* (2013) 13:745–51. doi:10.1016/S1473-3099(13)70154-3

10

The Drivers of Pathology in Zoonotic Avian Influenza: The Interplay Between Host and Pathogen

*William S. J. Horman[1,2], Thi H. O. Nguyen[1], Katherine Kedzierska[1], Andrew G. D. Bean[2] and Daniel S. Layton[2]**

[1] Department of Microbiology and Immunology, University of Melbourne at the Peter Doherty Institute for Infection and Immunity, Parkville, VIC, Australia, [2] Australian Animal Health Laboratory, Health and Biosecurity, Commonwealth Scientific and Industrial Research Organisation (CSIRO), East Geelong, VIC, Australia

***Correspondence:**
Daniel S. Layton
daniel.layton@csiro.au

The emergence of zoonotic strains of avian influenza (AI) that cause high rates of mortality in people has caused significant global concern, with a looming threat that one of these strains may develop sustained human-to-human transmission and cause a pandemic outbreak. Most notable of these viral strains are the H5N1 highly pathogenic AI and the H7N9 low pathogenicity AI viruses, both of which have mortality rates above 30%. Understanding of their mechanisms of infection and pathobiology is key to our preparation for these and future viral strains of high consequence. AI viruses typically circulate in wild bird populations, commonly infecting waterfowl and also regularly entering commercial poultry flocks. Live poultry markets provide an ideal environment for the spread AI and potentially the selection of mutants with a greater propensity for infecting humans because of the potential for spill over from birds to humans. Pathology from these AI virus infections is associated with a dysregulated immune response, which is characterized by systemic spread of the virus, lymphopenia, and hypercytokinemia. It has been well documented that host/pathogen interactions, particularly molecules of the immune system, play a significant role in both disease susceptibility as well as disease outcome. Here, we review the immune/virus interactions in both avian and mammalian species, and provide an overview or our understanding of how immune dysregulation is driven. Understanding these susceptibility factors is critical for the development of new vaccines and therapeutics to combat the next pandemic influenza.

Keywords: avian influenza virus, zoonosis, H7N9, H5N1, highly pathogenic avian influenza virus

EMERGENCE OF AVIAN INFLUENZA (AI) VIRUS INFECTION IN HUMANS

Influenza A viruses have consistently posed a major threat to human health, both through seasonal infections and pandemic outbreaks (1). AI viruses have contributed significantly to this, and in recent years, highly pathogenic AI (HPAI) viruses have emerged as a major zoonotic threat. AI viruses naturally circulate in wild bird populations, including but not limited to, ducks and waterfowl, and can spill over to poultry birds such as chickens. Other than a few novel strains isolated in bats, all influenza A subtypes have been found in aquatic birds, which act as natural reservoirs for the viruses (2). These viruses typically replicate in the gastrointestinal and upper respiratory tract of both these natural hosts and chickens, and typically present as subclinical to mild disease (3, 4). Based on these clinical signs in chickens, these influenza viruses are classified as "low pathogenicity AI" (LPAI) infections (5). Although many AI viruses circulate without causing serious disease, other viral subtypes can lead to more severe outbreaks within birds. Birds infected with these subtypes have more severe pathogenesis and rapid disease progression, often as the result of dissemination of the virus into tissues peripheral to the gastrointestinal and respiratory tracts. This type of infection in chickens defines the subtypes as HPAI (5). Highlighting the importance of HPAI viruses, recent outbreaks of HPAI H5N6 in China and the Philippines have caused approximately 37,000 bird deaths and 400,000 more culled at an economic cost of nearly $USD40 million (6, 7), and novel strains of H7 viruses such as H7N4 continue to cause sporadic outbreaks (8). While such outbreaks represent a significant economic burden to the poultry industry, of greater concern is the potential for HPAI viruses to cross the species barrier into mammals, especially humans.

Despite there being a broad range of AI subtypes, fortunately, only a very select subset of these have been shown to infect humans with highly pathogenic consequences (9). The first known HPAI infections in humans were highlighted by the outbreak of H5N1 avian-derived influenza in Hong Kong in 1997, leading to 6 deaths from 18 confirmed cases (10). Since then, sporadic outbreaks of H5N1 have had highly pathogenic consequences in humans, resulting in over 450 deaths from approximately 900 cases (11–13). The emergence of the avian-derived H7N9 strain infecting humans was first described in March 2013 in China's Yangtze River Delta, which has since caused 613 deaths out of 1,566 human cases throughout most of China as of January 2018 (14). This viral subtype is of a particular concern, as unlike H5N1, which is highly pathogenic in chickens and humans, H7N9 typically presents as an LPAI in chickens, but causes a high mortality rate in humans (40%), similar to that seen for H5N1 infections. H7N9 is one of several LPAI viruses in the H7 family capable of human infections, with viral transmission usually only acquired through close contact with host species (15–17). However, for reasons that are still unclear, H7N9 has greater transmissibility and more severe disease outcomes in humans than any other H7 viruses (18, 19). Thus, differences in clinical presentation across species, coupled with the potential of viruses such as H7N9 to cause a pandemic outbreak *via* evidence of human-to-human transmission (20), makes understanding the mechanisms by which these viruses cross the species barrier and become highly pathogenic in humans a critical area of investigation. Here, we discuss recent findings relating viral fitness to host susceptibility factors to understand how HPAI phenotypes are developed. We also outline how clinical manifestations following infection with LPAI or HPAI strains across different species provide further insights into the mechanisms underlying disease severity and susceptibility.

CLINICAL MANIFESTATIONS OF DISEASE IN DIFFERENT SPECIES

Human cases of AI infection have become increasingly common since outbreaks of H5N1 in the late 1990s and accentuated by a dramatic increase in H7N9 infections during the recent "fifth wave" of epidemic infections in China (21–23). These viruses were commonly contracted by people in regular close contact with live poultry markets (24, 25), where outbreaks of AI viruses in chickens can be common yet go largely unnoticed, especially in the case of H7N9 infections. Despite the vast diversity of AI viruses, predominantly only viruses from three hemagglutinin (HA) subtypes have been recorded to naturally infect humans: H5Nx viruses, most notably H5N1; H7Nx viruses such as H7N9; and H9Nx viruses, commonly H9N2. H9Nx strains present as LPAI infections in birds and have less severe symptoms in human hosts compared to H5 and H7 strains (26–29). Despite this, as H9N2 viruses are regularly found co-circulating with H5N1 and H7N9 with assortment frequently occurring between these viruses in poultry there is a real possibility of a novel HPAI strain emerging from these subtypes (30, 31). While there have been isolated cases of human infections with other subtypes, such as H10 (32), and H6 viruses which have been discussed as a potential precursor to H5N1 with pandemic potential (33–38), H5/H7/H9-subtypes of AI remain of greatest concern for human infections and potential pandemics. Thus, understanding the clinical manifestations of these viruses in avian hosts is needed for our understanding of why these viruses are considered such a threat.

In the case of LPAI, infections tend to localize in the mucosal surfaces of the gastrointestinal tract of infected birds and although often asymptomatic, chickens may present with mild clinical signs following infection. These include excess mucus and congested tracheae, watery droppings, and mild respiratory inflammation, with rarely any other signs of respiratory disease associated with influenza infections (3, 26, 39, 40). Highest viral titers typically occur 2–3 days after infection with limited gross lesions evident, allowing the virus to replicate and be excreted into the environment with little to no effect on the host animal (41, 42). Interestingly, ducks can exhibit even more limited clinical signs following LPAI infection than chickens (43). Thus, it is interesting to note that even in avian hosts, there is a range of clinical severity to LPAI viruses, with chickens showing more moderate/severe signs compared to waterfowl infected with LPAI.

In contrast to LPAI viruses, HPAI viruses have the ability to induce severe disease and cause devastating outbreaks with high mortality rates in poultry (44, 45). In chickens, H5N1 causes acute illness with high levels of viral shedding and clinical signs such as dehydration, nasal discharge, and lesions in many tissue types (46–48). While LPAI infections tend to remain within the fecal–oral tract of infected birds, HPAI infections are often identified by virus spreading systemically to multiple tissues (49). Suzuki and colleagues (50) described the pathology of H5N1 infections in chickens, finding that clinical signs progressed from milder signs such as feather ruffling and depression behavior, to the more severe outcomes of hemorrhaging and edema in multiple tissues. These birds also showed severe respiratory distress not seen in LPAI infections (50). By contrast, ducks can present with a wider range of symptoms following infection with HPAI H5N1, with experimentally infected ducks having clinical signs as mild as depressive behavior without any other complications (51). Ducks may also show severe signs such as those seen in chickens, with common outcomes including neurological spread and hemorrhaging in the body extremities. In addition, Yamamoto and colleagues have also found that domestic ducks, unlike chickens, show corneal opacity following H5N1 infection and less severe hemorrhaging compared to chickens (52, 53). Likewise, wild ducks have been shown to exhibit less severe signs following H5N1 infection compared to other gallinaceous birds including domestic ducks, despite showing high levels of viral shedding consistent with an HPAI infection, which may suggest their role as a key reservoir species (48).

Avian influenza viruses also have the ability to infect pigs, which are housed in close proximity to human populations. Pigs often act as a "mixing vessel" for influenza viruses, which are able to reassort and thus infect humans (54, 55). While this is particularly the case for low pathogenicity viruses, there has been little evidence to suggest that pigs can contract highly pathogenic strains such as H5N1 and H7N9 to any great level, with H5N1 strains isolated from pigs in China found to be attenuated from the HPAI form (56). Although there have been no confirmed cases of H7N9 infection in pigs (57), H7N9 can replicate, cause pathology, and transmit among pigs during *in vivo* studies at low levels (58–60), as well as replicate in swine respiratory tissue *in vitro*, reinforcing the idea that pigs could still act as an important reservoir species for mammalian-adapted H7N9 (61). Of particular concern, reports of H7N2 infection in pigs (62) suggest that as the frequency of H7Nx cases increases, the likelihood of an H7N9 virus infecting pigs and potentially gaining stable mammalian transmissibility is a genuine possibility.

Studies in ferrets as a model for human infection have shown that mammalian-adapted AI viruses typically localize to the respiratory tract (63), however, these viruses have can have a limited ability to transmit *via* droplets (64–66). H5N1 viruses cause acute illness in the upper respiratory tract of ferrets with symptoms such as nasal discharge, high temperatures, and weight loss due to dehydration, and worsened pathogenesis, as highlighted by lung damage due to extensive infiltration of the lung tissue by inflammatory cells (18, 67, 68). H7N9 can also cause severe respiratory distress in this way, with lengthened time until viral clearance contributing to viral transmission and the substantial inflammation in the lungs of ferrets (69). Severe infections may cause complications such as viral pneumonia due to the breakdown of lung endothelial barriers, which contributes to this systemic spread and may lead to encephalitis or other neurological issues (18, 70). However, systemic spread to the central nervous system is more commonly associated with HPAI H5N1 than LPAI H7N9 (68).

Symptoms following human infection with AI are similar to those observed in the ferret model. Less severe cases present as more typical influenza infections, with symptoms such as fever and coughing among those commonly associated with influenza-related illness (16, 71). However, these viruses can cause severe respiratory illness following infection in the lungs, which may manifest as atypical viral pneumonia and acute respiratory distress syndrome, and often patients who have contracted these infections die from respiratory failure (72, 73). Furthermore, much like in birds, dissemination of the virus away from the site of infection leads to other complications such as organ failure, encephalitis, and internal bleeding due to tissue destruction (10, 71, 74), all of which contribute to the lethal nature of these viruses. A summary of the varying degrees of clinical manifestations between the different species is depicted in **Figure 1**. These trends, including the ability for an LPAI AI viruses such as H7N9 to cause severe fatal disease in humans, is therefore of great importance to understand the pathology driving the variable signs and symptoms of these infections across species to best combat future infections.

PATHOGENESIS OF HPAI INFECTIONS

Several factors appear to contribute to the worsened pathology observed in HPAI infections when compared with LPAI infections. One hallmark of HPAI pathogenesis is a rapid and robust cytokine response, often referred to as a "cytokine storm" or hypercytokinemia. This build-up of cytokines causes an inflammatory environment at the site of infection, leading to immune cell infiltration. In addition to the hypercytokinemia, there is a well-established loss of leukocytes, leading to the severe pathogenesis seen in these infections (75). Recently, the main factors associated with pathology were further described by Kuchipudi and colleagues (76). Following infection with H5N1 *in vitro*, chicken lung cells had increased expression of specific pro-inflammatory cytokines, particularly interleukins (IL)-6 and IL-8 when compared to cells infected with LPAI H2N3, suggesting that IL-6 and IL-8 may be key regulators leading to worsened pathology of HPAI compared to LPAI (76). IL-6 and IL-8 were also found to be significantly upregulated in the lungs of H5N1 infected ferrets, as well as in peripheral tissues, including the spleen, heart, and liver (77). Interestingly, this study also found that IL-6 and IL-8 were downregulated in the nasal turbinates following infection with pandemic H1N1 virus, which produced a less severe clinical infection compared to the H5N1 in ferrets (77). These findings were consistent with studies completed in rhesus macaques, which similarly showed upregulation of tumor necrosis factor α (TNFα), IL-6, and IL-8 in response to experimentally induced H5N1 infection, along with an increase in the antiviral interferons (IFNs), findings which correlate to the severe fever symptoms observed in the macaques at the peak of the fever response at day six post-infection (78). Moreover, infections with the recently emerged HPAI H5N6 in chickens, which caused human fatalities, was shown to have a very distinct immune response compared to other H5N6 strains by producing much higher levels of IL-6, IL-8, and other pro-inflammatory mediators such as TNFα compared to previously identified strains (79). While chickens and ferrets show similar pathogenesis, conversely, duck lung cells infected with the same viruses showed a decrease in IL-6 expression compared to the LPAI viruses, while IL-8 remained unchanged. It suggests that IL-6 may play a pivotal role in the regulation of AI pathology in birds and, as previously discussed, ducks typically show lessened disease severity following H5N1 infection compared to chickens (**Figure 1**). Moreover in humans, H5N1 elicits a similarly robust cytokine response, with the upregulation of IL-6, IL-10, and TNFα in response to H5N1 (80).

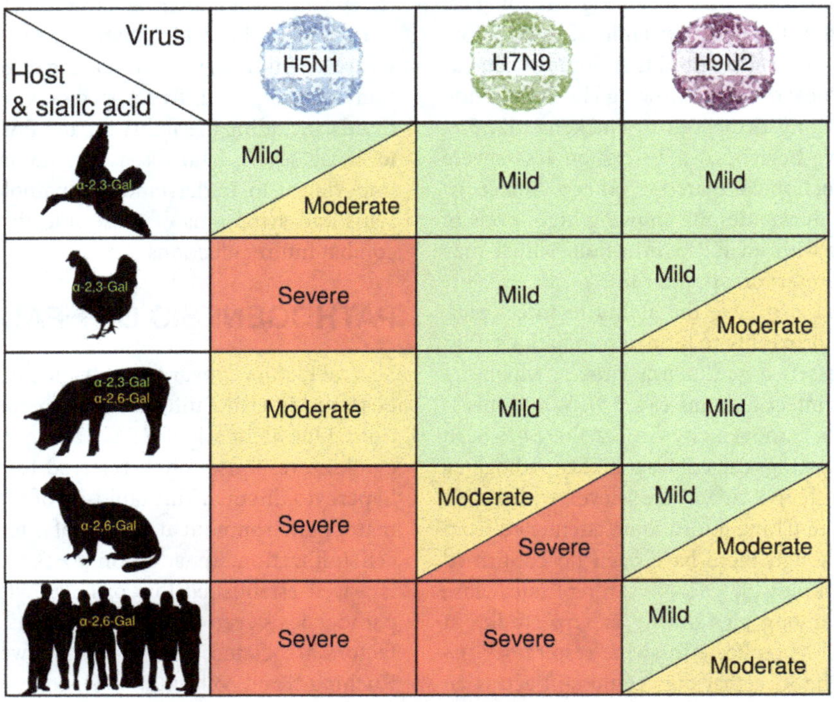

FIGURE 1 | Zoonotic influenza pathology is linked to host biology. H5N1, H7N9, and H9N2 avian influenza (AI) viruses causing varying degrees of clinical manifestations across different species is shown against different host and their sialic acid properties. AI viral hemagglutinin proteins selectively and preferentially bind to sialic residues with either an α-2,3-Gal or α-2,6-Gal terminating sequence on the host cell surface to allow for viral fusion and entry. This represents viral fitness and is a potential mechanism underlying the degree of disease severity and susceptibility in the different hosts.

As the H7N9 virus is classified as an LPAI in chickens, it is interesting to note that a similar trend was observed when H7N9 of human origin were shown to induce increased production of pro-inflammatory IL-6 and IL-8 cytokines when compared to H7N9 of chicken origin (81). In the same study, it was demonstrated that IFNλ1 production was reduced for the human isolate, suggesting a possible modulation of the immune response. In addition, Wu and colleagues also found that H7N9 patients had higher levels of C-reactive protein expression in their plasma compared to H1N1 patients, and as C-reactive protein is associated with broader inflammatory responses, it suggests that this may be yet another factor alongside these regulatory cytokines contributing to disease severity (82). A similar pro-inflammatory response was observed when alveolar macrophages were infected with H7N9, however, when compared to H5N1, this cytokine response was demonstrated to be milder (83). Downregulation of these inflammatory responses to infection confers a level of immunity to these viruses in pigs, which hints at how pigs can act as mixing vessel species for AI without succumbing to severe disease. Human lung epithelial cells can express 100-fold higher levels of TNFα compared to pig lung epithelia, with suppressor of cytokine signaling 3 (SOCS3) identified as a key factor in reducing levels of TNFα in pig cells (84).

The drivers of cytokine production are resident and infiltrating immune cells, which release these cytokines in response to the infection to recruit other immune cells and hinder viral replication. This occurs following cellular activation and results in further activation of leukocytes recruited to the area in a positive feedback loop (85). As pro-inflammatory molecules are associated with apoptotic pathways in humans, increased cytokine production is likely to be a contributing factor in the loss of immune cells, or leukopenia, observed in severe cases of HPAI infection (55). These pro-inflammatory regulators lead to upregulation of the death signaling molecule Fas-ligand on the infected host cell to initiate the caspase-mediated Fas-associated pathway, in which Fas receptors on the immune cell (part of the TNF-receptor family) bind to Fas-ligand and subsequently recruit the Fas-associated death domain (FADD) molecule (86). FADD interacts with caspase-8, which initiates a signaling cascade within the immune cell, resulting in the destruction of cellular components and thus cell death, which may be causative of the pathology seen in influenza patients (87). Indeed, both H5N1 and H7N9 have been observed to cause leukopenia in hospitalized patients (88–90). According to Boonnak and colleagues, $CD8^+$ T cells can be particularly affected by the Fas-ligand mediated pathway, where Fas-ligand was upregulated on plasmocytoid dendritic cells during lethal H5N1 infection in mice, which then lead to apoptosis of influenza-specific $CD8^+$ T cells in the lung draining lymph nodes (86). Furthermore, in hospitalized H7N9-infected patients during the emergence of H7N9 in 2013, the persistence of immune cell subsets within the blood contributed to disease severity and fatal outcomes, with the continuation of $CD38^+HLA\text{-}DR^+$ $CD8^+$ T cell responses shown to be predictive of fatal outcomes, possibly due to longer-lasting inflammatory responses in the peripheral blood and lung (91). Loss of peripheral blood lymphocytes was also observed in human seasonal influenza A infections, with these cell subsets succumbing to apoptosis by the same apoptotic pathways described for AI viruses (92). In summary, LPAI versus HPAI viral strains differentially promote the induction of pro-inflammatory cytokines, which then alter disease outcomes in different species. The potential mechanisms by which certain HPAI AI viruses cause more severe disease will be further discussed in the following sections.

VIRAL FITNESS ACROSS SPECIES

In order for AI viruses to be capable of infecting multiple host species they require viral adaptations allowing replication in different host cells, which ultimately increase their genetic fitness and create a sustainably replicating and transmitting virus (93). It is well established that for zoonotic transmission of AI viruses, the virus needs to present the appropriate HA binding specificity to allow viral fusion and entry. AI virus HA proteins typically have a binding preference for sialic acid residues with an α-2,3-Gal terminating sequence found on the surface of avian cells (**Figure 1**), resulting in restriction to avian cells (63, 94). Therefore, for AI viruses to gain entry into human cells displaying an α-2,6-Gal terminating sequence, modifications to the HA binding site may be required to allow this new interaction.

One of the commonly associated amino acid substitutions for LPAI strains converting from avian to mammalian receptor-specificity is a HA Q226L substitution (58, 95–97). For example, LPAI H9N2 isolates from birds can adopt a Q226L substitution, which increases its mammalian receptor binding affinity and potentially infect mammalian hosts (98, 99). However, with regards to H7N9 human isolates, Belser and colleagues described the Q226 bearing Shanghai/1 and the L226 bearing Anhui/1 as binding to largely avian α-2,3-Gal receptor analogs and mixed α-2,3/α-2,6-Gal receptors, respectively (64). Despite these differences, infections with each isolate produced effective replication in the lower respiratory tract of ferrets, suggesting additional factors are involved in mammalian adaptation. Similarly, this Q226L mutation has not been commonly observed in the HA of H5N1 HPAI viruses (100, 101). However, alternative substitutions, HA Q192H and HA I151T, can confer increased ability for replication in human hosts. Moreover, Herfst and colleagues demonstrated a closely related change to the HA of H5N1, HA Q222L, conferring more efficient replication and transmission in the ferret model (66). Additional to this HA mutation, an E627K change in the polymerase basic 2 (PB2) protein in H5N1 HPAI was also shown to be critical for transmission in ferrets (64, 102–105).

In addition to HA-sialic acid binding, key to viral fitness is the presence of a multi-basic cleavage site (MBCS), which has been shown extensively with H5N1, that the presence of an MBCS often dictates the use of the term HPAI (106, 107). The presence of an MBCS in the HA of influenza A viruses allows HA cleavage by additional enzymes such as furin-like proteases, whereas without an MBCS, the virus relies on only trypsin-like proteases (108). This flexible range of enzyme activity results in the virus being able to infect a greater range of cells and can lead to systemic infection (106, 107, 109). Though commonly associated with H5N1, this motif is seen in other avian-infecting HPAI viruses such as H7N3, however, these strains are less frequently transmitted to humans (19, 110). Interestingly, LPAI can also acquire MBCS motifs, changing the pathogenicity of the virus from low to high, such as in the case of an H7N8 outbreak in Turkey in 2016, where an LPAI virus caused a severe outbreak in the poultry due to the spontaneous addition of an MBCS, leading to over 800 bird deaths (111). However, the addition of an MBCS does not guarantee an LPAI virus to increase its pathogenicity, as recombinant H5 and H7 viruses do not exhibit HPAI pathology in chickens specifically due to the addition of an MBCS (112), which suggests that these motifs are one of many factors contributing to HPAI pathogenesis. H7N9 has also been shown to be able to obtain an MBCS to become highly pathogenic in chickens (113). Imai and colleagues showed increased disease severity of an MBCS-containing H7N9 virus in the ferret model compared to an LPAI H7N9 virus (18). However, H7N9 will still cause severe disease without an MBCS in most human cases, highlighting how unique this virus is in the AI landscape for its ability to show HPAI-like symptoms in mammals, while maintaining low pathogenicity in birds. Similarly for H5Nx viruses, several additional changes in the H5 HA protein, such as an N158D mutation, also allow greater replication of the virus in ferrets without the need for an MBCS, which combined with reassortment with human-adapted H1N1 gene segments shows the potential for these viruses to not only cross into humans but also cause severe, sustained human infection without systemic spread (114). This, coupled with H7N9's ability to cause severe disease without the requirement of an MBCS, suggests that while the MBCS still acts as a key virulence factor for AI viruses, it is not a sole-determining factor for HPAI in humans.

A key interaction between host and viral proteins is the interplay between Mx GTPases and viral nucleoprotein (NP), which may be pivotal in determining viral fitness. Human MxA and murine Mx1 protein have been shown to confer antiviral protection against influenza A viruses by interfering with the ability of NP to localize to the nucleus, inhibiting the viral replication cycle (115). While many influenza viruses are susceptible to Mx restriction, changes in the NP have been shown to confer resistance to this form of protection, particularly in the case of AI viruses such as H5N1 which shows greater susceptibility to MxA inhibition than pandemic H1N1 (116, 117). Moreover, LPAI H7N9 viruses were similarly shown to be affected by Mx1 in infected mice compared to H5N1 by Deeg and colleagues, who showed that these viruses required human adaptive motifs in their NPs to evade Mx restriction (118). Interestingly, avian species such as chickens have been found to have an Mx that does not display strong antiviral properties, suggestive of why these avian viruses do not commonly have NP capable of MxA evasion (119, 120). Therefore, while these AI viruses often appear to cause worsened disease progression due to their differences to human-infecting strains, in the case of Mx restriction it is a lack of human adaptation that may provide a level of protection to mammalian hosts.

Another key virulence factor elucidated in recent years is the ability of the non-structural protein 1 (NS1) to aid viral escape in the host immune system. In avian hosts, NS1 has been associated with worsened pathology through increases in iNOS and oxygen-reactive species for both LPAI H9N2 (121) and HPAI H5N1 (122). However, in contrast in mammals, the NS1 protein has been more closely associated with inhibition of host IFN responses. Jia and colleagues (123) showed that the H5N1 NS1 protein inhibits IFN production through interference with the JAK/STAT pathway. They found that expression of NS1 in HeLa cells prevented STAT phosphorylation and upregulated inhibitors of this pathway to prevent expression of IFNAR and SOCS3 proteins, which generally upregulate IFN expression (123). Furthermore, a naturally occurring deletion in the H5N1 NS1 effector domain can attenuate the virulence of the virus in both chickens and mice, suggesting that this protein is critical in the ability of H5N1 to suppress host immune antiviral responses across hosts (124). The pathogenicity of H5N1 in mice is also affected by the NS1 protein, as a single mutation (P42S) conferred greater pathogenicity to the virus by preventing nuclear factor-κB (NF-κB) and interferon-regulatory factor 3 (IRF3) signaling, and thus inhibiting IFN responses (125). Interestingly, in cats the NS1 protein can be associated with blocking NF-κB and IRF3 signaling in response to the emerging HPAI H5N6 virus, with inhibition of the IFN-β promoter blunting the feline IFN response (126), suggesting that NS1 may have different ways of interacting with influenza hosts across species to produce similar immune suppression. On the other hand, Thube and colleagues investigated the IFN responses of HPAI H5N1 compared to LPAI H11N1 and suggested that decreased IFN signaling occurred independently of NS1, suggesting other viral elements can also induce a reduced antiviral state in cells (127). It is worth noting that while the NS1 of LPAI H7N9 is inefficient at binding to CPSF30 (involved in pre-mRNA processing), a single I106M mutation restores CPSF30 binding to NS1 thereby blocking the expression of host antiviral genes. This renders the virus more virulent than other LPAI infections (128), which may explain why H7N9 causes more severe disease in humans compared to other LPAIs. These results also highlight inhibition of IFN-activation pathways as an important viral factor in preventing host immune responses to infection, allowing for more productive infection and potentially more severe clinical outcomes.

HOST SUSCEPTIBILITY FACTORS

In addition to the ability of the virus to gain function through mutation, in recent years there has been an increasing focus on how host genetic factors can lead to changes in resistance or susceptibility to influenza A viruses. While many factors have been identified in preventing influenza A infection, a key which has come to light for AI host/pathogen interactions is the interferon-induced transmembrane (IFITM) protein family, which unlike other factors such as MxA seems to be predominantly the host, rather than the virus, that seems to control whether the virus is able to replicate. IFITMs are family of transmembrane antiviral proteins that are stimulated by the presence of elevated IFN levels, giving another reason why so many AI viruses attempt to quash the IFN response (129, 130). The IFITM proteins can interfere with viral entry to the cytosol *via* cell membranes (131), with Brass and colleagues showing that overexpression of human IFITMs 1, 2, and 3 effectively blocked infection with several influenza A pseudoviruses (retroviruses expressing influenza surface proteins), including those enveloped with H5 and H7 proteins (132). Moreover, IFITM3 specifically localizes to the endosomes due to phosphorylation of the Y20 tyrosine residue, enabling these proteins to intrinsically target pH-dependent viral pathways such as that seen with influenza A viruses (133).

The IFITM3 molecule can play a significant role in mice and human influenza infections. Mice inoculated with influenza antigen showing higher IFITM3 expression in the lungs developed a more robust lung tissue-resident memory $CD8^{+}$ T cell response as well as a longer duration of response even following reduction of IFN-α, suggestive of this molecule playing a role in not only innate immunity but also adaptive immunity as well (134). Of particular note, a single-nucleotide polymorphism (SNP) in the IFITM3 gene, *rs12252-C*, has been shown to strongly correlate to worsened disease progression, as this SNP leads to a truncated splice-variant that affects the protein's ability to localize to the membrane (135, 136). IFITM3 protein dysfunction can be associated with severe hypercytokinemia and worsened disease progression in H7N9-infected hospitalized patients. In support, Zhang and colleagues showed that the *rs12252-C* mutation correlated to severe seasonal H1N1 influenza cases in Chinese populations where the mutation appeared in higher frequencies (136, 137). However, studies have shown that while this SNP does affect IFITM3′s ability to localize, restriction of the virus may continue with the variant protein or with a Y20A mutation to affect the localization of the full protein (138). Furthermore, a recent study by Makvandi-Nejad and colleagues found that primary cell lines homozygous for the *rs12252-C* SNP expressed the non-truncated mRNA transcript and thus expressed the wild-type IFITM3 protein at levels greater than 99% when compared to the truncated versions (139), which may provide insights into why the *rs12252-C* mutation appears not to act as a significant risk factor in Caucasian populations, but perhaps in the Chinese patients. Moreover, an additional SNP has recently been identified, *rs34481144-A,* which affects the promoter for the *IFITM3* gene, resulting in lower IFITM3 expression compared to hosts without the mutation. Interestingly, both the *rs12252-C* and *rs34481144-A* mutation were found to be non-overlapping, as the risk allele for one was inherited with the protective allele of the other, suggesting a multifaceted IFITM response to influenza A viruses (140).

IFITM1 and IFITM3 distribution in mice has been investigated in the context of H9N2 infection, with the distribution of these proteins correlating with increased restriction of the virus' entry into host tissues, due to upregulation in the lungs and peripheral tissues of BALB/c mice following inoculation. Interestingly, when infected with a H9N2 strain with higher pathogenicity and ability for systemic spread due to a K627E mutation (rV_{K627E}) in the viral PB2 protein, compared to the wild-type strain, IFITM3 was upregulated accordingly in the brain of rV_{K627E}-infected mice to combat this virus' ability to cause viral encephalitis (141). IFITM3 responses to H5 and H7 proteins have also been assessed in pigs and bats, with both these HA subtypes showing restricted entry due to the action of these IFITM3 proteins (142), suggestive of the broad action of IFITM molecules across species known to contract and potentially disseminate AI viruses. That IFITMs restrict AI viruses in "mixing vessel" species (i.e., pigs and bats) suggests that these proteins may have a key role in preventing the spread of human-infecting AI viruses through these routes, as well as contributing to these species showing lessened pathology compared to other mammalian species.

The role of IFITMs against AI viruses in avian species has not been clearly defined, though a study by Smith and colleagues has shown that chicken IFITM3 (which is "human IFITM1-like") similarly restricts H5 and H7 expressing viruses (143). However, when chickens were infected with H5N1, expression of IFITM molecules was not highly upregulated compared to other human-infecting seasonal strains such as H1N1, with IFITMs showing the weakest inhibiting effect against H7N9 (144). Hence, IFITM expression in chickens appears to be limited and does not vary greatly whether the virus is of low or high pathogenicity. Conversely, the IFITM expression profile observed in ducks is far more robust and variable between viral strains, whereby infection with LPAI H5N2 virus was reported to consistently cause a 3-fold increase in IFITM1, 2, and 3 expression levels in the lungs and ileum on day one post-inoculation, while infection with the HPAI H5N1 virus caused up to a 93-fold increase in IFITM3 expression in the lungs in a similar time frame (145). Therefore, understanding the differences in variable IFITM expression, and the reasons why chickens mount a lesser IFITM response to influenza viruses, may prove pivotal in understanding why some birds succumb to HPAI infection while others survive.

In addition to specific IFITM mutations, broad immunodeficiency can lead to worsened pathology and disease outcomes in humans and animals. For example, immunocompromised patients who contract LPAI viruses such as H9N2 suffer severe respiratory distress, and though many of these LPAI remain mild even in immunocompromised patients, H9N2 induces stronger cytokine responses than seasonal influenza viruses (146, 147). These trends are also observed in avian hosts, in which Nili and Asasi found that chickens co-infected with other pathogens such as *M. gallisepticum* showed worsened clinical signs such as severe necrotizing tracheitis, leading to a 19% mortality in the flock (148, 149). Therefore, it is apparent that both the host and pathogen can contribute to perturbed inflammation and severe disease outcomes. In addition, in humans, more severe AI subtypes have been associated with mortalities in very distinct age demographics when compared to seasonal influenza (**Figure 2**), and often manifest in age groups not commonly associated with immunodeficiency. Fatal cases in children (0–9 years) and younger adults (10–19 years) were predominantly caused by HPAI H5N1 infection, with 80.3% of H5N1 fatal cases seen in people aged 35 or under (12). Interestingly, a similar trend was observed with the pandemic [pdmH1N1(2009)] strain, which led to increased infection in younger age groups compared to other seasonal strains circulating at the same time (150). An interesting observation from the 2009 pandemic, however, was that disease outcomes were more mild in newly weaned ferrets infected with pdmH1N1(2009) as well as in younger children, suggesting the immune response in younger individuals may have a protective response to this strain (151, 152). Conversely, seasonal strains of influenza disproportionately impact older ferrets infected, which display a greater degree of morbidity and reduced HA and T cell responses (153). This is also true of human patients also whereby older patients (>60 years of age) are most susceptible to seasonal influenza strains (80% of mortality cases). With regards to H7N9 LPAI infections, the highest mortality was also skewed toward older people, which is likely due to the propensity for H7N9 cases to be found in live poultry farmers, typically older men (154, 155). This emphasizes the dynamic relationship between the pathogen and the human host, and how different strains of influenza viruses can lead to differential fatal outcomes across different ages, a concept further explored by Gostic and colleagues who suggest that pre-immunity to these viruses may confer differing levels of protection to AI based on whether they have been exposed to the viral HA class while still young (156).

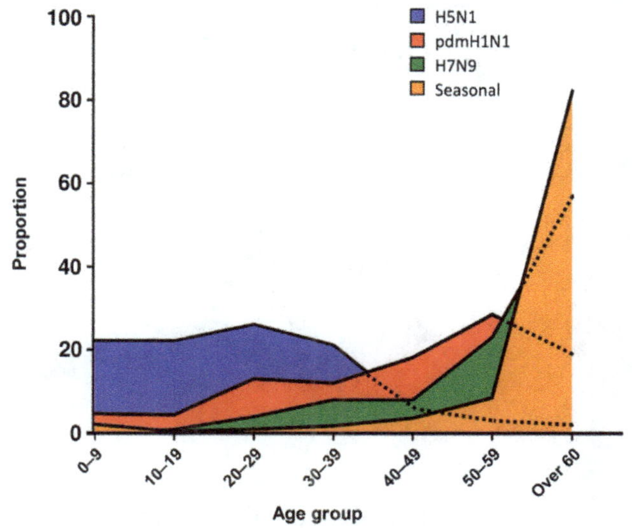

FIGURE 2 | Age-related mortality trends highlight impact of host–pathogen relationships. Frequency of age groups of patients who succumb to different strains of influenza is graphed as a proportion of total fatalities for a given strain. When we assessed the age of patients who succumb to different strains of influenza, as a proportion of the total mortalities for a given strain, trends emerge as to the host susceptibilities. For seasonal influenza, older patients (>60 years old) were the most susceptible, however, for a variation on seasonal influenza, pdmH1N1 2009, the age of patients who succumbed was reduced and included significant mortalities between 20 and 59 years old. Interestingly, the highly pathogenic AI H5N1 was predominantly fatal in those under 40 years old, whereas H7N9, a low pathogenicity AI strain, followed a similar trend to seasonal influenza.

While IFITM proteins aim to restrict viral entry, the interaction between influenza virus peptides and major histocompatibility complex (MHC) molecules is a key host–pathogen interaction affecting the outcome of disease following initial

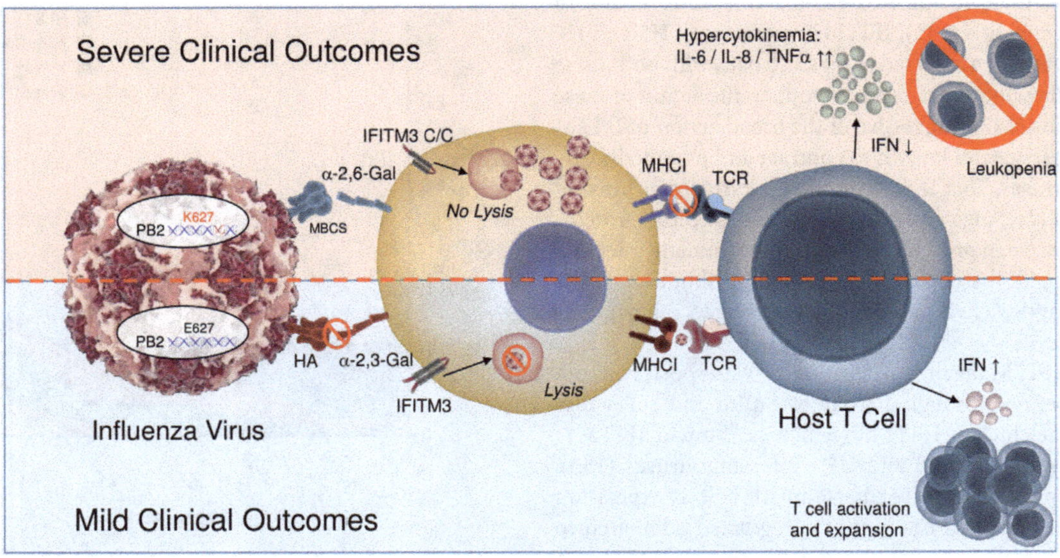

FIGURE 3 | Mechanisms leading to severe clinical outcomes involve both host and pathogen elements. A number of factors have been elucidated to contribute to the severity of influenza disease outcomes. This include viral fitness elements, such as the presence of a multi-basic cleavage site (MBCS), mutations to the polymerase basic 2 (PB2) genes, as well as the presentation of hemagglutinin (HA) protein capable of binding to human sialic acids. These viral fitness elements work in concert with host factors such as modified interferon-induced transmembrane (IFITM) proteins, with reduced ability to combat the virus and MHCI diversity which can or cannot present the antigen appropriately and efficiently to host T cells. Ultimately, these and other elements lead to changes in production of key cytokines as well as cellular activation that drives inflammation, cell death, and clinical manifestation of disease.

infection. In humans, MHC molecules are encoded for by the human leukocyte antigen (HLA) system, with a vast array of alleles in the genes encoding for the molecules responsible for the recognition of antigenic peptides. As such, different HLA subtypes confer different levels of susceptibility to influenza A viruses, as not all HLA subtypes respond to influenza peptides in the same way. For example, human populations expressing HLA-A*02:01 can elicit strong, cross-protective $CD8^+$ T cell responses following presentation of the internally conserved $M1_{58-66}$ epitope (157–160); this epitope is one of the most immunogenic influenza peptides observed in humans with HLA-A*02:01 being the most common HLA alleles expressed worldwide (157). Moreover, individuals lacking common HLA alleles may be at greater risk of influenza A infections, such as those carrying the HLA-A*24:02 allele, associated with increased mortality in individuals infected with pandemic H1N1 virus (161). Indigenous populations in particular are susceptible to influenza A due to a lowered prevalence of protective HLA variants toward these viruses (160). Wang and colleagues suggest that for AI viruses such as H7N9, MHC-interactions with internally conserved epitopes from other influenza A strains, such as pandemic H1N1, may explain why some populations show greater immunity through cross-reactive $CD8^+$ T cell responses than others (72). However, some H7N9 peptides may have cross-conservation with human host proteins that the immune system recognizes as "self," leading to an attenuated immune response to the virus and thus worsened disease progression due to T cell-mediated tolerance (162).

Interestingly, chickens show a restricted repertoire of MHC alleles compared to other species, and these haplotypes themselves are poorly characterized. As such, a few studies have been conducted into characterizing T cell epitopes in response to H5N1 infections, one such study predicting 25 potential T cell epitopes in the NP of H5N1 in four haplotypes (163). More recently, experiments into epitopes of a specific haplotype, BF2*15, further characterized NP epitopes that may lead to protective immunity against H5N1 (164). This limited repertoire may explain why chickens show more severe clinical outcomes due to HPAI such as H5N1 compared to waterfowl, as ducks show extensive diversity in their MHC class I alleles which allows the immune system greater coverage for viral variation (165). A recent investigation into duck MHC class I molecules found that the duck *Anpl*-UAA*01 complex showed similar peptide binding properties to HLA-A*02:01 in humans and as such appears to cover a greater array of influenza A virus epitopes compared to similar chicken MHC molecules such as BF2*2101 (166). Furthermore, migratory shorebirds which act as reservoirs for AI viruses (in particular LPAI H9N2) show increased diversity in their MHC alleles, likely as a mechanism for protecting against foreign pathogens that may be encountered during migration. A study in red knots found high MHC diversity with 36 alleles detected across eight birds, which when correlated to their low prevalence of shed AI virus and high antibody titers to AI viruses, they could mount effective immune responses toward these viruses, possibly *via* cytotoxic T lymphocyte responses recognizing novel peptide/MHC complexes (167). Based on a culmination of human and animal evidence, the interactions between the various pathogen and host factors contributing to human influenza severity are summarized in **Figure 3**.

CONCLUSION

The emergence of AI viruses is of major concern to the avian and human population. The lack of pre-existing antibody immunity and their ability to cause severe disease through multiple host and viral mechanisms makes these viruses difficult to counter. Currently, these viruses are yet to effectively replicate and transmit between humans, however, experiments in ferrets show that only a few mutations are needed for H5N1 and H7N9 viruses to quickly adapt and become a major pandemic threat (114, 168). Their ability to pass from birds to mammals commonly in contact with humans requires constant surveillance across all known bird reservoirs to limit the potential threat of an AI-derived pandemic. Characterization of the interactions between AI viruses and their hosts and how they illicit different degrees of clinical manifestations across species is of utmost importance. Here, we extend our current knowledge of the "cytokine storm" model of AI pathogenesis and delve into more complex underlying viral and host genetic factors that may also contribute greatly to disease severity and susceptibility outcomes.

AUTHOR CONTRIBUTIONS

WH and DL wrote and edited the manuscript. AB, TN, and KK edited the manuscript.

REFERENCES

1. Ehrhardt C, Seyer R, Hrincius ER, Eierhoff T, Wolff T, Ludwig S, et al. Interplay between influenza A virus and the innate immune signalling. *Microbes Infect* (2010) 12:81–7. doi:10.1016/j.micinf.2009.09.007
2. Tong S, Zhu X, Li Y, Shi M, Zhang J, Bourgeois M, et al. New world bats harbor diverse influenza A viruses. *PLoS Pathog* (2013) 9(10):e1003657. doi:10.1371/journal.ppat.1003657
3. Xing Z, Cardona CJ, Li J, Dao N, Tran T, Andrada J. Modulation of the immune response in chickens by low-pathogenicity avian influenza virus H9N2. *J Gen Virol* (2008) 89(5):1288–99. doi:10.1099/vir.0.83362-0
4. Daoust PY, Kibenge FS, Fouchier RA, van de Bildt MW, van Riel D, Kuiken T. Replication of low pathogenic avian influenza virus in naturally infected mallard ducks (*Anas platyrhynchos*) causes no morphologic lesions. *J Wildl Dis* (2011) 42(2):401–9. doi:10.7589/0090-3558-47.2.401
5. Alexander DJ. An overview of the epidemiology of avian influenza. *Vaccine* (2007) 25:5637–44. doi:10.1016/j.vaccine.2006.10.051
6. Du Y, Chen M, Yang J, Jia Y, Han S, Holmes EC, et al. Molecular evolution and emergence of H5N6 avian influenza virus in central China. *J Virol* (2017) 91(12):e00143-17. doi:10.1128/JVI.00143-17
7. Visperas E, Simeon LM. *First Bird Flu Outbreak: 400,000 to Be Culled*. Manila: The Philippine Star (2017).
8. World Health Organization. *Influenza at the Human-Animal Interface: Summary and Assessment, 26 January to 2 March 2018*. Geneva: World Health Organization (2018).
9. Wang Z, Loh L, Kedzierski L, Kedzierska K. Avian influenza viruses, inflammation, and CD8+ T cell immunity. *Front Immunol* (2016) 7:60. doi:10.3389/fimmu.2016.00060
10. Claas EC, Osterhaus AD, van Beek R, De Jong JC, Rimmelzwaan GF, Senne DA, et al. Human influenza A H5N1 virus related to a highly pathogenic avian influenza virus. *Lancet* (1998) 351:472–7. doi:10.1016/S0140-6736(97)11212-0
11. World Health Organization. *Cumulative Number of Confirmed Human Cases for Avian Influenza A(H5N1) Reported to WHO, 2003–2017*. Geneva: World Health Organization (2017). Available from: http://www.who.int/influenza/human_animal_interface/2017_10_30_tableH5N1.pdf?ua=1 (Accessed: March 21, 2018).
12. Lai S, Qin Y, Cowling BJ, Ren X, Wardrop NA, Gilbert M, et al. Global epidemiology of avian influenza A H5N1 virus infection in humans, 1997–2015: a systematic review of individual case data. *Lancet Infect Dis* (2016) 16:e108–18. doi:10.1016/S1473-3099(16)00153-5
13. World Health Organization. *Influenza at the Human-Animal Interface: Summary and Assessment, 28 September to 30 October 2017*. Geneva: World Health Organization (2017). Available from: http://www.who.int/influenza/human_animal_interface/Influenza_Summary_IRA_HA_interface_10_30_2017.pdf (Accessed: March 21, 2018).
14. World Health Organization. *Influenza at the Human-Animal Interface: Summary and Assessment, 8 December 2017 to 25 January 2018*. Geneva: World Health Organization (2018). Available from: http://www.who.int/influenza/human_animal_interface/Influenza_Summary_IRA_HA_interface_25_01_2018_FINAL.pdf?ua=1 (Accessed: March 21, 2018).
15. Teng Y, Bi D, Guo X, Hu D, Feng D, Tong Y. Contact reductions from live poultry market closures limit the epidemic of human infections with H7N9 influenza. *J Infect* (2018) 76:295–394. doi:10.1016/j.jinf.2017.12.015
16. Zaman M, Gasimov V, Oner AF, Dogan N, Adisasmito W, Coker R, et al. Recognizing true H5N1 infections in humans during confirmed outbreaks. *J Infect Dev Ctries* (2014) 8:202–7. doi:10.3855/jidc.3329
17. Farooqui A, Liu W, Zeng T, Liu Y, Zhang L, Khan A, et al. Probable hospital cluster of H7N9 influenza infection. *N Engl J Med* (2016) 374(6):596–8. doi:10.1056/NEJMc1505359
18. Imai M, Watanabe T, Kiso M, Nakajima N, Yamayoshi S, Iwatsuki-Horimoto K, et al. A highly pathogenic avian H7N9 influenza virus isolated from a human is lethal in some ferrets infected via respiratory droplets. *Cell Host Microbe* (2017) 22(5):615–26.e8. doi:10.1016/j.chom.2017.09.008
19. Lopez-Martinez I, Balish A, Barrera-Badillo G, Jones J, Nuñez-García TE, Jang Y, et al. Highly pathogenic avian influenza A(H7N3) virus in poultry workers, Mexico, 2012. *Emerg Infect Dis* (2013) 19(9):1531–4. doi:10.3201/eid1909.130087
20. Watanabe T, Kiso M, Fukuyama S, Nakajima N, Imai M, Yamada S, et al. Characterisation of H7N9 influenza A viruses isolated from humans. *Nature* (2013) 501(7468):551–5. doi:10.1038/nature12392
21. Huo X, Chen L, Qi X, Huang H, Dai Q, Yu H, et al. Significantly elevated number of human infections with H7N9 in Jiangsu in eastern China, October 2016 to January 2017. *Euro Surveill* (2017) 22(13):30496. doi:10.2807/1560-7917.ES.2017.22.13.30496
22. Su S, Gu M, Liu D, Cui J, Gao GF, Zhou J, et al. Epidemiology, evolution, and pathogenesis of H7N9 influenza viruses in five epidemic waves since 2013 in China. *Trends Microbiol* (2017) 25(9):713–28. doi:10.1016/j.tim.2017.06.008
23. Zhou L, Ren R, Yang L, Bao C, Wu J, Wang D, et al. Sudden increase in human infection with avian influenza A(H7N9) virus in China, September–December 2016. *Western Pac Surveill Response J* (2017) 8(1):6–14. doi:10.5365/WPSAR.2017.8.1.001
24. Pinsent A, Pepin KM, Zhu H, Guan Y, White MT, Riley S. The persistance of multiple strains of avian influenza in live bird markets. *Proc Biol Sci* (2017) 284(1868):20170715. doi:10.1098/rspb.2017.0715
25. Wan XF, Dong L, Lan Y, Long LP, Xu C, Zou S, et al. Indications that live poultry markets are a major source of human H5N1 influenza virus infection in China. *J Virol* (2011) 85(24):13432–8. doi:10.1128/JVI.05266-11
26. Bano S, Naeem K, Malik SA. Evaluation of pathogenic potential of avian influenza virus serotype H9N2 in chickens. *Avian Dis* (2003) 47(817):817–22. doi:10.1637/0005-2086-47.s3.817

27. Kalaiyarasu S, Kumar M, Senthil Kumar D, Bhatia S, Dash SK, Bhat S, et al. Highly pathogenic avian influenza H5N1 virus induces cytokine dysregulation with suppressed maturation of chicken monocyte-derived dendritic cells. *Microbiol Immunol* (2016) 60:687–93. doi:10.1111/1348-0421.12443
28. Huang Y, Li X, Zhang H, Chen B, Jiang Y, Yang L, et al. Human infection with an avian influenza A (H9N2) virus in the middle region of China. *J Med Virol* (2015) 87:1641–8. doi:10.1002/jmv.24231
29. Butt KM, Smith GJ, Chen H, Zhang LJ, Leung YH, Xu KM, et al. Human infection with an avian H9N2 influenza A virus in Hong Kong in 2003. *J Clin Microbiol* (2005) 43(11):5760–7. doi:10.1128/JCM.43.11.5760-5767.2005
30. Naguib MM, Arafa AS, El-Kady MF, Selim AA, Gunalan V, Maurer-Stroh S, et al. Evolutionary trajectories and diagnostic challenges of potentially zoonotic avian influenza viruses H5N1 and H9N2 co-circulating in Egypt. *Infect Genet Evol* (2015) 34:278–91. doi:10.1016/j.meegid.2015.06.004
31. Yu X, Jin T, Cui Y, Pu X, Li J, Xu J, et al. Influenza H7N9 and H9N2 viruses: coexistence in poultry linked to human H7N9 infection and genome characteristics. *J Virol* (2014) 88(6):3423–31. doi:10.1128/JVI.02059-13
32. Chen H, Yuan H, Gao R, Zhang J, Wang D, Xiong Y, et al. Clinical and epidemiological characteristics of a fatal case of avian influenza A H10N8 virus infection: a descriptive study. *Lancet* (2014) 383:714–21. doi:10.1016/S0140-6736(14)60111-2
33. Yuan J, Zhang L, Kan X, Jiang L, Yang J, Guo Z, et al. Origin and molecular characteristics of a novel 2013 avian influenza A(H6N1) virus causing human infection in Taiwan. *Clin Infect Dis* (2013) 57:1367–8. doi:10.1093/cid/cit479
34. Wei S-H, Yang JR, Wu HS, Chang MC, Lin JS, Lin CY, et al. Human infection with avian influenza A H6N1 virus: an epidemiological analysis. *Lancet Respir Med* (2013) 1(10):771–8. doi:10.1016/S2213-2600(13)70221-2
35. Ni F, Konrashkina E, Wang Q. Structural and functional studies of influenza virus A/H6 hemagglutinin. *PLoS One* (2015) 10(7):e0134576. doi:10.1371/journal.pone.0134576
36. Xin L, Bai T, Zhou JF, Chen YK, Li XD, Zhu WF, et al. Seropositivity for avian influenza H6 virus among humans, China. *Emerg Infect Dis* (2015) 21(7):1267–9. doi:10.3201/eid2107.150135
37. Hoffmann E, Stech J, Leneva I, Krauss S, Scholtissek C, Chin PS, et al. Characterization of the influenza A virus gene pool in avian species in Southern China: was H6N1 a derivative or a precursor of H5N1? *J Virol* (2000) 74(14):6309–15. doi:10.1128/JVI.74.14.6309-6315.2000
38. Chin PS, Hoffmann E, Webby R, Webster RG, Guan Y, Peiris M, et al. Molecular evolution of H6 influenza viruses from poultry in Southeastern China: prevalence of H6N1 influenza viruses possessing seven A/Hong Kong/156/97 (H5N1)-like genes in poultry. *J Virol* (2002) 76(2):507–16. doi:10.1128/JVI.76.2.507-516.2002
39. Lu H, Castro AE, Pennick K, Liu J, Yang Q, Dunn P, et al. Survival of avian influenza virus H7N2 in SPF chickens and their environments. *Avian Dis* (2003) 47(s3):1015–21. doi:10.1637/0005-2086-47.s3.1015
40. Gharaibeh S. Pathogenicity of an avian influenza serotype H9N2 in chickens. *Avian Dis* (2008) 52(1):106–10. doi:10.1637/8108-090907-Reg
41. França M, Stallknecht DE, Poulson R, Brown J, Howerth EW. The pathogenesis of low pathogenic avian influenza in mallards. *Avian Dis* (2012) 56:976–80. doi:10.1637/10153-040812-ResNote.1
42. Curran JM, Robertson ID, Ellis TM, Selleck PW, O'Dea MA. Variation in the responses of wild species of duck, gull, and wader to inoculation with a wild-bird-origin H6N2 low pathogenicity avain influenza virus. *Avian Dis* (2013) 57(3):581–6. doi:10.1637/10458-112712-Reg.1
43. Wang J, Li CC, Diao YX, Sun XY, Hao DM, Liu X, et al. Different outcomes of infection of chickens and ducks with duck-origin H9N2 influenza A virus. *Acta Virol* (2014) 58:223–30. doi:10.4149/av_2014_03_223
44. Aly MM, Arafa A-SA, Hassan MK. Epidemiological findings of outbreaks of disease caused by highly pathogenic H5N1 avian influenza virus in poultry in Egypt during 2006. *Avian Dis* (2008) 52(2):269–77. doi:10.1637/8166-103007-Reg.1
45. Perkins LEL, Swayne DE. Pathobiology of A/Chicken/Hong Kong/220/97 (H5N1) avian influenza virus in seven gallinaceous species. *Vet Pathol* (2001) 38(2):149–64. doi:10.1354/vp.38-2-149
46. Bingham J, Green DJ, Lowther S, Klippel J, Burggraaf S, Anderson DE, et al. Infection studies with two highly pathogenic avian influenza strains (Vietnamese and Indonesian) in Pekin ducks (*Anas platyrhynchos*), with particular reference to clinical disease, tissue tropism and viral shedding. *Avian Pathol* (2009) 38(4):267–78. doi:10.1080/03079450903055371
47. Acland HM, Silverman Bachin LA, Eckroade RJ. Lesions in broiler and layer chickens in an outbreak of highly pathogenic avian influenza virus infection. *Vet Pathol* (1984) 21:564–9. doi:10.1177/030098588402100603
48. Keawcharoen J, van Riel D, van Amerongen G, Bestebroer T, Beyer WE, van Lavieren R, et al. Wild ducks a long-distance vectors of highly pathogenic avian influenza virus (H5N1). *Emerg Infect Dis* (2008) 14(4):600–7. doi:10.3201/eid1404.071016
49. Pantin-Jackwood MJ, Swayne DE. Pathobiology of Asian highly pathogenic avian influenza H5N1 virus infections in ducks. *Avian Dis* (2007) 51(s1):250–9. doi:10.1637/7710-090606R.1
50. Suzuki K, Okada H, Itoh T, Tada T, Mase M, Nakamura K, et al. Association of increased pathogenicity of Asian H5N1 highly pathogenic avian influenza viruses in chickens with highly efficient viral replication accompanied by early destruction of innate immune responses. *J Virol* (2009) 83(15):7475–86. doi:10.1128/JVI.01434-08
51. Jeong O-M, Kim MC, Kim MJ, Kang HM, Kim HR, Kim YJ, et al. Experimental infection of chickens, ducks and quails with highly pathogenic H5N1 avian influenza virus. *J Vet Sci* (2009) 10(1):53–60. doi:10.4142/jvs.2009.10.1.53
52. Yamamoto Y, Nakamura K, Yamada M, Mase M. Corneal opacity in domestic ducks experimentally infected with H5N1 highly pathogenic avian influenza virus. *Vet Pathol* (2016) 53(1):65–76. doi:10.1177/0300985815591077
53. Yamamoto Y, Nakamura K, Yamada M, Mase M. Comparative pathology of chickens and domestic ducks experimentally infected with highly pathogenic avian influenza viruses (H5N1) isolated in Japan in 2007 and 2008. *Jpn Agric Res Q* (2010) 44(1):73–80. doi:10.6090/jarq.44.73
54. Ito T, Couceiro JN, Kelm S, Baum LG, Krauss S, Castrucci MR, et al. Molecular basis for the generation in pigs of influenza A viruses with pandemic potential. *J Virol* (1998) 72(9):7367–73.
55. Lipatov AS, Kwon YK, Sarmento LV, Lager KM, Spackman E, Suarez DL, et al. Domestic pigs have low susceptibility to H5N1 highly pathogenic avian influenza viruses. *PLoS Pathog* (2008) 4(7):e1000102. doi:10.1371/journal.ppat.1000102
56. Zhu Q, Yang H, Chen W, Cao W, Zhong G, Jiao P, et al. A naturally occurring deletion in its NS gene contributes to the attenuation of an H5N1 swine influenza virus in chickens. *J Virol* (2008) 82(1):220–8. doi:10.1128/JVI.00978-07
57. Zhou P, Hong M, Merrill MM, He H, Sun L, Zhang G. Serological report of influenza a (H7N9) infections among pigs in Southern China. *BMC Vet Res* (2014) 10:203. doi:10.1186/s12917-014-0203-x
58. Liu Q, Zhou B, Ma W, Bawa B, Ma J, Wang W, et al. Analysis of recombinant H7N9 wild-type and mutant viruses in pigs shows that the Q226L mutation in HA Is important for transmission. *J Virol* (2014) 88(14):8153–65. doi:10.1128/JVI.00894-14
59. Balzli C, Lager K, Vincent A, Gauger P, Brockmeier S, Miller L, et al. Susceptibility of swine to H5 and H7 low pathogenic avian influenza viruses. *Influenza Other Respi Viruses* (2016) 10(4):346–52. doi:10.1111/irv.12386
60. Yum J, Park EH, Ku KB, Kim JA, Oh SK, Kim HS, et al. Low infectivity of novel avian-origin H7N9 influenza virus in pigs. *Arch Virol* (2014) 159:2745–9. doi:10.1007/s00705-014-2143-y
61. Jones JC, Baranovich T, Zaraket H, Guan Y, Shu Y, Webby RJ, et al. Human H7N9 influenza A viruses replicate in swine respiratory tissue explants. *J Virol* (2013) 87(22):12496–8. doi:10.1128/JVI.02499-13
62. Kwon TY, Lee SS, Kim CY, Shin JY, Sunwoo SY, Lyoo YS. Genetic characterization of H7N2 influenza virus isolated from pigs. *Vet Microbiol* (2011) 153(3-4):393–7. doi:10.1016/j.vetmic.2011.06.011
63. van Riel D, Munster VJ, de Wit E, Rimmelzwaan GF, Fouchier RA, Osterhaus AD, et al. H5N1 virus attachment to lower respiratory tract. *Science* (2006) 312(5772):399. doi:10.1126/science.1125548
64. Belser JA, Gustin KM, Pearce MB, Maines TR, Zeng H, Pappas C, et al. Pathogenesis and transmission of avian influenza A (H7N9) virus in ferrets and mice. *Nature* (2013) 501:556–60. doi:10.1038/nature12391
65. Zhang Q, Shi J, Deng G, Guo J, Zeng X, He X, et al. H7N9 influenza viruses are transmissible in ferrets by respiratory droplet. *Science* (2013) 341(6144):410–4. doi:10.1126/science.1240532

66. Herfst S, Schrauwen EJ, Linster M, Chutinimitkul S, de Wit E, Munster VJ, et al. Airborne transmission of influenza A/H5N1 virus between ferrets. *Science* (2012) 336:1534–41. doi:10.1126/science.1213362
67. Zaraket H, Baranovich T, Kaplan BS, Carter R, Song MS, Paulson JC, et al. Mammalian adaptation of influenza A(H7N9) virus is limited by a narrow genetic bottleneck. *Nat Commun* (2015) 6:6553. doi:10.1038/ncomms7553
68. Edenborough KM, Lowther S, Laurie K, Yamada M, Long F, Bingham J, et al. Predicting disease severity and viral spread of H5N1 influenza virus in ferrets in the context of natural exposure routes. *J Virol* (2015) 90(4): 1888–97. doi:10.1128/JVI.01878-15
69. Zhu H, Wang D, Kelvin DJ, Li L, Zheng Z, Yoon SW, et al. Infectivity, transmission, and pathology of human-isolated H7N9 influenza virus in ferrets and pigs. *Science* (2013) 341(6142):183–6. doi:10.1126/science.1239844
70. Tundup S, Kandasamy M, Perez JT, Mena N, Steel J, Nagy T, et al. Endothelial cell tropism is a determinant of H5N1 pathogenesis in mammalian species. *PLoS Pathog* (2017) 13(3):e1006270. doi:10.1371/journal.ppat.1006270
71. Gao R, Cao B, Hu Y, Feng Z, Wang D, Hu W, et al. Human infection with a novel avian-origin influenza A (H7N9) virus. *N Engl J Med* (2013) 368(20):1888–97. doi:10.1056/NEJMoa1304459
72. Wang Z, Wan Y, Qiu C, Quiñones-Parra S, Zhu Z, Loh L, et al. Recovery from severe H7N9 disease is associated with diverse response mechanisms dominated by CD8+ T cells. *Nat Commun* (2015) 6:6833. doi:10.1038/ncomms7833
73. Hu Y, Lu S, Song Z, Wang W, Hao P, Li J, et al. Association between adverse clinical outcome in human disease caused by novel influenza A H7N9 virus and sustained viral shedding and emergence of antiviral resistance. *Lancet* (2013) 381(9885):2273–9. doi:10.1016/S0140-6736(13)61125-3
74. Zhang Z, Zhang J, Huang K, Li KS, Yuen KY, Guan Y, et al. Systemic infection of avian influenza A virus H5N1 subtype in humans. *Hum Pathol* (2009) 40:735–9. doi:10.1016/j.humpath.2008.08.015
75. To KF, Chan PK, Chan KF, Lee WK, Lam WY, Wong KF, et al. Pathology of fatal human infection associated with avian influenza A H5N1 virus. *J Med Virol* (2001) 63:242–6. doi:10.1002/1096-9071(200103)63:3<242::AID-JMV1007>3.0.CO;2-N
76. Kuchipudi SV, Tellabati M, Sebastian S, Londt BZ, Jansen C, Vervelde L, et al. Highly pathogenic avian influenza virus infection in chickens but not ducks is associated with elevated host immune and pro-inflammatory responses. *Vet Res* (2014) 45:118. doi:10.1186/s13567-014-0118-3
77. Short KR, Veeris R, Leijten LM, van den Brand JM, Jong VL, Stittelaar K, et al. Proinflammatory cytokine responses in extra-respiratory tissues during severe influenza. *J Infect Dis* (2017) 216:829–33. doi:10.1093/infdis/jix281
78. Shinya K, Gao Y, Cilloniz C, Suzuki Y, Fujie M, Deng G, et al. Integrated clinical, pathologic, virologic, and transcriptomic analysis of H5N1 influenza virus-induced viral pneumonia in the rhesus macaque. *J Virol* (2012) 86(11):6055–66. doi:10.1128/JVI.00365-12
79. Gao S, Kang Y, Yuan R, Ma H, Xiang B, Wang Z, et al. Immune responses of chickens infected with wild bird-origin H5N6 avian influenza virus. *Front Microbiol* (2017) 8:1081. doi:10.3389/fmicb.2017.01081
80. Meliopoulos VA, Karlsson EA, Kercher L, Cline T, Freiden P, Duan S, et al. Human H7N9 and H5N1 influenza viruses differ in induction of cytokines and tissue tropism. *J Virol* (2014) 88(22):12982–91. doi:10.1128/JVI.01571-14
81. To KK, Lau CC, Woo PC, Lau SK, Chan JF, Chan KH, et al. Human H7N9 virus induces a more pronounced pro-inflammatory cytokine but an attenuated interferon response in human bronchial epithelial cells when compared with an epidemiologically-linked chicken H7N9 virus. *Virol J* (2016) 13:42. doi:10.1186/s12985-016-0498-2
82. Wu W, Shi D, Fang D, Guo F, Guo J, Huang F, et al. A new perspective on C-reactive protein in H7N9 infections. *Int J Infect Dis* (2016) 44:31–6. doi:10.1016/j.ijid.2016.01.009
83. Zhao C, Qi X, Ding M, Sun X, Zhou Z, Zhang S, et al. Pro-inflammatory cytokine dysregulation is associated with novel avian influenza A (H7N9) virus in primary human macrophages. *J Gen Virol* (2016) 97(2):299–305. doi:10.1099/jgv.0.000357
84. Nelli RK, Dunham SP, Kuchipudi SV, White GA, Baquero-Perez B, Chang P, et al. Mammalian innate resistance to highly pathogenic avian influenza H5N1 virus infection is mediated through reduced proinflammation and infectious virus release. *J Virol* (2012) 86(17):9201–10. doi:10.1128/JVI.00244-12
85. Turner MD, Nedjai B, Hurst T, Pennington DJ. Cytokines and chemokines: at the crossroads of cell signalling and inflammatory disease. *Biochim Biophys Acta* (2014) 1843:2563–82. doi:10.1016/j.bbamcr.2014.05.014
86. Boonnak K, Vogel L, Feldmann F, Feldmann H, Legge KL, Subbarao K. Lymphopenia associated with highly virulent H5N1 virus infection due to plasmocytoid dendritic cell mediated apoptosis of T cells. *J Immunol* (2014) 192(12):5906–12. doi:10.4049/jimmunol.1302992
87. Waring P, Müllbacher A. Cell death induced by the Fas/Fas ligand pathway and its role in pathology. *Immunol Cell Biol* (1999) 77:312–7. doi:10.1046/j.1440-1711.1999.00837.x
88. Chen Y, Liang W, Yang S, Wu N, Gao H, Sheng J, et al. Human infections with the emerging avian influenza A H7N9 virus from wet market poultry: clinical analysis and characterisation of viral genome. *Lancet* (2013) 381:1916–25. doi:10.1016/S0140-6736(13)60903-4
89. Uiprasertkul M, Kitphati R, Puthavathana P, Kriwong R, Kongchanagul A, Ungchusak K, et al. Apoptosis and pathogenesis of avian influenza A (H5N1) virus in humans. *Emerg Infect Dis* (2007) 13(5):708–12. doi:10.3201/eid1305.060572
90. Wang C, Yu H, Horby PW, Cao B, Wu P, Yang S, et al. Comparison of patients hospitalized with influenza A subtypes H7N9, H5N1, and 2009 pandemic H1N1. *Clin Infect Dis* (2014) 58(8):1095–103. doi:10.1093/cid/ciu053
91. Wang Z, Zhu L, Nguyen THO, Wan Y, Sant S, Quiñones-Parra SM, et al. Clonally diverse CD38+HLA-DR+CD8+ T cells persist during fatal H7N9. *Nat Commun* (2018) 9:824. doi:10.1038/s41467-018-03243-7
92. Nichols JE, Niles JA, Roberts NJ Jr. Human lymphocyte apoptosis after exposure to influenza A virus. *J Virol* (2001) 73(13):5921–9. doi:10.1128/JVI.73.13.5921-5929.2001
93. Herfst S, Imai M, Kawaoka Y, Fouchier RA. Avian influenza virus transmission to mammals. *Curr Top Microbiol Immunol* (2014) 385:137–55. doi:10.1007/82_2014_387
94. Rogers GN, Pritchett TJ, Lane JL, Paulson JC. Differential sensitivity of human, avian, and equine influenza A viruses to a glycoprotein inhibitor of infection: selection of receptor specific variants. *Virology* (1983) 131(2):394–408. doi:10.1016/0042-6822(83)90507-X
95. de Vries RP, Peng W, Grant OC, Thompson AJ, Zhu X, Bouwman KM, et al. Three mutations switch H7N9 influenza to human-type receptor specificity. *PLoS Pathog* (2017) 13(6):e1006390. doi:10.1371/journal.ppat.1006390
96. Dortmans JC, Dekkers J, Wickramasinghe IN, Verheije MH, Rottier PJ, van Kuppeveld FJ, et al. Adaptation of novel H7N9 influenza virus to human receptors. *Sci Rep* (2013) 3:3058. doi:10.1038/srep03058
97. Chandrasekaran A, Srinivasan A, Raman R, Viswanathan K, Raguram S, Tumpey TM, et al. Glycan topology determines human adaptation of avian H5N1 virus hemagglutinin. *Nat Biotechnol* (2008) 26(1):107–13. doi:10.1038/nbt1375
98. Chrzastek K, Lee DH, Gharaibeh S, Zsak A, Kapczynski DR. Characterization of H9N2 avian influenza viruses from the Middle East demonstrates heterogeneity at amino acid position 226 in the hemagglutinin and potential for transmission to mammals. *Virology* (2018) 518:195–201. doi:10.1016/j.virol.2018.02.016
99. Li X, Shi J, Guo J, Deng G, Zhang Q, Wang J, et al. Genetics, receptor binding property, and transmissibility in mammals of naturally isolated H9N2 avian influenza viruses. *PLoS Pathog* (2014) 10(11):e1004508. doi:10.1371/journal.ppat.1004508
100. Watanabe Y, Arai Y, Daidoji T, Kawashita N, Ibrahim MS, El-Gendy E-D, et al. Characterization of H5N1 influenza virus variants with hemagglutinin mutations isolated from patients. *MBio* (2015) 6(2):e00081-15. doi:10.1128/mBio.00081-15
101. Watanabe Y, Ibrahim MS, Ellakany HF, Kawashita N, Mizuike R, Hiramatsu H, et al. Acquisition of human-type receptor binding specificity by new H5N1 influenza virus sublineages during their emergence in birds in Egypt. *PLoS Pathog* (2011) 7(5):e1002068. doi:10.1371/journal.ppat.1002068

102. Steel J, Lowen AC, Mubareka S, Palese P. Transmission of influenza virus in a mammalian host is increased by PB2 amino acids 627K or 627E/701N. *PLoS Pathog* (2009) 5(1):e1000252. doi:10.1371/journal.ppat.1000252
103. Labadie K, Dos Santos Afonso E, Rameix-Welti MA, van der Werf S, Naffakh N. Host-range determinants on the PB2 protein of influenza A viruses control the interaction between the viral polymerase and nucleoprotein in human cells. *Virology* (2007) 362:271–82. doi:10.1016/j.virol.2006.12.027
104. Yu K, Liu X, Qi T, Yang H, Whitfield DM, Y Chen Q, et al. General low-temperature reaction pathway from precursors to monomers before nucleation of compound semiconductor nanocrystals. *Nat Commun* (2016) 7:12223. doi:10.1038/ncomms12223
105. Zhang H, Li X, Guo J, Li L, Chang C, Li Y, et al. The PB2 E627K mutation contributes to the high polymerase activity and enhanced replication of H7N9 influenza virus. *J Gen Virol* (2014) 95:779–86. doi:10.1099/vir.0.061721-0
106. Schrauwen EJ, Herfst S, Leijten LM, van Run P, Bestebroer TM, Linster M, et al. The multibasic cleavage site in H5N1 virus is critical for systemic spread along the olfactory and hematogenous routes in ferrets. *J Virol* (2012) 86(7):3975–84. doi:10.1128/JVI.06828-11
107. Suguitan AL, Matsuoka Y, Lau YF, Santos CP, Vogel L, Cheng LI, et al. The multibasic cleavage site of hemagglutinin of highly pathogenic A/Vietnam/1203/2004 (H5N1) avian influenza virus acts as a virulence factor in a host-specific manner in mammals. *J Virol* (2012) 86(5):2706–14. doi:10.1128/JVI.05546-11
108. Stieneke-Gröber A, Vey M, Angliker H, Shaw E, Thomas G, Roberts C, et al. Influenza virus hemagglutinin with a multibasic cleavage site is activated by furin, a subtilisin-like endoprotease. *EMBO J* (1992) 11(7):2407–14.
109. Hagag IT, Mansour SM, Zhang Z, Ali AA, Ismaiel el-BM, Salama AA, et al. Pathogenicty of highly pathogenic avian influenza virus H5N1 in naturally infected poultry in Egypt. *PLoS One* (2015) 10(5):e0120061. doi:10.1371/journal.pone.0120061
110. Berhane Y, Hisanaga T, Kehler H, Neufeld J, Manning L, Argue C, et al. Highly pathogenic avian influenza virus A (H7N3) in domestic poultry, Saskatchewan, Canada, 2007. *Emerg Infect Dis* (2009) 15(9):1492–5. doi:10.3201/eid1509.080231
111. Killian ML, Kim-Torchetti M, Hines N, Yingst S, DeLiberto T, Lee DH. Outbreak of H7N8 low pathogenic avian influenza in commercial Turkeys with spontaneous mutation to highly pathogenic avian influenza. *Genome Announc* (2016) 4(3):e00457-16. doi:10.1128/genomeA.00457-16
112. Stech O, Veits J, Weber S, Deckers D, Schröer D, Vahlenkamp TW, et al. Acquisition of a polybasic hemagglutinin cleavage site by a low-pathogenic avian influenza virus is not sufficient for immediate transformation into a highly pathogenic strain. *J Virol* (2009) 83(11):5864–8. doi:10.1128/JVI.02649-08
113. Wang QM, Liu SL, Chen EF. [Advances on epidemiological research of human infections with novel avian influenza A (H7N9) virus]. *Zhonghua Yu Fang Yi Xue Za Zhi* (2017) 51(2):183–7. doi:10.3760/cma.j.issn.0253-9624.2017.02.017
114. Imai M, Watanabe T, Hatta M, Das SC, Ozawa M, Shinya K, et al. Experimental adaptation of an influenza H5 haemagglutinin (HA) confers respiratory droplet transmission to a reassortant H5 HA/H1N1 virus in ferrets. *Nature* (2012) 486:420–8. doi:10.1038/nature10831
115. Haller O, Gao S, von der Malsburg A, Daumke O, Kochs G. Dynamin-like MxA GTPase: structural insights into oligomerization and implications for antiviral activity. *J Biol Chem* (2010) 285(37):28419–24. doi:10.1074/jbc.R110.145839
116. Zimmermann P, Mänz B, Haller O, Schwemmle M, Kochs G. The viral nucleoprotein determines Mx sensitivity of influenza A viruses. *J Virol* (2011) 85(16):8133–40. doi:10.1128/JVI.00712-11
117. Mänz B, Dornfeld D, Götz V, Zell R, Zimmermann P, Haller O, et al. Pandemic influenza A viruses escape from restriction by human MxA though adaptive mutations in the nucleoprotein. *PLoS Pathog* (2013) 9(3):e1003279. doi:10.1371/journal.ppat.1003279
118. Deeg CM, Hassan E, Mutz P, Rheinemann L, Götz V, Magar L, et al. In vivo evasion of MxA by avian influenza viruses requires human signature in the viral nucleoprotein. *J Exp Med* (2017) 214(5):1239–48. doi:10.1084/jem.20161033
119. Schusser B, Reuter A, von der Malsburg A, Penski N, Weigend S, Kaspers B, et al. Mx Is dispensable for interferon-mediated resistance of chicken cells against influenza A virus. *J Virol* (2011) 85(16):8307–15. doi:10.1128/JVI.00535-11
120. Benfield CTO, Lyall JW, Tiley LS. The cytoplasmic location of chicken Mx is not the determining factor for its lack of antiviral activity. *PLoS One* (2010) 5(8):e12151. doi:10.1371/journal.pone.0012151
121. Qi X, Zhang H, Wang Q, Wang J. The NS1 protein of avian influenza virus H9N2 induces oxidative-stress-mediated chicken oviduct epithelial cells apoptosis. *J Gen Virol* (2016) 97:3183–92. doi:10.1099/jgv.0.000625
122. Burggraaf S, Bingham J, Payne J, Kimpton WG, Lowenthal JW, Bean AG. Increased inducible nitric oxide synthase expression in organs is associated with a higher severity of H5N1 influenza infection. *PLoS One* (2011) 6(1):e14561. doi:10.1371/journal.pone.0014561
123. Jia D, et al. Influenza virus non-structural protein 1 (NS1) disrupts interferon signalling. *PLoS One* (2010) 5(11):e13927. doi:10.1371/journal.pone.0013927
124. Wang J, Zeng Y, Xu S, Yang J, Wang W, Zhong B, et al. A naturally occurring deletion in the effector domain of H5N1 swine influenza virus nonstructural protein 1 regulates viral fitness and host innate immunity. *J Virol* (2018) 92(11):e00149-18. doi:10.1128/JVI.00149-18
125. Jiao P, Tian G, Li Y, Deng G, Jiang Y, Liu C, et al. A single-amino-acid substitution in the NS1 protein changes the pathogenicity of H5N1 avian influenza viruses in mice. *J Virol* (2008) 82(3):1146–54. doi:10.1128/JVI.01698-07
126. Wang L, Fu X, Zheng Y, Zhou P, Fang B, Huang S, et al. The NS1 protein of H5N6 feline influenza virus inhibits feline beta interfereon response by preventing NF-κB and IRF3 activation. *Dev Comp Immunol* (2017) 74:60–8. doi:10.1016/j.dci.2017.04.003
127. Thube MM, Shil P, Kasbe R, Patil AA, Pawar SD, Mullick J. Differences in Type I interferon response in human lung epithelial cells infected by highly pathogenic H5N1 and low pathogenic H11N1 avian influenza viruses. *Virus Genes* (2018) 54(3):414–23. doi:10.1007/s11262-018-1556-1
128. Ayllon J, Domingues P, Rajsbaum R, Miorin L, Schmolke M, Hale BG, et al. A single amino acid substitution in the novel H7N9 influenza A NS1 protein increases CPSF30 binding and virulence. *J Virol* (2014) 88(20):12146–51. doi:10.1128/JVI.01567-14
129. Bailey CC, Kondur HR, Huang IC, Farzan M. Interferon-induced transmembrane protein 3 is a type II transmembrane protein. *J Biol Chem* (2013) 288(45):32184–93. doi:10.1074/jbc.M113.514356
130. Bailey CC, Zhong G, Huang IC, Farzan M. IFITM-family proteins: the cell's first line of antiviral defense. *Annu Rev Virol* (2014) 1:261–83. doi:10.1146/annurev-virology-031413-085537
131. Feeley EM, Sims JS, John SP, Chin CR, Pertel T, Chen LM, et al. IFITM3 inhibits influenza A virus infection by preventing cytosolic entry. *PLoS Pathog* (2011) 7(10):e1002337. doi:10.1371/journal.ppat.1002337
132. Brass AL, Huang IC, Benita Y, John SP, Krishnan MN, Feeley EM, et al. The IFITM proteins mediate cellular resistance to influenza A H1N1 virus, West Nile virus, and dengue virus. *Cell* (2009) 139:1243–54. doi:10.1016/j.cell.2009.12.017
133. Jia R, Pan Q, Ding S, Rong L, Liu SL, Geng Y, et al. The N-terminal region of IFITM3 modulates its antiviral activity by regulating IFITM3 cellular localization. *J Virol* (2012) 86(24):13697–707. doi:10.1128/JVI.01828-12
134. Wakim LM, Gupta N, Mintern JD, Villadangos JA. Enhanced survival of tissue-resident memory CD8+ T cells during infection with influenza virus due to selective expression of IFITM3. *Nat Immunol* (2013) 14(3):238–46. doi:10.1038/ni.2525
135. Yang X, Tan B, Zhou X, Xue J, Zhang X, Wang P, et al. Interferon-inducible transmembrane protein 3 genetic variant rs12252 and influenza susceptibility and severity: a meta-analysis. *PLoS One* (2015) 10(5):e0124985. doi:10.1371/journal.pone.0124985
136. Zhang YH, Zhao Y, Li N, Peng YC, Giannoulatou E, Jin RH, et al. Interferon-induced transmembrane protein-3 genetic variant rs12252-C is associated with severe influenza in Chinese individuals. *Nat Commun* (2013) 4:1418. doi:10.1038/ncomms2433
137. Wang Z, Zhang A, Wan Y, Liu X, Qiu C, Xi X, et al. Early hypercytokinemia is associated with interferon-induced transmembrane protein-3

dysfunction and predictive of fatal H7N9 infection. *Proc Natl Acad Sci U S A* (2014) 111(2):769–74. doi:10.1073/pnas.1321748111

138. Williams DE, Wu WL, Grotefend CR, Radic V, Chung C, Chung YH, et al. IFITM3 polymorphism rs12252-C restricts influenza A viruses. *PLoS One* (2014) 9(10):e110096. doi:10.1371/journal.pone.0110096
139. Makvandi-Nejad S, Laurenson-Schafer H, Wang L, Wellington D, Zhao Y, Jin B, et al. Lack of truncated IFITM3 transcripts in cells homozygous for the rs12252-C variant that is associated with severe influenza infection. *J Infect Dis* (2018) 217:257–62. doi:10.1093/infdis/jix512
140. Allen EK, Randolph AG, Bhangale T, Dogra P, Ohlson M, Oshansky CM, et al. SNP-mediated disruption of CTCF binding at the IFITM3 promoter is associated with risk of severe influenza in humans. *Nat Med* (2017) 23:975–83. doi:10.1038/nm.4370
141. Yu M, Qi W, Huang Z, Zhang K, Ye J, Liu R, et al. Expression profile and histological distribution of IFITM1 and IFITM3 during H9N2 avian influenza virus infection in BALB/c mice. *Med Microbiol Immunol* (2015) 204:505–14. doi:10.1007/s00430-014-0361-2
142. Benfield CTO, Smith SE, Wright E, Wash RS, Ferrara F, Temperton NJ, et al. Bat and pig IFN-induced transmembrane protein 3 restrict cell entry by influenza virus and lyssavirus. *J Gen Virol* (2015) 96:991–1005. doi:10.1099/vir.0.000058
143. Smith SE, Gibson MS, Wash RS, Ferrara F, Wright E, Temperton N, et al. Chicken interferon-inducible transmembrane protein 3 restricts influenza viruses and lyssaviruses in vitro. *J Virol* (2013) 87(23):12957–66. doi:10.1128/JVI.01443-13
144. Cao Y, Huang Y, Xu K, Liu Y, Li X, Xu Y, et al. Differential responses of innate immunity triggered by different subtypes of influenza a viruses in human and avian hosts. *BMC Med Genomics* (2017) 10:70. doi:10.1186/s12920-017-0304-z
145. Smith J, Smith N, Yu L, Paton IR, Gutowska MW, Forrest HL, et al. A comparative analysis of host responses to avian influenza infection in ducks and chickens highlights a role for the interferon-induced transmembrane proteins in viral resistance. *BMC Genomics* (2015) 16:574. doi:10.1186/s12864-015-1778-8
146. Cheng VC, Chan JF, Wen X, Wu WL, Que TL, Chen H, et al. Infection of immunocompromised patients by avian H9N2 influenza A virus. *J Infect* (2011) 62:394–9. doi:10.1016/j.jinf.2011.02.007
147. Law AH, Lee DC, Yuen KY, Peiris M, Lau AS. Cellular response to influenza virus infection: a potential role for autophagy in CXCL10 and interferon-alpha induction. *Cell Mol Immunol* (2010) 7:263–70. doi:10.1038/cmi.2010.25
148. Nili H, Asasi K. Avian influenza (H9N2) outbreak in Iran. *Avian Dis* (2003) 47(s3):828–31. doi:10.1637/0005-2086-47.s3.828
149. Nili H, Asasi K. Natural cases and an experimental study of H9N2 avian influenza in commercial broiler chickens of Iran. *Avian Pathol* (2002) 31(3):247–52. doi:10.1080/03079450220136567
150. Simonsen L, Spreeuwenberg P, Lustig R, Taylor RJ, Fleming DM, Kroneman M, et al. Global mortality estimates for the 2009 influenza pandemic from the GLaMOR project: a modeling study. *PLoS Med* (2013) 10(11):e1001558. doi:10.1371/journal.pmed.1001558
151. Huang SS, Banner D, Degousee N, Leon AJ, Xu L, Paquette SG, et al. Differential pathological and immune responses in newly weaned ferrets are associated with a mild clinical outcome of pandemic 2009 H1N1 infection. *J Virol* (2012) 86(24):13187–201. doi:10.1128/JVI.01456-12
152. Helferty M, Vachon J, Tarasuk J, Rodin R, Spika J, Pelletier L. Incidence of hospital admissions and severe outcomes during the first and second waves of pandemic (H1N1) 2009. *CMAJ* (2010) 182(18):1981–7. doi:10.1503/cmaj.100746
153. Paquette SG, Huang SSH, Banner D, Xu L, León A, Kelvin AA, et al. Impaired heterologous immunity in aged ferrets during sequential influenza A H1N1 infection. *Virology* (2014) 46(4–465):177–83. doi:10.1016/j.virol.2014.07.013
154. Zhou L, Tan Y, Kang M, Liu F, Ren R, Wang Y, et al. Preliminary epidemiology of human infections with highly pathogenic avian influenza A(H7N9) virus, China, 2017. *Emerg Infect Dis* (2017) 23(8):1355–9. doi:10.3201/eid2308.170640
155. Mackay IM. *Influenza A(H7N9) Virus: Detection Numbers and Graphs….* VDU's blog (2014).
156. Gostic KM, Ambrose M, Worobey M, Lloyd-Smith JO. Potent protection against H5N1 and H7N9 influenza via childhood hemagglutinin imprinting. *Science* (2016) 354(6313):722–6. doi:10.1126/science.aag1322
157. Valkenburg SA, Josephs TM, Clemens EB, Grant EJ, Nguyen TH, Wang GC, et al. Molecular basis for universal HLA-A*0201-restricted CD8+ T-cell immunity against influenza viruses. *Proc Natl Acad Sci U S A* (2016) 113(16):4440–5. doi:10.1073/pnas.1603106113
158. Quiñones-Parra S, Grant E, Loh L, Nguyen TH, Campbell KA, Tong SY, et al. Preexisting CD8+ T-cell immunity to the H7N9 influenza A virus varies across ethnicities. *Proc Natl Acad Sci U S A* (2014) 111(3):1049–54. doi:10.1073/pnas.1322229111
159. Nguyen THO, Sant S, Bird NL, Grant EJ, Clemens EB, Koutsakos M, et al. Perturbed CD8+ T cell immunity across universal influenza epitopes in the elderly. *J Leukoc Biol* (2017) 103(2):321–39. doi:10.1189/jlb.5MA0517-207R
160. Clemens EB, Grant EJ, Wang Z, Gras S, Tipping P, Rossjohn J, et al. Towards identification of immune and genetic correlates of severe influenza disease in Indigenous Australians. *Immunol Cell Biol* (2016) 94:367–77. doi:10.1038/icb.2015.93
161. Hertz T, Oshansky CM, Roddam PL, DeVincenzo JP, Caniza MA, Jojic N, et al. HLA targeting efficiency correlates with human T-cell response magnitude and with mortality from influenza A infection. *Proc Natl Acad Sci U S A* (2013) 110(33):13492–7. doi:10.1073/pnas.1221555110
162. Liu R, Moise L, Tassone R, Gutierrez AH, Terry FE, Sangare K, et al. H7N9 T-cell epitopes that mimic human sequences are less immunogenic and may induce Treg-mediated tolerance. *Hum Vaccin Immunother* (2015) 11(9):2241–52. doi:10.1080/21645515.2015.1052197
163. Hou Y, Guo Y, Wu C, Shen N, Jiang Y, Wang J. Prediction and identification of T cell epitopes in the H5N1 influenza virus nucleoprotein in chicken. *PLoS One* (2012) 7(6):e39344. doi:10.1371/journal.pone.0039344
164. Zhang W, Huang Q, Lu M, Zhu F, Huang YY, Yang SH, et al. Exploration of the BF2*15 major histocompatibility complex class I binding motif and identification of cytotoxic T lymphocyte epitopes from the H5N1 influenza virus nucleoprotein in chickens. *Arch Virol* (2016) 161:3081–93. doi:10.1007/s00705-016-3013-6
165. Fleming-Canepa X, Jensen SM, Mesa CM, Diaz-Satizabal L, Roth AJ, Parks-Dely JA, et al. Extensive allelic diversity of MHC class I in wild mallard ducks. *J Immunol* (2016) 197:783–94. doi:10.4049/jimmunol.1502450
166. Wu Y, Wang J, Fan S, Chen R, Liu Y, Zhang J, et al. Structural definition of duck major histocompatibility complex class I molecules that might explain efficient cytotoxic T lymphocyte immunity to influenza A virus. *J Virol* (2017) 91(14):e02511-16. doi:10.1128/JVI.02511-16
167. Buehler DM, Verkuil YI, Tavares ES, Baker AJ. Characterization of MHC class I in a long-distance migrant shorebird suggests multiple transcribed genes and intergenic recombination. *Immunogenetics* (2013) 65:211–25. doi:10.1007/s00251-012-0669-2
168. Watanabe T, Zhong G, Russell CA, Nakajima N, Hatta M, Hanson A, et al. Circulating avian influenza viruses closely related to the 1918 virus have pandemic potential. *Cell Host Microbe* (2014) 15:692–705. doi:10.1016/j.chom.2014.05.006

11

Potential Role of MicroRNAs in the Regulation of Antiviral Responses to Influenza Infection

*Thi Hiep Nguyen[1,2], Xiaoming Liu[1,2], Zhen Zhong Su[3], Alan Chen-Yu Hsu[1,4], Paul S. Foster[1,2] and Ming Yang[1,2]**

[1] Priority Research Centre for Healthy Lungs, The University of Newcastle, Callaghan, NSW, Australia, [2] Faculty of Health and Medicine, School of Biomedical Sciences and Pharmacy, The University of Newcastle, Callaghan, NSW, Australia, [3] Department of Respiratory Medicine, The Second Hospital, Jilin University, ChangChun, China, [4] Faculty of Health and Medicine, School of Medicine and Public Health, The University of Newcastle, Callaghan, NSW, Australia

***Correspondence:**
Ming Yang
ming.yang@newcastle.edu.au

Influenza is a major health burden worldwide and is caused by influenza viruses that are enveloped and negative stranded RNA viruses. Little progress has been achieved in targeted intervention, either at a population level or at an individual level (to treat the cause), due to the toxicity of drugs and ineffective vaccines against influenza viruses. MicroRNAs (miRNAs) are small non-coding RNAs that play critical roles in gene expression, cell differentiation, and tissue development and have been shown to silence viral replication in a sequence-specific manner. Investigation of these small endogenous nucleotides may lead to new therapeutics against influenza virus infection. Here, we describe our current understanding of the role of miRNAs in host defense response against influenza virus, as well as their potential and limitation as new therapeutic approaches.

Keywords: microRNA, immune responses, influenza virus, infection, inflammation

INTRODUCTION

Influenza viruses belong to the *Orthomyxoviridae* family of single-stranded, negative sense RNA viruses with segmented RNA genomes (1, 2). There are three genera of influenza viruses including genus A, B, and C. Influenza A virus (IAV) causes significant respiratory infections in humans and global pandemics, while genus B virus can cause epidemics (but not pandemics) and genus C virus only leads to a mild disease (3).

Influenza viruses commonly cause acute respiratory infections and have posed serious threats to public health worldwide for many centuries due to their rapid and frequent mutation and recombination rate. Also, there is frequent and inevitable emergence of novel subtypes with unpredictable pathogenicity and transmissibility (4, 5). Each year, 3 to 5 million individuals experience severe influenza virus infections, with approximately 500,000 annual deaths worldwide (6–8). The clinical symptoms of acute respiratory infection by influenza viruses include high fever, body aches, headache, respiratory tract congestion, pharyngitis, and fatigue. In most cases, these symptoms are resolved in infected healthy subjects after 7–10 days. However, young children, elderly, and patients with chronic disorders such as asthma, chronic obstructive pulmonary disease (COPD), cardiovascular diseases, and diabetes are often at higher risk of developing complications such as severe bronchitis, pneumonia, or worsened medical conditions from influenza (9–14). Moreover, the severity of the disease differs between the virus subtypes (15). Although the pathogenesis and mechanisms of influenza virus infection are largely known, there is little progress in targeted intervention, either at a population level or at an individual level (to treat the cause). This is due to rapid and frequent mutations, and ineffective vaccines and antiviral drugs against influenza viruses. Furthermore, frequent antigenic changes (drift and shift) and constant emergence of drug resistant subtypes/strains also undermine the effectiveness of current anti-influenza approaches (16–20). Therefore, it is urgently required to develop more efficient approaches for prevention and treatment of the disease.

MICRORNAs (miRNAs)

MicroRNAs are a class of short non-coding single-stranded RNA sequences of about 20 bp first described two decades ago that negatively regulate gene expression in eukaryotes (21–24). These small RNAs are transcribed as long hairpin primary RNAs (pri-miRNAs) by RNA polymerase II. In nucleus, pri-miRNAs are cleaved by the microprocessor complex including Drosha ribonuclease III and the RNA-binding DGCR8 protein to form hairpin precursor miRNAs (pre-miRNAs, ~70 bp). Pre-miRNAs are exported to the cytoplasm by exportin-5 protein, belonging to the Ran-dependent nuclear transport receptor family, and are further cleaved by cytoplasmic endoribonuclease Dicer to form mature RNAs (**Figure 1**). Each miRNA gene has been recognized to generate two mature miRNAs that are designated as -3p miRNA and -5p miRNA (25–27). Both of them that can coexist are functional by associating with the RNA-Induced Silencing Complex. Mature miRNAs often are known to bind to 3-untranslated regions (UTRs) of target mRNAs to regulate gene expression. Most miRNA:mRNA interactions involve nucleotides 2–7 of miRNAs, a region called seed. Seed-based interactions lead to mRNA destabilization and/or translation inhibition.

Functional consequences of changed miRNA expression have been explored for diagnosis, prognosis, and severity of a wide range of diseases including infectious disease, autoimmune diseases, and cancer (28–31). Numerous investigations using anti-miRNA oligonucleotides, miRNA mimics/inhibitors, or mice deficient of a specific miRNA have demonstrated that a single miRNA can have extensive and crucial effects on the physiologic and pathological processes and that alterations in the function of miRNA can result in biological dysfunction and diseases (24, 31, 32). Despite the fact that the critical role of miRNAs in orchestrating cell differentiation, proliferation, and metabolism is well known (24, 33–35), we are only beginning to understand the contribution of these small RNAs to the innate immune responses to viral infections, to the regulation of gene expression programs, and immune cell activation (32, 34). In this review, we focus primarily on the role of miRNAs in regulating innate immune responses to IAV infections, and the potential use of miRNAs in the treatment of IAV infection.

MICRORNAs AS DIAGNOSIS MARKERS

MicroRNAs are found in the intracellular niche and the extracellular fluids encapsulated in exosomes including blood plasma, serum, urine, saliva, and semen (36–38). These small molecules are also detected in body fluids independently of intracellular and exosome compartments (38). Interestingly, the differential expression of miRNAs in these compartments is linked to the development of IAV infection (29, 39–42), indicating that these small RNAs can be used as the diagnosis markers for the disease (**Table 1**). Evaluation of peripheral blood mononuclear cells (PBMCs) from critically ill patients with swine-origin pandemic H1N1 infection by qRT-PCR and receiver operating characteristic (ROC)/area under ROC (AUC) curve analyze has revealed that increased levels of miR-148 (>2-fold) and decreased levels of miR-31 and miR-29a (>2-fold) are valuable biomarkers for severe influenza virus infections with the AUC value ranging from 0.881 to 0.951 (39). The ROC tool is commonly used to evaluate the diagnostic accuracy of differentially expressed

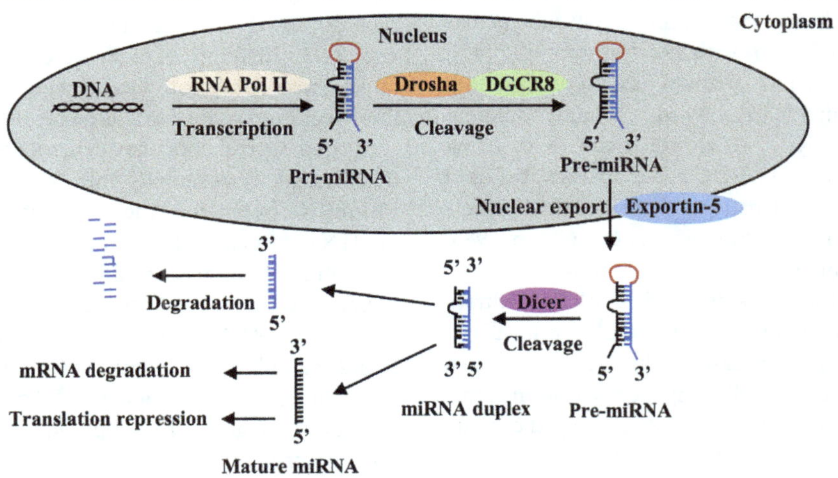

FIGURE 1 | MicroRNA (miRNA) processing and function. MiRNA is first transcribed as long hairpin primary RNA (pri-miRNA) by RNA polymerase II and cleaved into hairpin precursor miRNA (pre-miRNA) by the complex Drosha-DGCR8 in nucleus. This pre-miRNA then is exported to the cytoplasm by exportin-5 protein and cleaved to two strands by endoribonuclease Dicer, one strand becomes a mature miRNA and silence target mRNAs through mRNA degradation or translation repression and the other is degraded.

TABLE 1 | MicroRNAs (miRNAs) as diagnosis markers.

miRNAs	Regulation[a]	Study samples	Virus strains	Reference
miR-302a	↓	Throat swab, peripheral blood mononuclear cells (PBMCs)	H1N1	(71)
miR-30c-5p	↓	Throat swabs	H1N1, H3N2	(43)
miR-34c-3p	↑	Throat swabs	H1N1, H3N2	(43)
miR-181a-5p	↓	Throat swabs	H1N1, H3N2	(43)
miR-150	↑	Serum from critically ill patients	H1N1	(41)
miR-17, -20a, -106a, -376c	↑	Serum	H7N9	(42)
miR-148a	↑	PBMCs from critically ill patients	H1N1	(39)
miR-29a -3p	↓	PBMCs from critically ill patients, throat swaps	H1N1, H3N2	(39, 43, 44)
miR-31	↓	PBMCs from critically ill patients	H1N1	(39)
miR-122, -229-5p, -1260, -335, -664, -767-5p	↑	Whole blood	H1N1	(40)
miR-1285, -185, -18, -26a, -30a, -34b, -519e, -576-3p, -826-3p, -665, -765	↓	Whole blood	H1N1	(40)

[a]↓, *downregulation;* ↑, *upregulation.*

miRNAs for differentiating between IAV infection patients and healthy controls, and the accuracy is measured by AUC (39, 43). In another study, increased levels of miR-34c-3p (>4-fold) and decreased levels of miR-29a-3p, -30c-5p, and -181a-5p (>2-fold) have been demonstrated to be associated with the infection in the throat swab samples of H1N1-infected patients using qRT-PCR and ROC methods (43). The link between low levels of miR-29a-3p (threefold) and IAV infection has been further confirmed in the throat swabs of H1N1 infected patients using non-PCR MARS [microRNA-RNase-SPR (surface plasmon resonance)] assay (44). A similar study of peripheral blood samples from H3N2- or H1N1-infected patients using miRNA microarray and stem-loop PCR has identified that 14 miRNAs were linked to the pathogenesis of the disease (40). Among them, the levels of miR-229-5p, -335, -664, and -1260 were increased greater than twofold, while the levels of miR-18a, -26a, -30a, -34b, -185, -576-3p, -628-3p, -665, -765, and -1285 were decreased greater than fourfold. Expression of six (miR-26a, -335, -576-3p, -628-3p, -664, and -1260) of these miRNAs was confirmed in H1N1 infected A549 cells and Madin Darby Canine Kidney (MDCK) cells (40). Moreover, H7N9 has been demonstrated to cause more severe infection in humans, and to-date, this H7N9 subtype has resulted in 1,533 human infections with 592 deaths in 2017 (45). MiRNA microarray and qRT-PCR analyses using serum samples from H7N9 infected individuals showed a slightly different miRNA signature, with miR-17, -20a, -106a, and -376c being upregulated (>1.5-fold) (42). The ROC curve analysis was used to discriminate H7N9 infected patients from healthy controls for each miRNA with AUC values ranging from 0.622 to 0.988, while its value for a combination of these four miRNAs is 0.96 (42). Furthermore, miR-150 levels assessed by qRT-PCR have been found to be significantly higher (>1.5-fold) in critically ill patients than those with milder disease and healthy controls in a human study of H1N1 infection, indicating the association of this miRNA with poor disease outcome (41). Collectively, these earlier studies indicate that infection not only by different subtypes of IAVs but also by the different strains of the same IAV subtype with varying pathogenicity elicit different miRNA expression patterns in similar samples, which can be valuable diagnostic and/or prognostic markers for influenza infection and severity of the disease. Identification of these miRNAs may greatly aid the design of analytical kits for rapid and precise diagnosis of IAV subtypes of infection, and potentially to develop customized therapeutic approaches to control infection.

MICRORNAs DIRECTLY TARGET INFLUENZA VIRAL RNAs

Influenza A virus consists of eight gene segments that encode for 12 viral proteins including surface glycoprotein [hemagglutinin (HA) and neuraminidase (NA)], nucleoprotein (NP), two matrix proteins (M1 and M2), three polymerase complex proteins PB1, PB2, and PA, four non-structural proteins (NS1, NS2, PA-X, and PB1-F2) (2, 46, 47). HA and NA proteins predominantly regulate virus entry and exit from host cells, and their genes are the major genetic segments for influenza antigen drift and shift by genetic mutation and reassortment to create new strains/subtypes. In contrast, other IAV viral proteins are more conservative, which is essential for IAV replication. For example, viral polymerase complex proteins (PA, PB1, PB2) and NP form a viral ribonucleoprotein (vRNP), a minimal functional unit for influenza virus replication. M1 forms a coat inside the viral envelope and binds to viral RNA. Therefore, exploration of those miRNAs that directly target those conservative viral sequences could uncover novel therapeutics to control influenza replication and propagation.

Indeed, several lines of evidence have implied the feasibility of this concept. For example, miR -323, -491, and -654 destabilize PB1 mRNA by targeting the conservative region, as demonstrated in H1N1 infected cells that are treated with plasmids carrying those miRNA mimics or inhibitors, respectively (48). A similar investigation has shown that miR-485 directly binds to a conserved site of PB1 mRNA to regulate viral replication, in H5N1-infected HEK293T cells following miR-485 mimics or inhibitor treatment (49). Furthermore, multiple miRNAs may target the same seed sequence to regulate IAV replication. Khongnomnan and colleagues, through *in silico* analysis and a luciferase reporter assay have reported that the same conservative region of PB1 mRNAs of H1N1, H5N1, or H3N2 subtypes is targeted by miR-3145 (50). Neutralization of this miRNA by using plasmid encoded anti-miRNA oligonucleotides restored the expression of PB1 mRNA and miR-3145 mimics treatment reduced PB1 expression in

H5N1-, H1N1-, or H3N2-infected A549 cells (50). M1 is the most abundant protein in the IAV viral particle and regulates vRNP export, virus assembly and budding, and virus–host interactions (51, 52). Ma and colleagues have reported that let-7c precursor diminishes H1N1 replication by binding to the 3′-UTR of M1 mRNA and that let-7c inhibitor reinstates the expression of M1 protein and influenza infection in A549 cells (53). Certain microRNAs have also been shown to inhibit the expression of IAV viral proteins, not only in a direct manner but also through regulations of other host factors that affect viral replication. For example, miR-33a mimic suppressed the expression of NP and M1 proteins by directly binding to the 3′-UTR of Archain 1 (ARCN1) RNA in HEK293T, A549, and Hela cells infected with H1N1, H9N2, or H3N2, resulting in greatly decreased virus replication (54). ARCN1 is an important component of human coatomer protein complex, which regulates protein transport from the Golgi body to the endoplasmic reticulum and critically modulates influenza virus entry to host cells, viral membrane protein expression, and assembly (55, 56). Treatment with miR-33a inhibitor recovered the expression of ARCN1, NP, and M1 proteins, and thus increased H1N1, H9N2, or H3N2 replication (54). In the same study, miR-33a has also been shown to attenuate the replication of H1N1, H9N2, or H3N2 by reducing vRNP activity through an ARCN1-independent pathway in HEK293T cells (54), suggesting the multiple functions of this miRNA. A recent investigation has identified that miR-21 targets NP, PB1, PB2, PA, NA, and HA segments of H1N1, by using infected miR-21-deficient MDCK cells (28). It is promising that targeting NP segment or combination of both PA and NA segments of IAV simultaneously reduced IAV replication greater than twofold, as compared to other treatments (e.g., targeting sole segment and a combination of PA and HA) (28). Although the role of miRNAs in the pathogenesis of IAV infection should be further investigated, targeting these small viral RNAs may provide alternative approaches to reduce influenza infection by directly inhibiting expression of conserved viral proteins (e.g,. PB1, NP, or M1), regardless of the viral antigen drift and shift (**Figure 2** and **Table 2**).

MICRORNAs CONTROL IAV-INDUCED INFLAMMATORY RESPONSES

Bronchial epithelial cells and pulmonary innate immune cells such as alveolar macrophages, dendritic cells, and natural killer cells provide the first line of defense against influenza infection (57, 58). Upon infection, molecular patterns of influenza viruses are recognized by host molecular pattern recognition receptors (PPRs) including retinoic acid-inducible gene I (RIG-I)-like receptors and toll-like receptors (TLRs) (59–61). These pattern-recognition receptors are important sensors that recognize

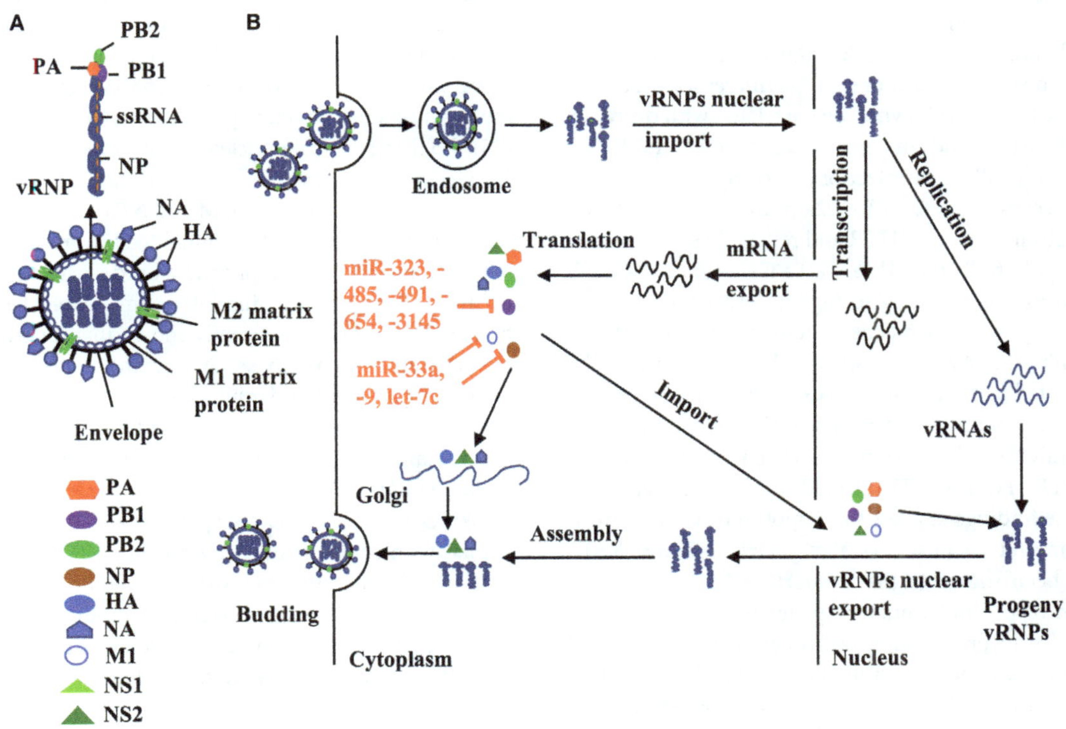

FIGURE 2 | (A) Influenza structure: a lipid bilayer envelope containing glycoproteins M1 and M2 ion channel. Hemagglutinin and neuraminidase proteins on the outside of the envelope. Eight RNA genome segments inside the envelope encoding for three polymerase complex proteins (PB1, PB2, and PA), nucleoproteins (NPs), M1 and M2 matrix proteins, and non-structural proteins (NS1, NS2, PA-X and PB1-F2). **(B)** Cellular microRNAs (miRNAs) modulate influenza replication. Host cellular miRNAs inhibit influenza replication through targeting viral RNAs and proteins that are essential for influenza replication and translation such as PB1, M1, and nucleoprotein.

TABLE 2 | MicroRNAs (miRNAs) target viral RNAs.

miRNAs	Cell types	Targets	Virus strains	Treatments	Reference
miR-485	HEK293T	PB1	H5N1	Mimic/inhibitor	(49)
miR-323, -491, -654	Madin Darby Canine Kidney (MDCK)	PB1	H1N1	Expression vectors/inhibitors	(48)
miR-3145	A549	PB1	H1N1, H5N1, H3N2	miRNA silencing vector	(50)
Let-7c	A549	M1	H1N1	Let-7c precursor/inhibitor	(53)
miR-33a	A549, HEK293T, Hela	ARCN1, viral ribonucleoprotein activity	H1N1, H9N2, H3N2	Mimic/inhibitor	(54)
miR-21	MDCK	nucleoprotein, hemagglutinin, neuraminidase	H1N1	miR-21 knockout cell	(28)

infectious pathogens and drive host defense responses. Among them, TLR3 and TLR7 induces the activation of interferon (IFN) regulatory transcription factor (IRF)-3 (IRF3)/IRF7 and TIR-domain containing adaptor inducing IFN-β (TRIF)/NF-κB signaling pathways after interacting with IAV RNAs, which leads to the production of type-I (IFN-α and IFN-β) and -III (IFN-λ) IFNs and proinflammatory cytokines and chemokines (58, 62–65). RIG-I is a cytoplasmic RNA helicase that recognizes short double-stranded RNA produced during viral replication (66), and viral genomic single-stranded RNA (ssRNA) bearing 5′ phosphates (67). By binding to IAV ssRNAs, RIG-I facilitates the activation of IRF3 that directly regulate the production of type-I and -III IFNs (58, 62, 68). IAV infections are known to cause severe pro-inflammatory cytokine storm in the lung by the induction of overproduced aforementioned cytokines, which can also spread into systemic circulation, leading to severe symptoms such as leukopenia (69).

MicroRNAs have been shown to play key roles in the regulation of pro-inflammatory intracellular signaling pathways during influenza infection (32, 70–73). For example, increased expression of the IRF5 gene has been shown to be correlated with decreased levels of miR-302a (2.5-fold) in throat swab samples and PBMCs from patients with influenza infection, as compared to healthy controls (71). Treatment with miR-302a mimics decreased IRF5 expression by binding to its 3′-UTR and reduced IRF5-regulated production of IFN-β, TNFα, IL-6, IL-8, CCL2, and CCL5 in H1N1-infected PBMCs, leading to higher H1N1 viral production (71). Recently, miR-144 has been demonstrated in a mouse model to inhibit anti-IAV host responses by targeting the TNF receptor-associated factor 6 (TRAF6)/IRF7 signaling axis, which underpins type-I IFN responses against H1N1 infection (72, 74, 75). Another miRNA, miR-146a, has also been shown to directly downregulate TRAF6 in H3N2 infected human nasal epithelial cells (73). These findings suggest the importance of those miRNAs in host immunity against IAV infection by targeting TRAF6.

NF-κB has been shown to play important roles not only in the production of pro-inflammatory genes in response to IAV infection but also in propagation of influenza viruses (76–79). Multiple miRNAs have been identified to regulate NF-κB activation, by targeting the 3′-UTRs of its components (80–82). NF-κB inhibitor β (NFKBIB, also known as IκBβ) is a regulatory protein for NF-κB that prevents nuclear translocation of NF-κB (RelA/p65), and subsequent transcription of its target genes (83, 84). Treatment of H1N1-infected human primary bronchial epithelial cells (pBECs) with miR-4776 inhibitor led to increased expression of NFKBIB, resulting in lower viral replication (82). In contrast, miR-4776 mimic decreased the expression of NFKBIB and increased viral replication (82). Gui and colleagues have shown that H3N2 infection suppresses miR-302c expression in A549 cells (80). MiR-302c inhibitor treatment restored the expression of its targeting molecule, NF-κB-inducing kinase (NIK) that is a critical component of NF-κB pathway. MiR-302c mimic treatment prevented the nuclear translocation of NF-κB and downregulated IRF3/7 expression, leading to decreased expression of IFN-β (80). In a study of H1N1- or H3N2-infected A549 cells, miR-132, -146a, and -1275 simultaneously decreased the transcription and expression of interleukin-1 receptor-associated kinase 1, a key component of NF-κB pathway (81). These three miRNAs also target mitogen-activated kinases (MAPK) 3 that plays an important role in the activation of pro-inflammatory MAPK pathway. Those miRNAs associated with pro-inflammatory signaling pathways are delineated in **Figure 3** and **Table 3**. Interestingly, miRNAs may contribute to virus replication by suppressing host antiviral responses. For example, Dong and colleagues recently have demonstrated with H1N1- or H3N2-infected A549 cells that miR-9 promotes IAV replication through the suppression of monocyte chemoattractant protein 1-induced protein (MCP1P1) (85). MCP1P1 is a ribonuclease that plays an important role in antiviral immune responses (86) and inhibits IAV replication by decreasing the production of M and NP proteins (85). Treatment with a miR-9 mimic greatly augmented the production of NP and M1 proteins and IAV replication by decreasing production of MCP1P1. By contrast, an inhibitor of miR-9 blocked IAV replication (85). We have also recently shown that miR-125a/b directly targets A20 deubiquitinase, an enzyme that degrades receptor interacting protein 1 and inhibits NF-κB activation (87). Infection with H3N2 or H1N1 led to increased expression of miR-125a/b, which suppressed A20 deubiquitinase production and resulted in elevated NF-κB activity and production of pro-inflammatory cytokines in pBECs of COPD patients and in *in vivo* model (87). Similarly, the association between miR-125a/b and the expression of A20 deubiquitinase was observed in the mouse model of COPD (87). Collectively, miRNAs with altered expression play important roles in IAV replication, demonstrating their potential roles of antiviral host defense responses.

MICRORNAs MEDIATE THE PRODUCTION OF ANTIVIRAL CYTOKINES

Three RIG-I like receptors are crucial in antiviral host defense and consists of RIG-I, melanoma differentiation-associated

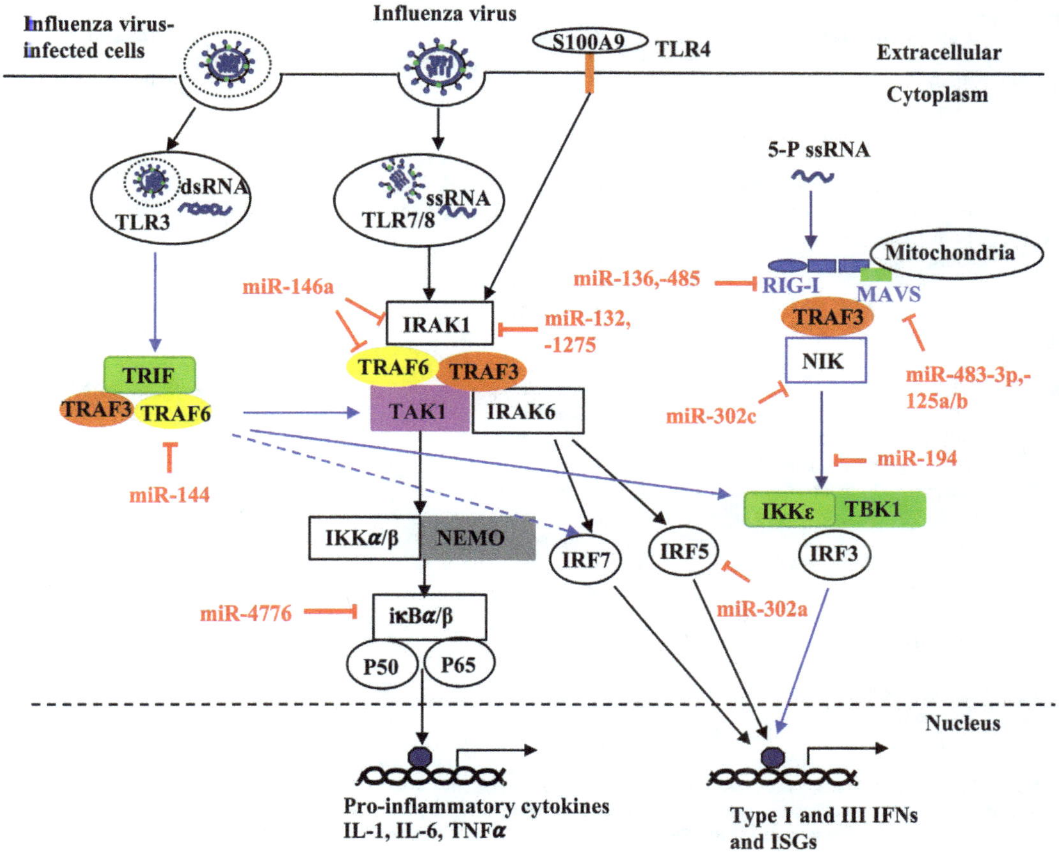

FIGURE 3 | MicroRNAs (miRNAs) regulate innate host immune response against influenza infection by targeting intracellular signaling pathways. Upon infection, influenza can activate different intracellular signaling pathways such as NF-κB, RIG-like receptor (RIG-I), TNF receptor-associated factors (TRAFs), and interferon regulatory factors (IRFs) through different pattern recognition receptors including TLR3, TLR4, TLR7/8. TLR3 and TR7/8 that recognize double stranded RNA and single-stranded RNA in the endosome, respectively. The ligand for TLR4 in influenza virus is unknown; however, it is thought to be activated by the damage-associated molecular patterns molecules released in influenza virus-infected cells and trigger TLR4-MyD88-signaling pathways. Induction of these TLRs can lead to activation of NF-κB, IRF 3, 5, and 7 and induce expression of type-I and -II IFN, IFN-stimulated genes, and inflammatory genes. Some miRNAs regulate these pathways through targeting critical components such as TRAF6, IRF3, IRF5, IFR7, interleukin-1 receptor-associated kinase 1, and IκBβ. Within the infected cells, RIG-I detects the 5-triphosphorylated RNA of replicating viral genomes in cytosol and associates with mitochondrial antiviral signaling protein (MAVS) to induce pro-inflammatory cytokines and type-I IFN. miRNAs can modulate this pathway by directly targeting RIG-I, MAVS, or NF-κB-inducing kinase.

protein 5 (MDA5), and laboratory of genetics and physiology 2 (LGP2) (88–90). RIG-I plays a central role in the induction of immune responses against IAV, by recognizing short RNA (67, 91). By contrast, MDA5 binds to long RNA and LGP2 acts as a positive regulator of RIG-I and MDA5 (92, 93). RIG-I recognizes viral RNA in the cytosol and interacts with the mitochondrial antiviral-signaling protein (MAVS), which is localized to the outer mitochondrial membrane (94). Aggregation of RIG-I, TRIM25, and MAVS then leads to the activation of IRF3/IRF7 by phosphorylation, which then induces the expression of type-I and -III IFNs (59, 94–96). These IFNs then bind to the respective IFN receptors on the same/neighboring cells and stimulate the expression of over 300 IFN-stimulated genes (ISGs), such as protein kinase R to limit viral replication. IAV-induced expression of miR-125a/b has also been shown to directly inhibit the expression of MAVs, leading to reduced production of type-I and III IFNs in pBECs of COPD patients and mouse model of COPD (87). Several miRNAs have been reported, either directly or indirectly, to regulate the RIG-I pathway for the antiviral response to IAV infection (97–99), this interaction is also shown in **Figure 3** and **Table 3**. For example, H1N5 or H1N1 infection increased the expression of miR-136 and miR-194 and both have been independently shown to suppress IFN-β expression by binding to the 3′-UTR of RIG-I transcript in IAV-infected A549 cells (97, 98). Furthermore, miR-483-3p, is highly expressed in the lung during infection of mice with H1N1, H5N1, or H7N9 (99). Transfection of H1N1-, H5N1-, or H7N9-infected MLE-12, a mouse cell line of lung epithelial cells, with miR-483-3p mimic led to decreased viral replication by targeting the transcript of RING-finger protein 5, which negatively regulates RIG-I signaling pathway (99). MiR-132 has also been shown to directly targets p300, an important component of IFN-β enhanceosome, which leads to reduced induction of IFN-β (100).

TABLE 3 | MicroRNAs (miRNAs) control influenza A virus-induced inflammatory and antiviral responses.

miRNAs	Cell type/models	Targets	Virus strains	Reference
miR-302a	A549	IRF5	H1N1	(71)
	Peripheral blood mononuclear cells	IFN-β, TNFα, IL-6, IL-8, CCL2, CCL5		
	Mouse			
miR-144	Mouse	TNF receptor-associated factor 6 (TRAF6)	H1N1	(72)
	Primary mouse lung epithelial cells	IRF7		
miR-146a	Human nasal epithelial cells	TRAF6	H3N2	(73)
miR-4776	Human pBECs	NFKBIB	H1N1	(82)
miR-302c	A549	NIK	H3N2	(80)
		NF-κB translocation		
		IRF3/7, IFN-β		
miR-132, -146a, -1275	A549	IRAK1	H3N2, H1N1	(81)
		MAPK 3		
miR-449b	A549	HDAC1, IFN-β	H3N2, H1N1	(102)
miR-9	A549	MCPIP1	H3N2, H1N1	(85)
miR-125a/b	pBECs of chronic obstructive pulmonary disease (COPD) patients	A20, MAVS	H3N2, H1N1	(87)
	Murine COPD model	IFN-β, p65, lung inflammation		
miR-136	A549	Retinoic acid-inducible gene I (RIG-I), IL-6, IFN-β	H5N1	(97)
miR-194	A549	FGF2, INFα, IFN-β	H1N1	(98)
	Mouse			
miR-483-3p	MLE-12	RNF5, IRF3, IFN-β, NF-κB	H1N1, H7N9, H5N1	(99)
	Mouse			
miR-132	HEK293T	P300	H5N1	(100)
		IFN-β		
miR-26a	A549, HEK293T	IFN-α/β, USP3	H1N1	(101)
miR-485	HEK293T	RIG-I	H5N1	(49)
miR-664	A549	LIF, NEK7	H7N9	(125)

NIK, NF-κB-inducing kinase; IRF, interferon regulatory factor; IRAK1, interleukin 1 receptor-associated kinase 1; MAPK3, mitogen-activated kinase 3; HDAC, histone deacetylase; MCPIP1, monocyte chemoattractant protein 1-induced protein 1; pBECs, primary bronchial epithelial cell; RNF5, RING-finger protein 5; NFKBIB, NF-κB inhibitor β; MLE-12, mouse cell line of lung epithelial cells; USP3, ubiquitin-specific protease 3; LIF, leukemia inhibitors factor; NEK7, NIMA-related kinase 7.

New evidence has emerged on the potential role of miRNAs in IAV-induced host defense responses and in the modulation of the production of cytokines. MiR-26a significantly inhibits IAV replication by promoting the type-I IFN production and subsequent expression of ISGs in H1N1-infected A549 cells (101). IAV infection decreases the expression of histone deacetylase 1 (HDAC1) that plays an important role in the activation of type-I IFN response against IAV infection (102, 103). Furthermore, H1N1 or H3N2 infection in A549 cells induced increased levels of miR-449b (>7-fold) (104). A recent investigation has also linked the increased expression of miR-449b (>6-fold) to the decreased expression of HDAC1 and the increased expression of IFN-β in H1N1- or H3N2-induced in A549 cells (102). Interestingly, treatment of miR-449b mimics further suppressed the expression of HDAC1 and enhanced the expression of IFN-β in H1N1- or H3N2-infected A549 cells (102), suggesting the important role of this miRNA in host defense against influenza virus infections.

Interestingly, certain miRNAs have been shown to have opposing effects on regulating the antiviral response when host cells are infected at different doses of specific viruses. MiR-485 is induced by IAV infection and inhibits RIG-I pathways at low levels of IAV infection, which suppresses host antiviral responses and enhances virus replication (49). By contrast, this miRNA abates virus replication by degrading PB1 transcripts at higher levels of IAV infection (49). It is likely that varying multiplicity of infection triggers slightly different antiviral signaling pathways. Although the regulatory targets of miR-485 are currently unclear, this miRNA likely regulates those factors that are highly expressed in these conditions. Hence, the miRNA biological function should be carefully and fully examined before developing therapeutic approaches.

MANIPULATION AND DELIVERY OF miRNA

Although miRNAs have been increasingly recognized in recent years as potential therapeutic targets for treating influenza infection, the successful miRNA manipulation can be difficult because of many factors such as short half-life of miRNAs, low cellular uptake and expression, pre-matured elimination by host immune cells, interruption of endogenous RNA processes and off-target effects. In particular, targeting a single miRNA may have limited success for treatment because an understanding of the molecular mechanisms underpinning many complex diseases (e.g., asthma, autoimmunity, and cancer) remains rudimentary. To elucidate the function of a miRNA family simultaneously, traditional antisense methods for a single miRNA are inadequate and laborious for targeting multiple miRNAs; to create genetically modified lab animals is even more arduous. As such, microRNA sponges have been designed to inhibit the function of a miRNA family by creating a single RNA sequence that consists of several tandem miRNA-binding sites for all the members (105). In fact, one of the unique features of miRNA function is that a family of miRNAs share an almost identical seed sequence, with often only a few nucleotides difference, although they may be expressed from different genomic loci (106–108). Therefore, targetting seed sequence may be particularly valuable using miRNA sponges to understand the pathogenesis of IAV infection and to treat the disease. A miRNA sponge could be designed to target those miRNAs that promote virus replication and IAV-induced inflammation.

How to effectively deliver miRNA sponges or mimics to manipulate host miRNAs is challenging for clinical application. For this reason, it is essential to carefully design and select candidate miRNA sequence. Non-specific responses induced by those molecules should also be examined with great caution. Any unexpected effect associated with miRNA's target should be quantified for the safety and success of miRNA manipulation approaches. Indeed, various types of strategies have been developed to optimize the delivery methods, including chemical modification of miRNA sponge molecules or to encapsulate them with macromolecules (e.g., polyamine, polyethylenimine, and basic complexes). Furthermore, the promoters used by miRNA sponge should be strongest and most suitable for the cells of interest to achieve highest efficacy. If the targeted miRNAs are expressed in many cell types in multiple tissues, the tissue- or cell-specific promoters could be employed to achieve precise expression, which could minimize potential side effects.

Many vectors that comprise plasmid, replication-deficient virus or transposons have been developed to accomplish successful gene interference *in vivo* (109–113, 124). Among these vectors, lentiviral vectors have been widely employed in the study of normal tissue physiology and processes of disease in animal models (114, 115). For example, lentiviral vectors carrying miR-30 mimic can inhibit viral replication in H1N1-infected MDCK cells by targeting viral NP and PB1 transcripts (116). IAV itself can also be modified to express exogenous miRNAs and modulate viral replication and for the treatment of the diseases (117), as incorporation of an artificial miRNA into IVA genome does not cause viral sequence instability or interfere with viral replication (117). Langlois and colleagues have shown that recombinant H1N1 expressing artificial miR-124 does not inhibit the function of other miRNAs only with limited repression of miR-124-star target by luciferase reporter system in transfected hamster kidney cells (118), suggesting the specificity of this delivery method. Indeed, live-attenuated IAV delivery has shown great potential in the development of more efficient IAV vaccine and in the treatment of infection respiratory diseases by carrying customized artificial miRNAs (119, 120). This notion is supported by a recent study, showing that exogenous miR-155 encoded by modified X31 IAV augments IAV-specific CD8^{+} T cell response and neutralizing antibody production in a mouse model of IAV infection (120).

Adenoviral and adenovirus-associated viral (AAV) vectors are also valuable to silence candidate miRNAs *in vivo*. Indeed, recent progresses have been made in delivering a miRNA mimic to explore the therapeutic potential of these vectors in animal models (121, 122). However, adenoviruses induce off-target host defense response because they infect a wide range of cells (123). On the other hand, AAV vectors cause very few side-effects to host because they integrate at limited and defined location in the genome of transfected targets (121, 123). This unique feature of AAV vectors thus minimizes the chance of mutational insertion and induces effective gene silencing following either systemic or tissue-specific injection (121, 123). Furthermore, non-viral transfection approaches using nanoparticles and liposome have also attracted attention in the establishment of miRNA intervention. Thus, although delivery strategies are far from being optimal yet, significant progress has been achieved recently toward targeted therapy with limited off-target effects.

LIMITATION

Current understanding of the roles of miRNAs in the pathogenesis of influenza is limited by a lack of sufficient characterization of the miRNA-associated molecular pathways in the context of influenza infection, IAV replication, and host immunity. Indeed, great challenge still exists in the field of the identification of miRNA targets within a living organism and in host defense processes that have many layers of molecular and cellular elements with specific spatiotemporal patterns. One of miRNA biological features is that they target multiple mRNAs; therefore, pathophysiological outcomes observed by modifying their function may correlate with subtle changes in the levels of diverse target mRNAs. Although *in vitro* assays using luciferase reporter system and miRNA mimics and inhibitors are usually employed to verify an interesting target transcript, caution should be taken to interpret the important biological function in dynamic living systems by exclusively relying on these methods. Furthermore, as miRNAs potentially act as master regulators of disease and inflammation, ill-designed manipulation of a miRNA may generate unexpected side-effects. This is particularly important when considering the observations that different species infected with different IAV strains/subtypes generate different miRNA signatures. In addition, delivery methods that limit miRNA mimics and inhibitors precisely to the infected and inflamed tissues are also needed to be further developed as it is essential for not causing any disruption to normal function of surrounding tissues.

Although many candidate miRNAs largely play suppressive roles in IAV infection, certain host miRNAs may assist viral replication. One example is that the miR-664 was highly upregulated approximately fourfold in H7N9-infected A549 cells, and treatment with miR-664 inhibitor reduced H7N9 replication (125). MiR-664 is predicted by *in silico* pathway analysis to target the 3′-UTRs of leukemia inhibitory factor (LIF) and NIMA-related kinase 7 (NEK7) whose activation leads to lower H7N9 replication (125). MiR-144 increased IAV infection by suppressing the activity of TRAF6-IRF6 axis posttranscriptionally as demonstrated in H1N1 infected miR-144 deficient mice and mouse lung epithelial cells (72). Although a specific miRNA may play either pro- or anti-IAV role, numerous investigation suggest that miRNAs have great potential as diagnostic biomarker and treatment of human diseases when considering the profound biological function regulated by these small RNAs and their extensive links to IAV infection.

CONCLUSION

Based on the unique features of miRNAs, a new generation of IAV vaccine may be developed by incorporating miRNA response elements (MRE, miRNA recognition sequences) into viral genomic segments such as NP, NS, or PB1. An attempt to generate novel attenuated IAV vaccine has yielded promising results by inserting a let-7b MRE into H1N1 PB1 gene, which significantly reduced viral replication in bronchial epithelial cells (126). Although preliminary, this method to generate attenuated IAV vaccine has been proven effective in a mouse model (122).

Manipulation of miRNAs needs to be approached with caution for the reason that intervention of miRNA function may predispose to impaired immunity, cancer, or other unforeseen biological abnormalities. However, miRNA has become more and more attractive as diagnostic biomarkers and potential clinical intervention targets as effective prevention and treatments for IAV infection is poorly available. Furthermore, direct targeting of key miRNAs that underpin IAV infection may lead to new and more specific therapeutic interventions as these small RNAs are implied in regulating specific gene clusters triggered by infection (e.g., cytokine driven inflammation). It is particularly important to explore those miRNAs that can both degrade IAV RNAs and alleviate virus-induced inflammation, as they may concurrently control both virus replication and over-reactive immune responses. Understanding the role of miRNA in fundamental processes associated with IAV infection is necessary to fully characterize their potential in disease diagnosis and prognosis and ultimately for the treatment of disease.

AUTHOR CONTRIBUTIONS

TN and MY wrote and edited the paper. XL, ZS, AH, and PF edited the paper.

REFERENCES

1. Bouvier NM, Palese P. The biology of influenza viruses. *Vaccine* (2008) 26(Suppl 4):D49–53. doi:10.1016/j.vaccine.2008.07.039
2. McCauley JW, Mahy BW. Structure and function of the influenza virus genome. *Biochem J* (1983) 211:281–94. doi:10.1042/bj2110281
3. Zambon MC. Epidemiology and pathogenesis of influenza. *J Antimicrob Chemother* (1999) 44(Suppl B):3–9. doi:10.1093/jac/44.suppl_2.3
4. Smith GJ, Vijaykrishna D, Bahl J, Lycett SJ, Worobey M, Pybus OG, et al. Origins and evolutionary genomics of the 2009 swine-origin H1N1 influenza A epidemic. *Nature* (2009) 459:1122–5. doi:10.1038/nature08182
5. Dawood FS, Iuliano AD, Reed C, Meltzer MI, Shay DK, Cheng PY, et al. Estimated global mortality associated with the first 12 months of 2009 pandemic influenza A H1N1 virus circulation: a modelling study. *Lancet Infect Dis* (2012) 12:687–95. doi:10.1016/S1473-3099(12)70121-4
6. Stohr K. Influenza – WHO cares. *Lancet Infect Dis* (2002) 2:517. doi:10.1016/S1473-3099(02)00366-3
7. Jernigan DB, Cox NJ. Chapter 1: Human influenza: one health, one world. In: Webster RG, Braciale TJ, Lamb RA, editors. *Textbook of Influenza*. Georgia, USA: Wiley Blackwell (2013). p. 3–19.
8. Lee N, Chan PK, Lui GC, Wong BC, Sin WW, Choi KW, et al. Complications and outcomes of pandemic 2009 Influenza A (H1N1) virus infection in hospitalized adults: how do they differ from those in seasonal influenza? *J Infect Dis* (2011) 203:1739–47. doi:10.1093/infdis/jir187
9. Hsu AC, Starkey MR, Hanish I, Parsons K, Haw TJ, Howland LJ, et al. Targeting PI3K-p110alpha suppresses influenza virus infection in chronic obstructive pulmonary disease. *Am J Respir Crit Care Med* (2015) 191:1012–23. doi:10.1164/rccm.201501-0188OC
10. Kloepfer KM, Olenec JP, Lee WM, Liu G, Vrtis RF, Roberg KA, et al. Increased H1N1 infection rate in children with asthma. *Am J Respir Crit Care Med* (2012) 185:1275–9. doi:10.1164/rccm.201109-1635OC
11. Allard R, Leclerc P, Tremblay C, Tannenbaum TN. Diabetes and the severity of pandemic influenza A (H1N1) infection. *Diabetes Care* (2010) 33:1491–3. doi:10.2337/dc09-2215
12. Nguyen JL, Yang W, Ito K, Matte TD, Shaman J, Kinney PL. Seasonal influenza infections and cardiovascular disease mortality. *JAMA Cardiol* (2016) 1:274–81. doi:10.1001/jamacardio.2016.0433
13. Hardelid P, Pebody R, Andrews N. Mortality caused by influenza and respiratory syncytial virus by age group in England and Wales 1999-2010. *Influenza Other Respir Viruses* (2013) 7:35–45. doi:10.1111/j.1750-2659.2012.00345.x
14. Cox NJ, Subbarao K. Influenza. *Lancet* (1999) 354:1277–82. doi:10.1016/S0140-6736(99)01241-6
15. Lewis DB. Avian flu to human influenza. *Annu Rev Med* (2006) 57:139–54. doi:10.1146/annurev.med.57.121304.131333
16. Kiso M, Mitamura K, Sakai-Tagawa Y, Shiraishi K, Kawakami C, Kimura K, et al. Resistant influenza A viruses in children treated with oseltamivir: descriptive study. *Lancet* (2004) 364:759–65. doi:10.1016/S0140-6736(04)16934-1
17. Hayden FG. Pandemic influenza: is an antiviral response realistic? *Pediatr Infect Dis J* (2004) 23:S262–9. doi:10.1097/01.inf.0000144680.39895.ce
18. Palese P. Influenza: old and new threats. *Nat Med* (2004) 10:S82–7. doi:10.1038/nm1141
19. Kandel R, Hartshorn KL. Novel strategies for prevention and treatment of influenza. *Expert Opin Ther Targets* (2005) 9:1–22. doi:10.1517/14728222.9.1.1
20. Smith DJ, Lapedes AS, de Jong JC, Bestebroer TM, Rimmelzwaan GF, Osterhaus AD, et al. Mapping the antigenic and genetic evolution of influenza virus. *Science* (2004) 305:371–6. doi:10.1126/science.1097211
21. Wightman B, Ha I, Ruvkun G. Posttranscriptional regulation of the heterochronic gene lin-14 by lin-4 mediates temporal pattern formation in *C. elegans*. *Cell* (1993) 75:855–62. doi:10.1016/0092-8674(93)90530-4
22. Lee RC, Feinbaum RL, Ambros V. The *C. elegans* heterochronic gene lin-4 encodes small RNAs with antisense complementarity to lin-14. *Cell* (1993) 75:843–54. doi:10.1016/0092-8674(93)90529-Y
23. Bartel DP. Metazoan MicroRNAs. *Cell* (2018) 173:20–51. doi:10.1016/j.cell.2018.03.006
24. Ha M, Kim VN. Regulation of microRNA biogenesis. *Nat Rev Mol Cell Biol* (2014) 15:509–24. doi:10.1038/nrm3838
25. Ro S, Park C, Young D, Sanders KM, Yan W. Tissue-dependent paired expression of miRNAs. *Nucleic Acids Res* (2007) 35:5944–53. doi:10.1093/nar/gkm641
26. Kuchenbauer F, Mah SM, Heuser M, McPherson A, Ruschmann J, Rouhi A, et al. Comprehensive analysis of mammalian miRNA* species and their role in myeloid cells. *Blood* (2011) 118:3350–8. doi:10.1182/blood-2010-10-312454
27. Kozomara A, Griffiths-Jones S. miRBase: annotating high confidence microRNAs using deep sequencing data. *Nucleic Acids Res* (2014) 42:D68–73. doi:10.1093/nar/gkt1181
28. Waring BM, Sjaastad LE, Fiege JK, Fay EJ, Reyes I, Moriarity B, et al. MicroRNA-based attenuation of influenza virus across susceptible hosts. *J Virol* (2018) 92:e01741-17. doi:10.1128/JVI.01741-17
29. Correia CN, Nalpas NC, McLoughlin KE, Browne JA, Gordon SV, MacHugh DE, et al. Circulating microRNAs as potential biomarkers of infectious disease. *Front Immunol* (2017) 8:118. doi:10.3389/fimmu.2017.00118
30. Qu Z, Li W, Fu B. MicroRNAs in autoimmune diseases. *Biomed Res Int* (2014) 2014:527895. doi:10.1155/2014/527895

31. Hosseinahli N, Aghapour M, Duijf PHG, Baradaran B. Treating cancer with microRNA replacement therapy: a literature review. *J Cell Physiol* (2018) 233:5574–88. doi:10.1002/jcp.26514
32. Nejad C, Stunden HJ, Gantier MP. A guide to miRNAs in inflammation and innate immune responses. *FEBS J* (2018). doi:10.1111/febs.14482
33. Bartel DP. MicroRNAs: genomics, biogenesis, mechanism, and function. *Cell* (2004) 116:281–97. doi:10.1016/S0092-8674(04)00045-5
34. He L, Hannon GJ. MicroRNAs: small RNAs with a big role in gene regulation. *Nat Rev Genet* (2004) 5:522–31. doi:10.1038/nrg1379
35. Flynt AS, Lai EC. Biological principles of microRNA-mediated regulation: shared themes amid diversity. *Nat Rev Genet* (2008) 9:831–42. doi:10.1038/nrg2455
36. Weber JA, Baxter DH, Zhang S, Huang DY, Huang KH, Lee MJ, et al. The microRNA spectrum in 12 body fluids. *Clin Chem* (2010) 56:1733–41. doi:10.1373/clinchem.2010.147405
37. Turchinovich A, Weiz L, Langheinz A, Burwinkel B. Characterization of extracellular circulating microRNA. *Nucleic Acids Res* (2011) 39:7223–33. doi:10.1093/nar/gkr254
38. Arroyo JD, Chevillet JR, Kroh EM, Ruf IK, Pritchard CC, Gibson DF, et al. Argonaute2 complexes carry a population of circulating microRNAs independent of vesicles in human plasma. *Proc Natl Acad Sci U S A* (2011) 108:5003–8. doi:10.1073/pnas.1019055108
39. Song H, Wang Q, Guo Y, Liu S, Song R, Gao X, et al. Microarray analysis of microRNA expression in peripheral blood mononuclear cells of critically ill patients with influenza A (H1N1). *BMC Infect Dis* (2013) 13:257. doi:10.1186/1471-2334-13-257
40. Tambyah PA, Sepramaniam S, Mohamed Ali J, Chai SC, Swaminathan P, Armugam A, et al. microRNAs in circulation are altered in response to influenza A virus infection in humans. *PLoS One* (2013) 8:e76811. doi:10.1371/journal.pone.0076811
41. Moran J, Ramirez-Martinez G, Jimenez-Alvarez L, Cruz A, Perez-Patrigeon S, Hidalgo A, et al. Circulating levels of miR-150 are associated with poorer outcomes of A/H1N1 infection. *Exp Mol Pathol* (2015) 99:253–61. doi:10.1016/j.yexmp.2015.07.001
42. Zhu Z, Qi Y, Ge A, Zhu Y, Xu K, Ji H, et al. Comprehensive characterization of serum microRNA profile in response to the emerging avian influenza A (H7N9) virus infection in humans. *Viruses* (2014) 6:1525–39. doi:10.3390/v6041525
43. Peng F, He J, Loo JF, Yao J, Shi L, Liu C, et al. Identification of microRNAs in throat swab as the biomarkers for diagnosis of influenza. *Int J Med Sci* (2016) 13:77–84. doi:10.7150/ijms.13301
44. Loo JF, Wang SS, Peng F, He JA, He L, Guo YC, et al. A non-PCR SPR platform using RNase H to detect microRNA 29a-3p from throat swabs of human subjects with influenza A virus H1N1 infection. *Analyst* (2015) 140:4566–75. doi:10.1039/c5an00679a
45. WHO. (2017). [cited 20017 15 Jun]. Available from: https://www.who.int/influenza/human_animal_interface/Influenza_Summary_IRA_HA_interface_06_15_2017.pdf?ua=1 (Accessed: 28 June, 2018).
46. Samji T. Influenza A: understanding the viral life cycle. *Yale J Biol Med* (2009) 82:153–9.
47. Te Velthuis AJ, Fodor E. Influenza virus RNA polymerase: insights into the mechanisms of viral RNA synthesis. *Nat Rev Microbiol* (2016) 14:479–93. doi:10.1038/nrmicro.2016.87
48. Song L, Liu H, Gao S, Jiang W, Huang W. Cellular microRNAs inhibit replication of the H1N1 influenza A virus in infected cells. *J Virol* (2010) 84:8849–60. doi:10.1128/JVI.00456-10
49. Ingle H, Kumar S, Raut AA, Mishra A, Kulkarni DD, Kameyama T, et al. The microRNA miR-485 targets host and influenza virus transcripts to regulate antiviral immunity and restrict viral replication. *Sci Signal* (2015) 8:ra126. doi:10.1126/scisignal.aab3183
50. Khongnomnan K, Makkoch J, Poomipak W, Poovorawan Y, Payungporn S. Human miR-3145 inhibits influenza A viruses replication by targeting and silencing viral PB1 gene. *Exp Biol Med (Maywood)* (2015) 240:1630–9. doi:10.1177/1535370215589051
51. Martin K, Helenius A. Nuclear transport of influenza virus ribonucleoproteins: the viral matrix protein (M1) promotes export and inhibits import. *Cell* (1991) 67:117–30. doi:10.1016/0092-8674(91)90576-K
52. Ciancanelli MJ, Abel L, Zhang SY, Casanova JL. Host genetics of severe influenza: from mouse Mx1 to human IRF7. *Curr Opin Immunol* (2016) 38:109–20. doi:10.1016/j.coi.2015.12.002
53. Ma YJ, Yang J, Fan XL, Zhao HB, Hu W, Li ZP, et al. Cellular microRNA let-7c inhibits M1 protein expression of the H1N1 influenza A virus in infected human lung epithelial cells. *J Cell Mol Med* (2012) 16:2539–46. doi:10.1111/j.1582-4934.2012.01572.x
54. Hu Y, Jiang L, Lai W, Qin Y, Zhang T, Wang S, et al. MicroRNA-33a disturbs influenza A virus replication by targeting ARCN1 and inhibiting viral ribonucleoprotein activity. *J Gen Virol* (2016) 97:27–38. doi:10.1099/jgv.0.000311
55. Sun E, He J, Zhuang X. Dissecting the role of COPI complexes in influenza virus infection. *J Virol* (2013) 87:2673–85. doi:10.1128/JVI.02277-12
56. Konig R, Stertz S, Zhou Y, Inoue A, Hoffmann HH, Bhattacharyya S, et al. Human host factors required for influenza virus replication. *Nature* (2010) 463:813–7. doi:10.1038/nature08699
57. Sanders CJ, Doherty PC, Thomas PG. Respiratory epithelial cells in innate immunity to influenza virus infection. *Cell Tissue Res* (2011) 343:13–21. doi:10.1007/s00441-010-1043-z
58. Iwasaki A, Pillai PS. Innate immunity to influenza virus infection. *Nat Rev Immunol* (2014) 14:315–28. doi:10.1038/nri3665
59. Kato H, Sato S, Yoneyama M, Yamamoto M, Uematsu S, Matsui K, et al. Cell type-specific involvement of RIG-I in antiviral response. *Immunity* (2005) 23:19–28. doi:10.1016/j.immuni.2005.04.010
60. Pang IK, Iwasaki A. Inflammasomes as mediators of immunity against influenza virus. *Trends Immunol* (2011) 32:34–41. doi:10.1016/j.it.2010.11.004
61. Goraya MU, Wang S, Munir M, Chen JL. Induction of innate immunity and its perturbation by influenza viruses. *Protein Cell* (2015) 6:712–21. doi:10.1007/s13238-015-0191-z
62. Le Goffic R, Pothlichet J, Vitour D, Fujita T, Meurs E, Chignard M, et al. Cutting edge: influenza A virus activates TLR3-dependent inflammatory and RIG-I-dependent antiviral responses in human lung epithelial cells. *J Immunol* (2007) 178:3368–72. doi:10.4049/jimmunol.178.6.3368
63. Guillot L, Le Goffic R, Bloch S, Escriou N, Akira S, Chignard M, et al. Involvement of toll-like receptor 3 in the immune response of lung epithelial cells to double-stranded RNA and influenza A virus. *J Biol Chem* (2005) 280:5571–80. doi:10.1074/jbc.M410592200
64. Lund JM, Alexopoulou L, Sato A, Karow M, Adams NC, Gale NW, et al. Recognition of single-stranded RNA viruses by Toll-like receptor 7. *Proc Natl Acad Sci U S A* (2004) 101:5598–603. doi:10.1073/pnas.0400937101
65. Meng D, Huo CY, Wang M, Xiao J, Liu B, Wei TT, et al. Influenza A viruses replicate productively in mouse mastocytoma cells (P815) and trigger pro-inflammatory cytokine and chemokine production through TLR3 signaling pathway. *Front Microbiol* (2017) 7:2130. doi:10.3389/fmicb.2016.02130
66. Yoneyama M, Kikuchi M, Natsukawa T, Shinobu N, Imaizumi T, Miyagishi M, et al. The RNA helicase RIG-I has an essential function in double-stranded RNA-induced innate antiviral responses. *Nat Immunol* (2004) 5:730–7. doi:10.1038/ni1087
67. Pichlmair A, Schulz O, Tan CP, Naslund TI, Liljestrom P, Weber F, et al. RIG-I-mediated antiviral responses to single-stranded RNA bearing 5'-phosphates. *Science* (2006) 314:997–1001. doi:10.1126/science.1132998
68. Kato H, Takeuchi O, Sato S, Yoneyama M, Yamamoto M, Matsui K, et al. Differential roles of MDA5 and RIG-I helicases in the recognition of RNA viruses. *Nature* (2006) 441:101–5. doi:10.1038/nature04734
69. Tisoncik JR, Korth MJ, Simmons CP, Farrar J, Martin TR, Katze MG. Into the eye of the cytokine storm. *Microbiol Mol Biol Rev* (2012) 76:16–32. doi:10.1128/MMBR.05015-11
70. Cullen BR. MicroRNAs as mediators of viral evasion of the immune system. *Nat Immunol* (2013) 14:205–10. doi:10.1038/ni.2537
71. Chen X, Zhou L, Peng N, Yu H, Li M, Cao Z, et al. MicroRNA-302a suppresses influenza A virus-stimulated interferon regulatory factor-5 expression and cytokine storm induction. *J Biol Chem* (2017) 292:21291–303. doi:10.1074/jbc.M117.805937
72. Rosenberger CM, Podyminogin RL, Diercks AH, Treuting PM, Peschon JJ, Rodriguez D, et al. miR-144 attenuates the host response to influenza virus by targeting the TRAF6-IRF7 signaling axis. *PLoS Pathog* (2017) 13:e1006305. doi:10.1371/journal.ppat.1006305
73. Deng Y, Yan Y, Tan KS, Liu J, Chow VT, Tao ZZ, et al. MicroRNA-146a induction during influenza H3N2 virus infection targets and regulates TRAF6 levels in human nasal epithelial cells (hNECs). *Exp Cell Res* (2017) 352:184–92. doi:10.1016/j.yexcr.2017.01.011

74. Honda K, Yanai H, Mizutani T, Negishi H, Shimada N, Suzuki N, et al. Role of a transductional-transcriptional processor complex involving MyD88 and IRF-7 in toll-like receptor signaling. *Proc Natl Acad Sci U S A* (2004) 101:15416–21. doi:10.1073/pnas.0406933101
75. Kawai T, Sato S, Ishii KJ, Coban C, Hemmi H, Yamamoto M, et al. Interferon-alpha induction through toll-like receptors involves a direct interaction of IRF7 with MyD88 and TRAF6. *Nat Immunol* (2004) 5:1061–8. doi:10.1038/ni1118
76. Schmolke M, Viemann D, Roth J, Ludwig S. Essential impact of NF-kappaB signaling on the H5N1 influenza A virus-induced transcriptome. *J Immunol* (2009) 183:5180–9. doi:10.4049/jimmunol.0804198
77. Wurzer WJ, Planz O, Ehrhardt C, Giner M, Silberzahn T, Pleschka S, et al. Caspase 3 activation is essential for efficient influenza virus propagation. *EMBO J* (2003) 22:2717–28. doi:10.1093/emboj/cdg279
78. Wurzer WJ, Ehrhardt C, Pleschka S, Berberich-Siebelt F, Wolff T, Walczak H, et al. NF-kappaB-dependent induction of tumor necrosis factor-related apoptosis-inducing ligand (TRAIL) and Fas/FasL is crucial for efficient influenza virus propagation. *J Biol Chem* (2004) 279:30931–7. doi:10.1074/jbc.M403258200
79. Nimmerjahn F, Dudziak D, Dirmeier U, Hobom G, Riedel A, Schlee M, et al. Active NF-kappaB signalling is a prerequisite for influenza virus infection. *J Gen Virol* (2004) 85:2347–56. doi:10.1099/vir.0.79958-0
80. Gui S, Chen X, Zhang M, Zhao F, Wan Y, Wang L, et al. Mir-302c mediates influenza A virus-induced IFNbeta expression by targeting NF-kappaB inducing kinase. *FEBS Lett* (2015) 589:4112–8. doi:10.1016/j.febslet.2015.11.011
81. Buggele WA, Johnson KE, Horvath CM. Influenza A virus infection of human respiratory cells induces primary microRNA expression. *J Biol Chem* (2012) 287:31027–40. doi:10.1074/jbc.M112.387670
82. Othumpangat S, Bryan NB, Beezhold DH, Noti JD. Upregulation of miRNA-4776 in influenza virus infected bronchial epithelial cells is associated with downregulation of NFKBIB and increased viral survival. *Viruses* (2017) 9(5):E94. doi:10.3390/v9050094
83. Palombella VJ, Rando OJ, Goldberg AL, Maniatis T. The ubiquitin-proteasome pathway is required for processing the Nf-Kappa-B1 precursor protein and the activation of Nf-Kappa-B. *Cell* (1994) 78:773–85. doi:10.1016/S0092-8674(94)90482-0
84. Ghosh S, May MJ, Kopp EB. NF-kappa B and Rel proteins: evolutionarily conserved mediators of immune responses. *Annu Rev Immunol* (1998) 16:225–60. doi:10.1146/annurev.immunol.16.1.225
85. Dong C, Sun X, Guan Z, Zhang M, Duan M. Modulation of influenza A virus replication by microRNA-9 through targeting MCPIP1. *J Med Virol* (2017) 89:41–8. doi:10.1002/jmv.24604
86. Lin RJ, Chien HL, Lin SY, Chang BL, Yu HP, Tang WC, et al. MCPIP1 ribonuclease exhibits broad-spectrum antiviral effects through viral RNA binding and degradation. *Nucleic Acids Res* (2013) 41:3314–26. doi:10.1093/nar/gkt019
87. Hsu AC, Dua K, Starkey MR, Haw TJ, Nair PM, Nichol K, et al. MicroRNA-125a and -b inhibit A20 and MAVS to promote inflammation and impair antiviral response in COPD. *JCI Insight* (2017) 2:e90443. doi:10.1172/jci.insight.90443
88. Loo YM, Gale M. Immune Signaling by RIG-I-like Receptors. *Immunity* (2011) 34:680–92. doi:10.1016/j.immuni.2011.05.003
89. Yoneyama M, Fujita T. Function of RIG-I-like receptors in antiviral innate immunity. *J Biol Chem* (2007) 282:15315–8. doi:10.1074/jbc.R700007200
90. Yoneyama M, Kikuchi M, Matsumoto K, Imaizumi T, Miyagishi M, Taira K, et al. Shared and unique functions of the DExD/H-box helicases RIG-I, MDA5, and LGP2 in antiviral innate immunity. *J Immunol* (2005) 175:2851–8. doi:10.4049/jimmunol.175.5.2851
91. Baum A, Garcia-Sastre A. Differential recognition of viral RNA by RIG-I. *Virulence* (2011) 2:166–9. doi:10.4161/viru.2.2.15481
92. Satoh T, Kato H, Kumagai Y, Yoneyama M, Sato S, Matsushita K, et al. LGP2 is a positive regulator of RIG-I- and MDA5-mediated antiviral responses. *Proc Natl Acad Sci U S A* (2010) 107:1512–7. doi:10.1073/pnas.0912986107
93. Rodriguez KR, Bruns AM, Horvath CM. MDA5 and LGP2: accomplices and antagonists of antiviral signal transduction. *J Virol* (2014) 88:8194–200. doi:10.1128/JVI.00640-14
94. Seth RB, Sun L, Ea CK, Chen ZJ. Identification and characterization of MAVS, a mitochondrial antiviral signaling protein that activates NF-kappaB and IRF 3. *Cell* (2005) 122:669–82. doi:10.1016/j.cell.2005.08.012
95. Matsumiya T, Stafforini DM. Function and regulation of retinoic acid-inducible gene-I. *Crit Rev Immunol* (2010) 30:489–513. doi:10.1615/CritRevImmunol.v30.i6.10
96. Sato M, Suemori H, Hata N, Asagiri M, Ogasawara K, Nakao K, et al. Distinct and essential roles of transcription factors IRF-3 and IRF-7 in response to viruses for IFN-alpha/beta gene induction. *Immunity* (2000) 13:539–48. doi:10.1016/S1074-7613(00)00053-4
97. Zhao L, Zhu J, Zhou H, Zhao Z, Zou Z, Liu X, et al. Identification of cellular microRNA-136 as a dual regulator of RIG-I-mediated innate immunity that antagonizes H5N1 IAV replication in A549 cells. *Sci Rep* (2015) 5:14991. doi:10.1038/srep14991
98. Wang K, Lai C, Gu H, Zhao L, Xia M, Yang P, et al. miR-194 inhibits innate antiviral immunity by targeting FGF2 in influenza H1N1 virus infection. *Front Microbiol* (2017) 8:2187. doi:10.3389/fmicb.2017.02187
99. Maemura T, Fukuyama S, Sugita Y, Lopes TJS, Nakao T, Noda T, et al. Lung-derived exosomal miR-483-3p regulates the innate immune response to influenza virus infection. *J Infect Dis* (2018) 217(9):1372–82. doi:10.1093/infdis/jiy035
100. Lagos D, Pollara G, Henderson S, Gratrix F, Fabani M, Milne RSB, et al. miR-132 regulates antiviral innate immunity through suppression of the p300 transcriptional co-activator. *Nat Cell Biol* (2010) 12:513–U232. doi:10.1038/ncb2054
101. Gao S, Li J, Song L, Wu J, Huang W. Influenza A virus-induced downregulation of miR-26a contributes to reduced IFNalpha/beta production. *Virol Sin* (2017) 32:261–70. doi:10.1007/s12250-017-4004-9
102. Buggele WA, Krause KE, Horvath CM. Small RNA profiling of influenza A virus-infected cells identifies miR-449b as a regulator of histone deacetylase 1 and interferon beta. *PLoS One* (2013) 8:e76560. doi:10.1371/journal.pone.0076560
103. Nagesh PT, Husain M. Influenza A virus dysregulates host histone Deacetylase 1 that inhibits viral infection in lung epithelial cells. *J Virol* (2016) 90:4614–25. doi:10.1128/JVI.00126-16
104. Buggele WA, Horvath CM. MicroRNA profiling of Sendai virus-infected A549 cells identifies miR-203 as an interferon-inducible regulator of IFIT1/ISG56. *J Virol* (2013) 87:9260–70. doi:10.1128/JVI.01064-13
105. Ebert MS, Neilson JR, Sharp PA. MicroRNA sponges: competitive inhibitors of small RNAs in mammalian cells. *Nat Methods* (2007) 4:721–6. doi:10.1038/nmeth1079
106. Vermeulen A, Robertson B, Dalby AB, Marshall WS, Karpilow J, Leake D, et al. Double-stranded regions are essential design components of potent inhibitors of RISC function. *RNA* (2007) 13:723–30. doi:10.1261/rna.448107
107. Pedersen IM, Cheng G, Wieland S, Volinia S, Croce CM, Chisari FV, et al. Interferon modulation of cellular microRNAs as an antiviral mechanism. *Nature* (2007) 449:919–22. doi:10.1038/nature06205
108. Bommer GT, Gerin I, Feng Y, Kaczorowski AJ, Kuick R, Love RE, et al. p53-mediated activation of miRNA34 candidate tumor-suppressor genes. *Curr Biol* (2007) 17:1298–307. doi:10.1016/j.cub.2007.06.068
109. Hommel JD, Sears RM, Georgescu D, Simmons DL, DiLeone RJ. Local gene knockdown in the brain using viral-mediated RNA interference. *Nat Med* (2003) 9:1539–44. doi:10.1038/nm964
110. Jacque JM, Triques K, Stevenson M. Modulation of HIV-1 replication by RNA interference. *Nature* (2002) 418:435–8. doi:10.1038/nature00896
111. Xia Y, Lin RX, Zheng SJ, Zhang ML, Wang SQ. Expression of siRNA target against human telomerase reverse transcriptase (hTERT) for gene silencing by constructing DNA-based plasmid vector. *Prog Biochem Biophys* (2004) 31:1079–84.
112. Rumpold H, Wolf AM, Gruenewald K, Gastl G, Gunsilius E, Wolf D. RNAi-mediated knockdown of P-glycoprotein using a transposon-based vector system durably restores imatinib sensitivity in imatinib-resistant CML cell lines. *Exp Hematol* (2005) 33:767–75. doi:10.1016/j.exphem.2005.03.014
113. Heggestad AD, Notterpek L, Fletcher BS. Transposon-based RNAi delivery system for generating knockdown cell lines. *Biochem Biophys Res Commun* (2004) 316:643–50. doi:10.1016/j.bbrc.2004.02.090
114. Szulc J, Wiznerowicz M, Sauvain MO, Trono D, Aebischer P. A versatile tool for conditional gene expression and knockdown. *Nat Methods* (2006) 3:109–16. doi:10.1038/nmeth846
115. Rubinson DA, Dillon CP, Kwiatkowski AV, Sievers C, Yang L, Kopinja J, et al. A lentivirus-based system to functionally silence genes in primary

mammalian cells, stem cells and transgenic mice by RNA interference. *Nat Genet* (2003) 33:401–6. doi:10.1038/ng1117

116. Xu F, Liu G, Liu Q, Zhou Y. RNA interference of influenza A virus replication by microRNA-adapted lentiviral loop short hairpin RNA. *J Gen Virol* (2015) 96:2971–81. doi:10.1099/jgv.0.000247
117. Varble A, Chua MA, Perez JT, Manicassamy B, Garcia-Sastre A, tenOever BR. Engineered RNA viral synthesis of microRNAs. *Proc Natl Acad Sci U S A* (2010) 107:11519–24. doi:10.1073/pnas.1003115107
118. Langlois RA, Shapiro JS, Pham AM, tenOever BR. In vivo delivery of cytoplasmic RNA virus-derived miRNAs. *Mol Ther* (2012) 20:367–75. doi:10.1038/mt.2011.244
119. Zeng Y, Wagner EJ, Cullen BR. Both natural and designed micro RNAs technique can inhibit the expression of cognate mRNAs when expressed in human cells. *Mol Cell* (2002) 9:1327–33. doi:10.1016/S1097-2765(02)00541-5
120. Izzard L, Dlugolenski D, Xia Y, McMahon M, Middleton D, Tripp RA, et al. Enhanced immunogenicity following miR-155 incorporation into the influenza A virus genome. *Virus Res* (2017) 235:115–20. doi:10.1016/j.virusres.2017.04.002
121. Zhang H, Tang X, Zhu C, Song Y, Yin J, Xu J, et al. Adenovirus-mediated artificial MicroRNAs targeting matrix or nucleoprotein genes protect mice against lethal influenza virus challenge. *Gene Ther* (2015) 22:653–62. doi:10.1038/gt.2015.31
122. Tan M, Sun W, Feng C, Xia D, Shen X, Ding Y, et al. The microRNA-let-7b-mediated attenuated strain of influenza A (H1N1) virus in a mouse model. *J Infect Dev Ctries* (2016) 10:973–81. doi:10.3855/jidc.6861
123. Thomas CE, Ehrhardt A, Kay MA. Progress and problems with the use of viral vectors for gene therapy. *Nat Rev Genet* (2003) 4:346–58. doi:10.1038/nrg1066
124. Boden D, Pusch O, Silbermann R, Lee F, Tucker L, Ramratnam B. Enhanced gene silencing of HIV-1 specific siRNA using microRNA designed hairpins. *Nucleic Acids Res* (2004) 32:1154–8. doi:10.1093/nar/gkh278
125. Wolf S, Wu WL, Jones C, Perwitasari O, Mahalingam S, Tripp RA. MicroRNA regulation of human genes essential for influenza A (H7N9) replication. *PLoS One* (2016) 11:e0155104. doi:10.1371/journal.pone.0155104
126. Shen X, Sun W, Shi Y, Xing Z, Su X. Altered viral replication and cell responses by inserting microRNA recognition element into PB1 in pandemic influenza A virus (H1N1) 2009. *Mediators Inflamm* (2015) 2015:976575. doi:10.1155/2015/976575

12

Influenza Virus: A Master Tactician in Innate Immune Evasion and Novel Therapeutic Interventions

Alan Chen-Yu Hsu[1,2]*

[1] *Viruses, Infections/Immunity, Vaccines & Asthma, Hunter Medical Research Institute, Newcastle, NSW, Australia,* [2] *Priority Research Centre for Healthy Lungs, Faculty of Health and Medicine, The University of Newcastle, Newcastle, NSW, Australia*

Correspondence:
Alan Chen-Yu Hsu
alan.hsu@newcastle.edu.au

Influenza is a contagion that has plagued mankind for many decades, and continues to pose concerns every year, with millions of infections globally. The frequent mutations and recombination of the influenza A virus (IAV) cast a looming threat that antigenically novel strains/subtypes will rise with unpredictable pathogenicity and fear of it evolving into a pandemic strain. There have been four major influenza pandemics, since the beginning of twentieth century, with the great 1918 pandemic being the most severe, killing more than 50 million people worldwide. The mechanisms of IAV infection, host immune responses, and how viruses evade from such defensive responses at the molecular and structural levels have been greatly investigated in the past 30 years. While this has advanced our understanding of virus–host interactions and human immunology, and has led to the development of several antiviral drugs, they have minimal impact on the clinical outcomes of infection. The heavy use of these drugs has also imposed selective pressure on IAV to evolve and develop resistance. Vaccination remains the cornerstone of public health efforts to protect against influenza; however, rapid mass-production of sufficient vaccines is unlikely to occur immediately after the beginning of a pandemic. This, therefore, requires novel therapeutic strategies against this continually emerging infectious virus with higher specificity and cross-reactivity against multiple strains/subtypes of IAVs. This review discusses essential virulence factors of IAVs that determine sustainable human-to-human transmission, the mechanisms of viral hijacking of host cells and subversion of host innate immune responses, and novel therapeutic interventions that demonstrate promising antiviral properties against IAV. This hopefully will promote discussions and investigations on novel avenues of prevention and treatment strategies of influenza, that are effective and cross-protective against multiple strains/subtypes of IAV, in preparation for the advent of future IAVs and pandemics.

Keywords: influenza, influenza A virus, virulence factors, hemagglutinin, polymerase acidic 1-F2, NS1, therapeutics

INTRODUCTION

Influenza A viruses (IAVs) and their continuous emergence/re-emergence are undoubtedly an important cause of global concern, morbidity and mortality, clinical, and socio-economical burden in humans. The emergence of highly pathogenic avian influenza virus H5N1 in 1997 and 2003, H7N7 in 2003, recent influenza H1N1 pandemic in 2009 (H1N1pdm09), and H7N9 in 2013 have caused tremendous mortality in the affected populations, and in our current inter-connected world, the concerns and impact of potential pandemics are truly global.

The ongoing circulation of IAVs in their natural hosts and the ever-mutating antigenicity frequently leads to the appearance of novel viruses with the ability to cross species barriers and infect humans with unpredictable pathogenicity. Furthermore, effective immuno-evasive and modulatory strategies employed by IAVs have made it difficult for both the innate and acquired immunity to combat the infections without the help of vaccination.

The early innate immune responses to IAV infections are essential in the immediate control of viral replication and spread. However, IAVs have also evolved to produce only a handful, but multi-functional proteins to combat the intricate layers of human innate immune signaling pathways. These virulence factors inhibit host antiviral immunity, while stimulating inflammatory responses in the airways (cytokine storm) that cause severe symptoms. It is, therefore, imperative to understand the molecular mechanisms of IAV-mediated modulation of innate immunity by these viral factors in order to identify potential therapeutic options.

While antiviral drugs are mostly used either prophylactically or in treatment, they have minimal impact on the course of the disease. Heavy reliance on antiviral drugs has also placed a strong selective pressure on IAVs to mutate and develop resistance (1, 2). The unpredictable nature of novel IAVs and limited prevention and treatment options, therefore, urges the research and development of novel approaches against IAVs. This review summarizes the current understanding of the mechanisms of IAV infection in humans, the ways by which IAV suppresses antiviral immunity and causes the inflammatory cytokine storm, and novel peptide-based anti-influenza drugs that may potentially be beneficial as preventative and treatment strategies in current and future IAV pandemics.

IAV—SIMPLE AND ELEGANT

IAVs is a negative sense, single-stranded RNA virus (~80–120 nm in diameter) (3). The viral envelope features two surface glycoproteins, hemaglutinin (HA) and neuraminidase (NA), at a ratio of four HA to one NA (4). A small number of M2 ion channel is also embedded in the viral envelope at a ratio of one M2 channel to 10^1–10^2 HA molecules (5) (**Figure 1**).

Within the envelope are the eight segments of influenza RNA, which are presented in a form of helical hairpin structure, each of which is coated with arginine-rich nucleoprotein (NP) (6–8). NP-RNA is complexed with heterotrimeric RNA-dependent RNA polymerase, which consists of three subunits, polymerase basic (PB)1, PB2, and polymerase acidic (PA) (3). Segment 1, 3, 4, 5, and 6 encodes for PB2, PA, HA, NP, and NA, respectively. Segment 2 encodes for PB1 and *via* a different reading frame an accessory protein PB1-F2 is expressed in most influenza A strains. Segment 7 encodes for matrix 1 (M1) protein and also M2 ion channel *via* alternative splicing. Segment 8 encodes for non-structural protein (NS)-1 and nuclear export protein. At

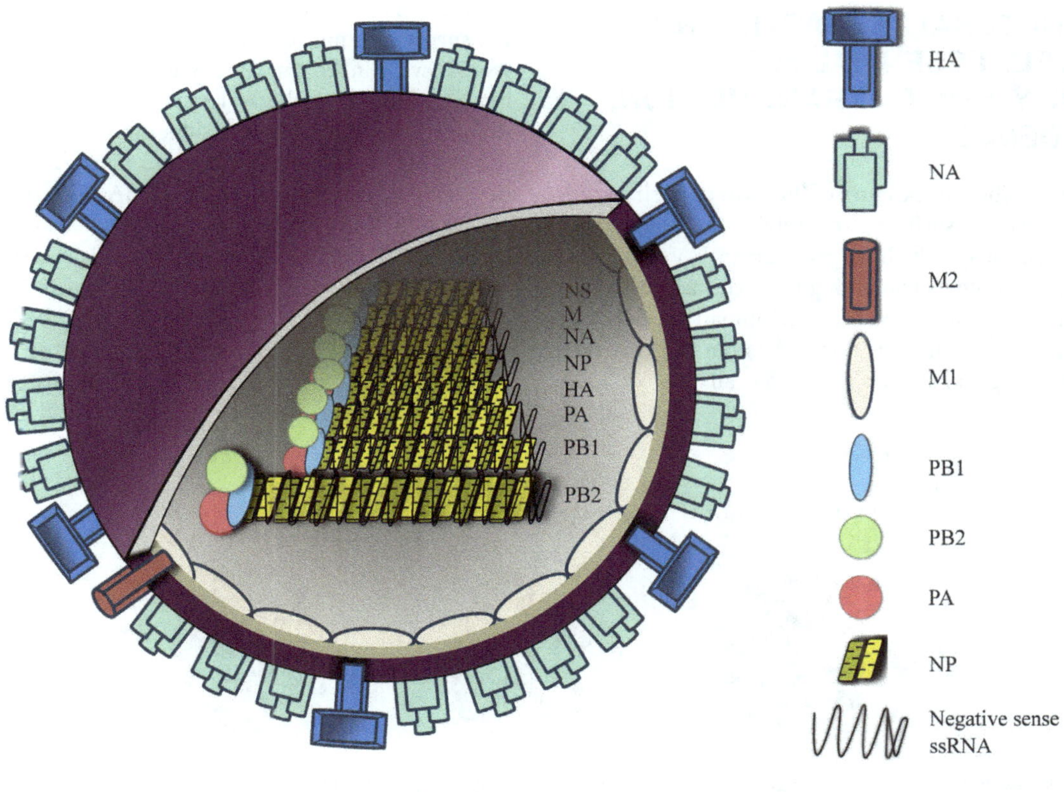

FIGURE 1 | Influenza A virus (IAV) structure. IAV contains an outer membrane envelope with hemaglutinin (HA), neuraminidase (NA), and matrix 2 (M2) ion channels, and an inner M1 protein layer that encloses an eight segmented RNA genome. The RNA segments are folded into a helical hairpin structure with nucleoprotein, which are complexed with heterotrimeric RNA-dependent RNA polymerase [polymerase basic (PB1), PB2, and polymerase acidic (PA)].

both 3′ and 5′ ends of each segment lies a non-coding region of varying length that acts as a promoter site for viral polymerase complex to initiate transcription. This region also contains an mRNA polyadenylation signal and a signal for virus assembly.

The primary site of infection by IAVs are epithelial cells of the respiratory mucosa. Airway epithelial cells are both susceptible and permissive to IAV infection. This occurs by the binding of HA to the sialyl sugar chain receptors on the host cell surface, allowing the virus to be internalized into endosomes in the host epithelial cells. The low pH environment of the endosome promotes HA to undergo conformational change that liberates and inserts a fusion peptide from the amino terminus of HA into the endosomal membrane. This spring-loaded mechanism fuses the viral envelope and the membrane together, thereby releasing viral RNP into the host cytoplasm (9, 10). The M2 ion channel also allows an influx of H^+ ions into the virion, and lowers the intra-virionic pH. This in turn disrupts the viral RNP-M1 protein interaction and subsequently releases viral RNP into host cellular cytoplasm (11–14). Released IAV RNAs and polymerases are then translocated into the nucleus where viral replication occurs. The newly synthesized viral structural proteins and viral segments then traffic to lipid rafts on the plasma membrane to be released (15, 16). Since the viral envelope is derived from the host membrane, which contains sialic acid glycoproteins, the newly formed virion remains intact on the host cell surface. The viral NA cleaves the host cell surface sialic acid residues, releasing the newly formed virions free from the host cell surface.

HA—STRUCTURALLY PLASTIC AND ABSOLUTELY ESSENTIAL FOR INFECTIVITY, HUMAN TRANSMISSION, AND PANDEMIC

IAVs HA is responsible for the entry of the virus in the host cells by binding to host cell surface glycoproteins terminated with sialic acid residues at specific linkages. Human IAVs preferentially bind to glycoproteins containing the terminal SAα2,6Gal linkage, which are predominately found in human upper airway epithelium (17–19). In contrast, avian IAVs bind to that with terminal SAα2,3Gal linkage in the lower airways (17–21). This difference in binding specificity and distribution of sialic acid residues may in part explain why highly pathogenic avian influenza virus H5N1 is currently incapable of transmitting from human to human in a sustainable manner. In contrast, pig trachea contains both SAα2,6Gal and SAα2,3Gal linkages, indicating that pigs can act as an intermediate mixing host (22–24), allowing the reassortment of both avian and human viruses to occur. The prime example is the emergence of the 2009 H1N1 pandemic, which was the result of triple reassortment between avian, swine, and human IAVs in pigs (25, 26). The difference in their binding specificity can be explained by the amino acid residue at position 226 of HA glycoprotein. HA of human influenza viruses contains a Leu226 that results in the preferential binding to SAα2,6Gal linkage. In contrast, HA of avian influenza viruses have a Gln226, which binds to SAα2,3Gal-linked glycoproteins (27, 28).

Two recent important investigations further characterized the molecular changes that are required for H5N1 to become transmissible among humans. Imai et al. showed that Gln226Leu/Gly228Ser increased the binding of H5 HA to SAα2,6Gal while retaining the binding capacity to SAα2,3Gal. When Asn158Asp/Asn224Lys/Thr318Ile was introduced with Gln226Leu/Gly228Ser, this fully converted the virus with H5 HA in an H1N1pdm09 backbone to achieve sustainable aerosol transmission in a ferret model (29). In addition, Herfst et al. also demonstrated that mutant H5N1 containing His103Tyr, Thr156Ala, and Gln222Leu in the HA protein, and Glu627Lys in the viral polymerase protein PB2 was able to efficiently transmit between ferret models *via* aerosols (30). Interestingly, although not surprising, most of these residues (Asn158Asp; Gln222Leu; Asn224Lys; Gln226Leu; Gly228Ser) are at the sialic acid residue binding site of the globular domain.

When these amino acid residues in H5N1 HA were changed *in silico* to the ones in the airborne-capable HA, and structurally modelled using the wild-type H5N1 HA as a template in SWISS-MODEL (31), the binding cavity in the mutant, surrounded by the 130-, 190-, and 220-loop, may potentially be lengthened and result in a slightly larger binding cavity (**Figure 2**). Furthermore, Asn158Asp is also likely to make the receptor binding pocket slightly more acidic, further facilitating a more efficient airborne transmission. A mutant H1N1 with Tyr17His (pH 6.0) in HA

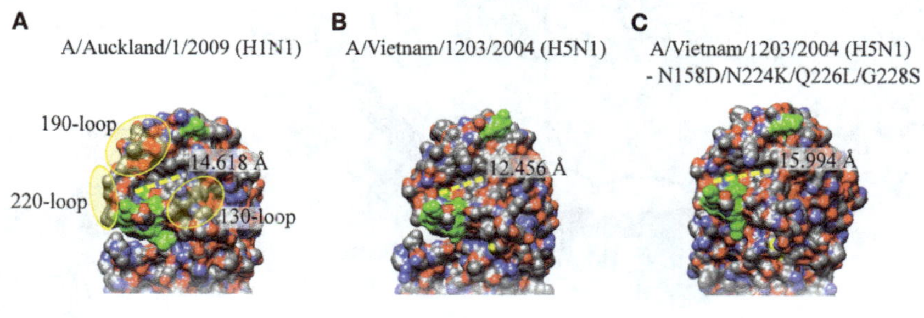

FIGURE 2 | Crystal structure of hemaglutinin (HA) sialic acid residue binding site of H1N1pdm09, H5N1, and airborne-transmissible H5N1. The sialic acid residue binding site on the HA of **(A)** A/Washington/5/2011 (H1N1pdm09; PDB: 4LKX), **(B)** A/Vietnam/1203/2004 (H5N1; PDB: 2FK0), and **(C)** H5N1 with Asn148Asp, Gln222Leu Asn224Lys Gln226Leu, and Gly228Ser. These amino acid residues were changed *in silico* and modeled using HA of H5N1(PDB: 2FK0) as a template in SWISS-MODEL. Protein visualization and distance calculation was performed in UCSF Chimera molecular visualization application.

showed loss of airborne transmission, and was less efficient in contact transmission with reduced pathogenicity in mice, and His17Tyr (pH 5.3) revertant virus regained the airborne transmissibility and pathogenicity (32). This may also widen the binding capacity toward moieties with other linkages/modifications. While changes in these residues are important in airborne transmission in ferret models, it remains unclear whether similar or other changes in HA need to occur for a sustainable airborne transmission in humans, these studies provide valuable insight into cause of efficient human transmission, surveillance for potential human transmissible IAVs, and new approach into therapeutic designs.

Epidermal growth factor receptor, a glycoprotein with potential terminal SAα2,6Gal and SAα2,3Gal linkages (33, 34), has been shown to be important in IAV entry into host cells in a ligand (EGF)-independent, and phosphoinositide-3 kinase (PI3K)-activation-dependent manner (35–37). However, IAV has also been demonstrated to cause infection in the absence of its respective receptors. H3N2 and H1N1 was able to infect and replicate to the similar titer in the lung of the mice lacking receptors with SAα2,6Gal linkages compared to wild type mice (38). Consistent with this finding, while human bronchial epithelial cells showed higher levels of SAα2,6Gal compared with SAα2,3Gal linkages, human IAV H3N2, and a low pathogenic avian H11N9 have been shown to enter into bronchial epithelial cells at a similar rate (39). This indicates that sialic acid residues may not be absolutely essential in influenza virus entry, and other moieties, such as sulfonated or fucosylated glycoproteins may also be targeted by HA protein (40, 41).

THE POLYMERASE CONSTELLATION

IAV RNA is always packaged in a heterotrimeric RNA-dependent RNA polymerase complex with viral polymerase basic (PB)1, PB2, polymerase acidic (PA), and nucleoprotein (NP), and upon successful entry into epithelial cells, this complex translocates to the nucleus where replication occurs. As IAV viral RNA does not contain a 5′ cap as they do on host RNAs, PB2 contains a cap-binding domain that binds to the 5′ cap of nascent host RNAs, and PA then "steals" the cap off the host RNA by cleavage, which is then used as primers to initiate transcription of viral mRNAs. This process is called cap-snatching. This polymerase complex, therefore, is critical in the survival of IAVs, and has been implicated in the host range determination. Clements et al. demonstrated that the reassortment virus containing the PB2 gene of avian origin and all other genes from human IAV is able to replicate efficiently in the avian host, while showing restricted replication in the mammalian respiratory tract (42). This reassortment virus was then progressively passaged to generate mutant viruses that were able to replicate in mammalian tissues. Nucleotide sequence analysis revealed that this phenotype of the reassortment virus was due to the Glu627 of the PB2 gene (43). A single amino acid substitution to a lysine residue allowed this mutant reassortment virus to replicate efficiently with increased pathogenicity in the mammalian system (44–47). All the avian IAVs analyzed to date have a Glu627 in the PB2, whereas human IAVs have a Lys627, indicating this residue at position 627 of PB2 is an important host range determinant of IAVs (43). Furthermore, Glu627Lys substitution being a prerequisite for aerosol to airborne transmissibility switch is troubling, as the viruses isolated from the recent fatal cases of H7N9 infection in China carried Glu627Lys substitution, but the viruses isolated from poultry did not (48, 49).

The compatibility of other subunits of the polymerase complex is also involved in the host range specificity (50, 51). Reassortment viruses with human PA and avian PB1 and PB2, or with human PA and PB2 and avian PB1 showed a restricted viral replication in mammalian cells, indicating that a specific constellation of polymerase genes may be involved in the host range specificities (51).

PB1-F2—A PYROGENIC DEATH DEALER

In the middle of searching for an IAV-derived out-of-frame polypeptide that can be recognized by $CD8^+$ T lymphocytes, an 11th gene, PB1-F2, was serendipitously discovered (52). PB1-F2 is an accessory protein that is translated from an alternative +1 open reading frame of PB1. It modulates innate immune responses at multiple signaling levels, leading to increased inflammatory and impaired antiviral responses. PB1-F2 contains a mitochondrial targeting sequence at the carboxyl-terminus and has a pro-apoptotic effect on immune cells (53). By binding to the inner and outer mitochondrial membrane transport protein adenine nucleotide translocator 3 and voltage-dependent anion channel 1 (VDAC1), PB1-F2 disrupts mitochondrial integrity, releasing cytochrome C, and leading to apoptosis. Another study also demonstrated that PB1-F2 can be translocated into the inner mitochondrial space in a TOM40-dependent manner, and impair mitochondrial function (54).

Host innate immune response is triggered by the pattern recognition receptors including retinoic acid inducible gene 1 (RIG-I). RIG-I binds to IAV RNAs and forms a complex with the adaptor protein tripartite motif-containing protein (TRIM)25 (55). This complex interacts with mitochondrial antiviral signaling (MAVS) protein to induce the activation of interferon (IFN)-regulatory factor (IRF) 3, which initiates the induction of important antiviral cytokines including type I and III IFNs (56, 57). These IFNs then stimulate the expression of over 300 IFN-stimulated genes (ISGs) such as protein kinase R (PKR) to limit viral replication (58). Toll-like receptor 3 also recognizes IAV RNAs and activates an important transcription factor nuclear-factor-kappa-B (NF-κB), which stimulates the expression of predominantly inflammatory cytokines, including interleukin (IL)-6 and IL-1β (59–61).

PB1-F2 has also been shown to inhibit RIG-I-TRIM25-mediated antiviral signaling pathway by direct interaction with MAVS (62, 63). Furthermore, this inhibition of type I and III IFNs was enhanced with Asn66Ser substitution. Intriguingly, PB1-F2 can also be expressed as a truncated (57 amino acids) protein devoid of the carboxyl terminus, which failed to translocate into the mitochondria (54). The full length PB1-F2 is mostly expressed by highly pathogenic viruses, such as H5N1, whereas low pathogenic subtypes, such as H1N1 (except PB1-F2 of 1918 H1N1) tend to express this truncated form. PB1-F2 also enhances the development of secondary bacterial pneumonia in mice with reduced survival rate. When PB1-F2 of A/PR/8 was engineered to become that of 1918 H1N1 by mutagenesis, the resulting mutant virus became more pathogenic with and without secondary bacterial infection (64). Surprisingly, this increased pathogenicity by PB1-F2 of 1918 H1N1 was also attributed to Asn66Ser (65). A mutant virus carrying H5N1 PB1-F2 gene with Asn66Ser in A/WSN/33 background led to increased pathogenicity with 100-fold increase in viral replication compared with wild-type virus in mice. Similarly, when the 1918 H1N1 virus was reconstructed to carry a pathogenicity-reducing substitution (Ser66Asn), the resulting virus led to attenuated viral replication and reduced mortality.

PB1-F2-mediated IAV pathogenicity could be the result of its interaction with NLRP3-inflammasome. PB1-F2 of H7N9 has been shown to form fibrillar higher molecular weight aggregates that were incorporated into the phagolysosome and induced ASC speck formation upon acidification (66). This resulted in the activation of NLRP3-mediated inflammasome, leading to increased production of pyrogenic cytokine IL-1β and enhance the pathogenesis of influenza viral pneumonia in mouse models (66, 67). PB1-F2 of avian H7N9 has also been shown to increase mitochondrial reactive oxygen species (ROS) and calcium (Ca^{2+}) efflux, which contributed to the activation of NLRP3 inflammasome (68).

PB1-F2, therefore, appears to be a major driving force for excessive pro-inflammatory cytokine storm and pathogenesis (**Figure 3**), and Asn66 is important in the function of PB1-F2. Nevertheless, how IAV-mediated inflammatory cytokine storm holds an advantage in IAV survival remains elusive. The formation of this fibrillary PB1-F2 aggregate is consistent with the crystal structural data that indicated a strong propensity for PB1-F2 to adopt an oligomerization structure and form membrane pores in planar lipid bilayers (69, 70). However, it remains unknown whether it is a requirement for PB1-F2 to form this fibrillar structure to interact with all of its binding targets, and while the oligomerization domain is located in carboxyl-terminal α-helix, it is unknown if oligomerization is dependent on Asn66. It is also unclear if this structure is unique to highly pathogenic strains or is present in all subtypes/strains.

NS1—THE INVERSE INTERFERON

When IFNs were first described by Isaacs and Lindenmann, it was found that cells treated with heat-inactivated, but not live IAV could produce these antiviral cytokines, an immuno-inhibitory phenomenon he described as "inverse interference" (71, 72). The identity of Lindenmann's inverse interferon was later revealed to be NS1 protein. NS1 protein is encoded by the NS gene together with nuclear export protein *via* alternative splicing. As NS1 is encoded by the shortest gene of all, NS1 protein is rapidly expressed to high levels in the infected epithelial cells (73, 74).

NS1 is a multi-functional protein with a RNA-binding domain at its amino-terminus (residue 1–73), and an effector domain (residue 74–230) at the carboxyl-terminus (73, 75, 76). The RNA-binding domain of NS1 recognizes dsRNA sequences and blocks the host RNA detection system. The effector domain of NS1 can stabilize the RNA-binding domain, but it predominantly interacts with host cellular proteins and interferes with host mRNA processing and host innate immune responses (**Figure 4**). NS1 inhibits host pre-mRNA endonucleolytic cleavage and poly-adenylation by direct interaction and inhibition of cleavage and

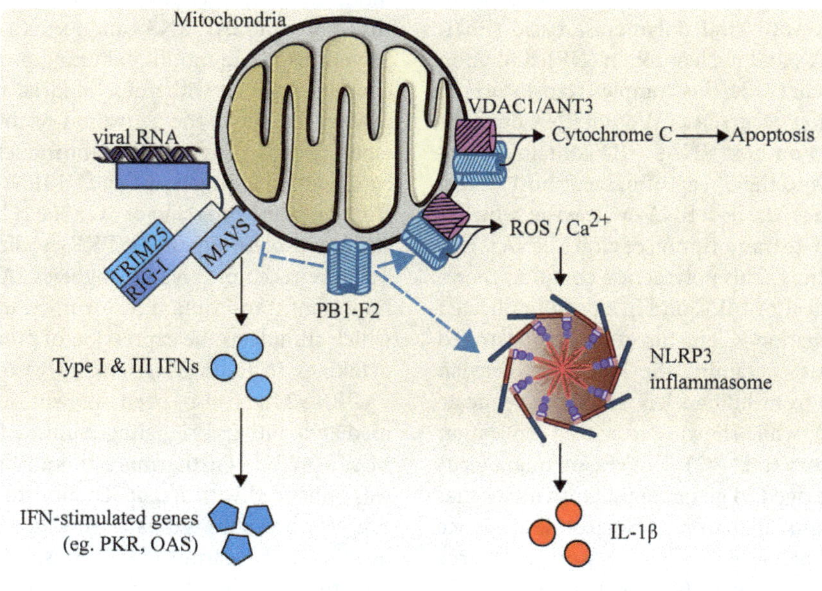

FIGURE 3 | PB1-F2 and its multi-functional functions. PB1-F2 binds and inhibits RIG-I/TRIM25/MAVS-mediated signaling activity, reduces the transcription of type I, III interferon (IFNs), and the downstream induction of antiviral responses. PB1-F2 also forms fibrillar higher molecular weight aggregates that facilitate the release of pyrogenic IL-1β by activating NLRP3-dependent inflammasome. Outer mitochondrial membrane ion channel voltage-dependent anion channel 1 (VDAC1) and adenine nucleotide translocator 3 (ANT3) are also targeted by PB1-F2, leading to increased release of cytochrome C, reactive oxygen species (ROS), and Ca^{2+}. These result in apoptosis and NLRP3-inflammasome activation.

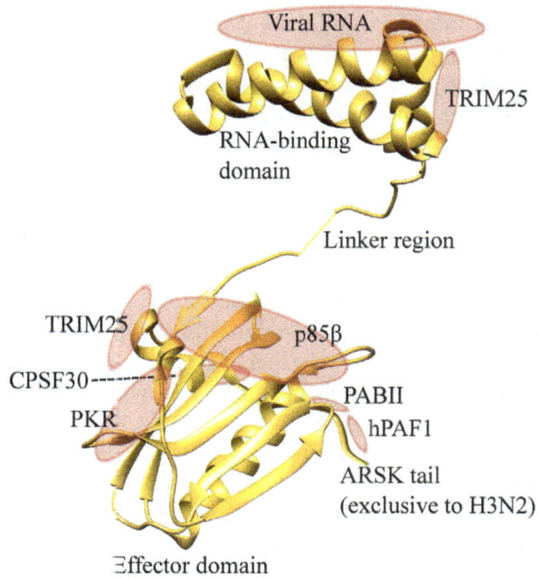

FIGURE 4 | NS1 is an effective suppressor of host antiviral immunity. NS1 protein contains an amino-terminal RNA binding domain and carboxyl-terminal effector domain. RNA binding domain binds to viral RNAs and prevents detection by the host pattern recognition system. The effector domain binds to TRIM25, and inhibits RIG-I-MAVS interaction and downstream induction of type I and III IFNs. This domain also interacts with protein kinase R (PKR), therefore, inhibiting its pro-apoptotic activities. PI3K-p85β subunit is also targeted by the effector domain to inhibit apoptosis. NS1 binds with CPSF30 and poly A binding protein II (PABII), inhibiting host protein synthesis and facilitating viral protein synthesis. The ARSK tail is exclusively found in H3N2, and directly binds with hPAF1 complex and inhibits the transcription of antiviral genes. Protein visualization was performed in UCSF chimera molecular visualization application.

polyadenylation specificity factor –30 subunit (CPSF30) and poly A binding protein II (77–79). By shutting down the host cellular protein synthesis in the infected cells, this helps the virus to gain control of the host machineries required for efficient viral protein synthesis.

The major function of NS1 is to antagonize host innate immune responses during infection, and this occurs at multiple stages of the IFN signalling cascade. In the nucleus, NS1 of human IAV H3N2 was recently shown to contain carboxyl-terminal ARSK tail sequence (amino acids 226–229), which is analogous to the ARTK sequence on the lysine 4 of histone H3 (H3K4) (80). This ARSK tail could act as a H3K4 histone mimic that directly interacts with human polymerase II-associated factor 1 complex and impairs the transcription of antiviral genes. However, this ARSK tail appears to be unique to H3N2, and is absent in H5N1, H7N9, and H1N1pdm09. In the cytoplasmic space, NS1 inhibits RIG-I-mediated signaling and subsequent induction of type I IFNs (81, 82). Specifically, the NS1 protein inhibits RIG-I ubiquitination mediated by TRIM25, which is crucial for maximal type I and III IFNs expression during viral infection (83). This NS1-TRIM25 binding event is dependent on the Arg38 and Lys41 in the RNA binding domain, and Glu96 and Glu97 in the effector domain of NS1 (84, 85). NS1 protein also interferes with functions of important intracellular antiviral ISGs, including PKR and oligoadenylate synthase (OAS). The RNA-binding domain of NS1 can bind to viral RNA and avoid detection by PKR (86). It also binds to PKR itself via the effector domain (residue 123–127) and inhibits PKR-mediated viral mRNA suppression and apoptosis (87–90). OAS, which detects and cleaves viral RNA by activating RNase L, can also be blocked by influenza NS1. The RNA-binding domain of NS1 can out-compete the RNA binding capacity of OAS, thereby inhibiting the antiviral response (91). Another important target of NS1 is the PI3K signaling pathway. NS1 activates PI3K pathway by direct interaction with p85β subunit, thereby increasing the rate of viral internalization and inhibition of apoptosis. NS1-p85β interaction is dependent on Tyr89/Met93 (92), Leu141/Glu142 (93), and Pro164/Pro167 (94) of the effector domain, all of which are located adjacent to each other within a cleft between the two NS1 monomers. The anti-apoptotic effect of NS1-PKR and NS1-p85β interaction, however, appears to conflict with the pro-apoptotic function of PB1-F2. The molecular equipoise of pro- and anti-apoptotic response by these two contradicting signals and the timing of apoptosis remain elusive.

The carboxyl-terminus of the effector domain is essential in the NS1-mediated inhibition of antiviral responses. A mutant H7N7 virus that lacked NS1 gene or with a large carboxyl-terminus deletion showed impaired IFN suppression activity and attenuated replication in mammalian and avian epithelial cells (95). Similar findings were also observed with influenza viruses of different species. Both swine and turkey influenza virus with NS1 carboxyl-terminal truncation showed attenuated replication and an increase in IFN response compared to the wild type infection in its respective epithelial cells (96, 97). When the NS1 gene of high pathogenic avian H5N1 was replaced with the one that had a natural deletion of residues 191–195 from low pathogenic swine H5N1, the resulting virus was attenuated in viral replication and its IFNs inhibition in chickens (98). The deleted residues were then engineered into this NS1 and the resulting virus gained virulence, demonstrating the importance of these residues at 191–195 in IFN inhibition. The overall suppression of host antiviral immunity by the NS1 protein appears to be more effective with human IAV H3N2 compared with a low pathogenic subtype (39). This difference in the levels of inhibition by the NS1 proteins was likely due to differences in the amino acid residues discussed previously, which might be driven by the selective pressure and the long evolution of the virus in human populations. The H5N1 NS1 was able to dramatically reduce the induction of antiviral cytokines, leading to much higher viral replication (99, 100). Influenza NS1 is no doubt a powerful and fast-deployable antagonist that rapidly controls critical host immune infrastructure (**Figures 3** and **4**). The dual wields of NS1 and PB1-F2 thus allow for maximal viral replication with minimal interference from the host immune system, while causing severe disease in the infected individuals.

NOVEL THERAPEUTIC STRATEGIES

Influenza vaccination remains the cornerstone of efforts to protect against influenza, however, there are serious concerns regarding current vaccine prediction and manufacturing process. Mis-match or unforeseeable mutations between the circulating strain and the vaccine strain often results in compromised herd immunity and increased infections in that year (101). Vaccine manufacturing is a slow and problematic process, and this issue became evident during the 2009 H1N1 pandemic. The first vaccines only became available 5 months after the identification of the virus, and mutations can occur during the vaccine manufacturing period, leading to reduced effectiveness than anticipated. Antiviral drugs, such as M2 channel and neuraminidase inhibitors, are mostly used as treatment for influenza. However, these drugs were mostly given to patients who had symptoms after the virus had shed, therefore, had limited effect. Neuraminidase inhibitors have been shown to be more effective in reducing length of hospital stay than a reduction of mortality rate (102, 103). Heavy use of these drugs has also resulted in a massive development of resistance, including the emergence of oseltamivir-resistant H1N1pdm09 (A/Newcastle/1/2011) in Newcastle, NSW, Australia (2). There is, therefore, an urgent need to identify and develop novel therapeutic targets for influenza, in preparation for future emergence of influenza viruses and pandemics.

The peptide-based therapeutics is an ideal approach that offers specificity with relatively minor side-effects, and can be administered directly to the lung *via* the pulmonary delivery route. This delivery route also increases the adsorption area in the lung by the therapeutic peptides. For these reasons, a number of peptides have been discovered to inhibit IAV replication at different stages of infection.

IAV HA represents an initial and critical step to a successful infection, and would be an ideal target for drug design as a preventative strategy. By screening a HA fragment peptide library, Chen and Guo identified a HA-targeting peptide, HA-pep25, that inhibited influenza virus binding and infection, including human H1N1, human and avian H5N1, and avian H7N9 (104). HA-pep25 is an 18-mer mimicking peptide that corresponds to the sialic acid residue binding site ($HA_{221-238}$), and specifically binds to the sialic acid residues, thereby shielding the cells from the viral attachment. Jones et al. also demonstrated that a 20-amino acid peptide derived from fibroblast growth factor 4 was able to inhibit viral binding to sialic acid residues by several IAVs, including H1N1, H3N2, and H5N1 (105). Prophylactic treatment in mice substantially reduced viral replication, and post-infection treatment was also as effective as rimantadine in protection against H5N1 in mice. Other peptide-based inhibitors, such as Flupep and Flufirvitide, have also been shown to be effective in inhibiting viral attachment to the cells. Flupep interacts with HA and inhibits viral binding (H1N1pdm09, H3N2, and H5N1) to the cell membrane (106). Flufirvitide is a mixture of hydrophobic α-helical peptides that also binds with HA and blocks viral internalization and infection, and is currently being tested in clinical trials (107).

A class of synthetic anti-lipopolysaccharide peptides (SALPs) has been reported to also inhibit IAV attachment to cell surface. SALPs were originally designed to inhibit bacteria-mediated lethal septic shock in mice (108), but also possess antiviral activities against IAVs. Specifically, SALP PEP19-2.5 peptide showed high binding affinity toward the sialic acid residues, and led to reduced viral attachment and internalization, including human H3N2, H1N1pdm09, and high pathogenic H7N7 (109). Given that primary IAV infection is frequently followed by secondary bacterial infection, this class of peptides would be an ideal therapeutic approach for IAVs as a preventative or post-infection treatment. IAV polymerase complex is also an ideal therapeutic target due to its importance in viral protein synthesis in the host cells. $PB1_{1-25}$ and $PB1_{715-740}$ (110), and $PB1_{731-757}$ (111) mimicking peptides have been separately shown to bind to a conserved PB1 binding site on PA subunit, and substantially reduced viral replication of a panel of viruses, including H1N1 and H5N1.

Advances in structural interactions between human broadly neutralizing antibodies and HA have directed several synthetic proteins and peptides that inhibit fusogenic conformational changes in the endosome. A panel of synthetic HA binder (HB) scaffold proteins have been shown to bind with the conserved region of the stems of HA protein (112, 113). HB36 and HB80 were shown to bind H1 and H5 HA stem with nanomolar affinity, and inhibited low-pH-induced conformational changes. HB80 also displayed similar levels of neutralization compared with the broadly neutralizing antibodies. Furthermore, Kadam et al. recently constructed a series of small cyclic peptides that resemble the epitopes of the stem-targeting broadly neutralizing antibodies (114). These peptidic fusion inhibitors bound to the conserved HA stem epitope at nanomolar affinity, and inhibited HA conformational change at low pH. Similar design strategies could also be applied to other conserved sites on HA, or to other virulence factors of IAV.

As PB1-F2 and NS1 are two major virulence factors that promote pro-inflammatory cytokine storm and inhibit important antiviral immunity, it is interesting to note that there has been no progress in identifying peptides that specifically target these two factors. Ideal therapeutic peptides need to either shield hosts from IAV internalization, or have anti-inflammatory properties without affecting or even increasing antiviral immune responses to infection. These peptides, therefore, are an attractive direction for therapeutics against IAVs, and may be combined with current antiviral drugs to increase the effectiveness of the anti-influenza treatment. The efficacy of peptide-based drugs as preventive agents, however, needs to be further explored, particularly in transmission models such as ferrets.

CONCLUSION

The constant genetic mutations, recombination, and selection pressure ensure the survival of IAV and its continued threat to mankind. This rapid and threatening evolution of IAV enables the virus to infect multiple species, and with its superior immunomodulatory tactics, the emergence of novel IAVs is unpredictable and inevitable.

HA is the key for the virus to infect, spread, and to create a pandemic. Understanding the absolute molecular requirements for IAV to cross species barriers and achieve sustainable human transmission, and/or aerosol-airborne transmissibility switch will be vital in the development of next-generation virus-targeted therapeutics. This is crucial as the potential scenario of future IAV pandemics is likely to start with a lack of an IAV-specific vaccine, and current antiviral drugs would be available, but with questionable beneficial effect. The efficacy of peptide-based antiviral drugs as preventative agents will be an important first line of defense. However, when infection occurs, inhibiting viral polymerases with specific anti-PB1/2/PA peptides may also be feasible.

The dynamic duet of PB1-F2 and NS1 effectively controls the host cellular machineries for efficient viral replication, while instigating severe cytokine storm and disarming the host innate antiviral immunity in the infected individuals. Neutralization of their functions would be desirable to reduce infection and potentially fatal symptoms. By the time the infected individuals are admitted to hospital with symptoms, the virus would have shed. Future therapeutics will, therefore, also need to be host-targeted to treat symptoms such as the exaggerated airway or systemic inflammation that is left behind by the virus.

Peptide-based therapeutics may be the new generation of antiviral drugs, and would be protective against multiple strains/subtypes of IAV if targeted at the essential and conserved regions. This together with ever-improving nanoparticle delivery technologies could be the future of drug design and intracellular delivery system, and must be explored in the calm before the storm.

The great 1918 influenza pandemic happened before, and it will happen again.

AUTHOR CONTRIBUTIONS

AH conceptualized and wrote the manuscript.

REFERENCES

1. Hurt AC, Hardie K, Wilson NJ, Deng YM, Osbourn M, Leang SK, et al. Characteristics of a widespread community cluster of H275Y oseltamivir-resistant A(H1N1)pdm09 influenza in Australia. *J Infect Dis* (2012) 206(2):148–57. doi:10.1093/infdis/jis337
2. Hurt AC, Hardie K, Wilson NJ, Deng YM, Osbourn M, Gehrig N, et al. Community transmission of oseltamivir-resistant A(H1N1)pdm09 influenza. *N Engl J Med* (2011) 365(26):2541–2. doi:10.1056/NEJMc1111078
3. Lamb RA, Choppin PW. The gene structure and replication of influenza virus. *Annu Rev Biochem* (1983) 52:467–506. doi:10.1146/annurev.bi.52.070183.002343
4. Palese P, Shaw ML, editors. *Orthomyxoviridae: The Viruses and Their Replication*. Philadelphia: Lippincott Williams & Wilkins (2007).
5. Zebedee SL, Lamb RA. Influenza A virus M2 protein: monoclonal antibody restriction of virus growth and detection of M2 in virions. *J Virol* (1988) 62(8):2762–72.
6. Baudin F, Bach C, Cusack S, Ruigrok RW. Structure of influenza virus RNP. I. Influenza virus nucleoprotein melts secondary structure in panhandle RNA and exposes the bases to the solvent. *EMBO J* (1994) 13(13):3158–65.
7. Compans RW, Content J, Duesberg PH. Structure of the ribonucleoprotein of influenza virus. *J Virol* (1972) 10(4):795–800.
8. Murti KG, Webster RG, Jones IM. Localization of RNA polymerases on influenza viral ribonucleoproteins by immunogold labeling. *Virology* (1988) 164(2):562–6. doi:10.1016/0042-6822(88)90574-0
9. Carr CM, Kim PS. Flu virus invasion: halfway there. *Science* (1994) 266(5183):234–6. doi:10.1126/science.7939658
10. Hernandez LD, Hoffman LR, Wolfsberg TG, White JM. Virus-cell and cell-cell fusion. *Annu Rev Cell Dev Biol* (1996) 12:627–61. doi:10.1146/annurev.cellbio.12.1.627
11. Whittaker GR, Helenius A. Nuclear import and export of viruses and virus genomes. *Virology* (1998) 246(1):1–23. doi:10.1006/viro.1998.9165
12. Zhirnov OP. Isolation of matrix protein M1 from influenza viruses by acid-dependent extraction with nonionic detergent. *Virology* (1992) 186(1):324–30. doi:10.1016/0042-6822(92)90090-C
13. Bui M, Whittaker G, Helenius A. Effect of M1 protein and low pH on nuclear transport of influenza virus ribonucleoproteins. *J Virol* (1996) 70(12):8391–401.
14. Martin K, Helenius A. Transport of incoming influenza virus nucleocapsids into the nucleus. *J Virol* (1991) 65(1):232–44.
15. Scheiffele P, Roth MG, Simons K. Interaction of influenza virus haemagglutinin with sphingolipid-cholesterol membrane domains via its transmembrane domain. *EMBO J* (1997) 16(18):5501–8. doi:10.1093/emboj/16.18.5501
16. Zhang J, Pekosz A, Lamb RA. Influenza virus assembly and lipid raft microdomains: a role for the cytoplasmic tails of the spike glycoproteins. *J Virol* (2000) 74(10):4634–44. doi:10.1128/JVI.74.10.4634-4644.2000
17. Ito T, Suzuki Y, Mitnaul L, Vines A, Kida H, Kawaoka Y. Receptor specificity of influenza A viruses correlates with the agglutination of erythrocytes from different animal species. *Virology* (1997) 227(2):493–9. doi:10.1006/viro.1996.8323
18. Ito T, Suzuki Y, Suzuki T, Takada A, Horimoto T, Wells K, et al. Recognition of N-glycolylneuraminic acid linked to galactose by the alpha2,3 linkage is associated with intestinal replication of influenza A virus in ducks. *J Virol* (2000) 74(19):9300–5. doi:10.1128/JVI.74.19.9300-9305.2000
19. Ryan-Poirier K, Suzuki Y, Bean WJ, Kobasa D, Takada A, Ito T, et al. Changes in H3 influenza A virus receptor specificity during replication in humans. *Virus Res* (1998) 56(2):169–76. doi:10.1016/S0168-1702(98)00067-7
20. Rogers GN, Paulson JC. Receptor determinants of human and animal influenza virus isolates: differences in receptor specificity of the H3 hemagglutinin based on species of origin. *Virology* (1983) 127(2):361–73. doi:10.1016/0042-6822(83)90150-2
21. Baum LG, Paulson JC. Sialyloligosaccharides of the respiratory epithelium in the selection of human influenza virus receptor specificity. *Acta Histochem* (1990) 40:35–8.
22. Suzuki Y, Matsunaga M, Matsumoto M. N-Acetylneuraminyllactosylceramide, GM3-NeuAc, a new influenza A virus receptor which mediates the adsorption-fusion process of viral infection. Binding specificity of influenza virus A/Aichi/2/68 (H3N2) to membrane-associated GM3 with different molecular species of sialic acid. *J Biol Chem* (1985) 260(3):1362–5.
23. Ito T, Suzuki Y, Takada A, Kawamoto A, Otsuki K, Masuda H, et al. Differences in sialic acid-galactose linkages in the chicken egg amnion and allantois influence human influenza virus receptor specificity and variant selection. *J Virol* (1997) 71(4):3357–62.
24. Ito T, Couceiro JN, Kelm S, Baum LG, Krauss S, Castrucci MR, et al. Molecular basis for the generation in pigs of influenza A viruses with pandemic potential. *J Virol* (1998) 72(9):7367–73.
25. Shinde V, Bridges CB, Uyeki TM, Shu B, Balish A, Xu X, et al. Triple-reassortant swine influenza A (H1) in humans in the United States, 2005-2009. *N Engl J Med* (2009) 360(25):2616–25. doi:10.1056/NEJMoa0903812
26. Trifonov V, Khiabanian H, Rabadan R. Geographic dependence, surveillance, and origins of the 2009 influenza A (H1N1) virus. *N Engl J Med* (2009) 361(2):115–9. doi:10.1056/NEJMp0904572
27. Connor RJ, Kawaoka Y, Webster RG, Paulson JC. Receptor specificity in human, avian, and equine H2 and H3 influenza virus isolates. *Virology* (1994) 205(1):17–23. doi:10.1006/viro.1994.1615
28. Rogers GN, D'Souza BL. Receptor binding properties of human and animal H1 influenza virus isolates. *Virology* (1989) 173(1):317–22. doi:10.1016/0042-6822(89)90249-3
29. Imai M, Watanabe T, Hatta M, Das SC, Ozawa M, Shinya K, et al. Experimental adaptation of an influenza H5 HA confers respiratory droplet transmission to a reassortant H5 HA/H1N1 virus in ferrets. *Nature* (2012) 486(7403):420–8. doi:10.1038/nature10831
30. Herfst S, Schrauwen EJ, Linster M, Chutinimitkul S, de Wit E, Munster VJ, et al. Airborne transmission of influenza A/H5N1 virus between ferrets. *Science* (2012) 336(6088):1534–41. doi:10.1126/science.1213362
31. Biasini M, Bienert S, Waterhouse A, Arnold K, Studer G, Schmidt T, et al. SWISS-MODEL: modelling protein tertiary and quaternary structure using evolutionary information. *Nucleic Acids Res* (2014) 42(Web Server issue):W252–8. doi:10.1093/nar/gku340

32. Russier M, Yang G, Rehg JE, Wong SS, Mostafa HH, Fabrizio TP, et al. Molecular requirements for a pandemic influenza virus: an acid-stable hemagglutinin protein. *Proc Natl Acad Sci U S A* (2016) 113(6):1636–41. doi:10.1073/pnas.1524384113
33. Cummings RD, Soderquist AM, Carpenter G. The oligosaccharide moieties of the epidermal growth factor receptor in A-431 cells. Presence of complex-type N-linked chains that contain terminal N-acetylgalactosamine residues. *J Biol Chem* (1985) 260(22):11944–52.
34. Yen HY, Liu YC, Chen NY, Tsai CF, Wang YT, Chen YJ, et al. Effect of sialylation on EGFR phosphorylation and resistance to tyrosine kinase inhibition. *Proc Natl Acad Sci U S A* (2015) 112(22):6955–60. doi:10.1073/pnas.1507329112
35. Hsu AC, Starkey MR, Hanish I, Parsons K, Haw TJ, Howland LJ, et al. Targeting PI3K-p110alpha suppresses influenza virus infection in chronic obstructive pulmonary disease. *Am J Respir Crit Care Med* (2015) 191(9):1012–23. doi:10.1164/rccm.201501-0188OC
36. Kedzierski L, Tate MD, Hsu AC, Kolesnik TB, Linossi EM, Dagley L, et al. Suppressor of cytokine signaling (SOCS)5 ameliorates influenza infection via inhibition of EGFR signaling. *Elife* (2017) 6:e20444. doi:10.7554/eLife.20444
37. Eierhoff T, Hrincius ER, Rescher U, Ludwig S, Ehrhardt C. The epidermal growth factor receptor (EGFR) promotes uptake of influenza A viruses (IAV) into host cells. *PLoS Pathog* (2010) 6(9):e1001099. doi:10.1371/journal.ppat.1001099
38. Glaser L, Conenello G, Paulson J, Palese P. Effective replication of human influenza viruses in mice lacking a major alpha2,6 sialyltransferase. *Virus Res* (2007) 126(1-2):9–18. doi:10.1016/j.virusres.2007.01.011
39. Hsu AC, Barr I, Hansbro PM, Wark PA. Human influenza is more effective than avian influenza at antiviral suppression in airway cells. *Am J Respir Cell Mol Biol* (2011) 44(6):906–13. doi:10.1165/rcmb.2010-0157OC
40. Nunes-Correia I, Eulalio A, Nir S, Pedroso de Lima MC. Caveolae as an additional route for influenza virus endocytosis in MDCK cells. *Cell Mol Biol Lett* (2004) 9(1):47–60.
41. Rapoport EM, Mochalova LV, Gabius HJ, Romanova J, Bovin NV. Search for additional influenza virus to cell interactions. *Glycoconj J* (2006) 23(1-2):115–25. doi:10.1007/s10719-006-5444-x
42. Clements ML, Subbarao EK, Fries LF, Karron RA, London WT, Murphy BR. Use of single-gene reassortant viruses to study the role of avian influenza A virus genes in attenuation of wild-type human influenza A virus for squirrel monkeys and adult human volunteers. *J Clin Microbiol* (1992) 30(3):655–62.
43. Subbarao EK, London W, Murphy BR. A single amino acid in the PB2 gene of influenza A virus is a determinant of host range. *J Virol* (1993) 67(4):1761–4.
44. de Wit E, Munster VJ, van Riel D, Beyer WE, Rimmelzwaan GF, Kuiken T, et al. Molecular determinants of adaptation of highly pathogenic avian influenza H7N7 viruses to efficient replication in the human host. *J Virol* (2010) 84(3):1597–606. doi:10.1128/JVI.01783-09
45. Li Z, Chen H, Jiao P, Deng G, Tian G, Li Y, et al. Molecular basis of replication of duck H5N1 influenza viruses in a mammalian mouse model. *J Virol* (2005) 79(18):12058–64. doi:10.1128/JVI.79.18.12058-12064.2005
46. Gabriel G, Dauber B, Wolff T, Planz O, Klenk HD, Stech J. The viral polymerase mediates adaptation of an avian influenza virus to a mammalian host. *Proc Natl Acad Sci U S A* (2005) 102(51):18590–5. doi:10.1073/pnas.0507415102
47. Le QM, Sakai-Tagawa Y, Ozawa M, Ito M, Kawaoka Y. Selection of H5N1 influenza virus PB2 during replication in humans. *J Virol* (2009) 83(10):5278–81. doi:10.1128/JVI.00063-09
48. Kageyama T, Fujisaki S, Takashita E, Xu H, Yamada S, Uchida Y, et al. Genetic analysis of novel avian A(H7N9) influenza viruses isolated from patients in China, February to April 2013. *Euro Surveill* (2013) 18(15):20453.
49. Gao R, Cao B, Hu Y, Feng Z, Wang D, Hu W, et al. Human infection with a novel avian-origin influenza A (H7N9) virus. *N Engl J Med* (2013) 368(20):1888–97. doi:10.1056/NEJMoa1304459
50. Kawaoka Y, Krauss S, Webster RG. Avian-to-human transmission of the PB1 gene of influenza A viruses in the 1957 and 1968 pandemics. *J Virol* (1989) 63(11):4603–8.
51. Snyder MH, Buckler-White AJ, London WT, Tierney EL, Murphy BR. The avian influenza virus nucleoprotein gene and a specific constellation of avian and human virus polymerase genes each specify attenuation of avian-human influenza A/Pintail/79 reassortant viruses for monkeys. *J Virol* (1987) 61(9):2857–63.
52. Chen W, Calvo PA, Malide D, Gibbs J, Schubert U, Bacik I, et al. A novel influenza A virus mitochondrial protein that induces cell death. *Nat Med* (2001) 7(12):1306–12. doi:10.1038/nm1201-1306
53. Zamarin D, Garcia-Sastre A, Xiao X, Wang R, Palese P. Influenza virus PB1-F2 protein induces cell death through mitochondrial ANT3 and VDAC1. *PLoS Pathog* (2005) 1(1):e4. doi:10.1371/journal.ppat.0010004
54. Yoshizumi T, Ichinohe T, Sasaki O, Otera H, Kawabata S, Mihara K, et al. Influenza A virus protein PB1-F2 translocates into mitochondria via Tom40 channels and impairs innate immunity. *Nat Commun* (2014) 5:4713. doi:10.1038/ncomms5713
55. Gack MU, Shin YC, Joo CH, Urano T, Liang C, Sun L, et al. TRIM25 RING-finger E3 ubiquitin ligase is essential for RIG-I-mediated antiviral activity. *Nature* (2007) 446(7138):916–20. doi:10.1038/nature05732
56. Seth RB, Sun L, Ea CK, Chen ZJ. Identification and characterization of MAVS, a mitochondrial antiviral signaling protein that activates NF-kappaB and IRF 3. *Cell* (2005) 122(5):669–82. doi:10.1016/j.cell.2005.08.012
57. Fitzgerald KA, McWhirter SM, Faia KL, Rowe DC, Latz E, Golenbock DT, et al. IKKepsilon and TBK1 are essential components of the IRF3 signaling pathway. *Nat Immunol* (2003) 4(5):491–6. doi:10.1038/ni921
58. Stark GR, Kerr IM, Williams BR, Silverman RH, Schreiber RD. How cells respond to interferons. *Annu Rev Biochem* (1998) 67:227–64. doi:10.1146/annurev.biochem.67.1.227
59. Alexopoulou L, Holt AC, Medzhitov R, Flavell RA. Recognition of double-stranded RNA and activation of NF-kappaB by toll-like receptor 3. *Nature* (2001) 413(6857):732–8. doi:10.1038/35099560
60. Chaouat A, Savale L, Chouaid C, Tu L, Sztrymf B, Canuet M, et al. Role for interleukin-6 in COPD-related pulmonary hypertension. *Chest* (2009) 136(3):678–87. doi:10.1378/chest.08-2420
61. Takeda K, Kaisho T, Akira S. Toll-like receptors. *Annu Rev Immunol* (2003) 21:335–76. doi:10.1146/annurev.immunol.21.120601.141126
62. Varga ZT, Grant A, Manicassamy B, Palese P. Influenza virus protein PB1-F2 inhibits the induction of type I interferon by binding to MAVS and decreasing mitochondrial membrane potential. *J Virol* (2012) 86(16):8359–66. doi:10.1128/JVI.01122-12
63. Varga ZT, Ramos I, Hai R, Schmolke M, Garcia-Sastre A, Fernandez-Sesma A, et al. The influenza virus protein PB1-F2 inhibits the induction of type I interferon at the level of the MAVS adaptor protein. *PLoS Pathog* (2011) 7(6):e1002067. doi:10.1371/journal.ppat.1002067
64. McAuley JL, Hornung F, Boyd KL, Smith AM, McKeon R, Bennink J, et al. Expression of the 1918 influenza A virus PB1-F2 enhances the pathogenesis of viral and secondary bacterial pneumonia. *Cell Host Microbe* (2007) 2(4):240–9. doi:10.1016/j.chom.2007.09.001
65. Conenello GM, Zamarin D, Perrone LA, Tumpey T, Palese P. A single mutation in the PB1-F2 of H5N1 (HK/97) and 1918 influenza A viruses contributes to increased virulence. *PLoS Pathog* (2007) 3(10):1414–21. doi:10.1371/journal.ppat.0030141
66. McAuley JL, Tate MD, MacKenzie-Kludas CJ, Pinar A, Zeng W, Stutz A, et al. Activation of the NLRP3 inflammasome by IAV virulence protein PB1-F2 contributes to severe pathophysiology and disease. *PLoS Pathog* (2013) 9(5):e1003392. doi:10.1371/journal.ppat.1003392
67. Zamarin D, Ortigoza MB, Palese P. Influenza A virus PB1-F2 protein contributes to viral pathogenesis in mice. *J Virol* (2006) 80(16):7976–83. doi:10.1128/JVI.00415-06
68. Pinar A, Dowling JK, Bitto NJ, Robertson AA, Latz E, Stewart CR, et al. PB1-F2 peptide derived from avian influenza A virus H7N9 induces inflammation via activation of the NLRP3 inflammasome. *J Biol Chem* (2017) 292(3):826–36. doi:10.1074/jbc.M116.756379
69. Chanturiya AN, Basanez G, Schubert U, Henklein P, Yewdell JW, Zimmerberg J. PB1-F2, an influenza A virus-encoded proapoptotic mitochondrial protein, creates variably sized pores in planar lipid membranes. *J Virol* (2004) 78(12):6304–12. doi:10.1128/JVI.78.12.6304-6312.2004
70. Bruns K, Studtrucker N, Sharma A, Fossen T, Mitzner D, Eissmann A, et al. Structural characterization and oligomerization of PB1-F2, a proapoptotic influenza A virus protein. *J Biol Chem* (2007) 282(1):353–63. doi:10.1074/jbc.M606494200
71. Isaacs A, Lindenmann J, Valentine RC. Virus interference. II. Some properties of interferon. *Proc R Soc Lond B Biol Sci* (1957) 147(927):268–73. doi:10.1098/rspb.1957.0049

72. Isaacs A, Lindenmann J. Virus interference. I. The interferon. *Proc R Soc Lond B Biol Sci* (1957) 147(927):258–67. doi:10.1098/rspb.1957.0048
73. Hatada E, Fukuda R. Binding of influenza A virus NS1 protein to dsRNA in vitro. *J Gen Virol* (1992) 73(Pt 12):3325–9. doi:10.1099/0022-1317-73-12-3325
74. Privalsky ML, Penhoet EE. The structure and synthesis of influenza virus phosphoproteins. *J Biol Chem* (1981) 256(11):5368–76.
75. Chien CY, Xu Y, Xiao R, Aramini JM, Sahasrabudhe PV, Krug RM, et al. Biophysical characterization of the complex between double-stranded RNA and the N-terminal domain of the NS1 protein from influenza A virus: evidence for a novel RNA-binding mode. *Biochemistry* (2004) 43(7):1950–62. doi:10.1021/bi030176o
76. Qian XY, Chien CY, Lu Y, Montelione GT, Krug RM. An amino-terminal polypeptide fragment of the influenza virus NS1 protein possesses specific RNA-binding activity and largely helical backbone structure. *RNA* (1995) 1(9):948–56.
77. Chen Z, Li Y, Krug RM. Influenza A virus NS1 protein targets poly(A)-binding protein II of the cellular 3'-end processing machinery. *EMBO J* (1999) 18(8):2273–83. doi:10.1093/emboj/18.8.2273
78. Nemeroff ME, Barabino SM, Li Y, Keller W, Krug RM. Influenza virus NS1 protein interacts with the cellular 30 kDa subunit of CPSF and inhibits 3' end formation of cellular pre-mRNAs. *Mol Cell* (1998) 1(7):991–1000. doi:10.1016/S1097-2765(00)80099-4
79. Noah DL, Twu KY, Krug RM. Cellular antiviral responses against influenza A virus are countered at the posttranscriptional level by the viral NS1A protein via its binding to a cellular protein required for the 3' end processing of cellular pre-mRNAS. *Virology* (2003) 307(2):386–95. doi:10.1016/S0042-6822(02)00127-7
80. Marazzi I, Ho JS, Kim J, Manicassamy B, Dewell S, Albrecht RA, et al. Suppression of the antiviral response by an influenza histone mimic. *Nature* (2012) 483(7390):428–33. doi:10.1038/nature10892
81. Mibayashi M, Martinez-Sobrido L, Loo YM, Cardenas WB, Gale M Jr, Garcia-Sastre A. Inhibition of retinoic acid-inducible gene I-mediated induction of beta interferon by the NS1 protein of influenza A virus. *J Virol* (2007) 81(2):514–24. doi:10.1128/JVI.01265-06
82. Talon J, Horvath CM, Polley R, Basler CF, Muster T, Palese P, et al. Activation of interferon regulatory factor 3 is inhibited by the influenza A virus NS1 protein. *J Virol* (2000) 74(17):7989–96. doi:10.1128/JVI.74.17.7989-7996.2000
83. Gack MU, Albrecht RA, Urano T, Inn KS, Huang IC, Carnero E, et al. Influenza A virus NS1 targets the ubiquitin ligase TRIM25 to evade recognition by the host viral RNA sensor RIG-I. *Cell Host Microbe* (2009) 5(5):439–49. doi:10.1016/j.chom.2009.04.006
84. Bornholdt ZA, Prasad BV. X-ray structure of NS1 from a highly pathogenic H5N1 influenza virus. *Nature* (2008) 456(7224):985–8. doi:10.1038/nature07444
85. Wang X, Basler CF, Williams BR, Silverman RH, Palese P, Garcia-Sastre A. Functional replacement of the carboxy-terminal two-thirds of the influenza A virus NS1 protein with short heterologous dimerization domains. *J Virol* (2002) 76(24):12951–62. doi:10.1128/JVI.76.24.12951-12962.2002
86. Lu Y, Wambach M, Katze MG, Krug RM. Binding of the influenza virus NS1 protein to double-stranded RNA inhibits the activation of the protein kinase that phosphorylates the elF-2 translation initiation factor. *Virology* (1995) 214(1):222–8. doi:10.1006/viro.1995.9937
87. Bergmann M, Garcia-Sastre A, Carnero E, Pehamberger H, Wolff K, Palese P, et al. Influenza virus NS1 protein counteracts PKR-mediated inhibition of replication. *J Virol* (2000) 74(13):6203–6. doi:10.1128/JVI.74.13.6203-6206.2000
88. Dauber B, Schneider J, Wolff T. Double-stranded RNA binding of influenza B virus nonstructural NS1 protein inhibits protein kinase R but is not essential to antagonize production of alpha/beta interferon. *J Virol* (2006) 80(23):11667–77. doi:10.1128/JVI.01142-06
89. Li S, Min JY, Krug RM, Sen GC. Binding of the influenza A virus NS1 protein to PKR mediates the inhibition of its activation by either PACT or double-stranded RNA. *Virology* (2006) 349(1):13–21. doi:10.1016/j.virol.2006.01.005
90. Min JY, Li S, Sen GC, Krug RM. A site on the influenza A virus NS1 protein mediates both inhibition of PKR activation and temporal regulation of viral RNA synthesis. *Virology* (2007) 363(1):236–43. doi:10.1016/j.virol.2007.01.038
91. Min JY, Krug RM. The primary function of RNA binding by the influenza A virus NS1 protein in infected cells: inhibiting the 2'-5' oligo (A) synthetase/RNase L pathway. *Proc Natl Acad Sci U S A* (2006) 103(18):7100–5. doi:10.1073/pnas.0602184103
92. Hale BG, Jackson D, Chen YH, Lamb RA, Randall RE. Influenza A virus NS1 protein binds p85beta and activates phosphatidylinositol-3-kinase signaling. *Proc Natl Acad Sci U S A* (2006) 103(38):14194–9. doi:10.1073/pnas.0606109103
93. Li Y, Anderson DH, Liu Q, Zhou Y. Mechanism of influenza A virus NS1 protein interaction with the p85beta, but not the p85alpha, subunit of phosphatidylinositol 3-kinase (PI3K) and up-regulation of PI3K activity. *J Biol Chem* (2008) 283(34):23397–409. doi:10.1074/jbc.M802737200
94. Shin YK, Li Y, Liu Q, Anderson DH, Babiuk LA, Zhou Y. SH3 binding motif 1 in influenza A virus NS1 protein is essential for PI3K/Akt signaling pathway activation. *J Virol* (2007) 81(23):12730–9. doi:10.1128/JVI.01427-07
95. Kochs G, Koerner I, Thiel L, Kothlow S, Kaspers B, Ruggli N, et al. Properties of H7N7 influenza A virus strain SC35M lacking interferon antagonist NS1 in mice and chickens. *J Gen Virol* (2007) 88(Pt 5):1403–9. doi:10.1099/vir.0.82764-0
96. Cauthen AN, Swayne DE, Sekellick MJ, Marcus PI, Suarez DL. Amelioration of influenza virus pathogenesis in chickens attributed to the enhanced interferon-inducing capacity of a virus with a truncated NS1 gene. *J Virol* (2007) 81(4):1838–47. doi:10.1128/JVI.01667-06
97. Solorzano A, Webby RJ, Lager KM, Janke BH, Garcia-Sastre A, Richt JA. Mutations in the NS1 protein of swine influenza virus impair anti-interferon activity and confer attenuation in pigs. *J Virol* (2005) 79(12):7535–43. doi:10.1128/JVI.79.12.7535-7543.2005
98. Zhu Q, Yang H, Chen W, Cao W, Zhong G, Jiao P, et al. A naturally occurring deletion in its NS gene contributes to the attenuation of an H5N1 swine influenza virus in chickens. *J Virol* (2008) 82(1):220–8. doi:10.1128/JVI.00978-07
99. Twu KY, Kuo RL, Marklund J, Krug RM. The H5N1 influenza virus NS genes selected after 1998 enhance virus replication in mammalian cells. *J Virol* (2007) 81(15):8112–21. doi:10.1128/JVI.00006-07
100. Hsu AC, Parsons K, Barr I, Lowther S, Middleton D, Hansbro PM, et al. Critical role of constitutive type I interferon response in bronchial epithelial cell to influenza infection. *PLoS One* (2012) 7(3):e32947. doi:10.1371/journal.pone.0032947
101. Chambers BS, Parkhouse K, Ross TM, Alby K, Hensley SE. Identification of hemagglutinin residues responsible for H3N2 antigenic drift during the 2014-2015 influenza season. *Cell Rep* (2015) 12(1):1–6. doi:10.1016/j.celrep.2015.06.005
102. Nguyen-Van-Tam JS, Venkatesan S, Muthuri SG, Myles PR. Neuraminidase inhibitors: who, when, where? *Clin Microbiol Infect* (2015) 21(3):222–5. doi:10.1016/j.cmi.2014.11.020
103. Wolkewitz M, Schumacher M. Neuraminidase inhibitors and hospital mortality in British patients with H1N1 influenza A: a re-analysis of observational data. *PLoS One* (2016) 11(9):e0160430. doi:10.1371/journal.pone.0160430
104. Chen Q, Guo Y. Influenza viral hemagglutinin peptide inhibits influenza viral entry by shielding the host receptor. *ACS Infect Dis* (2016) 2(3):187–93. doi:10.1021/acsinfecdis.5b00139
105. Jones JC, Turpin EA, Bultmann H, Brandt CR, Schultz-Cherry S. Inhibition of influenza virus infection by a novel antiviral peptide that targets viral attachment to cells. *J Virol* (2006) 80(24):11960–7. doi:10.1128/JVI.01678-06
106. Nicol MQ, Ligertwood Y, Bacon MN, Dutia BM, Nash AA. A novel family of peptides with potent activity against influenza A viruses. *J Gen Virol* (2012) 93(Pt 5):980–6. doi:10.1099/vir.0.038679-0
107. Cederlund A, Gudmundsson GH, Agerberth B. Antimicrobial peptides important in innate immunity. *FEBS J* (2011) 278(20):3942–51. doi:10.1111/j.1742-4658.2011.08302.x
108. Gutsmann T, Razquin-Olazaran I, Kowalski I, Kaconis Y, Howe J, Bartels R, et al. New antiseptic peptides to protect against endotoxin-mediated shock. *Antimicrob Agents Chemother* (2010) 54(9):3817–24. doi:10.1128/AAC.00534-10
109. Hoffmann J, Schneider C, Heinbockel L, Brandenburg K, Reimer R, Gabriel G. A new class of synthetic anti-lipopolysaccharide peptides inhibits influenza A virus replication by blocking cellular attachment. *Antiviral Res* (2014) 104:23–33. doi:10.1016/j.antiviral.2014.01.015
110. Ghanem A, Mayer D, Chase G, Tegge W, Frank R, Kochs G, et al. Peptide-mediated interference with influenza A virus polymerase. *J Virol* (2007) 81(14):7801–4. doi:10.1128/JVI.00724-07
111. Li C, Ba Q, Wu A, Zhang H, Deng T, Jiang T. A peptide derived from the C-terminus of PB1 inhibits influenza virus replication by interfering with viral polymerase assembly. *FEBS J* (2013) 280(4):1139–49. doi:10.1111/febs.12107

112. Fleishman SJ, Whitehead TA, Ekiert DC, Dreyfus C, Corn JE, Strauch EM, et al. Computational design of proteins targeting the conserved stem region of influenza hemagglutinin. *Science* (2011) 332(6031):816–21. doi:10.1126/science.1202617
113. Whitehead TA, Chevalier A, Song Y, Dreyfus C, Fleishman SJ, De Mattos C, et al. Optimization of affinity, specificity and function of designed influenza inhibitors using deep sequencing. *Nat Biotechnol* (2012) 30(6):543–8. doi:10.1038/nbt.2214
114. Kadam RU, Juraszek J, Brandenburg B, Buyck C, Schepens WBG, Kesteleyn B, et al. Potent peptidic fusion inhibitors of influenza virus. *Science* (2017) 358(6362):496–502. doi:10.1126/science.aan0516

13

A Review of DNA Vaccines Against Influenza

*Leo Yi Yang Lee, Leonard Izzard and Aeron C. Hurt**

World Health Organisation Collaborating Centre for Reference and Research on Influenza at the Peter Doherty Institute, Melbourne, VIC, Australia

***Correspondence:**
Aeron C. Hurt
aeron.hurt@influenzacentre.org

The challenges of effective vaccination against influenza are gaining more mainstream attention, as recent influenza seasons have reported low efficacy in annual vaccination programs worldwide. Combined with the potential emergence of novel influenza viruses resulting in a pandemic, the need for effective alternatives to egg-produced conventional vaccines has been made increasingly clear. DNA vaccines against influenza have been in development since the 1990s, but the initial excitement over success in murine model trials has been tempered by comparatively poor performance in larger animal models. In the intervening years, much progress has been made to refine the DNA vaccine platform—the rational design of antigens and expression vectors, the development of novel vaccine adjuvants, and the employment of innovative gene delivery methods. This review discusses how these advances have been applied in recent efforts to develop an effective influenza DNA vaccine.

Keywords: DNA vaccine, influenza, adjuvant, hemagglutinin, immunization

INTRODUCTION

Seasonal influenza epidemics continue to challenge public health systems worldwide, causing 3–5 million cases of severe respiratory disease and 290–650 thousand deaths annually (1). Despite annual updates to the seasonal vaccine, in 2017 overall vaccine effectiveness for Australia was estimated to be only 33% (2), and interim estimates from the United States were similarly low for the 2017–2018 influenza seasons (36%) (3). In addition, current seasonal vaccines provide little or no protection against novel pandemic viruses of animal origin (4). Consequently, research efforts have increased to improve seasonal vaccines and develop new vaccine platforms to achieve better protection against both seasonal and potentially pandemic influenza A viruses.

DNA vaccines possess numerous properties ideal for influenza control and have been trialled for a range of diseases, including viral and bacterial infections, and some cancers (5–7). Whilst inactivated influenza vaccines (IIVs) largely rely on antibody production to achieve effective protection (8), DNA vaccines can efficiently engage both humoral and cell-mediated immune responses (9). Their production does not require the growth of live virus and can be rapidly upscaled in response to emerging pandemic influenza (10, 11). Despite these advantages, promising immunogenic responses achieved in small animal models, predominantly mice, are rarely replicated in larger animals (12, 13). Murine model data are based on immune responses in highly inbred animals to mouse-adapted influenza viruses—an unreliable comparison to vaccination in the outbred human population against circulating influenza viruses (14, 15). Larger animal models susceptible to human influenza virus provide more relevant data—ferrets exhibit clinical signs, lung pathology, and transmission similar to humans (16, 17), whist human-like immune responses to influenza in cynomolgus macaques are good predictors of vaccine efficacy in humans (15, 18). As such, achieving sufficient immunogenicity in larger animals has required the development of potent delivery systems and adjuvants (19, 20). This review summarises innovations in the design, formulation, and delivery of DNA vaccines against influenza, and the major obstacles impeding their implementation (**Figure 1**).

INFLUENZA VACCINES: PRODUCTION AND MECHANISMS OF PROTECTION

Inactivated influenza vaccines and live attenuated influenza vaccines (LAIV) are the most widely used forms of influenza vaccine, and are generated by harvesting viruses grown in embryonated hen's eggs (21). The delivery of viral antigens derived from this process induces the production of antigen-specific antibodies, particularly against the haemagglutinin (HA) surface glycoprotein, to protect against future infections (22). However, egg-based vaccine production is time-consuming and resource-intensive, and manufacturing delays have previously caused severe vaccine shortages (23, 24). The overall vaccine effectiveness against seasonal influenza ranges from 40 to 60% during typical seasons, but is significantly reduced when antigenic mismatch occurs (25, 26). Furthermore, antigenic mismatch can be exacerbated by mutations which allow vaccine viruses to grow in eggs, which may also alter antigenic sites (27).

DNA vaccines are able to avoid many issues associated with egg-based vaccine production by generating viral proteins within host cells. To create a DNA vaccine, an antigen-encoding gene is cloned into a non-replicative expression plasmid, which is delivered to the host by traditional vaccination routes (28). Host cells which take up the plasmid express the vaccine antigen which can be presented to immune cells *via* the major histocompatibility complex (MHC) pathways. CD4+ T helper cell activation following MHC class II presentation of secreted DNA vaccine protein is critical for the production of antigen-specific antibodies (29),

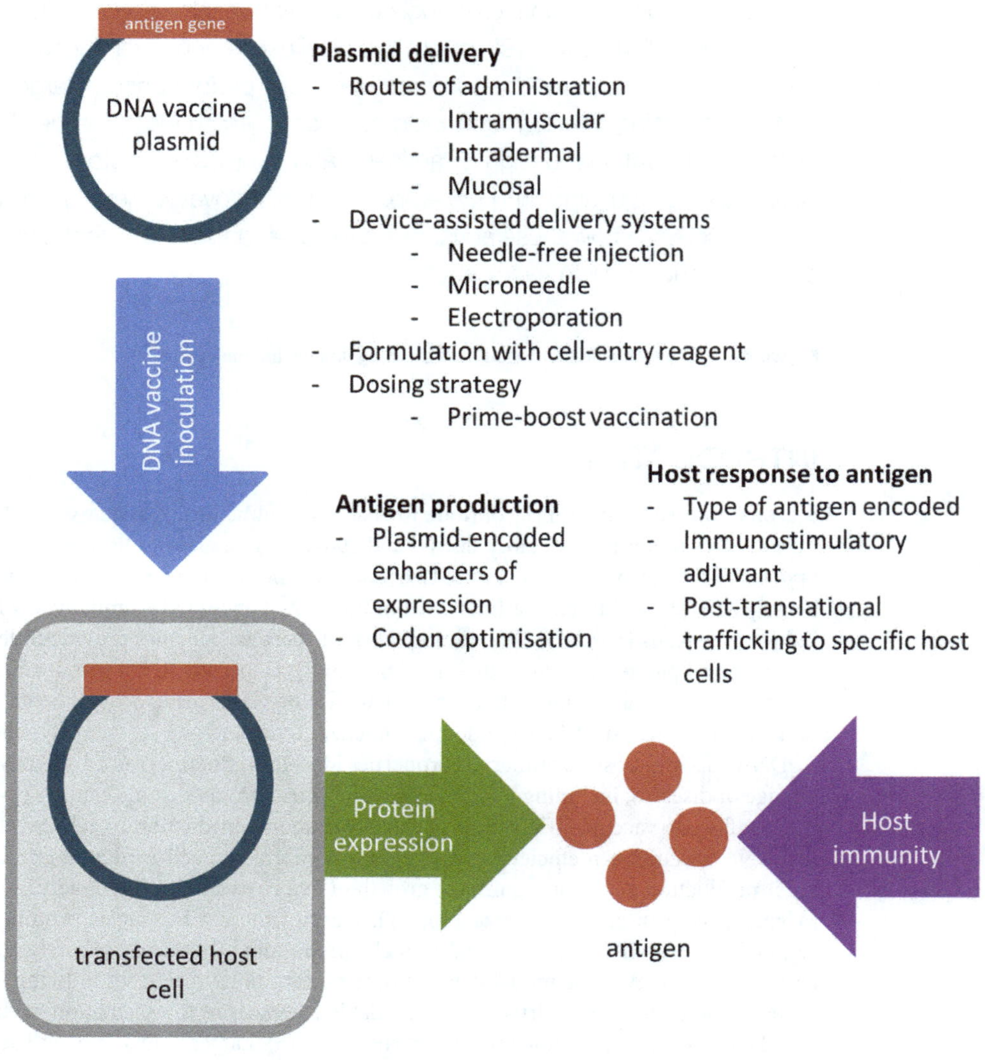

FIGURE 1 | Key factors considered in the design, formulation, and inoculation of DNA vaccines to improve *in vivo* transfection efficiency and antigen immunogenicity.

whist CD8+ T cell immunity, important for viral clearance, is predominantly activated by endogenously expressed antigens presented on MHC class I molecules (30).

DESIGNING ANTIGENS FOR INFLUENZA DNA VACCINES

The protection conferred by conventional IIV is based on the induction of HA-specific serum antibodies, which interfere with virus attachment to inhibit cell entry and limit infection (8, 31). Early mouse studies using DNA vaccines encoding H1 HA genes reported that protection against lethal homologous challenge correlated with increasing titres of HA-specific serum antibody (32, 33). As observed in LAIV, other correlates of immunity are less well defined, but the induction of local inflammation and cytotoxic T cell responses have been implicated as key mechanisms to enhance vaccine cross-reactivity and reduce the severity of infections (34, 35). As such, the nature of the host response to influenza DNA vaccination can be manipulated by the encoded antigen.

"Universal" influenza vaccines are being developed to induce broadly protective responses against drifted variant viruses and animal-origin strains that may result in a pandemic. Protection induced by evolutionarily stable influenza antigens is associated with viral clearance mediated by broadly reactive cytotoxic CD8+ T cells, reducing the severity of clinical disease (36). Candidate universal influenza vaccine targets include the nucleoprotein (NP), matrix proteins (M1 and M2), and the RNA-directed RNA polymerase catalytic subunit (PB1). Individual plasmids encoding NP (37) and M2 (38) have each been reported to decrease viral load and enhance survival against lethal heterologous challenge viruses in BALB/c mice. Combined immunisation with matrix protein, NP, and PB1 plasmids has been reported to induce protection against heterologous challenge in mice (39), pigs (40), ferrets (41), and macaques (42). Chimeric protein antigens designed to increase the breadth of host responses can be delivered by DNA vaccines. Plasmid-encoded fusion proteins of H1N1 HA and the conserved M2-ectodomain improved the cross-reactivity of antibody responses to drifted H1N1 viruses compared to a plasmid encoding HA alone in mice (43).

Attempts to create HA-based universal influenza vaccines have targeted the conserved stem region of the HA protein (31). Mice vaccinated with plasmids encoding a PR8 "headless HA" antigen developed serum antibody responses to a greater range of influenza viruses than wild-type HA DNA-vaccinated animals (44). The expression of consensus HA sequences has also increased the cross-reactivity of antibody responses (45–47). Chen et al. (48) constructed a plasmid encoding a consensus H5 HA generated from 467 HA sequences, which induced protection against a wide spectrum of lethal H5N1 reassortant challenge viruses in mice. Broadly reactive responses have also been induced using polyvalent formulations similar to currently available trivalent and quadrivalent IIVs (26). Huber et al. (49) generated cross-reactive antibodies against multiple H3 drift variants in mice by vaccinating with three different H3-expressing plasmids. Rao et al. (50) achieved similar success against several variant H5N1 viruses in chickens using vaccines containing up to 10 different H5 HA plasmids.

Efficient antigen expression *in situ* is a key factor for DNA vaccine effectiveness which can be modulated by altering the antigen coding sequence. Encoding antigens using codons optimised for expressing within the host species is a commonly used strategy to enhance influenza DNA vaccine expression (51–53). Jiang et al. (54) used a lethal H5N1 challenge model in chickens to compare the protective efficacy of DNA vaccines encoding either the wild-type HA or HA codon-optimised for chickens. Chickens receiving the codon-optimised HA plasmid demonstrated up to fourfold increases in antibody titre compared to animals inoculated with wild-type HA plasmids, resulting in greater survival rates during viral challenge.

DNA vaccine antigen design can direct the post-translational trafficking of expressed proteins to influence the development of host immunity. The human tissue plasminogen activator leader sequence promotes high levels of protein secretion and has improved antibody responses to an H5 HA DNA vaccine in rabbits (55). Grodeland et al. (29) encoded DNA vaccine antigens consisting of H1 HA linked to MHC class II-targeting units which enhanced its delivery to antigen-presenting cells (APCs). Ferrets and pigs vaccinated with plasmids expressing the targeted H1 fusion protein generated significant antibody titres, whereas H1 DNA alone failed to cause seroconversion. A similar DNA vaccine strategy expressing APC-targeted H7 fusion proteins was found to improve anti-HA serum antibody and cytotoxic T cell responses to highly pathogenic avian influenza (56).

DNA VACCINE DELIVERY PLATFORMS

For influenza DNA vaccines, the route of administration is critical to vaccine effectiveness as it dictates the cell types that will be transfected. DNA vaccines were initially tested in the murine model using intramuscular injection of naked plasmids to produce antigens in passively transfected myocytes (muscle cells) (57). This method relies on the influx of leucocytes following local inflammation to expose the immune system to DNA vaccine antigens (58). Outside of the murine model, effective intramuscular administration of plasmids depends on adjuvants and delivery systems to achieve sufficient immunogenicity (59). More recently, cutaneous delivery has become a highly desirable route for DNA vaccines, as the epidermis is abundant in Langerhans cells, which can efficiently transport and present DNA vaccine-encoded antigens in the lymph node (58).

Alternative delivery devices have been developed to improve upon traditional needle and syringe inoculation for parenteral administration. In small animal models, the gene gun induces immune responses successfully with low doses of DNA by delivering gas-propelled plasmid-coated gold microparticles directly into epidermal cells (60, 61). Human clinical trials of influenza DNA vaccines have successfully employed the Biojector system (iHealthNet, GA, USA), which uses pressurised CO_2 to transport a liquid inoculum to the intradermal or intramuscular layer (62–64). Recently, the development of patches composed of micron-length needles has enabled the dermal delivery of lyophilised DNA vaccine (65–67). HA DNA vaccination in mice using dry-coated microneedle patches were reported to induce antibody titres and T cell responses up to five times higher than an equivalent intramuscular dose (68).

Parenteral gene delivery has been further enhanced by electroporation, which temporarily increases the permeability of local cell membranes with electrical pulses (69). Its early use alongside intramuscular delivery required highly invasive electrodes associated with excessive inflammation and the production of lesions (70). Updated devices such as the CELLECTRA system (Inovio, PA, USA) can target the dermal and subcutaneous layers and are optimised to be minimally invasive for clinical use (71). Electroporation has been reported to enable influenza DNA vaccines to generate robust antibody titres and T cell responses in guinea pigs (72), swine (73), and macaques (47, 74).

The mucosa is an appealing site of inoculation for influenza vaccines as it is easily accessible and is the clinical site of entry for influenza viruses (75). Existing mucosal influenza vaccines such as FluMist (MedImmune, MD, USA) mediate protection through local mucosal inflammation and the production of secretory IgA (34, 76). The enrichment of dendritic cells and M cells at mucosal surfaces is ideal for the immune presentation of DNA vaccine antigens (77, 78). However, successful mucosal delivery of plasmids in large animal models requires specialised adjuvants or highly optimised delivery systems (79, 80). Torrieri-Dramard et al. (81) reported that an intranasal HA DNA vaccine failed to elicit detectable IgA titres unless the plasmid was complexed with a polyethylenimine nanocarrier. To induce detectable seroconversion in sheep, Rajapaksa et al. (82) used a novel acoustic nebuliser to produce aerosols of an optimal size to deliver HA plasmids to deep lung tissue.

ADJUVANTS

The co-administration of adjuvants with influenza DNA vaccines is a common strategy to elicit adequate levels of protection *in vivo*. The mechanisms of action for licensed conventional adjuvants include the formation of antigen depot at the inoculation site, the activation of inflammatory pathways, and the recruitment of APCs (83).

The goal of adjuvant design is to increase the immune response to vaccine antigens, a critical hurdle in the DNA vaccine field. Mineral salts such as alum are widely used in human vaccines and have resulted in up to fivefold increase in HA DNA vaccine-induced antibody titres (84). Cytokine expression vectors exploit host signalling pathways to heighten immune stimulation (85). IL-6 is an important inflammatory mediator involved in B cell stimulation and the recruitment of leucocytes (86, 87). Co-administration of an IL-6-expressing plasmid in HA DNA-vaccinated mice has been reported to reduce the duration of influenza illness (88). Lee et al. (60) reported that only 50% of HA and NP DNA-vaccinated mice survived a lethal homologous challenge, whereas mice receiving the additional IL-6-expressing plasmid were fully protected. The cytokine activity of high mobility group box 1 protein has been shown to increase the survival of mice vaccinated with NP DNA in a homologous viral challenge, and has been found to enhance antibody production induced by HA DNA vaccines by twofold (89). Cytokine adjuvants have also demonstrated effectiveness in large animal models such as macaques, where the use of adjuvant plasmids encoding GM-CSF, a potent immune cell proliferation and differentiation factor, resulted in up to fivefold increases in the serum antibody titre compared to a HA DNA vaccine delivered alone (90).

Adjuvant compounds developed as delivery reagents aim to improve the transfection efficiency of DNA vaccine plasmids. The efficiency of the cellular uptake of DNA vaccines is determined by cell membrane permeability and the susceptibility of foreign DNA to host enzymes. It is estimated that only 1% of a naked plasmid inoculation is able to reach the nuclei of target cells for protein expression—most plasmids remain in the extracellular space to be cleared by host processes (91). Synthetic nanocarriers form structures that protect DNA from host enzymes and facilitate its entry through the cell membrane lipid bilayer (85). Cationic lipids form vesicles known as liposomes, which interact electrostatically with negatively charged DNA to form lipoplexes that efficiently enter host cells through endocytosis (92). Vaxfectin (Vical, San Diego) is a cationic lipid-based system that has boosted influenza DNA vaccine immunogenicity in numerous large animal models (93–95). Other nanoparticle-forming polymers have been reported to enhance influenza DNA vaccine formulation including poly(lactic-co-glycolic) acid (96, 97), chitosan (98), and polyethylenimine (81).

PRIME-BOOST STRATEGIES

The administration of novel vaccine types including adenovirus vectors (99, 100), subviral particles (101), and recombinant protein antigens (102) in combination with conventional influenza vaccines has been reported to enhance seroconversion and antibody cross-reactivity. Wang et al. (103) demonstrated that a primary HA DNA vaccine followed by a seasonal trivalent inactivated vaccine (TIV) boost induced significantly higher antibody titres compared to two doses of either DNA vaccine or TIV in rabbits. Similar results have reported using DNA vaccines to prime LAIV in ferrets (104) and recombinant HA-protein vaccine in chickens (105). However, human trials applying this strategy against circulating seasonal influenza failed to significantly improve seroconversion compared to TIV alone (106, 107).

Despite this, studies have indicated that DNA vaccines may have a clinical application in pandemic settings. Chang et al. (108) demonstrated that mice which had been pre-exposed to H1N1 were significantly protected from lethal H5N1 challenge after DNA vaccination with H5N1 NP- and M1-expressing plasmids. Given the commonality of H1N1 exposure amongst the public, this suggests DNA vaccines could be rapidly deployed to protect a large susceptible population against H5N1 outbreaks. During the 2009 pandemic, a Phase 1 human clinical trial was conducted using an A(H1N1)pdm09 DNA vaccine produced 2 months before the licensed monovalent inactivated vaccine (MIV) (64). Seroconversion was observed in 30% of recipients after three doses of DNA vaccine delivered by Biojector, and the response rate rose to 72% after a booster dose of MIV. Similar human trials of DNA prime-MIV boost vaccines against H5N1 (109) and H7N9 (110) have reported significant improvements in antibody responses compared to MIV alone, indicating that DNA vaccines can effectively prime the immune system against viruses where there is low pre-existing immunity in the population. These recent developments indicate the potential for further research into combined DNA vaccine/IIV strategies as viable control measures against novel influenza outbreaks.

FUTURE PROSPECTS

After two decades of research, DNA vaccine technology is gaining maturity—several veterinary DNA vaccines are currently licensed for West Nile virus and melanoma (111), and significantly, the first commercial DNA vaccine against H5N1 in chickens has recently been conditionally approved by the USDA (112). In addition ongoing large animal trials of DNA vaccines against other diseases such as against HIV (6, 113, 114), hepatitis (115, 116), and Zika virus (117, 118) offer valuable insights that can be applied to influenza DNA vaccine design. Promising approaches have arisen from the numerous studies evaluating different DNA vaccine formulations and delivery systems, but a strategy that consistently elicits protection against influenza in large animal models has not yet emerged. Successful plasmid delivery and the use of appropriate adjuvants remain key challenges that need to be addressed before influenza DNA vaccines become effective for human use.

AUTHOR CONTRIBUTIONS

All authors listed have made a substantial, direct, and intellectual contribution to the work and approved it for publication.

ACKNOWLEDGMENTS

We would like to thank Paulina Koszalka for editing and critiquing early drafts of this review.

REFERENCES

1. WHO. *Influenza (Seasonal) – Fact Sheet.* Geneva: World Health Organisation Media Centre (2018). Available from: http://www.who.int/mediacentre/factsheets/fs211/en/ (Accessed: April 17, 2018).
2. Sullivan SG, Chilver MB, Carville KS, Deng YM, Grant KA, Higgins G, et al. Low interim influenza vaccine effectiveness, Australia, 1 May to 24 September 2017. *Euro Surveill* (2017) 22(43):17-00707. doi:10.2807/1560-7917.ES.2017.22.43.17-00707
3. Flannery B, Chung JR, Belongia EA, Mclean HQ, Gaglani M, Murthy K, et al. Interim estimates of 2017–18 seasonal influenza vaccine effectiveness – United States, February 2018. *MMWR Morb Mortal Wkly Rep* (2018) 67:180–5. doi:10.15585/mmwr.mm6706a2
4. Dos Santos G, Neumeier E, Bekkat-Berkani R. Influenza: can we cope better with the unpredictable? *Hum Vaccin Immunother* (2016) 12:699–708. doi:10.1080/21645515.2015.1086047
5. Bruffaerts N, Huygen K, Romano M. DNA vaccines against tuberculosis. *Expert Opin Biol Ther* (2014) 14:1801–13. doi:10.1517/14712598.2014.951630
6. Mann JF, Mckay PF, Fiserova A, Klein K, Cope A, Rogers P, et al. Enhanced immunogenicity of an HIV-1 DNA vaccine delivered with electroporation via combined intramuscular and intradermal routes. *J Virol* (2014) 88:6959–69. doi:10.1128/JVI.00183-14
7. Yang B, Jeang J, Yang A, Wu TC, Hung C-F. DNA vaccine for cancer immunotherapy. *Hum Vaccin Immunother* (2014) 10:3153–64. doi:10.4161/21645515.2014.980686
8. Rimmelzwaan GF, McElhaney JE. Correlates of protection: novel generations of influenza vaccines. *Vaccine* (2008) 26:D41–4. doi:10.1016/j.vaccine.2008.07.043
9. Stachyra A, Gora-Sochacka A, Sirko A. DNA vaccines against influenza. *Acta Biochim Pol* (2014) 61:515–22.
10. Williams JA. Vector design for improved DNA vaccine efficacy, safety and production. *Vaccines (Basel)* (2013) 1:225–49. doi:10.3390/vaccines1030225
11. Xenopoulos A, Pattnaik P. Production and purification of plasmid DNA vaccines: is there scope for further innovation? *Expert Rev Vaccines* (2014) 13:1537–51. doi:10.1586/14760584.2014.968556
12. Gerdts V, Wilson HL, Meurens F, Van Drunen Littel-Van Den Hurk S, Wilson D, Walker S, et al. Large animal models for vaccine development and testing. *ILAR J* (2015) 56:53–62. doi:10.1093/ilar/ilv009
13. Porter KR, Raviprakash K. DNA vaccine delivery and improved immunogenicity. *Curr Issues Mol Biol* (2017) 22:129–38. doi:10.21775/cimb.022.129
14. van der Laan JW, Herberts C, Lambkin-Williams R, Boyers A, Mann AJ, Oxford J. Animal models in influenza vaccine testing. *Expert Rev Vaccines* (2008) 7:783. doi:10.1586/14760584.7.6.783
15. Bodewes R, Rimmelzwaan GF, Osterhaus ADME. Animal models for the preclinical evaluation of candidate influenza vaccines. *Expert Rev Vaccines* (2010) 9:59–72. doi:10.1586/erv.09.148
16. Munster VJ, De Wit E, Van Den Brand JMA, Herfst S, Schrauwen EJA, Bestebroer TM, et al. Pathogenesis and transmission of Swine-Origin 2009 A(H1N1) influenza virus in ferrets. *Science* (2009) 325:481–3. doi:10.1126/science.1177127
17. Belser JA, Katz JM, Tumpey TM. The ferret as a model organism to study influenza A virus infection. *Dis Model Mech* (2011) 4:575–9. doi:10.1242/dmm.007823
18. Rimmelzwaan GF, Katz JM. Immune responses to infection with H5N1 influenza virus. *Virus Res* (2013) 178:44–52. doi:10.1016/j.virusres.2013.05.011
19. Grunwald T, Ulbert S. Improvement of DNA vaccination by adjuvants and sophisticated delivery devices: vaccine-platforms for the battle against infectious diseases. *Clin Exp Vaccine Res* (2015) 4:1–10. doi:10.7774/cevr.2015.4.1.1
20. Li L, Petrovsky N. Molecular mechanisms for enhanced DNA vaccine immunogenicity. *Expert Rev Vaccines* (2016) 15:313–29. doi:10.1586/14760584.2016.1124762
21. Wong S-S, Webby RJ. Traditional and new influenza vaccines. *Clin Microbiol Rev* (2013) 26:476–92. doi:10.1128/CMR.00097-12
22. Schultz-Cherry S, Jones JC. Influenza vaccines: the good, the bad, and the eggs. *Adv Virus Res* (2010) 77:63–84. doi:10.1016/B978-0-12-385034-8.00003-X
23. Kempe A, Daley MF, Stokley S, Crane LA, Beaty BL, Barrow J, et al. Impact of a severe influenza vaccine shortage on primary care practice. *Am J Prev Med* (2007) 33:486–91. doi:10.1016/j.amepre.2007.07.038
24. Uscher-Pines L, Barnett DJ, Sapsin JW, Bishai DM, Balicer RD. A systematic analysis of influenza vaccine shortage policies. *Public Health* (2008) 122:183–91. doi:10.1016/j.puhe.2007.06.005
25. Tewawong N, Prachayangprecha S, Vichiwattana P, Korkong S, Klinfueng S, Vongpunsawad S, et al. Assessing antigenic drift of seasonal influenza A(H3N2) and A(H1N1)pdm09 viruses. *PLoS One* (2015) 10:e0139958. doi:10.1371/journal.pone.0139958
26. Zimmerman RK, Nowalk MP, Chung J, Jackson ML, Jackson LA, Petrie JG, et al. 2014–2015 influenza vaccine effectiveness in the United States by vaccine type. *Clin Infect Dis* (2016) 63:1564–73. doi:10.1093/cid/ciw635

27. Parker L, Wharton SA, Martin SR, Cross K, Lin Y, Liu Y, et al. Effects of egg-adaptation on receptor-binding and antigenic properties of recent influenza A (H3N2) vaccine viruses. *J Gen Virol* (2016) 97:1333–44. doi:10.1099/jgv.0.000457
28. Leitner WW, Ying H, Restifo NP. DNA and RNA-based vaccines: principles, progress and prospects. *Vaccine* (1999) 18:765–77. doi:10.1016/S0264-410X(99)00271-6
29. Grodeland G, Fredriksen AB, Løset GÅ, Vikse E, Fugger L, Bogen B. Antigen targeting to human HLA class II molecules increases efficacy of DNA vaccination. *J Immunol* (2016) 197:3575–85. doi:10.4049/jimmunol.1600893
30. Rush C, Mitchell T, Garside P. Efficient priming of CD4+ and CD8+ T cells by DNA vaccination depends on appropriate targeting of sufficient levels of immunologically relevant antigen to appropriate processing pathways. *J Immunol* (2002) 169:4951. doi:10.4049/jimmunol.169.9.4951
31. Wiersma LCM, Rimmelzwaan GF, De Vries RD. Developing universal influenza vaccines: hitting the nail, not just on the head. *Vaccines (Basel)* (2015) 3:239–62. doi:10.3390/vaccines3020239
32. Robinson HL, Hunt LA, Webster RG. Protection against a lethal influenza virus challenge by immunization with a haemagglutinin-expressing plasmid DNA. *Vaccine* (1993) 11:957–60. doi:10.1016/0264-410X(93)90385-B
33. Robinson HL, Boyle CA, Feltquate DM, Morin MJ, Santoro JC, Webster RG. DNA immunization for influenza virus: studies using hemagglutinin- and nucleoprotein-expressing DNAs. *J Infect Dis* (1997) 176:S50–5. doi:10.1086/514176
34. Barría MI, Garrido JL, Stein C, Scher E, Ge Y, Engel SM, et al. Localized mucosal response to intranasal live attenuated influenza vaccine in adults. *J Infect Dis* (2013) 207:115–24. doi:10.1093/infdis/jis641
35. Sridhar S, Begom S, Bermingham A, Hoschler K, Adamson W, Carman W, et al. Cellular immune correlates of protection against symptomatic pandemic influenza. *Nat Med* (2013) 19:1305. doi:10.1038/nm.3350
36. Berlanda Scorza F, Tsvetnitsky V, Donnelly JJ. Universal influenza vaccines: shifting to better vaccines. *Vaccine* (2016) 34:2926–33. doi:10.1016/j.vaccine.2016.03.085
37. Ulmer JB, Donnelly JJ, Parker SE, Rhodes GH, Felgner PL, Dwarki VJ, et al. Heterologous protection against influenza by injection of DNA encoding a viral protein. *Science* (1993) 259:1745–9. doi:10.1126/science.8456302
38. Tompkins SM, Zhao ZS, Lo CY, Misplon JA, Liu T, Ye Z, et al. Matrix protein 2 vaccination and protection against influenza viruses, including subtype H5N1. *Emerg Infect Dis* (2007) 13:426–35. doi:10.3201/eid1303.061125
39. Wang W, Li R, Deng Y, Lu N, Chen H, Meng X, et al. Protective efficacy of the conserved NP, PB1, and M1 proteins as immunogens in DNA- and vaccinia virus-based universal influenza A virus vaccines in mice. *Clin Vaccine Immunol* (2015) 22:618–30. doi:10.1128/CVI.00091-15
40. Bragstad K, Vinner L, Hansen MS, Nielsen J, Fomsgaard A. A polyvalent influenza A DNA vaccine induces heterologous immunity and protects pigs against pandemic A(H1N1)pdm09 virus infection. *Vaccine* (2013) 31:2281–8. doi:10.1016/j.vaccine.2013.02.061
41. Price GE, Soboleski MR, Lo C-Y, Misplon JA, Pappas C, Houser KV, et al. Vaccination focusing immunity on conserved antigens protects mice and ferrets against virulent H1N1 and H5N1 influenza A viruses. *Vaccine* (2009) 27:6512–21. doi:10.1016/j.vaccine.2009.08.053
42. Koday MT, Leonard JA, Munson P, Forero A, Koday M, Bratt DL, et al. Multigenic DNA vaccine induces protective cross-reactive T cell responses against heterologous influenza virus in nonhuman primates. *PLoS One* (2017) 12:e0189780. doi:10.1371/journal.pone.0189780
43. Park KS, Seo YB, Lee JY, Im SJ, Seo SH, Song MS, et al. Complete protection against a H5N2 avian influenza virus by a DNA vaccine expressing a fusion protein of H1N1 HA and M2e. *Vaccine* (2011) 29:5481–7. doi:10.1016/j.vaccine.2011.05.062
44. Steel J, Lowen AC, Wang TT, Yondola M, Gao Q, Haye K, et al. Influenza virus vaccine based on the conserved hemagglutinin stalk domain. *MBio* (2010) 1(1):e00018-10. doi:10.1128/mBio.00018-10
45. Wang B, Yu H, Yang FR, Huang M, Ma JH, Tong GZ. Protective efficacy of a broadly cross-reactive swine influenza DNA vaccine encoding M2e, cytotoxic T lymphocyte epitope and consensus H3 hemagglutinin. *Virol J* (2012) 9:127. doi:10.1186/1743-422X-9-127
46. Choi EJ, Lee HS, Noh JY, Song JY, Cheong HJ, Shin OS, et al. Humoral and cellular immunogenicity induced by avian influenza A (H7N9) DNA vaccine in mice. *Infect Chemother* (2017) 49:117–22. doi:10.3947/ic.2017.49.2.117
47. Yan J, Morrow MP, Chu JS, Racine T, Reed CC, Khan AS, et al. Broad cross-protective anti-hemagglutination responses elicited by influenza microconsensus DNA vaccine. *Vaccine* (2018) 36(22):3079–89. doi:10.1016/j.vaccine.2017.09.086
48. Chen M-W, Cheng T-JR, Huang Y, Jan J-T, Ma S-H, Yu AL, et al. A consensus–hemagglutinin-based DNA vaccine that protects mice against divergent H5N1 influenza viruses. *Proc Natl Acad Sci USA* (2008) 105:13538–43. doi:10.1073/pnas.0806901105
49. Huber VC, Thomas PG, Mccullers JA. A multi-valent vaccine approach that elicits broad immunity within an influenza subtype. *Vaccine* (2009) 27:1192–200. doi:10.1016/j.vaccine.2008.12.023
50. Rao S, Kong WP, Wei CJ, Yang ZY, Nason M, Styles D, et al. Multivalent HA DNA vaccination protects against highly pathogenic H5N1 avian influenza infection in chickens and mice. *PLoS One* (2008) 3:e2432. doi:10.1371/journal.pone.0002432
51. Wang S, Taaffe J, Parker C, Solorzano A, Cao H, Garcia-Sastre A, et al. Hemagglutinin (HA) proteins from H1 and H3 serotypes of influenza A viruses require different antigen designs for the induction of optimal protective antibody responses as studied by codon-optimized HA DNA vaccines. *J Virol* (2006) 80:11628–37. doi:10.1128/JVI.01065-06
52. Tenbusch M, Grunwald T, Niezold T, Bonsmann MSG, Hannaman D, Norley S, et al. Codon-optimization of the hemagglutinin gene from the novel swine origin H1N1 influenza virus has differential effects on CD4+ T-cell responses and immune effector mechanisms following DNA electroporation in mice. *Vaccine* (2010) 28:3273–7. doi:10.1016/j.vaccine.2010.02.090
53. Stachyra A, Redkiewicz P, Kosson P, Protasiuk A, Gora-Sochacka A, Kudla G, et al. Codon optimization of antigen coding sequences improves the immune potential of DNA vaccines against avian influenza virus H5N1 in mice and chickens. *Virol J* (2016) 13:143. doi:10.1186/s12985-016-0599-y
54. Jiang Y, Yu K, Zhang H, Zhang P, Li C, Tian G, et al. Enhanced protective efficacy of H5 subtype avian influenza DNA vaccine with codon optimized HA gene in a pCAGGS plasmid vector. *Antiviral Res* (2007) 75:234–41. doi:10.1016/j.antiviral.2007.03.009
55. Wang S, Hackett A, Jia N, Zhang C, Zhang L, Parker C, et al. Polyvalent DNA vaccines expressing HA antigens of H5N1 influenza viruses with an optimized leader sequence elicit cross-protective antibody responses. *PLoS One* (2011) 6:e28757. doi:10.1371/journal.pone.0028757
56. Andersen TK, Zhou F, Cox R, Bogen B, Grødeland G. A DNA vaccine that targets hemagglutinin to antigen presenting cells protects mice against H7 influenza. *J Virol* (2017) 91(23):e01340–17. doi:10.1128/JVI.01340-17
57. Wolff JA, Malone RW, Williams P, Chong W, Acsadi G, Jani A, et al. Direct gene transfer into mouse muscle in vivo. *Science* (1990) 247:1465–8. doi:10.1126/science.1690918
58. Combadiere B, Liard C. Transcutaneous and intradermal vaccination. *Hum Vaccin* (2011) 7:811–27. doi:10.4161/hv.7.8.16274
59. Widera G, Austin M, Rabussay D, Goldbeck C, Barnett SW, Chen M, et al. Increased DNA vaccine delivery and immunogenicity by electroporation in vivo. *J Immunol* (2000) 164:4635–40. doi:10.4049/jimmunol.164.9.4635
60. Lee SW, Youn JW, Seong BL, Sung YC. IL-6 induces long-term protective immunity against a lethal challenge of influenza virus. *Vaccine* (1999) 17:490–6. doi:10.1016/S0264-410X(98)00223-0
61. Yager EJ, Stagnar C, Gopalakrishnan R, Fuller JT, Fuller DH. Optimizing particle-mediated epidermal delivery of an influenza DNA vaccine in ferrets. *Methods Mol Biol* (2013) 940:223–37. doi:10.1007/978-1-62703-110-3_19
62. Ledgerwood JE, Hu Z, Gordon IJ, Yamshchikov G, Enama ME, Plummer S, et al. Influenza virus h5 DNA vaccination is immunogenic by intramuscular and intradermal routes in humans. *Clin Vaccine Immunol* (2012) 19:1792–7. doi:10.1128/CVI.05663-11
63. Graham BS, Enama ME, Nason MC, Gordon IJ, Peel SA, Ledgerwood JE, et al. DNA vaccine delivered by a needle-free injection device improves potency of priming for antibody and CD8+ T-cell responses after rAd5 boost in a randomized clinical trial. *PLoS One* (2013) 8:e59340. doi:10.1371/journal.pone.0059340
64. Crank MC, Gordon IJ, Yamshchikov GV, Sitar S, Hu Z, Enama ME, et al. Phase 1 study of pandemic H1 DNA vaccine in healthy adults. *PLoS One* (2015) 10:e0123969. doi:10.1371/journal.pone.0123969
65. Raphael AP, Prow TW, Crichton ML, Chen X, Fernando GJ, Kendall MA. Targeted, needle-free vaccinations in skin using multilayered, densely-packed

dissolving microprojection arrays. *Small* (2010) 6:1785–93. doi:10.1002/smll.201000326

66. Kim YC, Song JM, Lipatov AS, Choi SO, Lee JW, Donis RO, et al. Increased immunogenicity of avian influenza DNA vaccine delivered to the skin using a microneedle patch. *Eur J Pharm Biopharm* (2012) 81:239–47. doi:10.1016/j.ejpb.2012.03.010
67. Fernando GJ, Zhang J, Ng HI, Haigh OL, Yukiko SR, Kendall MA. Influenza nucleoprotein DNA vaccination by a skin targeted, dry coated, densely packed microprojection array (Nanopatch) induces potent antibody and CD8(+) T cell responses. *J Control Release* (2016) 237:35–41. doi:10.1016/j.jconrel.2016.06.045
68. Song J-M, Kim Y-C, Eunju O, Compans RW, Prausnitz MR, Kang S-M. DNA vaccination in the skin using microneedles improves protection against influenza. *Mol Ther* (2012) 20:1472–80. doi:10.1038/mt.2012.69
69. Smith TRF, Schultheis K, Kiosses WB, Amante DH, Mendoza JM, Stone JC, et al. DNA vaccination strategy targets epidermal dendritic cells, initiating their migration and induction of a host immune response. *Mol Ther Methods Clin Dev* (2014) 1:14054. doi:10.1038/mtm.2014.54
70. Hartikka J, Sukhu L, Buchner C, Hazard D, Bozoukova V, Margalith M, et al. Electroporation-facilitated delivery of plasmid DNA in skeletal muscle: plasmid dependence of muscle damage and effect of poloxamer 188. *Mol Ther* (2001) 4:407–15. doi:10.1006/mthe.2001.0483
71. Diehl MC, Lee JC, Daniels SE, Tebas P, Khan AS, Giffear M, et al. Tolerability of intramuscular and intradermal delivery by CELLECTRA(®) adaptive constant current electroporation device in healthy volunteers. *Hum Vaccin Immunother* (2013) 9:2246–52. doi:10.4161/hv.24702
72. Schultheis K, Schaefer H, Yung BS, Oh J, Muthumani K, Humeau L, et al. Characterization of guinea pig T cell responses elicited after EP-assisted delivery of DNA vaccines to the skin. *Vaccine* (2017) 35:61–70. doi:10.1016/j.vaccine.2016.11.052
73. Borggren M, Nielsen J, Bragstad K, Karlsson I, Krog JS, Williams JA, et al. Vector optimization and needle-free intradermal application of a broadly protective polyvalent influenza A DNA vaccine for pigs and humans. *Hum Vaccin Immunother* (2015) 11:1983–90. doi:10.1080/21645515.2015.1011987
74. Laddy DJ, Yan J, Khan AS, Andersen H, Cohn A, Greenhouse J, et al. Electroporation of synthetic DNA antigens offers protection in nonhuman primates challenged with highly pathogenic avian influenza virus. *J Virol* (2009) 83:4624–30. doi:10.1128/JVI.02335-08
75. Zanin M, Baviskar P, Webster R, Webby R. The interaction between respiratory pathogens and mucus. *Cell Host Microbe* (2016) 19:159–68. doi:10.1016/j.chom.2016.01.001
76. Gould VMW, Francis JN, Anderson KJ, Georges B, Cope AV, Tregoning JS. Nasal IgA provides protection against human influenza challenge in volunteers with low serum influenza antibody titre. *Front Microbiol* (2017) 8:900. doi:10.3389/fmicb.2017.00900
77. Zaman M, Chandrudu S, Toth I. Strategies for intranasal delivery of vaccines. *Drug Deliv Transl Res* (2013) 3:100–9. doi:10.1007/s13346-012-0085-z
78. Loh L, Wang Z, Sant S, Koutsakos M, Jegaskanda S, Corbett AJ, et al. Human mucosal-associated invariant T cells contribute to antiviral influenza immunity via IL-18-dependent activation. *Proc Natl Acad Sci U S A* (2016) 113: 10133–8. doi:10.1073/pnas.1610750113
79. Xu Y, Yuen PW, Lam JK. Intranasal DNA vaccine for protection against respiratory infectious diseases: the delivery perspectives. *Pharmaceutics* (2014) 6:378–415. doi:10.3390/pharmaceutics6030378
80. Savelkoul HF, Ferro VA, Strioga MM, Schijns VE. Choice and design of adjuvants for parenteral and mucosal vaccines. *Vaccines (Basel)* (2015) 3:148–71. doi:10.3390/vaccines3010148
81. Torrieri-Dramard L, Lambrecht B, Ferreira HL, Van Den Berg T, Klatzmann D, Bellier B. Intranasal DNA vaccination induces potent mucosal and systemic immune responses and cross-protective immunity against influenza viruses. *Mol Ther* (2011) 19:602–11. doi:10.1038/mt.2010.222
82. Rajapaksa AE, Ho JJ, Qi A, Bischof R, Nguyen T-H, Tate M, et al. Effective pulmonary delivery of an aerosolized plasmid DNA vaccine via surface acoustic wave nebulization. *Respir Res* (2014) 15:60–60. doi:10.1186/1465-9921-15-60
83. He P, Zou Y, Hu Z. Advances in aluminum hydroxide-based adjuvant research and its mechanism. *Hum Vaccin Immunother* (2015) 11:477–88. doi:10.1080/21645515.2014.1004026
84. Ulmer JB, Dewitt CM, Chastain M, Friedman A, Donnelly JJ, Mcclements WL, et al. Enhancement of DNA vaccine potency using conventional aluminum adjuvants. *Vaccine* (1999) 18:18–28. doi:10.1016/S0264-410X(99)00151-6
85. Li L, Petrovsky N. Molecular adjuvants for DNA vaccines. *Curr Issues Mol Biol* (2017) 22:17–40. doi:10.21775/cimb.022.017
86. Silver JS, Hunter CA. gp130 at the nexus of inflammation, autoimmunity, and cancer. *J Leukoc Biol* (2010) 88:1145–56. doi:10.1189/jlb.0410217
87. Rose-John S. IL-6 trans-signaling via the soluble IL-6 receptor: importance for the pro-inflammatory activities of IL-6. *Int J Biol Sci* (2012) 8:1237–47. doi:10.7150/ijbs.4989
88. Larsen DL, Dybdahl-Sissoko N, Mcgregor MW, Drape R, Neumann V, Swain WF, et al. Coadministration of DNA encoding interleukin-6 and hemagglutinin confers protection from influenza virus challenge in mice. *J Virol* (1998) 72:1704–8.
89. Fagone P, Shedlock DJ, Bao H, Kawalekar OU, Yan J, Gupta D, et al. Molecular adjuvant HMGB1 enhances anti-influenza immunity during DNA vaccination. *Gene Ther* (2011) 18:1070–7. doi:10.1038/gt.2011.59
90. Loudon PT, Yager EJ, Lynch DT, Narendran A, Stagnar C, Franchini AM, et al. GM-CSF increases mucosal and systemic immunogenicity of an H1N1 influenza DNA vaccine administered into the epidermis of non-human primates. *PLoS One* (2010) 5:e11021. doi:10.1371/journal.pone.0011021
91. Babiuk LA, Pontarollo R, Babiuk S, Loehr B, Van Drunen Littel-Van Den Hurk S. Induction of immune responses by DNA vaccines in large animals. *Vaccine* (2003) 21:649–58. doi:10.1016/S0264-410X(02)00574-1
92. Hoekstra D, Rejman J, Wasungu L, Shi F, Zuhorn I. Gene delivery by cationic lipids: in and out of an endosome. *Biochem Soc Trans* (2007) 35:68–71. doi:10.1042/BST0350068
93. Jimenez GS, Planchon R, Wei Q, Rusalov D, Geall A, Enas J, et al. Vaxfectin-formulated influenza DNA vaccines encoding NP and M2 viral proteins protect mice against lethal viral challenge. *Hum Vaccin* (2007) 3:157–64. doi:10.4161/hv.3.5.4175
94. Lalor PA, Webby RJ, Morrow J, Rusalov D, Kaslow DC, Rolland A, et al. Plasmid DNA-based vaccines protect mice and ferrets against lethal challenge with A/Vietnam/1203/04 (H5N1) influenza virus. *J Infect Dis* (2008) 197:1643–52. doi:10.1086/588431
95. Smith LR, Wloch MK, Ye M, Reyes LR, Boutsaboualoy S, Dunne CE, et al. Phase 1 clinical trials of the safety and immunogenicity of adjuvanted plasmid DNA vaccines encoding influenza A virus H5 hemagglutinin. *Vaccine* (2010) 28:2565–72. doi:10.1016/j.vaccine.2010.01.029
96. Wang G, Pan L, Zhang Y, Wang Y, Zhang Z, Lu J, et al. Intranasal delivery of cationic PLGA nano/microparticles-loaded FMDV DNA vaccine encoding IL-6 elicited protective immunity against FMDV challenge. *PLoS One* (2011) 6:e27605. doi:10.1371/journal.pone.0027605
97. Seok H, Noh JY, Lee DY, Kim SJ, Song CS, Kim YC. Effective humoral immune response from a H1N1 DNA vaccine delivered to the skin by microneedles coated with PLGA-based cationic nanoparticles. *J Control Release* (2017) 265:66–74. doi:10.1016/j.jconrel.2017.04.027
98. Sawaengsak C, Mori Y, Yamanishi K, Srimanote P, Chaicumpa W, Mitrevej A, et al. Intranasal chitosan-DNA vaccines that protect across influenza virus subtypes. *Int J Pharm* (2014) 473:113–25. doi:10.1016/j.ijpharm.2014.07.005
99. Khurana S, Coyle EM, Manischewitz J, King LR, Ishioka G, Alexander J, et al. Oral priming with replicating adenovirus serotype 4 followed by subunit H5N1 vaccine boost promotes antibody affinity maturation and expands H5N1 cross-clade neutralization. *PLoS One* (2015) 10:e0115476. doi:10.1371/journal.pone.0115476
100. Wu Y, Yang D, Xu B, Liang W, Sui J, Chen Y, et al. Immune efficacy of an adenoviral vector-based swine influenza vaccine against antigenically distinct H1N1 strains in mice. *Antiviral Res* (2017) 147:29–36. doi:10.1016/j.antiviral.2017.09.009
101. Elaish M, Ngunjiri JM, Ali A, Xia M, Ibrahim M, Jang H, et al. Supplementation of inactivated influenza vaccine with norovirus P particle-M2e chimeric vaccine enhances protection against heterologous virus challenge in chickens. *PLoS One* (2017) 12:e0171174. doi:10.1371/journal.pone.0171174
102. Zhu W, Pewin W, Wang C, Luo Y, Gonzalez GX, Mohan T, et al. A boosting skin vaccination with dissolving microneedle patch encapsulating M2e vaccine broadens the protective efficacy of conventional influenza vaccines. *J Control Release* (2017) 261:1–9. doi:10.1016/j.jconrel.2017.06.017
103. Wang S, Parker C, Taaffe J, Solórzano A, García-Sastre A, Lu S. Heterologous HA DNA vaccine prime – inactivated influenza vaccine boost is more

effective than using DNA or inactivated vaccine alone in eliciting antibody responses against H1 or H3 serotype influenza viruses. *Vaccine* (2008) 26:3626–33. doi:10.1016/j.vaccine.2008.04.073

104. Suguitan AL Jr, Cheng X, Wang W, Wang S, Jin H, Lu S. Influenza H5 hemagglutinin DNA primes the antibody response elicited by the live attenuated influenza A/Vietnam/1203/2004 vaccine in ferrets. *PLoS One* (2011) 6: e21942. doi:10.1371/journal.pone.0021942
105. Stachyra A, Pietrzak M, Macioła A, Protasiuk A, Olszewska M, Śmietanka K, et al. A prime/boost vaccination with HA DNA and Pichia-produced HA protein elicits a strong humoral response in chickens against H5N1. *Virus Res* (2017) 232:41–7. doi:10.1016/j.virusres.2017.01.025
106. Ledgerwood JE, Bellamy AR, Belshe R, Bernstein DI, Edupuganti S, Patel SM, et al. DNA priming for seasonal influenza vaccine: a phase 1b double-blind randomized clinical trial. *PLoS One* (2015) 10:e0125914. doi:10.1371/journal.pone.0125914
107. Ledgerwood JE, Hu Z, Costner P, Yamshchikov G, Enama ME, Plummer S, et al. Phase I clinical evaluation of seasonal influenza hemagglutinin (HA) DNA vaccine prime followed by trivalent influenza inactivated vaccine (IIV3) boost. *Contemp Clin Trials* (2015) 44:112–8. doi:10.1016/j.cct.2015.08.006
108. Chang H, Huang C, Wu J, Fang F, Zhang W, Wang F, et al. A single dose of DNA vaccine based on conserved H5N1 subtype proteins provides protection against lethal H5N1 challenge in mice pre-exposed to H1N1 influenza virus. *Virol J* (2010) 7:197–197. doi:10.1186/1743-422X-7-197
109. Ledgerwood JE, Zephir K, Hu Z, Wei CJ, Chang L, Enama ME, et al. Prime-boost interval matters: a randomized phase 1 study to identify the minimum interval necessary to observe the H5 DNA influenza vaccine priming effect. *J Infect Dis* (2013) 208:418–22. doi:10.1093/infdis/jit180
110. DeZure AD, Coates EE, Hu Z, Yamshchikov GV, Zephir KL, Enama ME, et al. An avian influenza H7 DNA priming vaccine is safe and immunogenic in a randomized phase I clinical trial. *NPJ Vaccines* (2017) 2:15. doi:10.1038/s41541-017-0016-6
111. Myhr AI. DNA vaccines: regulatory considerations and safety aspects. *Curr Issues Mol Biol* (2017) 22:79–88. doi:10.21775/cimb.022.079
112. AgriLabs. *First DNA Vaccine Licensed for Chickens*. PR Newswire: Cision (2017). Available: https://www.prnewswire.com/news-releases/first-dna-vaccine-licensed-for-chickens-300554855.html (Accessed: January 14, 2018).
113. Takeda A, Igarashi H, Nakamura H, Kano M, Iida A, Hirata T, et al. Protective efficacy of an AIDS vaccine, a single DNA priming followed by a single booster with a recombinant replication-defective Sendai virus vector, in a macaque AIDS model. *J Virol* (2003) 77:9710–5. doi:10.1128/JVI.77.17.9710-9715.2003
114. Yu S, Feng X, Shu T, Matano T, Hasegawa M, Wang X, et al. Potent specific immune responses induced by prime-boost-boost strategies based on DNA, adenovirus, and Sendai virus vectors expressing gag gene of Chinese HIV-1 subtype B. *Vaccine* (2008) 26:6124–31. doi:10.1016/j.vaccine.2008.09.017
115. Grubor-Bauk B, Yu W, Wijesundara D, Gummow J, Garrod T, Brennan AJ, et al. Intradermal delivery of DNA encoding HCV NS3 and perforin elicits robust cell-mediated immunity in mice and pigs. *Gene Ther* (2016) 23:26–37. doi:10.1038/gt.2015.86
116. Lee H, Jeong M, Oh J, Cho Y, Shen X, Stone J, et al. Preclinical evaluation of multi antigenic HCV DNA vaccine for the prevention of hepatitis C virus infection. *Sci Rep* (2017) 7:43531. doi:10.1038/srep43531
117. Gaudinski MR, Houser KV, Morabito KM, Hu Z, Yamshchikov G, Rothwell RS, et al. Safety, tolerability, and immunogenicity of two Zika virus DNA vaccine candidates in healthy adults: randomised, open-label, phase 1 clinical trials. *Lancet* (2017) 391:552–62. doi:10.1016/S0140-6736(17)33105-7
118. Tebas P, Roberts CC, Muthumani K, Reuschel EL, Kudchodkar SB, Zaidi FI, et al. Safety and immunogenicity of an anti-Zika virus DNA vaccine – preliminary report. *N Engl J Med* (2017). doi:10.1056/NEJMoa1708120

14

Highly Pathogenic H5N1 Influenza A Virus Spreads Efficiently in Human Primary Monocyte-Derived Macrophages and Dendritic Cells

Veera Westenius[1]*, *Sanna M. Mäkelä*[1], *Ilkka Julkunen*[2] *and Pamela Österlund*[1]

[1] *Expert Microbiology Unit, Department of Health Security, National Institute for Health and Welfare, Helsinki, Finland,*
[2] *Institute of Biomedicine, University of Turku, Turku, Finland*

Correspondence:
Veera Westenius
veera.westenius@thl.fi

Influenza A viruses cause recurrent epidemics and occasional global pandemics. Wild birds are the natural reservoir of influenza A virus from where the virus can be transmitted to poultry or to mammals including humans. Mortality among humans in the highly pathogenic avian influenza H5N1 virus infection is even 60%. Despite intense research, there are still open questions in the pathogenicity of the H5N1 virus in humans. To characterize the H5N1 virus infection in human monocyte-derived macrophages (Mϕs) and dendritic cells (DCs), we used human isolates of highly pathogenic H5N1/2004 and H5N1/1997 and low pathogenic H7N9/2013 avian influenza viruses in comparison with a seasonal H3N2/1989 virus. We noticed that the H5N1 viruses have an overwhelming ability to replicate and spread in primary human immune cell cultures, and even the addition of trypsin did not equalize the infectivity of H7N9 or H3N2 viruses to the level seen with H5N1 virus. H5N1 virus stocks contained more often propagation-competent viruses than the H7N9 or H3N2 viruses. The data also showed that human DCs and Mϕs maintain 1,000- and 10,000-fold increase in the production of infectious H5N1 virus, respectively. Both analyzed highly pathogenic H5N1 viruses showed multi-cycle infection in primary human DCs and Mϕs, whereas the H3N2 and H7N9 viruses were incapable of spreading in immune cells. Interestingly, H5N1 virus was able to spread extremely efficiently despite the strong induction of antiviral interferon gene expression, which may in part explain the high pathogenicity of H5N1 virus infection in humans.

Keywords: influenza A virus, avian influenza, macrophages, dendritic cells, viral replication, innate immunity

INTRODUCTION

Influenza A viruses are one of the most important viral pathogens annually infecting even 5–10% of the human population and causing an estimated 250,000–500,000 deaths worldwide. Occasionally, influenza A viruses cause global pandemics of which the most devastating one was the pandemic caused by Spanish flu in 1918 leading up to 50 million deaths (1). The segmented genome of influenza A viruses confers evolutionary advantages and influenza A viruses have a great ability to evolve by two different mechanisms, antigenic drift and shift. All pandemics in the twentieth century have been of avian origin (2, 3). Avian influenza A viruses circulate continuously in birds and occasionally they have caused infections in humans. The highly pathogenic avian influenza (HPAI) H5N1 viruses have caused almost 900 human infections from 2003 until today and the mortality among humans has been over 50% (4). The H7N9 virus, which emerged in humans in 2013, has a surprising character as it causes only a mild infection in domestic poultry but an HPAI-like disease in humans. In the beginning of 2017, a human infection was detected with H7N9 virus possessing a multi-basic HA1-HA2 cleavage site motif in the hemagglutinin (HA) molecule characteristic of HPAI viruses (5). Thus far, there have been over 1,500 human infections caused by the H7N9 virus with a mortality rate reaching 40% (4, 6). Therefore, these avian influenza virus strains pose a serious risk for a pandemic. Despite active research, it is not completely clear which factors in H5N1 or H7N9 viruses or in host responses contribute to a severe disease in humans.

After infecting the epithelial cells of respiratory tract, influenza A viruses can spread to alveolar dendritic cells (DCs) and macrophages (Mϕs) which reside in the immediate proximity of the epithelium (7). DCs and Mϕs are the key cell types to orchestrate host immune responses (8, 9). Typically influenza A virus induces antiviral responses in immune cells by inducing type I and III interferons (IFNs) which are known to inhibit virus replication and propagation (10–12). Both alveolar and monocyte-derived Mϕs as well as DCs, including monocyte-derived DCs (moDCs), express receptors for both avian-adapted (α-2,3-linked sialic acids) and human-adapted (α-2,6-linked sialic acids) influenza A viruses (13–16). The viral HA binds to sialylated host cell surface receptor molecules and mediates virus entry. Influenza viruses enter the cells mainly *via* endocytosis and the fusion of viral and endosomal membranes. For the fusion to happen the precursor form of the HA, HA0 has to be cleaved into HA1 and HA2 subunits by host cells proteases. The membrane fusion mediated by the mature form of the HA occurs at low pH which enables the release of the segmented viral genome into the cytoplasm. The genome of the influenza virus is structured in eight separate viral ribonucleoprotein (vRNP) complexes which are transported into the nucleus for the transcription and replication of the virus. The viral proteins are translated in the cytoplasm but the viral proteins are assembled into vRNPs in the nucleus. Newly synthesized vRNPs are exported to the cytoplasm, virus particles are assembled at the cell membrane, and progeny virus particles bud out of the cell. All eight vRNAs have to be packed into a virion to produce infective progeny viruses and the infection to be productive. The mechanism behind the genome packaging is not fully understood but it is believed that influenza A virus packs its vRNAs in a specific manner by a selective packaging mechanism (17). Some studies suggest that most influenza A virus particles are noninfectious since they express incomplete set of viral gene segments and are incapable of inducing a secondary infection (18). However, three-dimensional analysis of the virions has shown that at least 80% of virions have all eight RNPs packaged (19). In addition, it is known that there are differences between various seasonal influenza virus strains in their ability to cause a productive infection (18) but the comparison between avian influenza and seasonal influenza virus strains in primary human cells have remained poorly characterized.

Previously, we have shown that human moDCs are susceptible to the avian influenza virus infection (12, 20). In this study, we show that the highly pathogenic H5N1 influenza A viruses can efficiently replicate and produce new infective particles in human primary moDCs and Mϕs and, despite the strong IFN-mediated antiviral responses induced by the infection, be able to spread throughout the whole immune cell culture. These results suggest that the excessive cytokine production ("cytokine storm") induced by H5N1 infection may in fact be due to extremely efficient spread of the virus infection in the infection site leading to greatly enhanced cytokine gene expression.

MATERIALS AND METHODS

Ethics Statement

The permission to import the human isolates of avian virus strains for research purposes was obtained from the Finnish Food Safety Authority (permission no 8634/0527/2012). Infective H5N1 and H7N9 viruses were handled strictly under Biosafety Level (BSL) 3 laboratory conditions at the National Institute for Health and Welfare (THL), Finland. Different virus subtypes were always handled in separate biosafety cabinets to avoid any possible creation of recombinant viruses. Adult human blood was obtained from anonymous healthy blood donors through the Finnish Red Cross Blood Transfusion Service (permission no 37/2016, renewed annually). Animal immunizations related to this study were approved by the Ethical Committee of the National Institute for Health and Welfare (permission no. KTL 2008-02).

Cell Cultures

The buffy coats were obtained from healthy blood donors (Finnish Red Cross Blood Transfusion Service, Helsinki, Finland). Monocytes were purified from buffy coats as described previously (21). Human peripheral blood mononuclear cells were isolated by density gradient centrifugation over a Ficoll-Paque gradient (Amersham Biosciences).

To obtain monocytes for Mϕ differentiation, mononuclear cells were allowed to adhere onto plates or glass coverslips for 1 h at +37°C in RPMI 1640 (Sigma-Aldrich) supplemented with 0.6 μg/ml penicillin, 60 μg/ml streptomycin, 2 mM L-glutamine, and 20 mM HEPES. Nonadherent cells were removed by washing with phosphate-buffered saline (PBS), and the remaining monocytes were cultured in Mϕ serum-free medium (Life Technologies) supplemented with streptomycin and human recombinant granulocyte-macrophage colony-stimulating factor (rGM-CSF) (10 ng/ml; Nordic Biosite). The cells were differentiated into Mϕs for 7 days, with a change to fresh culture medium every 2 days.

To obtain moDCs, Percoll gradient (Amersham Biosciences) centrifugation was done after Ficoll-Paque gradient centrifugation. The fraction containing monocytes were collected and remaining T and B cells were depleted by using anti-CD3 and anti-CD19 magnetic beads (Dynal). Monocytes were allowed to adhere to plates (Sarstedt) for 1 h at +37°C in RPMI 1640 supplemented as described above. Non-adherent cells were removed by washing with PBS, and immature moDCs were generated by cultivating adherent monocytes in RPMI 1640 supplemented as described above and with 10% fetal calf serum (Integro), 10 ng/ml human rGM-CSF, and 20 ng/ml human recombinant interleukin-4 (R&D Systems). The cells were cultivated for 6 days, and fresh medium was added every 2 days.

In each experiment, cells from three to four different donors were cultured and used separately for infection experiments.

Viruses

Human influenza A/Beijing/353/89 (H3N2) virus (originates from WHO Collaborating Centre for Reference and Research on Influenza, The Francis Crick Institute, UK) and human isolates of the avian influenza viruses A/Vietnam/1194/2004 (H5N1) and A/Hong Kong/156/1997 (H5N1) (Molecular Virology, Erasmus MC—Department of Viroscience, Rotterdam, Netherlands) and A/Anhui/1/2013 (H7N9) (WHO Collaborating Centre for Reference and Research on Influenza, The Francis Crick Institute, UK) were grown in the allantoic cavity of 10- to 11-day-old embryonated chicken eggs at +36°C for 2–3 days. Since the infectivity of influenza A viruses vary from one type of cell to another, the virus titers were determined by different assays. A hemagglutination titration was done with standard protocol using 0.5% turkey or guinea pig red blood cells. The infective virus titer in Madin–Darby Canine Kidney (MDCK) cells were determined by plaque assay. The viruses were serially diluted and inoculated to confluent MDCK cells on the 6-well plates for 1 h at 37°C. After incubation, cells were washed with PBS and covered with Avicel microcrystalline cellulose [Eagle-MEM containing 1.2% Avicel (#RC-591 NF, FMC BioPolymers)], 0.3% BSA, 2 μg/ml *N*-tosyl-L-phenylalanine chloromethyl ketone (TPCK) treated trypsin, 60 μg/ml streptomycin, 2 mM L-glutamine, and 20 mM HEPES. After incubation at 37°C for 1 day for supernatant samples and for 2 days for virus stocks Avicel was removed, cells washed with PBS, fixed with 4% paraformaldehyde (PFA), and stained with diluted crystal violet. The plaques were counted to obtain the concentration of infective viruses as plaque forming units (PFU)/ml.

The infectivity of the viruses was determined in Mϕs by immunofluorescence microscopy and in moDCs by flow cytometry. The number of infected cells with different virus dilutions was counted to obtain the concentration of infective virus particles as focus forming units per milliliter (FFU/ml). The multiplicity of infection (MOI) in Mϕs or moDCs is given according to the titers determined in Mϕs or moDCs, respectively (**Table 1**).

Virus Infection Experiments

Macrophages and moDCs were infected with different MOI values of virus for different times, as indicated in the figures. Mϕs were differentiated on glass coverslips or cell culture plates, growth medium was removed, and virus dilution was added on cells. After 1 h at 37°C incubation, cells were washed with PBS, and fresh medium was added. For infection experiments in moDCs, the virus dilutions were added into cell cultures medium without changing the growth medium. For 6 h infectivity experiments in Mϕs and moDCs, cells were incubated with neuraminidase inhibitor, 20 nM oseltamivir carboxylate which is an active metabolite of oseltamivir phosphate (#RO0640802-002, Roche). All infection experiments with H5N1 and H7N9 viruses were performed in BSL-3 facility and only samples inactivated with validated methods were brought out from the BSL-3 laboratory.

Immunofluorescence Microscopy

Macrophages were differentiated on glass coverslips, infected with different influenza A viruses at MOI values as indicated in the figures, incubated for 1 h at 37°C, washed with PBS, fresh Mϕ medium was added and incubated at 37°C with 5% CO_2. At different times after infection, cells were washed, fixed with 4% PFA for 30 min at room temperature, washed, permeabilized with 0.1% Triton X-100 for 5 min, washed, and blocked with 0.5% BSA for 30 min. A/Beijing/353/89 (H3N2) virus-infected cells were stained with guinea pig antibody against influenza A virus H3N2 nucleoprotein (NP) (22). To visualize A/Vietnam/1194/2004(H5N1) or A/Anhui/1/2013(H7N9) virus-infected cells, guinea pig antibodies against H5N1 viral glycoproteins were used. Antibodies were prepared by immunizing guinea pigs and rabbits for four times every 2 weeks with A/Indonesia/5/2005 vaccine antigen (2 + 6 in PR8) (4 μg of HA/immunization) mixed with AS03 adjuvant (GlaxoSmithKline, Rixenart, Belgium) according to the instructions by the manufacturer. Secondary antibodies were fluorescein isothiocyanate (FITC)-labeled goat anti-guinea pig antibodies. In infectivity experiments, NucBlue Fixed Cell Ready Probes reagent (Life Technologies, DAPI) was added to secondary antibody staining solutions. Incubation time in every staining was 30 min in 0.5% BSA in PBS at 37°C and coverslips were washed three times with 0.5% Tween 20 (VWR) in PBS in every step. Finally, cells were washed with water and mounted in 25% Mowiol (Polysciences) in a solution containing 25 mM Tris–HCl (pH 7.5), 50% glycerol, and 2.5% 1,4-diazabicyclo(2,2,2)octane.

TABLE 1 | Quantitation of H3N2, H5N1/1997, H5N1/2004, and H7N9 virus stocks.

	HA (turkey)	HA (guinea pig)	PFU/ml [Madin–Darby Canine Kidney (MDCK)]	FFU/ml [macrophage (Mϕ)]	FFU/ml [monocyte-derived DC (moDC)]
A/Beijing/353/89 (H3N2)	128	256	2×10^7	3×10^7	5×10^6
A/Hong Kong/156/97 (H5N1)	256	256	2×10^8	2.8×10^8	1.2×10^8
A/Vietnam/1194/04 (H5N1)	128	256	1×10^7	7.8×10^8	7.8×10^7
A/Anhui/1/13 (H7N9)	1,024	1,024	2×10^8	4.7×10^8	1×10^7

The infectivity titers of viral stocks propagated in chicken eggs were determined in turkey and guinea pig red blood cells by hemagglutination assay (HA), in MDCK cells by the plaque forming assay (PFU), in human macrophages (Mϕs) and dendritic cells (moDC) by focus forming assay (FFU) with microscopy and flow cytometry, respectively.

The cells were imaged with Leica TCS SPE confocal microscope with a 63 1.40-numerical-aperture (NA) oil objective maintaining the same image acquisition settings for all acquired images. In the infectivity experiments, the cells were imaged with a Zeiss Stallion fluorescence microscope with a Hamamatsu ORCA-Flash 4.0 LT sCMOS camera and a 20 0.4-NA objective by using Slidebook 6 software (Intelligent Imaging Innovations). In the productivity assay, cells were calculated with 20 0.6-NA air objective with Leica TCS SPE confocal microscope.

Flow Cytometry

For determining the infectivity of viruses in moDCs, the cells were differentiated on 6-well plates. Cells were infected with different virus dilutions and times as indicated in the figures. After different times of infection, cells from four different blood donors were harvested and handled separately. Cells were fixed with 4% PFA for 30 min, permeabilized with 0.1% Triton X-100 for 5 min, and stored with 0.5% BSA in PBS. A/Beijing/353/89 (H3N2) virus-infected cells were stained with rabbit antibodies against H3N2 glycoproteins (23). To visualize A/Vietnam/1194/2004 (H5N1) or A/Anhui/1/2013 (H7N9) virus-infected cells, antibodies against A/Indonesia/5/2005 (H5N1) vaccine antigen were used (see above). The secondary antibody was FITC-labeled goat anti-rabbit IgG (H + L) (Invitrogen, #F2765). In all antibody stainings, the cells were stained at RT for 1 h and washed twice with 0.5% BSA in PBS. The samples were analyzed with a FACSCanto II (BD) device using FACSDiva software.

Western Blotting

For protein analysis, Mϕs or moDCs from four blood donors were harvested and pooled. We pooled the donors to be able to analyze higher amount of donors to get a more global and general view of the protein expression changes. Cell pellets were lysed with passive lysis buffer (Promega) containing 1 mM Na_3VO_4. Total cellular proteins were boiled in a Laemmli sample buffer, proteins were separated in SDS-PAGE gels and transferred onto Hybond-P polyvinylidene difluoride membranes (Amersham Biosciences). The membranes were blocked with 5% milk protein (Valio Co., Helsinki) in PBS. Anti-influenza A virus NP and M1 and MxA protein-specific antibodies were prepared as described previously (12, 24). Monoclonal anti-influenza A virus H7 HA antibody was obtained through BEI Resources, NIAID, NIH and anti-H3N2 glycoprotein antibodies and anti H5N1 virus antibodies were produced as described above. Antibody stainings for phosphorylated form of IRF3 (P-IRF3), P-STAT2, STAT2, and GAPDH proteins (Cell Signaling Technology) were performed according to the manufacturer's instructions. For secondary antibodies, anti-rabbit or anti-mouse HRP-conjugated antibodies (Dako) were used. Protein bands were visualized on HyperMax films using a Pierce® ECL Western Blotting substrate (Thermo Fisher Scientific).

qRT-PCR

Infected Mϕs or moDCs from four blood donors were pooled (25), and total cellular RNA was isolated using the RNEasy Mini kit (Qiagen) and DNase digestion was performed with RNasefree DNase kit (Qiagen). 0.5 μg of total cellular RNA was transcribed to cDNA using TaqMan Reverse Transcriptase kit (Applied Biosystems) with random hexamers as primers. cDNAs were amplified by PCR using TaqMan Universal PCR Mastermix and Gene Expression Assays for IFN-λ1 (Hs00601677_g1), IFN-α1 (Hs00256882_s1),IFN-β1(Hs00277188_s1),TNF-α(Hs01113624_g1), IL-1β (Hs00174097_m1), CXCL10 (Hs00171042_m1), CCL5 (Hs00174575_m1) (Applied Biosystems) or with primers and probes for influenza A virus M1 (12). The data were normalized to 18S rRNA with TaqMan Endogenous Control kit (Applied Biosystems). The relative gene expression in relation to an unstimulated sample was calculated with the ΔΔCT method according to instructions provided by Applied Biosystems.

To quantify viral RNA from the supernatant samples, moDCs and Mϕs were infected as described above and the supernatant samples were collected at 1 and 24 h after the infection. RNA was isolated using RNEasy Mini kit (Qiagen) with Qiacube (Qiagen). cDNA synthesis was done with RevertAid H Minus Reverse Transcriptase (Thermo Fisher Scientific) kit according to the manufacturer's instructions with RiboLock RNase inhibitor (Thermo Fisher Scientific) and random hexamers (Roche) as primers. qRT-PCR was performed using QIAGEN® QuantiTect™ Multiplex PCR NoRox Kit (Qiagen) with the same influenza A virus M1 primer–probe pair as above. The relative viral gene expression in relation to a 1-h sample was calculated with the ΔCT method according to the instructions provided by Applied Biosystems.

Quantitation of Propagation-Competent Virus Particles

Macrophages were grown on glass coverslips and infected with MOI of 0.01. After 1 h incubation, virus dilution was removed, and cells were washed with PBS. Cells were overlaid with 1.2% Avicel in E-MEM (containing 2 μg/ml TPCK-trypsin, 0.3% BSA, 60 μg/ml streptomycin, 2 mM L-glutamine, and 20 mM HEPES) and incubated for 15 h. After incubation, the cells were washed two times with PBS, fixed with 4% PFA for 30 min, washed with PBS, permeabilized with 0.1% triton X-100 for 5 min, and stained with antibodies of different specificity (above-mentioned) followed by immunofluorescence analysis [adapted from Ref. (18)]. The percentage of productive vs. total infection events was determined by eye using confocal microscope with 20× objective and cells were imaged with 40× objective (Figures 7A,B).

Statistical Analysis

The data was analyzed with the Student's *t*-test to determine the statistical significance of differences between H5N1 virus and H3N2 or H7N9 viruses. Values of $p < 0.05$ were considered significant.

RESULTS

Highly Pathogenic H5N1 Virus Has an Ability to Efficiently Spread in Primary Human Immune Cell Cultures

To determine the infectivity of influenza A/Beijing/353/89 (H3N2), A/Vietnam/1194/2004 (H5N1), and A/Anhui/1/2013

(H7N9) viruses in human Mϕs and dendritic cells (moDCs), we infected the cells with different virus doses for 6 h. We determined the number of infective units [focus forming units per milliliter (FFU/ml), **Table 1**] in virus stocks for both cell models separately from the dilution where approximately 50% of the cells were infected (**Figures 1A,C,E**). We used the FFU/ml values to determine the actual MOI. In the single-cycle infection (6 h), the infectivity curves with different doses of H5N1, H7N9, or H3N2 viruses both in Mϕs (**Figure 1A**) and moDCs (**Figure 1C**) corresponded well to the determined FFU/ml values. However, during a multi-cycle infection (24 h), H5N1 virus was able to efficiently spread in the culture and the virus infected all cells even with the very low MOI value in the beginning of the infection (**Figures 1B,D**).

All virus stocks were propagated in low passages in chicken eggs and the stock virus infectivity titers in different cell types were assessed. To determine the titers of infective units in the virus stocks, we performed a plaque forming assay in MDCK cells. In these cells, the H5N1 strain from 2004 gave the lowest titers when compared with those of H7N9 and H3N2 viruses (**Table 1**). The reason for this could be that the H7N9 virus has a high affinity to both α-2,3- (avian type) and α-2,6-linked (human type) sialic acids whereas usually the avian type H5N1 viruses prefer the α-2,3-type receptor (26). However, in moDCs and Mϕs where both α-2,3- and α-2,6-linked sialic acids are expressed (14, 15), the infectivity titer of H5N1 stock was the highest when compared with H3N2 or H7N9 viruses. Moreover, it seems that human Mϕs are more permissive than moDCs to all of these viruses (**Table 1**).

Besides primary infectivity in Mϕs and moDCs, we investigated the replication of these viruses in Mϕs and moDCs by analyzing the expression of viral M1 RNA with qRT-PCR. During the first 6 h of infection, we did not observe any clear differences in M1 gene expression between H3N2, H5N1, or H7N9 viruses, which indicate that the rate of viral replication is similar between the viruses during the primary infection. In the secondary infection phase (24 h time point) in H5N1-infected cells, the expression of M1 gene reached the same submaximal levels regardless of the MOI values used (0.01–10) (**Figures 2A,B**). In H3N2 and H7N9 virus-infected cells, instead, there was a clear dose-dependent expression of viral M1 RNA in different time points (**Figures 2A,B**). In addition, there was a clear difference in the production of viral NP and M proteins between H5N1 and H7N9 or H3N2 virus-infected cells. In H5N1 virus-infected cells viral protein expression was high, independent of the MOI value used in the beginning of the infection, while in H3N2 or H7N9-infected cells viral protein levels depended on the virus dose at the beginning of the infection (**Figures 2C,D**).

The HA of H5N1 Virus Is Efficiently Cleaved in Human Immune Cells

For the newly produced viruses to be infective, their HA precursor (HA0) has to be cleaved to HA1 and HA2 subunits by cellular proteases. Thus, we next analyzed how efficiently the HA molecule of H5N1, H7N9, and H3N2 viruses is cleaved in human immune cells. As visualized by immunoblotting in H3N2 virus-infected Mϕs, there was only some or none of the HA2 subunit detectable (**Figure 3A**). The A/Vietnam/1194/04 (H5N1) strain has multiple arginine and lysine residues at the HA1–HA2 cleavage site as a marker for a highly pathogenic form of an avian influenza virus. This multi-basic cleavage site can be cleaved by ubiquitous cellular proteases and, indeed, we noticed that in H5N1-infected human Mϕs a great amount of the HA0 protein produced at 24 h even with very low MOI was efficiently cleaved to HA1 and HA2 subunits (**Figure 3B**). However, like in H3N2 infection, in H7N9 virus-infected Mϕs, there was only some or none of the HA2 subunit detectable (**Figure 3C**). The HA of the different viruses was cleaved in similar fashion also in moDCs (**Figures 3D–F**).

Addition of Trypsin Does Not Increase the Infectivity of H3N2 or H7N9 Viruses to the Levels Seen With the H5N1 Virus

Next we investigated whether the trypsin-induced cleavage of HA contributes to influenza virus spread in immune cells. Human Mϕs and moDCs were infected with H3N2, H5N1, and H7N9 viruses in the presence of TPCK-trypsin to induce the cleavage of HA0 into HA1 and HA2 subunits and the number of virus-infected cells was analyzed by immunofluorescence or flow cytometry, respectively. We noticed that trypsin increased the infectivity of the H3N2 and H7N9 viruses to some extent at the 24-h time point (compared **Figures 4A,B** with **Figures 1B,D**) but yet the infectivity of H3N2 and H7N9 remained at a much lower level when compared with that of the H5N1 virus. In Mϕs, even at a MOI of 0.004 nearly 100% of cells were infected by the H5N1 virus while in H3N2 or H7N9 infection less than 40% of the cells were infected (**Figure 4A**). In moDCs, the difference was equally clear and in H3N2 or H7N9 infection with the lowest MOI values only ca. 20% of the cells were infected while with similar H5N1 virus dose most cells were infected (**Figure 4B**). Unexpectedly, the infectivity of H3N2 or H7N9 virus, even with added trypsin, did not become as effective as was seen with H5N1 virus. This suggests that H5N1 can spread in human immune cells extremely efficiently and this spread is not solely dependent on the effective cleavage of HA.

H5N1 Virus Is Able to Spread in Immune Cell Starting From Only a Few Infectious Virus Particles

Next, we analyzed how low amount of the H5N1 virus was sufficient to infect the whole immune cell culture. To do this, we made dilutions series of the stock virus and infected moDCs with MOI values ranging from 1 to 10^{-12} for 48 h. Interestingly, most moDCs were infected even at a MOI 10^{-5} of H5N1 virus and the infectivity decreased to background levels at a MOI of 10^{-8}, where there should not be any viral particles left (**Figure 5**). The findings suggest that the H5N1 virus is able to start a productive infection and spread eventually to the whole cell culture even from one infectious virus particle.

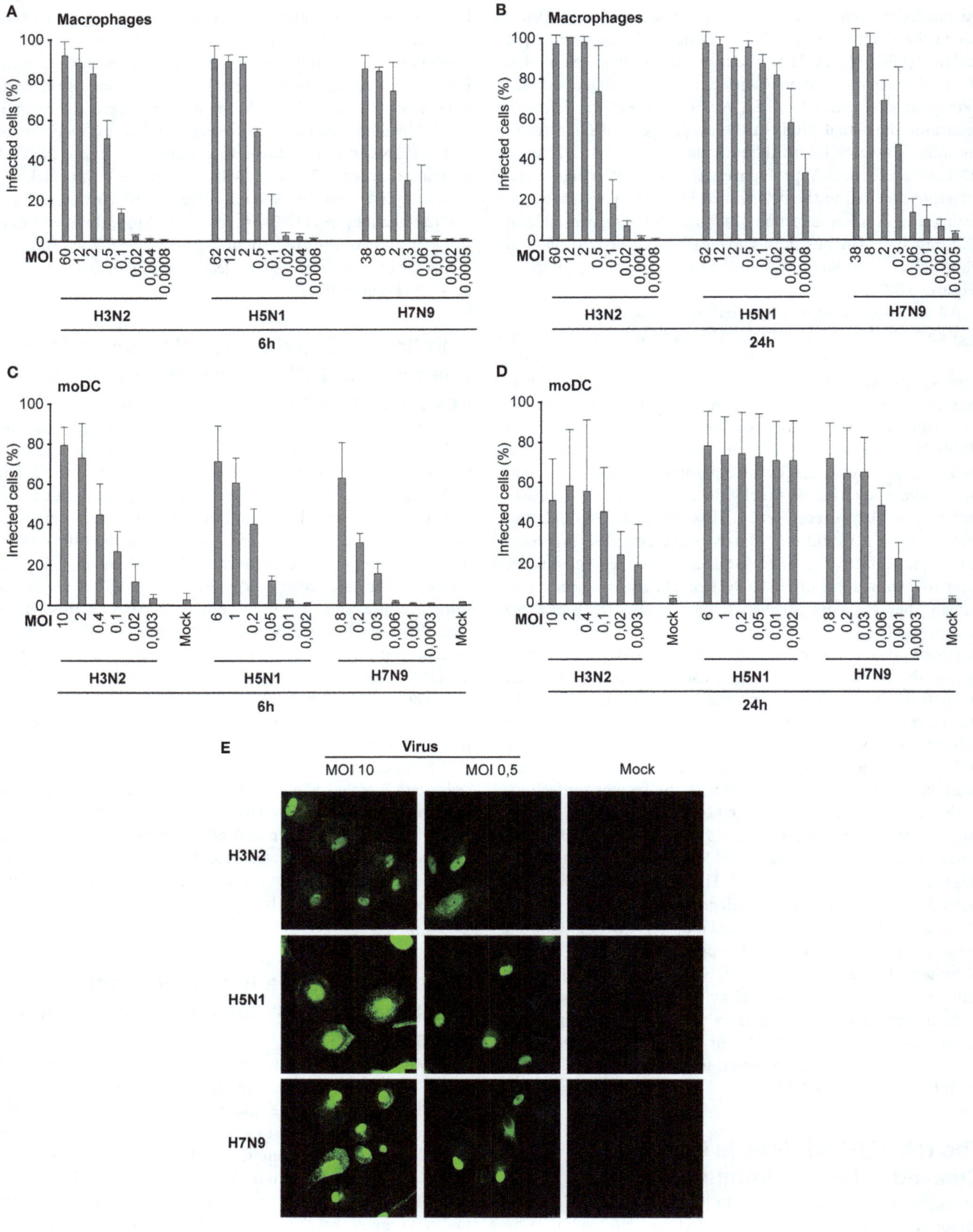

FIGURE 1 | Continued

FIGURE 1 | Infectivity of the H3N2, H5N1, and H7N9 influenza A viruses in human immune cells. **(A)** Human monocyte-derived macrophages (Mϕs) were infected with different doses of a seasonal influenza virus A/Beijing/353/89 (H3N2) or human isolates of avian influenza viruses A/Vietnam/1194/2004 (H5N1) or A/Anhui/1/2013 (H7N9) **(A)** for 6 h in the presence of oseltamivir carboxylate to prevent the spread of viruses, or **(B)** for 24 h in the absence of oseltamivir carboxylate. Infected Mϕs were detected with virus protein-specific antibodies by immunofluorescence microscopy. Results represent the mean values of three **(A)** or four **(B)** donors. From each donor at least 200 cells (average ca. 330) **(A)** or 300 cells (average ca. 840) **(B)** were counted. Human dendritic cells [monocyte-derived DCs (moDCs)] were infected with different virus doses **(C)** for 6 h in the presence of oseltamivir carboxylate, or **(D)** for 24 h in the absence of oseltamivir carboxylate. The proportion of infected moDCs was determined after staining the cells with antibodies against respective viral proteins for flow cytometry. From each donor, 10,000 events were analyzed. The mock sample (uninfected cells) was used to separate the uninfected and infected cells. Results are the mean values of four donors **(C,D)** analyzed separately. The infective particles per ml (FFU/ml) were calculated for Mϕs and moDCs separately, and multiplicity of infection (MOI) values was determined afterward. The MOI values in each experiment were calculated based on FFU/ml values determined in panels **(A,C)**. **(E)** Representative images of Mϕs infected with H3N2, H5N1, or H7N9 viruses at MOI 10 or 0.5 stained with virus-specific antibodies and secondary fluorescein isothiocyanate-labeled antibodies.

An Efficient Spread in Human Immune Cells and Efficient HA Cleavage Are General Features of HPAI H5N1 Viruses

Our next question was, whether the ability to spread in human immune cells is only associated with this specific HPAI H5N1 strain A/Vietnam/1194/04 or whether it is a more universal feature of all highly pathogenic avian-origin H5N1 viruses. Thus, we included another highly pathogenic H5N1 strain into the study. This A/Hong Kong/156/1997 H5N1 virus gave almost an equally high titer in MDCK cells than the H7N9 virus, whereas the other H5N1/2004 strain gave the lowest PFU titer (**Table 1**). It may be that the H5N1/1997 virus is already adapted to the mammalian MDCK cells, because H5N1/1997 virus has been cultivated at least four passages in MDCK cells before the propagation in chicken eggs. This likely explains the high PFU/ml titer of H5N1/1997 virus. The infectivity of A/Hong Kong/156/1997 (H5N1) virus was also determined in Mϕs and moDCs at 6 and 24 h by immunofluorescence microscopy and flow cytometry, respectively (**Figures 6A,B**), and calculated the FFU/ml values (**Table 1**) for virus stocks as was done for H3N2, H5N1/2004, and H7N9 viruses (**Figures 1A,C**). In multi-cyclic infection at 24 h, H5N1/1997 virus was spreading efficiently in Mϕs and moDCs (**Figures 6A,B**) in a similar fashion as the H5N1/2004 virus (**Figures 1B,D**). Infection with H5N1/1997 virus at MOI value of 10^{-5} reached over 60% infection rate in moDCs at 48 h. In addition, 10% of the cells got infected from the virus dose of MOI 10^{-6} where theoretically only one infectious virus particle was added into the culture (**Figure 6C**). Furthermore, the HA of the H5N1/1997 virus was efficiently cleaved from HA0 to HA1 and HA2 subunits as was also the case with the HA of the H5N1/2004 virus (**Figure 6D**). These data show that the H5N1/1997 virus has a similar ability to spread in human Mϕs and moDCs as the H5N1/2004 virus and the cleavage of HA is extremely efficient in these cell types suggesting that these features are general to HPAI H5N1 viruses.

Primary Infective Units of H5N1 Virus Are More Often Propagation-Competent and Productive Than Those of H3N2 or H7N9 Viruses in Human Immune Cells

We assumed that one reason for the efficient spread of H5N1 virus may be that H5N1 virus particles are more often packed with a complete set of gene segments and therefore these virus particles are propagation-competent and infection events are productive. To investigate this possibility, we set up the propagation-competent virus particle test (18). Human primary Mϕs were plated on coverslips followed by infection with H3N2, H5N1 from 2004 and H7N9 viruses at MOI of 0.01, overlaid with Avicel cellulose, incubated 15 h, fixed, and the infected cells stained for fluorescent microscopic analysis. Infection events were considered productive when three or more adjacent cells were infected. Our results show that significantly more infection events were productive with H5N1 virus, with almost 30% of the total infection events being productive, when compared with the 12 and 8% of events with H3N2 and H7N9 viruses, respectively (**Figure 7A**). We also noticed that the clusters of H5N1 virus-infected cells were larger and consisted of even 10 cells while those with H7N9 or H3N2 viruses were smaller and consisted of only a few cells (**Figure 7B**). Next, we analyzed whether the H3N2, H5N1, or H7N9 virus infections were productive by propagating new infectious virions in human Mϕs and moDC. For that, we performed plaque assays from the supernatant samples collected at 1 or 24 h after the infection. We noticed that the amount of infectious virus in the Mϕ cell culture supernatant was increased with all the studied viruses but H5N1 was superior, producing approximately 1,000-fold higher virus titers (**Figure 8A**). In moDCs, the virus titers increased even 10,000-fold in H5N1 virus infection after 24 h (**Figure 8B**). In contrast to the H5N1 virus infection, in infections with H3N2 or H7N9 viruses, the virus titers had a tendency to decrease (**Figure 8B**). In addition to analyzing the amount of secreted infectious virus, we investigated the viral RNA levels at 1 and 24 h in the Mϕs and moDCs supernatants of H3N2, H5N1, and H7N9 virus-infected cells. In H5N1 virus-infected Mϕs and moDC supernatants, total viral RNA levels increased over 100,000- and 100-fold, respectively, whereas in H3N2 or H7N9 virus-infected cells, viral RNA levels increased ca 10,000-fold in Mϕs and 10-fold in moDCs (**Figures 8C,D**). The data indicate that the H5N1 virus spreads more efficiently than H3N2 or H7N9 viruses in human immune cell cultures leading to efficient secretion of newly produced infectious H5N1 viruses.

H5N1 Virus Infection Is Able to Spread in Human Immune Cell Cultures Irrespective of Induced IFN Responses

Influenza virus infection induces type I and III IFN production in response to the recognition of viral RNAs by host receptors.

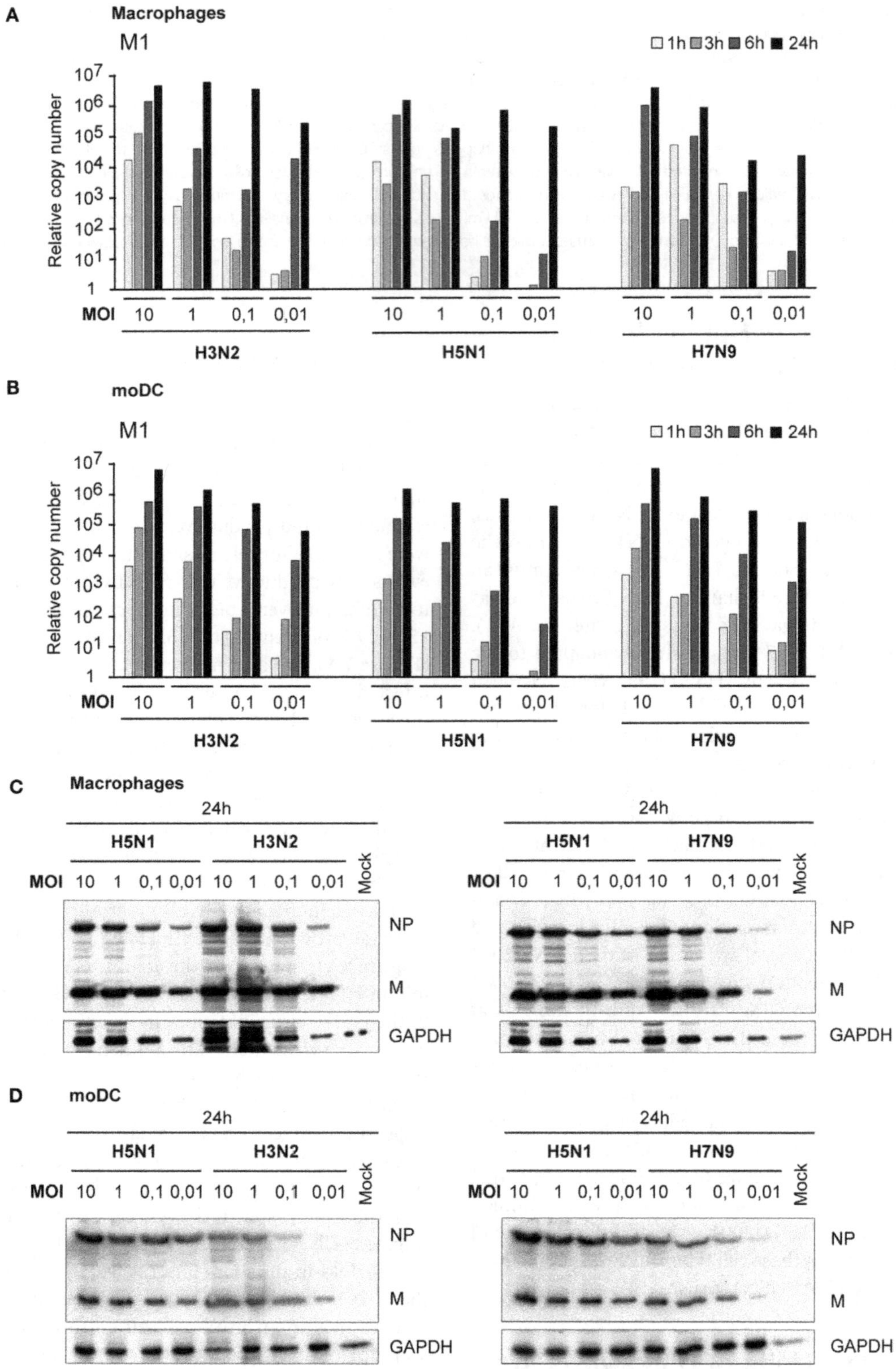

FIGURE 2 | Viral RNA expression and protein synthesis in H3N2, H5N1, and H7N9 virus-infected monocyte-derived macrophages (Mϕs) and monocyte-derived DCs (moDCs). Mϕs and moDCs from four different blood donors were separately infected with A/Beijing/353/89 (H3N2), A/Vietnam/1194/2004 (H5N1), and A/Anhui/1/2013 (H7N9) influenza viruses at different multiplicity of infection (MOI) values for up to 24 h. **(A)** Mϕs and **(B)** moDCs were collected at 1, 3, 6, and 24 h after infection, cells from different donors were pooled and total cellular RNA was isolated for measuring of viral M1 RNA expression by qRT-PCR. The fold induction was calculated over mock sample. The data shown are representative of three independent experiments. **(C,D)** Cellular protein lysates from **(C)** Mϕs or **(D)** moDCs were collected at 24 h after infection, samples from different donors were pooled and viral NP and M1 protein expression was analyzed using Western blotting. GAPDH levels were analyzed to control the equal loading of the samples. A representative experiment out of two (Mϕs) or three (moDC) is shown.

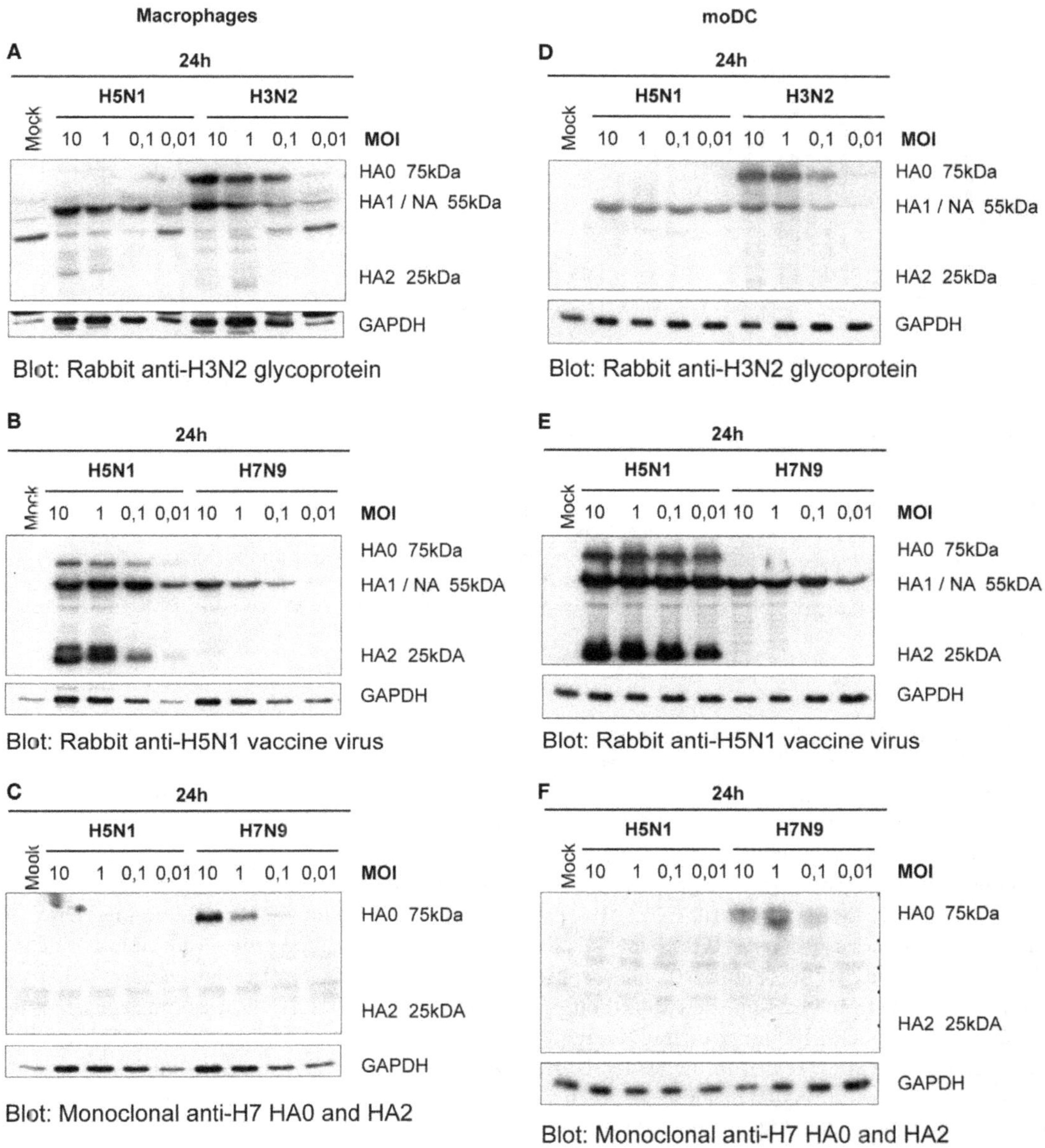

FIGURE 3 | Cleavage of the hemagglutinin (HA) protein of the influenza viruses in infected **(A–C)** monocyte-derived macrophages (Mϕs) and **(D–F)** monocyte-derived DCs (moDCs). Mϕs and moDCs from four blood donor were infected with A/Beijing/353/89 (H3N2), A/Vietnam/1194/2004 (H5N1), and A/Anhui/1/2013 (H7N9) influenza viruses at indicated multiplicity of infection (MOI) values for 24 h. Cellular lysates for protein samples were collected, the samples of different donors were pooled, and HA proteins were analyzed by Western blotting. The membranes were stained **(A,D)** with antibodies against glycoproteins of H3N2 virus to detect the HA0, HA1, and HA2 of the H3N2 virus, **(B,E)** against the glycoproteins of H5N1 virus to detect the HA0, HA1 and HA2 of the H5N1 virus, or **(C,F)** against the HA of H7 virus to detect HA0 and HA2 of the H7N9 virus. In panels **(A,B)**, HA1 and NA co-migrate and thus the heterologous signal is due to cross-reactivity of the NA protein. The levels of GAPDH were used as an internal loading control. A representative experiment out of two is shown.

We and others have previously shown that IFN-α can inhibit H3N2, H5N1, and H7N9 virus replication (12, 27). Here, we show that the H5N1/2004 avian influenza strain replicates and spreads efficiently in Mϕs and moDCs even at very low multiplicity infection (MOI 0.01) (**Figures 2A,B**), although the host cells respond to the infection with maximal cytokine gene expression (**Figures 9** and **10**). The H5N1/2004 virus induced strong IFN-λ1, IFN-α1, and IFN-β gene expression in Mϕs (**Figures 9A–C**). This suggests that the H5N1 virus is able to spread irrespective of the activation of antiviral immune responses since otherwise IFNs should inhibit virus replication. Lower virus doses in H3N2 or H7N9-infected moDCs led to clearly weaker IFN responses when compared with H5N1-infected cells at the 24 h time point (**Figures 9A–C**) suggesting that there are likely less infected cells that produce IFNs. To get further view of H5N1/2004 virus induced "cytokine storm," we investigated the expression of chemokine CXCL10 and CCL5 and pro-inflammatory cytokine IL-1β and TNF-α genes in H3N2, H5N1/2004, or H7N9

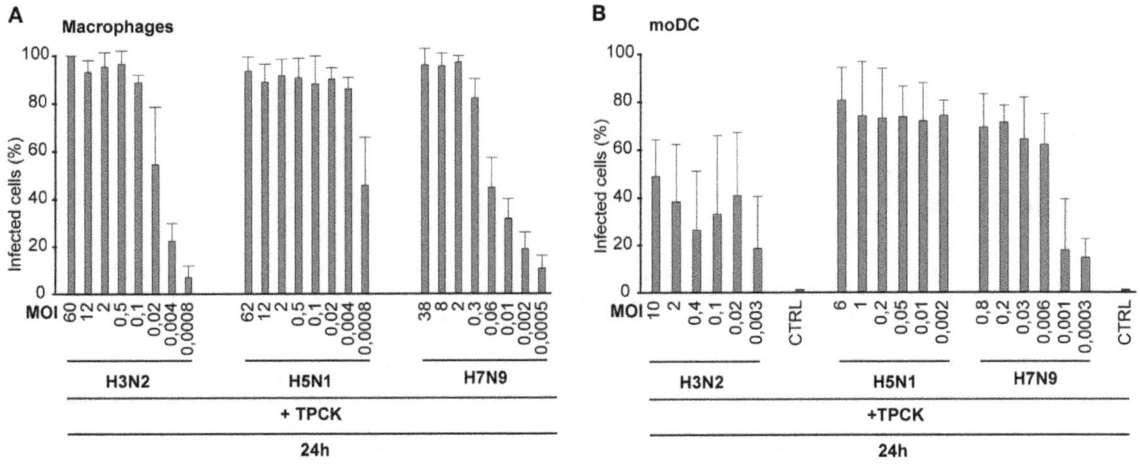

FIGURE 4 | Infectivity of the H3N2, H5N1, and H7N9 viruses in the presence of trypsin. Monocyte-derived macrophages (Mϕs) **(A)** or monocyte-derived DCs (moDCs) **(B)** were infected with externally added TPCK-trypsin with A/Beijing/353/89 (H3N2), A/Vietnam/1194/2004 (H5N1), and A/Anhui/1/2013 (H7N9) influenza viruses with indicated multiplicity of infection (MOI) values and the samples were collected at 24 h after infection. **(A)** The proportion of infected Mϕs was analyzed with immunofluorescence microscopy by staining the cells with antibody against respective virus proteins. From each donor at least 300 cells (average ca. 550) were counted. **(B)** moDCs were stained with antibody against virus proteins and infected cells were analyzed with flow cytometry. From each donor 10,000 events were analyzed.

virus-infected Mϕs (**Figures 9D–G**). Like IFN responses, with low MOI value, also CXCL10, CCL5, and TNF-α responses were higher in H5N1-infected Mϕs with low MOI value than with low MOI values in H3N2 or H7N9 virus infection. Induction of IL-1β gene expression is very low with H3N2, H5N1, and H7N9 viruses (**Figure 9F**) as we have also previously shown in moDCs (12). IFN-λ1, IFN-α1, IFN-β, CXCL10, CCL5, IL-1β, and TNF-α gene expression was also investigated in H3N2, H5N1, and H7N9 virus-infected moDCs (**Figure 10**). Data from moDCs correlate with the data from virus-infected Mϕs though CXCL10 mRNA induction was clearly higher in moDCs than in Mϕs, whereas CCL5 gene was expressed in higher levels in Mϕs. Thus, we next analyzed the expression of antiviral proteins in H3N2, H5N1, and H7N9-infected Mϕs (**Figure 11A**) and moDCs (**Figure 11B**). With all analyzed viruses, the expression of IFN-induced antiviral MxA protein was the strongest at the 24-h time point (**Figures 10A,B**). We also analyzed the expression of phosphorylated transcription factors IRF3 (P-IRF3) and STAT2 (P-STAT2) and noticed that the protein expression of these proteins was weaker in H7N9-infected cells compared with those seen in H5N1 or H3N2 infected cells (**Figures 11A,B**) which correlates well with the gene expression of IFNs (**Figures 9** and **10**) as well as with our previous study (12). The data show that in a multi-cyclic infection the H5N1 virus is able to induce very strong IFN gene expressions and antiviral MxA protein expression.

DISCUSSION

In 1997, a direct transmission of an avian influenza H5N1 virus from poultry to humans was documented for the first time (28). After that many subtypes of avian influenza A viruses have been reported to cause infections in humans, among them the H7N9 influenza type (4). High prevalence of influenza viruses in birds, the possibility of formation of new highly pathogenic reassortants and the ability of these viruses to spread to humans makes avian influenza A viruses of great global concern and emphasize the importance of virus–host cell interaction studies in human cell systems. In this study, we wanted to characterize different steps of H5N1 virus infection in human immune cells to reveal potential mechanisms explaining the severe clinical outcome of the H5N1 virus infection. In our previous study, we have shown that the avian H5N1 and H7N9 viruses can replicate in human moDCs (12). Here, we show that, unlike the H7N9 or seasonal influenza A viruses, the H5N1 virus is efficiently spreading in human immune cell cultures leading to a productive infection and robust IFN response. The remarkable ability of H5N1 virus to spread in human immune cells and likely other human cell types can be one explanation for the severe disease seen in humans with H5N1 virus infection. Here, we show that this ability is associated with at least two different HPAI H5N1 virus strains, and it may be a universal feature for all highly pathogenic avian-origin influenza A virus subtypes. There may be other viral or host factors regulating avian influenza pathogenicity in humans, since the LPAI H7N9 virus (LPAI in birds) has caused more human infections and deaths than the H5N1 subtype (4). In addition, there is now evidence that the H7N9 subtype has evolved to a HPAI H7N9 strain in birds, and this type of virus has already caused infections in humans (5).

Human infections with the HPAI H5N1 viruses are associated with a high viral load (29), and our data presented in this study confirm that the ability of the H5N1 virus to replicate and spread in immune cell culture is completely different from those of the LPAI H7N9 and seasonal H3N2 influenza A virus infections (**Figures 1, 2** and **6A,B**). The efficacy of systemic spread of influenza viruses depends on the cleavage of HA0 into HA1

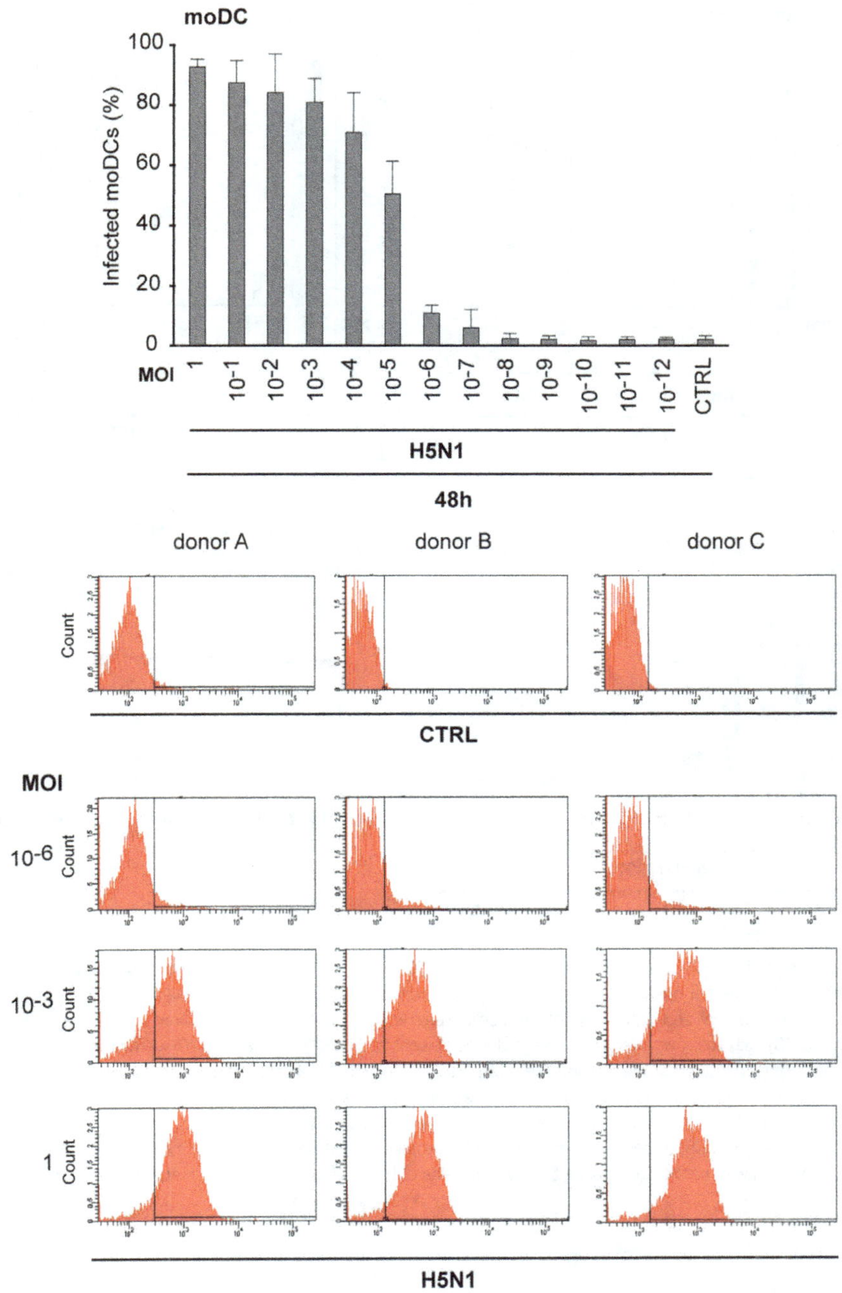

FIGURE 5 | Infectivity of H5N1 virus with serial dilutions in monocyte-derived DCs (moDCs). To titrate the infectivity and the spread of infection, A/Vietnam/1194/2004 (H5N1) virus stock was diluted in 1:10 series from multiplicity of infection (MOI) 1 to MOI 10–12 and moDCs from 3 different donors were infected for 48 h. Cells were collected and the percentage of infected cells was analyzed with flow cytometry. From each donor 10,000 events were analyzed.

and HA2 subunits and the distribution of appropriate proteases in host tissues. We noticed that the HA0 of H5N1 virus is cleaved very efficiently in human immune cells while the cleavage of the HA0 of H3N2 or H7N9 viruses is inefficient (**Figures 3** and **6D**). However, externally added TPCK-trypsin, which cleaves the HA0 precursor to HA1 and HA2 subunits, increases the proportion of infected cells in H3N2 and H7N9 infection (**Figures 4A,B**). There is clear evidence that the multi-basic HA1–HA2 cleavage site constituting of several lysine or/and arginine residues in the HA molecule of the HPAI strains, in contrast to a mono-basic cleavage site in LPAI and seasonal influenza viruses, regulate the pathogenesis of influenza A viruses. The multi-basic cleavage site in the HA has been shown to be a critical determinant of systemic spread of HPAI H5N1 virus (30). The emerged HPAI form of the H7N9 virus expressing the multi-basic site in HA is showing mammalian adaptation with increased pathogenicity and

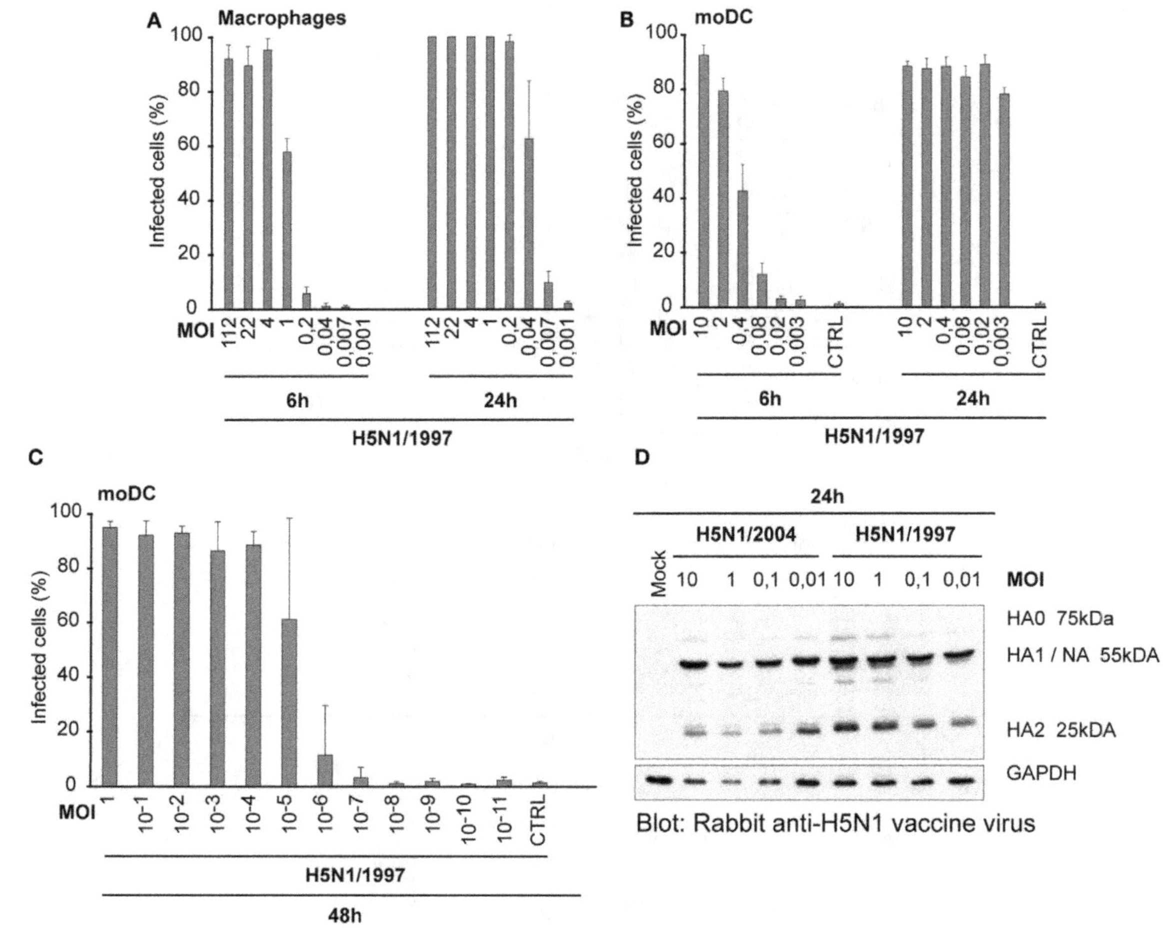

FIGURE 6 | Infectivity and the cleavage of the HA protein of A/Hong Kong/156/1997 (H5N1) virus. **(A)** Monocyte-derived macrophages (Mφs) or **(B)** monocyte-derived DCs (moDCs) were infected with different doses of a human isolate of avian influenza A/Hong Kong/156/1997 (H5N1) virus for 6 or 24 h. Results are the mean values from four donors infected and analyzed separately. Infected cells were detected with antibodies against H5N1 vaccine antigens **(A)** using immunofluorescence microscopy or **(B)** with flow cytometry. From each donor, at least 200 cells (average ca. 420) were counted **(A)** or 10,000 events were analyzed **(B)**. The titers for infective particles per ml (FFU/ml) and representative multiplicity of infection (MOI) values were calculated for Mφs and moDCs. **(C)** moDCs were infected with H5N1/1997 virus at different MOI values for 48 h. The cells were stained with virus-specific antibodies and analyzed with flow cytometry. From each donor, 10,000 events were analyzed. Results are the mean values of four donors analyzed separately. **(D)** moDCs from four donors were infected with indicated MOI values of H5N1/1997 virus for 24 h with or without added TPCK-trypsin and for protein samples cellular lysates from different donors were pooled. Cleavage of HA protein was detected by Western blotting with antibodies against the glycoproteins of H5N1 virus to detect the HA0, HA1, and HA2 of the H5N1 virus.

respiratory droplet transmission in ferrets (31). Yet, there must be other factors besides the multi-basic cleavage site that contribute to virus replication and spreading in mammals. Schrauwen and coworkers (32) have shown that the insertion of a multi-basic cleavage site in the HA of H3N2 virus enhances the cleavage of HA and replication in MDCK cells, but it did not increase the pathogenicity in ferrets. In addition, the study by Matthaei et al. (27) shows that the human H5N1 isolates replicate more efficiently in human epithelial cells than the avian H5N1 isolates, suggesting that there must be other differences in addition to multi-basic HA0 cleavage site between human and avian isolates that contribute to the pathogenicity of the virus. Zhao and coworkers have shown that a G158N mutation in HA (H3 numbering) of an avian HPAI H5N1 isolate enhanced viral production and induced stronger host immune responses in mammalian cells (33) which indicates that multi-basic HA1–HA2 cleavage site is not the only factor affecting virulence. Also, our results are consistent with this study of Zhao et al. since both A/Hong Kong/156/1997 and A/Vietnam/1194/2004 H5N1 viruses have asparagine residue at position 158.

It is generally accepted that influenza A virus infection in epithelial cells is productive leading to the release of a great number of progeny viruses from these cells. There is, however, a controversy whether human DCs and Mφs can efficiently produce infectious influenza A viruses. Bender and coworkers showed that a seasonal H1N1 influenza A virus infection in human DCs is abortive (34). Tate et al. (35) and Ioannidis et al. (36) obtained very similar results in mouse Mφ and DC model systems with both seasonal H1N1 and H3N2 influenza A viruses. On the other hand, the study by Yu et al. (16) indicates that the

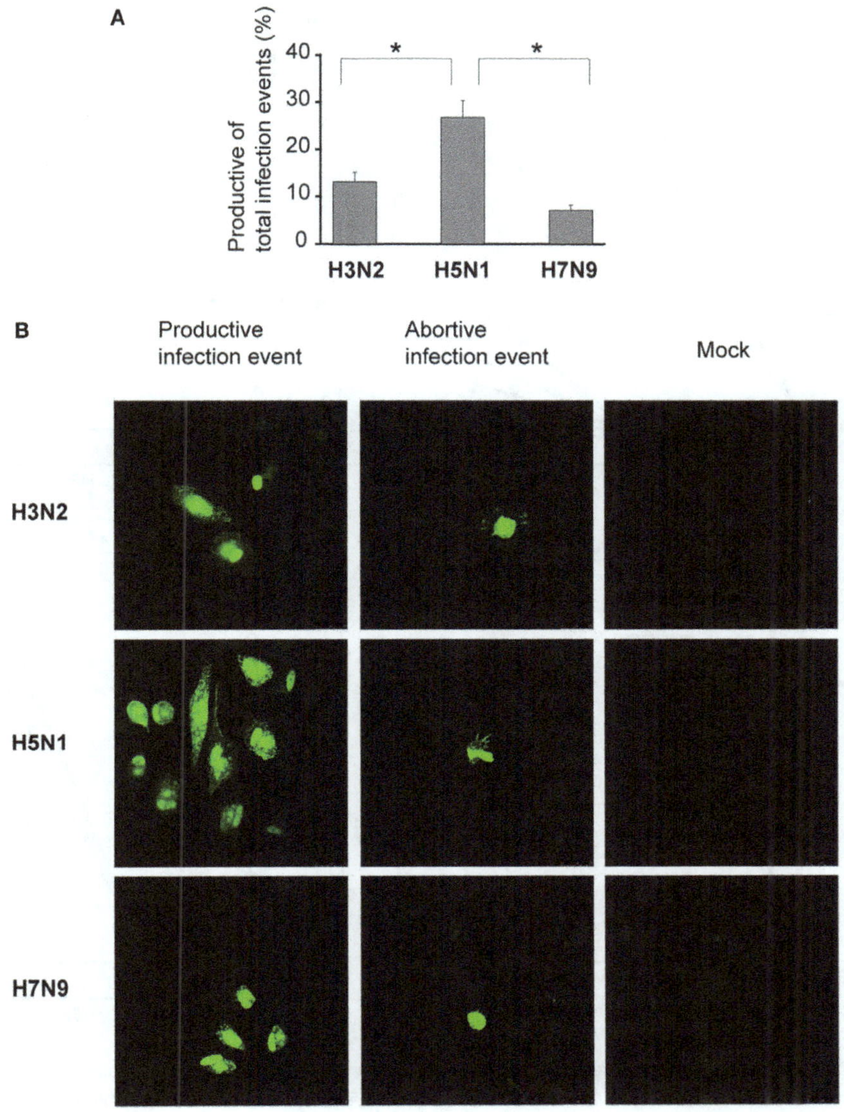

FIGURE 7 | Proportion of the propagation-competent virus particles in virus stocks. Monocyte-derived macrophages (Mϕs) were grown on glass coverslips, infected with A/Beijing/353/89 (H3N2), A/Vietnam/1194/2004 (H5N1), or A/Anhui/1/2013 (H7N9) influenza viruses at multiplicity of infection (MOI) of 0.01. After 1 h incubation, cells were washed and overlaid with 1.2% Avicel in E-MEM with added trypsin. After 15 h incubation, cells were fixed, permeabilized, and stained for viral protein expression. **(A)** Productive and abortive infection events were calculated. The results represent the mean values + SDs of the means from the cells of four different donors. From each donor, four coverslips with 80 to 500 infection events were counted. The statistical significance of differences between H5N1 and H3N2 or H7N9 was determined by Student's *t*-test, *<0.05. **(B)** Representative immunofluorescence images of infection events for each virus. Infection events were considered productive if three or more adjacent cells were infected. If two or less adjacent cells were infected, the infection event was considered abortive. Immunofluorescence images from one representative donor are shown.

HPAI H5N1 virus can replicate productively in human alveolar Mϕs but the infection with seasonal H1N1 virus was abortive. Also, several other studies show that an infection in monocyte-derived Mϕs with seasonal H3N2 or HPAI H5N1 viruses seems to be productive (7, 14, 37, 38). In conclusion, it seems that a H1N1 type influenza A virus infection is likely abortive and, consistent with our results, HPAI H5N1 virus infection is productive (**Figures 8A,B**) in human immune cells. Nonetheless, there are inconsistent results on the productivity of seasonal H3N2 influenza A virus infection in human cells. In our analyses, a H3N2 influenza A virus as well as the LPAI human isolate of H7N9 virus appeared to cause abortive infection in human moDCs (**Figure 8B**). Instead, H3N2 and H7N9 virus infections seemed to be productive in Mϕs (**Figure 8A**). However, the productivity of these viruses was clearly lower when compared with that of the HPAI H5N1 virus. We used another way, namely analyzing the relative amount of virus-specific RNA from cell culture supernatants, to indirectly quantitate the amount of secreted influenza virus into cell culture supernatant. Based on this analysis, there was a good correlation between the amount of infectious virus

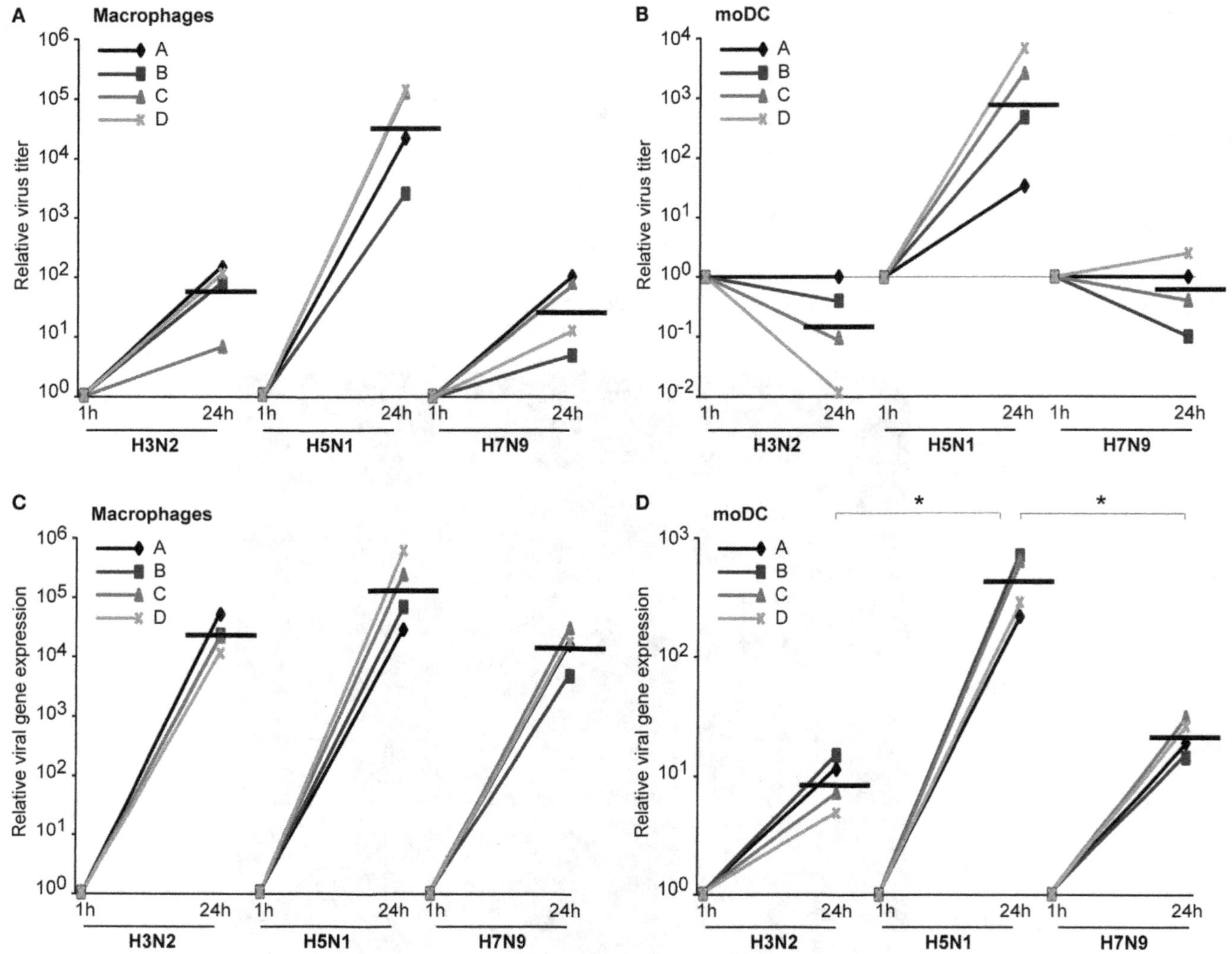

FIGURE 8 | The productivity of H3N2, H5N1, and H7N9 infections in human innate immune cells. Monocyte-derived macrophages (Mϕs) or monocyte-derived DCs (moDCs) from four different donors were infected with A/Beijing/353/89 (H3N2), A/Vietnam/1194/2004 (H5N1), or A/Anhui/1/2013 (H7N9) influenza viruses at multiplicity of infection (MOI) of 0.01 and after 1 and 24 h of infection the supernatant samples were collected. **(A,B)** The infective viral titers produced from Mϕs **(A)** or moDCs **(B)** were determined by plaque assay in Madin–Darby Canine Kidney cells. The relative virus titers were calculated over 1 h samples. The horizontal lines represent the geometric means of the results from four blood donors. **(C,D)** The RNA was isolated from the supernatant samples from Mϕs **(C)** and moDCs **(D)** and the viral RNA levels were detected by qRT-PCR. The relative viral RNA expressions were calculated over 1 h samples with ΔCT method. The horizontal lines represent the geometric means from different donors. The statistical significance of differences between H5N1 and H3N2 or H7N9 was determined by Student's *t*-test, *<0.05.

and the viral RNA levels in the supernatants of H3N2, H5N1, and H7N9-infected Mϕs and moDCs (**Figures 8C,D**). A technical detail may, however, confound the results since in moDC infections the input virus was not washed away. It may be that, since in the plaque assay of the supernatant samples the background is relative high and H3N2 or H7N9 infections are only weakly productive, we are unable to clearly see an increase in the virus titers. The productivity of influenza virus infections in human DCs and Mϕs have remained poorly investigated and thus our result is a significant addition to the present knowledge.

There is limited amount of information of how many new influenza virus particles or infective units a single-infected cell can produce. Baccam et al. (39) estimated that a single H1N1 virus-infected cell of the upper respiratory tract can produce up to 22 new infectious virus particles leading to a productive infection. It is possible that a single H5N1 virus-infected cell produces even more infective progeny viruses, which may explain the fast and efficient spread of the H5N1 virus in our experimental systems. This study shows that in human immune cells the HPAI H5N1 virus can spread faster than the H3N2 or H7N9 viruses. This may contribute to the ability of H5N1 virus to cause a systemic infection associated with a fatal outcome in H5N1 virus-infected humans.

It is commonly thought that the IFN system is the key factor regulating the efficacy of host antiviral responses and the clearance of the virus. However, the high mortality in H5N1

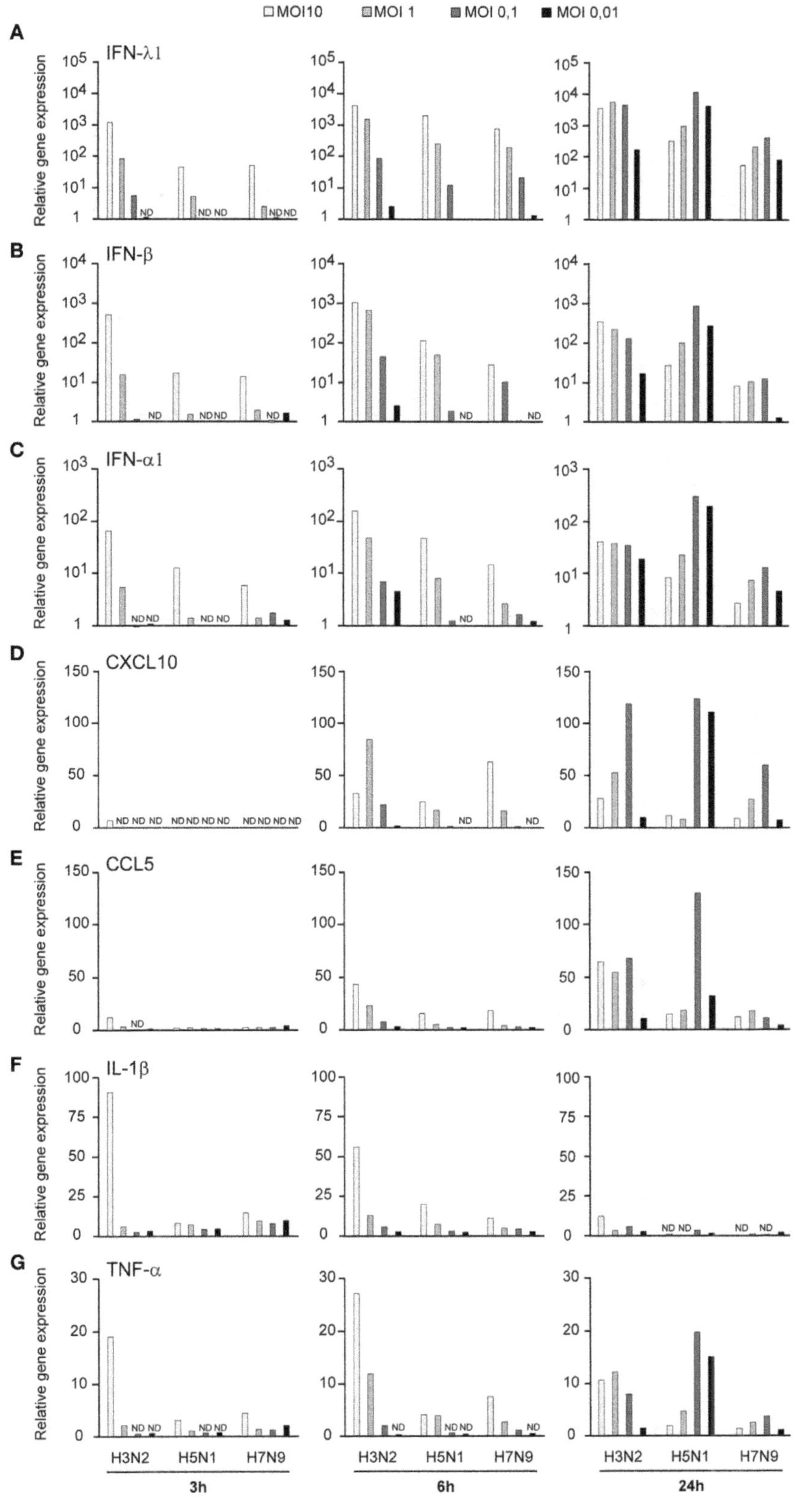

FIGURE 9 | Innate immune responses in H3N2, H5N1, and H7N9 influenza virus-infected human monocyte-derived macrophages (Mϕs). Mϕs were infected with A/Beijing/353/89 (H3N2), A/Vietnam/1194/2004 (H5N1), or A/Anhui/1/2013 (H7N9) influenza viruses at multiplicity of infection (MOI) values of 10 to 0.01 for 24 h. **(A)** Cells from four donors were collected at different time points after infection as indicated in the figure, cells from different donors were pooled and total cellular RNA was isolated. **(A)** IFN-λ1, **(B)** IFN-β, **(C)** IFN-α1, **(D)** CXCL10, **(E)** CCL5, **(F)** IL-1β, and **(G)** TNF-α gene expression was analyzed by qRT-PCR. Gene expression < 1 is defined as not detected (ND). A representative experiment out of two is shown.

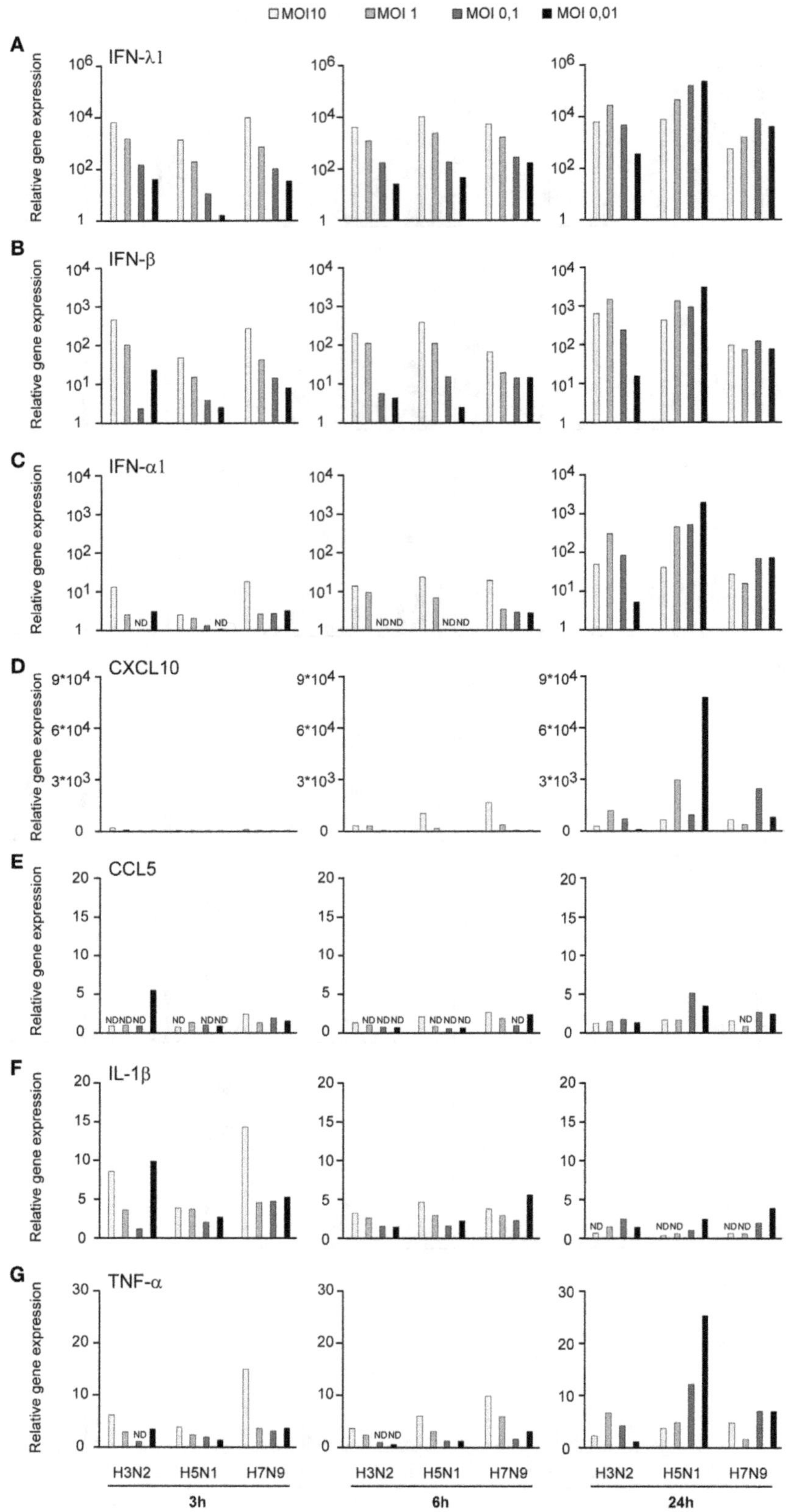

FIGURE 10 | Innate immune responses in H3N2, H5N1, and H7N9 influenza virus-infected human monocyte-derived DCs (moDCs). moDCs were infected with A/Beijing/353/89 (H3N2), A/Vietnam/1194/2004 (H5N1), or A/Anhui/1/2013 (H7N9) influenza viruses at multiplicity of infection (MOI) values of 10 to 0.01 for 24 h. **(A)** Cells from four donors were collected at different time points after infection as indicated in the figure, cells from different donors were pooled and total cellular RNA was isolated. **(A)** IFN-λ1, **(B)** IFN-β, **(C)** IFN-α1, **(D)** CXCL10, **(E)** CCL5, **(F)** IL-1β, and **(G)** TNF-α gene expression was analyzed by qRT-PCR. Gene expression < 1 is defined as not detected (ND). A representative experiment out of three is shown.

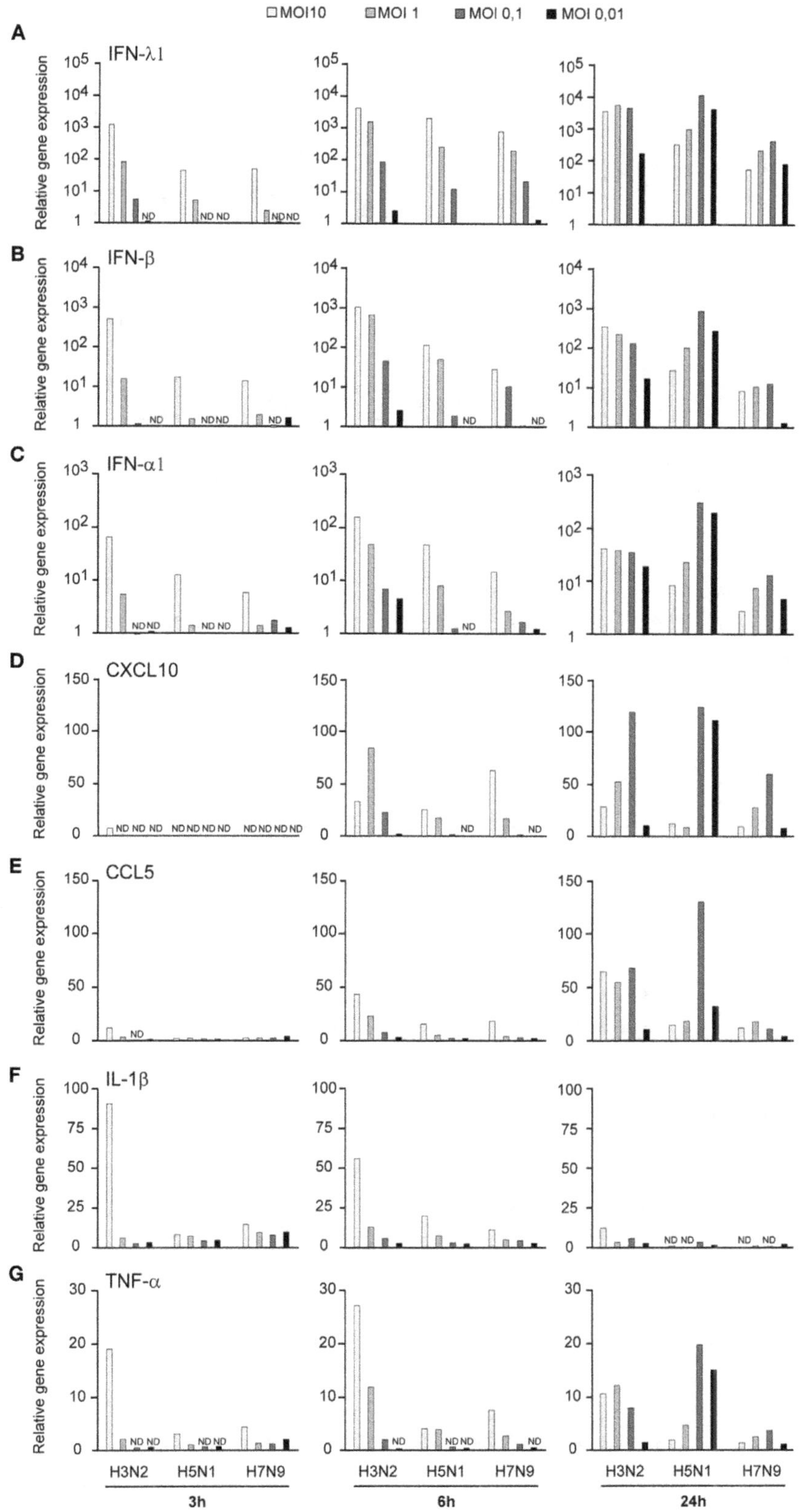

FIGURE 9 | Innate immune responses in H3N2, H5N1, and H7N9 influenza virus-infected human monocyte-derived macrophages (Mϕs). Mϕs were infected with A/Beijing/353/89 (H3N2), A/Vietnam/1194/2004 (H5N1), or A/Anhui/1/2013 (H7N9) influenza viruses at multiplicity of infection (MOI) values of 10 to 0.01 for 24 h. **(A)** Cells from four donors were collected at different time points after infection as indicated in the figure, cells from different donors were pooled and total cellular RNA was isolated. **(A)** IFN-λ1, **(B)** IFN-β, **(C)** IFN-α1, **(D)** CXCL10, **(E)** CCL5, **(F)** IL-1β, and **(G)** TNF-α gene expression was analyzed by qRT-PCR. Gene expression < 1 is defined as not detected (ND). A representative experiment out of two is shown.

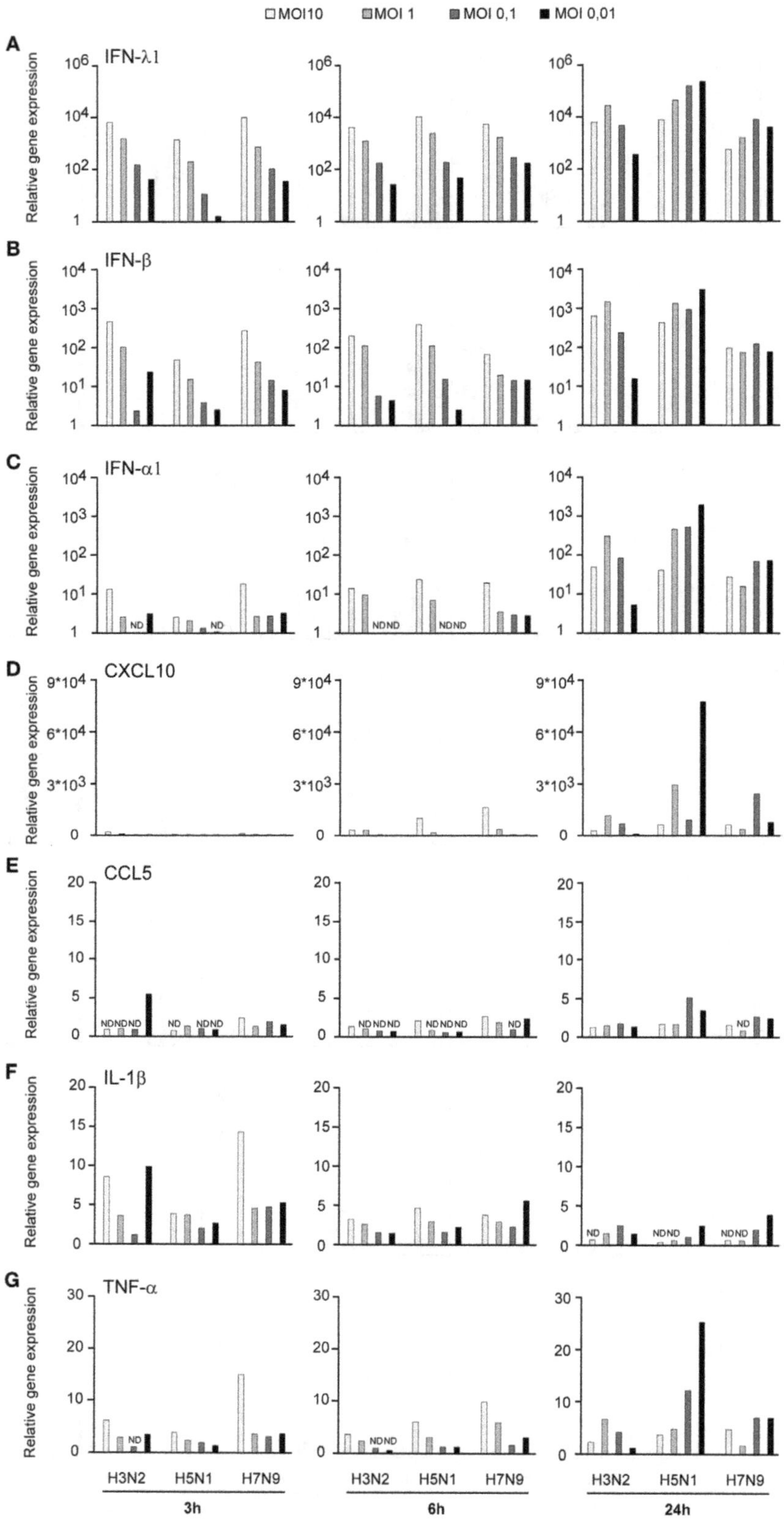

FIGURE 10 | Innate immune responses in H3N2, H5N1, and H7N9 influenza virus-infected human monocyte-derived DCs (moDCs). moDCs were infected with A/Beijing/353/89 (H3N2), A/Vietnam/1194/2004 (H5N1), or A/Anhui/1/2013 (H7N9) influenza viruses at multiplicity of infection (MOI) values of 10 to 0.01 for 24 h. **(A)** Cells from four donors were collected at different time points after infection as indicated in the figure, cells from different donors were pooled and total cellular RNA was isolated. **(A)** IFN-λ1, **(B)** IFN-β, **(C)** IFN-α1, **(D)** CXCL10, **(E)** CCL5, **(F)** IL-1β, and **(G)** TNF-α gene expression was analyzed by qRT-PCR. Gene expression < 1 is defined as not detected (ND). A representative experiment out of three is shown.

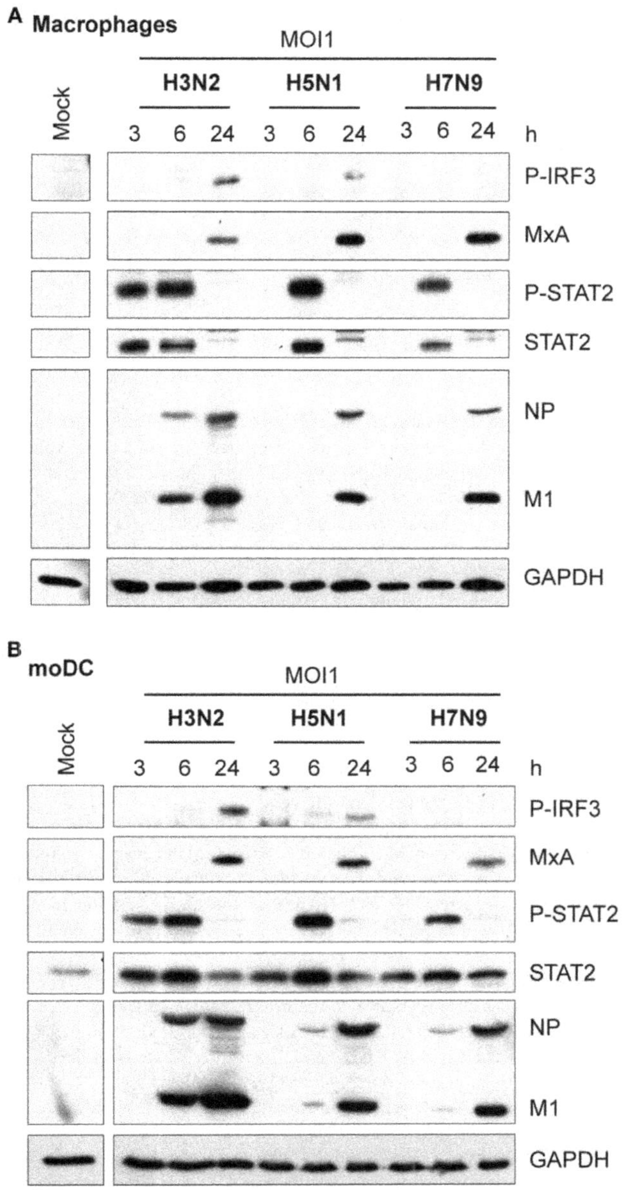

FIGURE 11 | Activation of transcription factors and expression of antiviral MxA protein in H3N2, H5N1, and H7N9 influenza virus-infected human monocyte-derived macrophages (Mϕs) and monocyte-derived DCs (moDCs). **(A)** Mϕs and **(B)** moDCs were infected with A/Beijing/353/89 (H3N2), A/Vietnam/1194/2004 (H5N1), or A/Anhui/1/2013 (H7N9) influenza viruses at multiplicity of infection (MOI) values of 1. Cellular protein lysates were collected at 3, 6, and 24 h after infection, samples from four donors were pooled and P-IRF3, MxA, P-STAT2, STAT2, and viral NP and M1 protein expression was analyzed by Western blotting using specific antisera. GAPDH protein expression was analyzed to control equal loading of the samples. A representative experiment out of two (Mϕs) or three (moDCs) is shown.

infection has been associated with an excessive inflammatory response in the lungs of virus-infected individuals (29). Our study shows that the H5N1 virus grows extremely well in human immune cells and it induces strong IFN responses (**Figures 1**, **2**, **9A–C** and **10A–C**), both of which may contribute to the clinical outcome of the H5N1 infection. Our data show that IFN and also pro-inflammatory cytokine and chemokine responses are higher in infection with H5N1 than with H3N2 or H7N9 viruses at low MOI at the 24 h time point after infection. At the same time, we see that after 24 h infection with the H5N1 virus all cells are infected whereas with the H3N2 or H7N9 virus only proportion of the cells is infected. This suggests that there is a positive correlation between the spread of infection and the cytokine responses. Thus, the strong IFN responses and virus replication are not exclusive of each other; for instance, Ngunjiri et al. (40) have shown that the highly pathogenic H5N1 virus is sensitive to the antiviral actions of IFNs. There is also evidence that H5N1 viruses with high replication competency can ultimately overcome the antiviral effects induced by IFN-α and IFN-β (41). Bordi et al. (42) have shown that IFN-λ and IFN-α have antagonistic antiviral activity against Crimean-Congo hemorrhagic fever virus. However, in our previous study (43) in influenza A virus infection, we did not see any antagonistic activity between IFN-α and IFN-λ, or IFN-λ and IFN-γ, or IFN-α and IFN-γ. We have shown that in H5N1 virus infection IFN-α is produced leading to strong MxA protein expression in the cells which proves that IFN signaling is intact in H5N1-infected cells (12). Still, in this study, we clearly show that HPAI H5N1 virus can replicate and spread extremely efficiently in human innate immune cells despite of strong activation of IFN gene expression and MxA protein expression (**Figure 11**). This indicates that due to efficient spread of H5N1 virus and high infectivity in the cell cultures there are more cells which can produce IFNs leading to a cytokine storm associated with H5N1-infected patients. This may in part explain the fatal outcome of a H5N1 virus infection in humans. Although the clinical outcome in humans is similar in H5N1 and H7N9 virus infections, surprisingly the antiviral IFN and pro-inflammatory cytokine gene expression is impaired in H7N9 virus-infected immune cells (**Figures 9** and **10**). Thus, it seems that the mechanism behind the pathogenicity is different in H5N1 and H7N9 virus infection which still demands further investigations.

In this study, we have shown that different types of influenza A viruses may behave very differently in immune cells, primary human monocyte-derived Mϕs and DCs functioning as our model cell systems. While HPAI H5N1 virus efficiently replicated and spread in immune cell cultures seasonal H3N2 and surprisingly LPAI H7N9 viruses showed reduced ability to establish a productive infection. More studies are clearly warranted to further reveal the mechanistic details regulating the ability of HPAI avian influenza viruses to replicate in human primary immune cells and to understand the relationship between the virus and host innate immune system.

AUTHOR CONTRIBUTIONS

VW performed most of the experiments, analyzed the data, and wrote the manuscript. SM and PÖ helped with experiments. IJ and PÖ together with VW designed the experiments and wrote the manuscript.

ACKNOWLEDGMENTS

We are grateful to Professor Ron A. M. Fouchier and Dr. John McCauley for providing the H5N1 and H7N9 viruses, respectively. The following reagent was obtained through BEI Resources, NIAID, NIH: Monoclonal Anti-Influenza A Virus H7 Hemagglutinin (HA) Protein, A/Netherlands/219/2003 (H7N7), Clone AT241.375.173 (produced *in vitro*), NR-48980. We thank our technical assistants Johanna Rintamäki, Teija Aalto, Nina Aho, Svetlana Kaijalainen, and especially Hanna Valtonen and Riitta Santanen for assistance in BSL-3 work, and we appreciate the help from the biosafety officer Susanna Sissonen at THL. We also thank our trainees Riia Järvi and Olga Jänisniemi for their assistance in laboratory work.

REFERENCES

1. Johnson NP, Mueller J. Updating the accounts: global mortality of the 1918-1920 "Spanish" influenza pandemic. *Bull Hist Med* (2002) 76(1):105–15. doi:10.1353/bhm.2002.0022
2. Novel Swine-Origin Influenza A (H1N1) Virus Investigation Team, Dawood FS, Jain S, Finelli L, Shaw MW, Lindstrom S, et al. Emergence of a novel swine-origin influenza A (H1N1) virus in humans. *N Engl J Med* (2009) 360(25): 2605–15. doi:10.1056/NEJMoa0903810
3. Horimoto T, Kawaoka Y. Influenza: lessons from past pandemics, warnings from current incidents. *Nat Rev Microbiol* (2005) 3(8):591–600. doi:10.1038/nrmicro1208
4. WHO. *Latest Risk Assessment Summary of Influenza at the Human-Animal Interface*. Available from: http://www.who.int/influenza/human_animal_interface/Influenza_Summary_IRA_HA_interface_02_03_2018.pdf?ua=1 (Accessed: March 2, 2018).
5. Zhang F, Bi Y, Wang J, Wong G, Shi W, Hu F, et al. Human infections with recently-emerging highly pathogenic H7N9 avian influenza virus in china. *J Infect* (2017) 75(1):71–5. doi:10.1016/j.jinf.2017.04.001
6. Morens DM, Taubenberger JK, Fauci AS. H7N9 avian influenza A virus and the perpetual challenge of potential human pandemicity. *MBio* (2013) 4(4):13. doi:10.1128/mBio.00445-13
7. Perrone LA, Plowden JK, Garcia-Sastre A, Katz JM, Tumpey TM. H5N1 and 1918 pandemic influenza virus infection results in early and excessive infiltration of macrophages and neutrophils in the lungs of mice. *PLoS Pathog* (2008) 4(8):e1000115. doi:10.1371/journal.ppat.1000115
8. Moltedo B, López C, Pazos M, Becker M, Hermesh T, Moran T. Cutting edge: stealth influenza virus replication precedes the initiation of adaptive immunity. *J Immunol* (2009) 183:3569–73. doi:10.4049/jimmunol.0900091
9. Seo SH, Webby R, Webster RG. No apoptotic deaths and different levels of inductions of inflammatory cytokines in alveolar macrophages infected with influenza viruses. *Virology* (2004) 329(2):270–9. doi:10.1016/j.virol.2004.08.019
10. Garcia-Sastre A, Biron CA. Type 1 interferons and the virus-host relationship: a lesson in detente. *Science* (2006) 312(5775):879–82. doi:10.1126/science.1125676
11. Osterlund PI, Pietila TE, Veckman V, Kotenko SV, Julkunen I. IFN regulatory factor family members differentially regulate the expression of type III IFN (IFN-lambda) genes. *J Immunol* (2007) 179(6):3434–42. doi:10.4049/jimmunol.179.6.3434
12. Arilahti V, Mäkelä S, Tynell J, Julkunen I, Osterlund P. Novel avian influenza A (H7N9) virus induces impaired interferon responses in human dendritic cells. *PLoS One* (2014) 9:e96350. doi:10.1371/journal.pone.0096350
13. Shinya K, Ebina M, Yamada S, Ono M, Kasai N, Kawaoka Y. Avian flu: influenza virus receptors in the human airway. *Nature* (2006) 440(7083):435–6. doi:10.1038/440435a
14. Thitithanyanont A, Engering A, Ekchariyawat P, Wiboon-ut S, Limsalakpetch A, Yongvanitchit K, et al. High susceptibility of human dendritic cells to avian influenza H5N1 virus infection and protection by IFN-alpha and TLR ligands. *J Immunol* (2007) 179(8):5220–7. doi:10.4049/jimmunol.179.8.5220
15. Sakabe S, Iwatsuki-Horimoto K, Takano R, Nidom CA, Le Mt, Nagamura-Inoue T, et al. Cytokine production by primary human macrophages infected with highly pathogenic H5N1 or pandemic H1N1 2009 influenza viruses. *J Gen Virol* (2011) 92(Pt 6):1428–34. doi:10.1099/vir.0.030346-0
16. Yu WC, Chan RW, Wang J, Travanty EA, Nicholls JM, Peiris JS, et al. Viral replication and innate host responses in primary human alveolar epithelial cells and alveolar macrophages infected with influenza H5N1 and H1N1 viruses. *J Virol* (2011) 85(14):6844–55. doi:10.1128/JVI.02200-10
17. Gerber M, Isel C, Moules V, Marquet R. Selective packaging of the influenza A genome and consequences for genetic reassortment. *Trends Microbiol* (2014) 22(8):446–55. doi:10.1016/j.tim.2014.04.001
18. Brooke CB, Ince WL, Wrammert J, Ahmed R, Wilson PC, Bennink JR, et al. Most influenza a virions fail to express at least one essential viral protein. *J Virol* (2013) 87(6):3155–62. doi:10.1128/JVI.02284-12
19. Nakatsu S, Sagara H, Sakai-Tagawa Y, Sugaya N, Noda T, Kawaoka Y. Complete and incomplete genome packaging of influenza A and B viruses. *MBio* (2016) 7(5):16. doi:10.1128/mBio.01248-16
20. Westenius V, Mäkelä SM, Ziegler T, Julkunen I, Österlund P. Efficient replication and strong induction of innate immune responses by H9N2 avian influenza virus in human dendritic cells. *Virology* (2014) 471–473:38–48. doi:10.1016/j.virol.2014.10.002
21. Veckman V, Miettinen M, Pirhonen J, Sirén J, Matikainen S, Julkunen I. *Streptococcus pyogenes* and *Lactobacillus rhamnosus* differentially induce maturation and production of Th1-type cytokines and chemokines in human monocyte-derived dendritic cells. *J Leukoc Biol* (2004) 75:764–71. doi:10.1189/jlb.1003461
22. Mäkelä SM, Österlund P, Westenius V, Latvala S, Diamond MS, Gale M Jr, et al. RIG-I signaling is essential for influenza B virus-induced rapid interferon gene expression. *J Virol* (2015) 89(23):12014–25. doi:10.1128/JVI.01576-15
23. Julkunen I, Hautanen A, Keski-Oja J. Interaction of viral envelope glycoproteins with fibronectin. *Infect Immun* (1983) 40(3):876–81.
24. Ronni T, Melén K, Malygin A, Julkunen I. Control of IFN-inducible MxA gene expression in human cells. *J Immunol* (1993) 150:1715–26.
25. Pietilä T, Latvala S, Österlund P, Julkunen I. Inhibition of dynamin-dependent endocytosis interferes with type III IFN expression in bacteria-infected human monocyte-derived DCs. *J Leukoc Biol* (2010) 88:665–74. doi:10.1189/jlb.1009651
26. Shi Y, Zhang W, Wang F, Qi J, Wu Y, Song H, et al. Structures and receptor binding of hemagglutinins from human-infecting H7N9 influenza viruses. *Science* (2013) 342(6155):243–7. doi:10.1126/science.1242917
27. Matthaei M, Budt M, Wolff T. Highly pathogenic H5N1 influenza A virus strains provoke heterogeneous IFN-alpha/beta responses that distinctively affect viral propagation in human cells. *PLoS One* (2013) 8(2):e56659. doi:10.1371/journal.pone.0056659
28. de Jong JC, Claas EC, Osterhaus AD, Webster RG, Lim WL. A pandemic warning? *Nature* (1997) 389(6651):554. doi:10.1038/39221
29. de Jong MD, Simmons CP, Thanh TT, Hien VM, Smith GJ, Chau TN, et al. Fatal outcome of human influenza A (H5N1) is associated with high viral load and hypercytokinemia. *Nat Med* (2006) 12:1203–7. doi:10.1038/nm1477
30. Schrauwen EJ, Herfst S, Leijten LM, van Run P, Bestebroer TM, Linster M, et al. The multibasic cleavage site in H5N1 virus is critical for systemic spread along the olfactory and hematogenous routes in ferrets. *J Virol* (2012) 86: 3975–84. doi:10.1128/JVI.06828-11
31. Imai M, Watanabe T, Kiso M, Nakajima N, Yamayoshi S, Iwatsuki-Horimoto K, et al. A highly pathogenic avian H7N9 influenza virus isolated from A human is lethal in some ferrets infected via respiratory droplets. *Cell Host Microbe* (2017) 22(5):626.e8. doi:10.1016/j.chom.2017.09.008

32. Schrauwen EJ, Bestebroer TM, Munster VJ, de Wit E, Herfst S, Rimmelzwaan GF, et al. Insertion of a multibasic cleavage site in the haemagglutinin of human influenza H3N2 virus does not increase pathogenicity in ferrets. *J Gen Virol* (2011) 92:1410–5. doi:10.1099/vir.0.030379-0
33. Zhao D, Liang L, Wang S, Nakao T, Li Y, Liu L, et al. Glycosylation of the hemagglutinin protein of H5N1 influenza virus increases its virulence in mice by exacerbating the host immune response. *J Virol* (2017) 91(7):16. doi:10.1128/JVI.02215-16
34. Bender A, Albert M, Reddy A, Feldman M, Sauter B, Kaplan G, et al. The distinctive features of influenza virus infection of dendritic cells. *Immunobiology* (1998) 198(5):552–67. doi:10.1016/S0171-2985(98)80078-8
35. Tate MD, Pickett DL, van Rooijen N, Brooks AG, Reading PC. Critical role of airway macrophages in modulating disease severity during influenza virus infection of mice. *J Virol* (2010) 84(15):7569–80. doi:10.1128/JVI.00291-10
36. Ioannidis LJ, Verity EE, Crawford S, Rockman SP, Brown LE. Abortive replication of influenza virus in mouse dendritic cells. *J Virol* (2012) 86(10):5922–5. doi:10.1128/JVI.07060-11
37. Hoeve MA, Nash AA, Jackson D, Randall RE, Dransfield I. Influenza virus A infection of human monocyte and macrophage subpopulations reveals increased susceptibility associated with cell differentiation. *PLoS One* (2012) 7(1):e29443. doi:10.1371/journal.pone.0029443
38. van Riel D, Leijten LM, van der Eerden M, Hoogsteden HC, Boven LA, Lambrecht BN, et al. Highly pathogenic avian influenza virus H5N1 infects alveolar macrophages without virus production or excessive TNF-alpha induction. *PLoS Pathog* (2011) 7(6):e1002099. doi:10.1371/journal.ppat.1002099
39. Baccam P, Beauchemin C, Macken CA, Hayden FG, Perelson AS. Kinetics of influenza A virus infection in humans. *J Virol* (2006) 80(15):7590–9. doi:10.1128/JVI.01623-05
40. Ngunjiri JM, Mohni KN, Sekellick MJ, Schultz-Cherry S, Webster RG, Marcus PI. Lethal H5N1 influenza viruses are not resistant to interferon action in human, simian, porcine or chicken cells. *Nat Med* (2012) 18(10):1456–7. doi:10.1038/nm.2879
41. Szretter KJ, Gangappa S, Belser JA, Zeng H, Chen H, Matsuoka Y, et al. Early control of H5N1 influenza virus replication by the type I interferon response in mice. *J Virol* (2009) 83(11):5825–34. doi:10.1128/JVI.02144-08
42. Bordi L, Lalle E, Caglioti C, Travaglini D, Lapa D, Marsella P, et al. Antagonistic antiviral activity between IFN-lambda and IFN-alpha against lethal Crimean-Congo hemorrhagic fever virus in vitro. *PLoS One* (2015) 10(2): e0116816. doi:10.1371/journal.pone.0116816
43. Osterlund P, Veckman V, Sirén J, Klucher KM, Hiscott J, Matikainen S, et al. Gene expression and antiviral activity of alpha/beta interferons and interleukin-29 in virus-infected human myeloid dendritic cells. *J Virol* (2005) 79(15):9608–17. doi:10.1128/JVI.79.15.9608-9617.2005

15

Infuenza A Virus Cell Entry, Replication, Virion Assembly and Movement

Dan Dou, Rebecca Revol, Henrik Östbye, Hao Wang and Robert Daniels*

Department of Biochemistry and Biophysics, Stockholm University, Stockholm, Sweden

***Correspondence:**
Robert Daniels
robertd@dbb.su.se

Influenza viruses replicate within the nucleus of the host cell. This uncommon RNA virus trait provides influenza with the advantage of access to the nuclear machinery during replication. However, it also increases the complexity of the intracellular trafficking that is required for the viral components to establish a productive infection. The segmentation of the influenza genome makes these additional trafficking requirements especially challenging, as each viral RNA (vRNA) gene segment must navigate the network of cellular membrane barriers during the processes of entry and assembly. To accomplish this goal, influenza A viruses (IAVs) utilize a combination of viral and cellular mechanisms to coordinate the transport of their proteins and the eight vRNA gene segments in and out of the cell. The aim of this review is to present the current mechanistic understanding for how IAVs facilitate cell entry, replication, virion assembly, and intercellular movement, in an effort to highlight some of the unanswered questions regarding the coordination of the IAV infection process.

Keywords: influenza A virus, viral ribonucleoprotein, hemagglutinin, viral entry mechanism, viral envelope proteins, HA and NA, viral replication, neuraminidase

INFLUENZA VIRUSES

Influenza viruses belong to the *Orthomyxoviridae* family and are classified as either type A, B, C, or the recently identified type D (1, 2). Influenza A viruses (IAVs) and type B viruses (IBVs) contain 8, negative-sense, single-stranded viral RNA (vRNA) gene segments (**Figure 1A**) (3, 4), which encode transcripts for 10 essential viral proteins, as well as several strain-dependent accessory proteins (**Figure 1B**). In comparison, influenza type C and D viruses only possess seven vRNA gene segments, as the hemagglutinin–esterase fusion protein vRNA replaces the hemagglutinin (HA or H) and the neuraminidase (NA or N) vRNAs (1, 2). IAVs will be the main focus of this review since they are the primary agents responsible for influenza pandemics, and a major contributor to the annual influenza epidemics in the human population (5).

The natural reservoir for IAVs is wild aquatic birds, but they commonly infect other species, including humans, and have even been isolated from penguins in Antarctica (12–15). The ability to adapt to multiple species is a major reason why IAVs are more diverse than IBVs, which are essentially exclusive to humans. Despite the host-range differences, many similarities do exist between these two viruses. Both possess a host-derived lipid membrane, referred to as an envelope, which is decorated on the surface with the viral membrane proteins HA, NA, and to a lesser extent the matrix 2 (M2) protein (**Figure 1C**) (16–18). The envelope is supported underneath by the matrix 1 (M1) protein, and inside, the eight vRNAs are found as individual viral ribonucleoprotein (vRNP) complexes (**Figure 1C**, bottom). Each vRNP is comprised of a vRNA that is wrapped around numerous

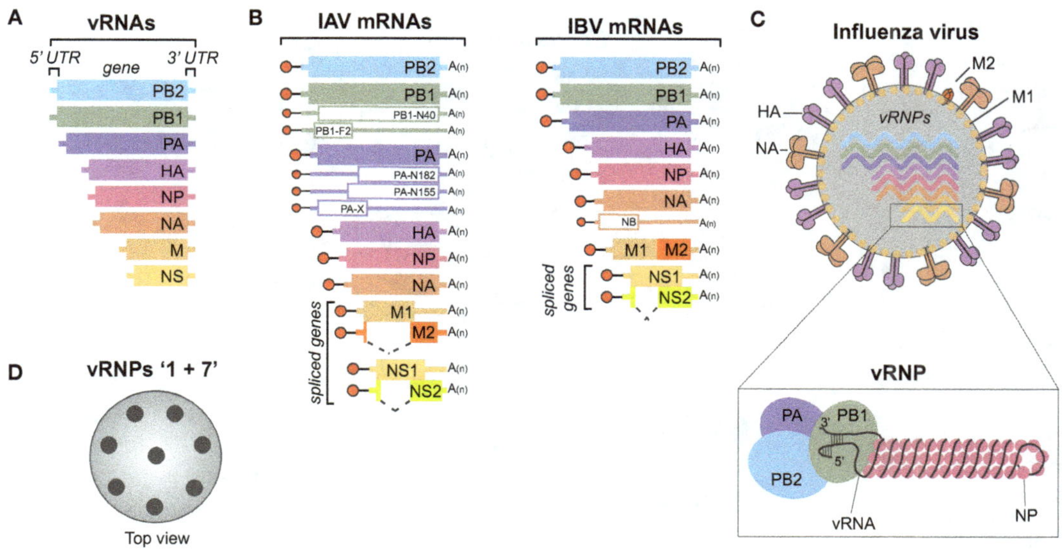

FIGURE 1 | Influenza A and B viruses. **(A)** Schematic of the eight viral RNA (vRNA) gene segments that comprise the influenza A and B genomes. The 5′ and 3′ untranslated regions (UTRs), which contain the viral promoters, are represented with a line, and the box corresponds to the coding region within each vRNA. **(B)** Diagram of the viral mRNAs that are transcribed from the IAV (left) and IBV (right) vRNA templates. Boxes indicate the viral gene product encoded by each mRNA and the dashed lines show the alternative splicing of the IAV M and NS transcripts, as well as the IBV NS transcript. Red circles represent the 5′ M^7pppG cap, black lines denote the 10–13 nucleotide, host-derived primers that are obtained by the cap-snatching mechanism of the viral polymerase. A(n) corresponds to the 3′ poly-A tail produced by reiterative stuttering of the viral polymerase. The smaller mRNAs (empty boxes) represent transcripts that encode nonessential accessory proteins found in many strains, whereas those that are less prevalent (PB2-S1, M42, and NS3) are not illustrated (6–11). **(C)** Diagram of an influenza A or B virus. The viral membrane proteins HA, NA, and M2 are shown, along with the eight viral ribonucleoproteins (vRNPs), and the matrix protein M1 that supports the viral envelope. To highlight the vRNP components, the illustration beneath the virus is not to scale. A single vRNA gene segment is shown wrapped around multiple nucleoprotein (NP) copies with the conserved promoter regions in the 5′ and 3′ UTRs forming a helical hairpin, which is bound by a single heterotrimeric viral RNA-dependent RNA polymerase (PB1, PB2, and PA). **(D)** Top view of an influenza virus cross-section showing the vRNP "1 + 7" configuration. vRNPs are depicted with black circles as it is not known if the positioning of a particular vRNP is conserved or interchangeable.

copies of the viral nucleoprotein (NP) and bound by a single copy of the heterotrimeric viral polymerase, consisting of PB1, PB2, and PA (19–21). The polymerase binds the vRNAs at a helical hairpin that results from the base pairing between the conserved semi-complimentary 5′ and 3′ ends (21–23).

Morphologically, IAVs can either form spheres with a diameter of ~100 nm or filaments that can reach up to 20 μm in length [reviewed in Ref. (24)]. However, upon passaging in eggs, or MDCK cells, the filamentous form is generally lost (25, 26). Several studies have attributed the morphology change to M1, presumably through its function in supporting the envelope (27–29). Regardless of the virion shape, HA is the most abundant viral envelope protein, followed by NA, and M2 (30). Recent work has shown that the viral envelope also contains host membrane proteins (30, 31). These proteins are likely recruited based on the lipid composition at the plasma membrane budding site, which can differ between cell types (32, 33). Through possible interactions with each other and M1, the eight vRNPs typicallly form a 1 + 7 configuration inside the virus (**Figure 1D**) (34, 35). The 1 + 7 configuration may have a mechanistic function, as it is also conserved in type C and D viruses that only possess 7 vRNAs (36). Further supporting the mechanistic concept, it was recently shown that IAVs can package cellular ribosomal RNA (as a vRNP) when one of the vRNAs is made unavailable (37), possibly explaining how type C and D viruses acquire their "eighth" vRNA.

The classification of IAVs into subtypes is based on the genetic and antigenic properties of the surface antigens HA and NA, which mediate viral entry and release, respectively (17, 18). To date, 16 HA (H1-16) and 9 NA subtypes (N1-9) have been found in IAVs isolated from aquatic birds (13). Two additional subtypes for HA (H17 and H18) and NA (N10 and N11) have recently been identified in bats (38, 39), but in contrast to the HA and NA subtypes from the more traditional avian IAVs, these do not appear to recognize sialic acid (SA) (40–42). Despite the numerous possible subtype combinations, only three have consistently persisted in the human population, causing the following pandemics in the process: 1918 and 2009 (H1N1), 1957 (H2N2), and 1968 (H3N2) (43). Currently, only the H1N1 and H3N2 subtypes, as well as the two antigenically distinct IBV lineages (Victoria and Yamagata), are endemic in the human population (44), which is why many IAV vaccines include two representative IAV and IBV strains (5).

A significant challenge in battling IAVs is the constant evolution of the surface antigens (HA and NA) in response to pressure from the host immune system, which is referred to as antigenic drift and antigenic shift. Antigenic drift is most evident in circulating seasonal IAVs, where substitutions by the polymerase that cause mutations in the surface antigen epitopes have continuously been selected to enable reinfection of the same host (45). Antigenic shift is responsible for the development of the IAV pandemics, and it relies on the less

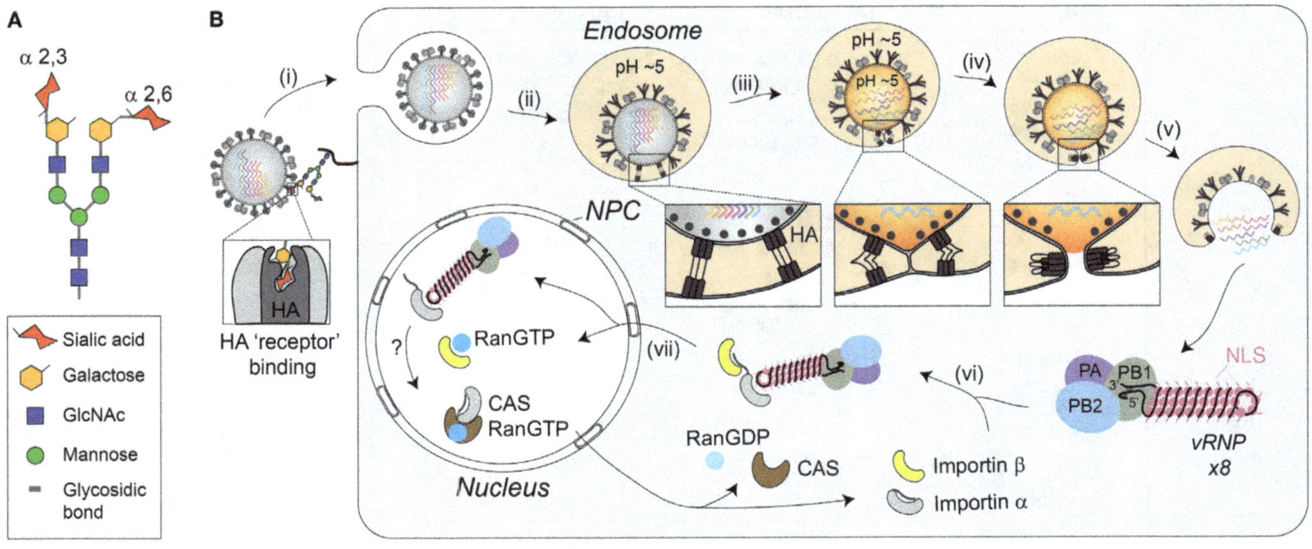

FIGURE 2 | Receptor-mediated cell entry of IAVs. **(A)** Diagram of a bi-antennary N-linked glycan. The terminal sialic acid residues are displayed with an α-2,3 linkage, as well as an α-2,6 linkage, to illustrate the "linear" and "bent" presentations. **(B)** Illustration of IAV cell entry. (i) IAVs initiate cell entry by using the HA receptor-binding domain (located in the HA1 region) to associate with sialylated glycoconjugates on a host "receptor." Binding to the "receptor" triggers endocytosis. (ii) The virus then traffics to the endosome where the lower pH facilitates a conformational change in HA, exposing the fusion peptide (located in the HA2 region) for insertion into the endosomal membrane. (iii) The HA pre-hairpin conformation begins to collapse, forming a six-helix bundle that promotes hemifusion of the viral envelop with the endosomal membrane. At some point, the M2 channel opens to release the viral ribonucleoproteins (vRNPs) from M1 by acidifying the viral interior. (iv) HA further collapses into a trimer of hairpins to promote the formation of the fusion pore, which (v) releases the vRNPs into the cytosol. (vi) The exposed nuclear localization signals (NLS) on the vRNPs are recognized by the adaptor protein importin-α, leading to the recruitment of importin-β that (vii) facilitates the transport through the nuclear pore complex (NPC) and into the nucleus.

frequent process of reassortment, which involves the exchange of vRNAs between two IAVs during co-infection of a cell (43, 46, 47). While reassortment can happen between two related IAVs, antigenic shift occurs when the reassortment process yields a new IAV subtype.

IAVs are also under constant negative selection due to the functional requirements of the viral proteins, and the constraints of the limited genome. Several roles have been reported for most of the IAV proteins. These include the function of HA in receptor binding, as well as membrane fusion, and viral release by the sialidase activity of NA. To perform these functions, the proteins need to correctly fold, oligomerize, and as for the genome itself, they have to be properly trafficked and packaged into new virions. Thus mutations that benefit one property may hinder another. The goal of this review is to highlight these functional requirements by providing a summary of the mechanisms IAVs have evolved to facilitate cell entry, replication, virion assembly and movement, with particular attention to how IAVs coordinate the infection process.

IAV CELL BINDING AND FUSION

IAVs initiate the infection process by using the HA molecules on the viral envelope. Upon reaching a potential host cell, the HA receptor-binding site attaches the virus to surface glycoconjugates that contain terminal SA residues (**Figure 2A**) (18, 48, 49). IAVs then scan the cell surface for the proper sialylated "receptor" by using the sialidase function of NA to remove local SAs and liberate nonproductive HA associations (50). Currently, the "receptor's" identity remains unknown, but it is generally thought that HAs from avian IAVs have higher specificity for receptors with α-2,3-linked SAs that have a "linear" presentation (51, 52), whereas HAs from human IAVs prefer an α-2,6 linkage, which results in a more "bent" presentation (**Figure 2A**) (53, 54). While these preferences correlate with SA linkages in the respective hosts (55), several studies have shown that matching HA receptor binding preferences with the SA linkages in a particular host is not essential for infection, but is more critical for transmission (56–59). This implies that the IAV "receptor" either displays significant cell tropism in the airways or that IAVs can potentially use more than one receptor.

Despite the unknown identity of the receptor, it is clear that HA-mediated binding to the receptor triggers endocytosis of the virion (**Figure 2B**, step i). The endocytosis can either occur in a clathrin-dependent manner, involving dynamin and the adaptor protein Epsin-1 (60–62), or by macropinocytosis (61, 63, 64). Once inside the cell, the virus is trafficked to the endosome, where the low pH activates the M2 ion channel (61, 65, 66), and causes a large conformational change in HA that exposes the fusion peptide (**Figure 2B**, step ii) (67–69). Opening of the M2 ion channel acidifies the inside of the viral particle, releasing the packaged vRNPs from M1 (**Figure 2B**, step iii), which enables the transfer of the vRNPs to the host cytoplasm following HA-mediated fusion (70, 71).

Fusion of the viral-endosomal membranes by HA occurs through multiple steps [reviewed in Refs. (72, 73), and requires cleavage of HA by host cell proteases into two subunits, HA1 and HA2 (55, 74, 75)]. The cleavage (see HA Proteolytic Activation at the *Golgi* or Plasma Membrane) is required to enable the exposure of the fusion peptide on the N-terminus of the HA2 upon the pH change in the endosome (69). Once exposed, the fusion peptide inserts into the endosomal membrane, while the C-terminal transmembrane domain (TMD) anchors HA2 in the viral membrane, creating a pre-hairpin conformation (see **Figure 2B**, step ii "box"). The HA2 trimers then fold back on themselves creating a hairpin that begins to position the two membranes in close proximity to each other (see **Figure 2B**, step iii "box"). The hairpin bundles then further collapse into a six-helix bundle, and in doing so, the two membranes come closer together enabling the formation of the lipid stalk, and the subsequent fusion of the two membranes (**Figure 2B**, step iv). To date, not all of these stages have been observed with HA and some have been inferred based on observations of related fusogens from other viruses.

IAV GENOME TRAFFICKING TO THE HOST CELL NUCLEUS

In contrast to the early steps in IAV entry, vRNP trafficking to the nucleus following the fusion event is highly dependent on the host cell machinery and transport pathways [reviewed in Ref. (76)]. Supported by numerous studies, the current model is that the newly released cytoplasmic vRNPs use the importin-α–importin-β nuclear import pathway to gain entry to the host cell nucleoplasm (**Figure 2B**, steps vi and vii) (77–83). To initially engage this pathway, it is thought that the vRNPs use the surface exposed nuclear localization sequences from the numerous NP molecules to recruit the adapter protein importin-α (80–82). Upon binding to the vRNP, importin-α is recognized by the importin-β transport receptor, which directs the vRNP to the nuclear pore complex, where it is transported into the nucleoplasm.

Recent improvements in imaging and RNA labeling techniques have made it possible to monitor the entire entry process in single cells (61, 62, 83–85). The cumulative results from these studies show that IAVs can deliver their vRNPs from the cell surface to

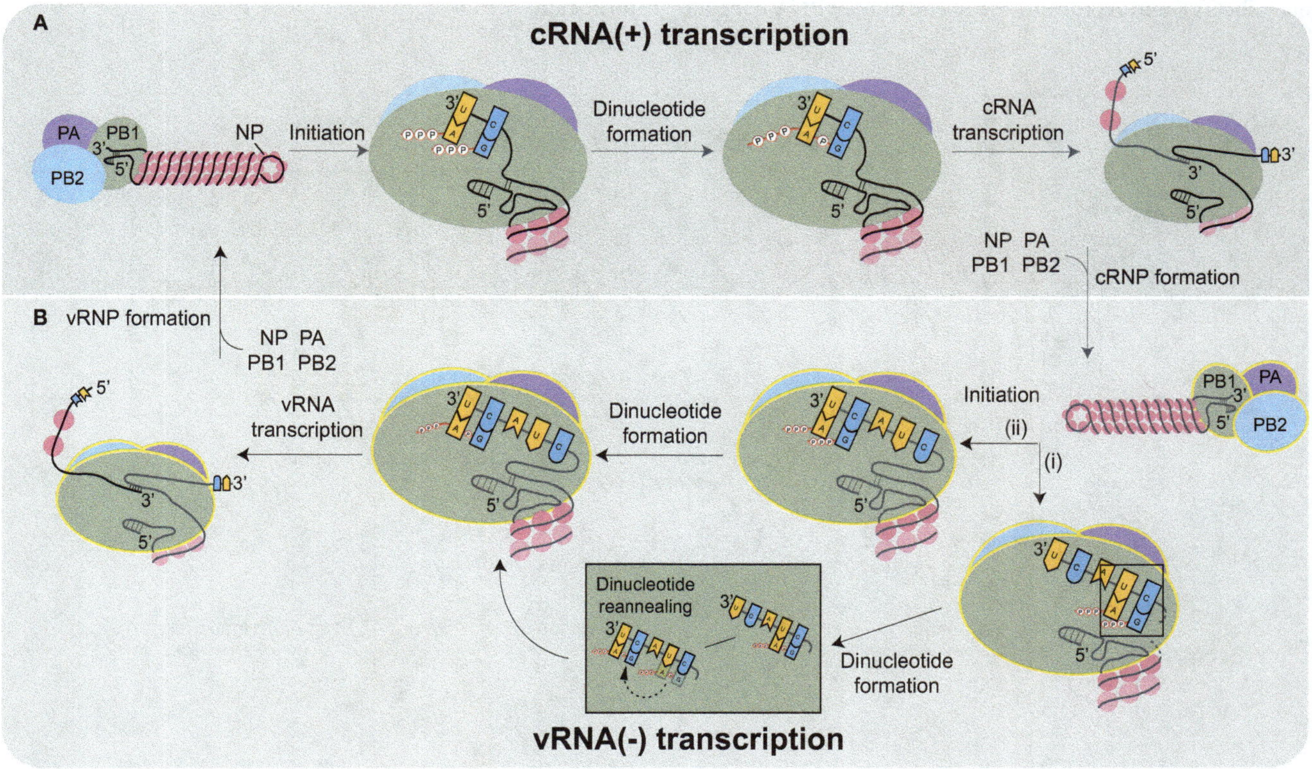

FIGURE 3 | Transcription of the complimentary RNA (cRNA) and viral RNA (vRNA) by the heterotrimeric viral RNA-dependent RNA polymerase (PB2, PB1, and PA). **(A)** The viral polymerase initiates transcription of the positive-sense cRNA upon base-pairing of ATP and GTP with the complimentary nucleotides in the 3′ end of the vRNA. The subsequent formation of the A-G dinucleotide is followed by elongation of the cRNA transcript. Nucleoprotein (NP) molecules successively bind to the cRNA as it exits the polymerase, promoting cRNP assembly. cRNP formation is completed upon the termination of transcription and with the binding of a newly synthesized viral polymerase (yellow outline). **(B)** vRNA transcription proceeds in a similar manner as cRNA synthesis. Recent structures support a model where (i) ATP and GTP base pair to the nucleotides located 4 and 5 bases from the cRNA 3′ end, and there form a dinucleotide, which then disassociates and reanneals with the bases at positions 1 and 2. (ii) Alternatively, ATP and GTP could bind directly to the terminal nucleotides and form a dinucleotide. Both mechanisms would position the dinucleotide at the cRNA 3′ end, which is necessary to transcribe a full-length vRNA. Similar to cRNP formation, multiple NPs and a viral polymerase bind to the newly transcribed vRNA to produce a new viral ribonucleoprotein (vRNP).

the nucleus in approximately 1 h, with entry and fusion occurring rather quickly (~10 min), and nuclear import requiring the bulk of the time (85). A striking observation from these studies is the efficiency with which the eight vRNAs reach the nucleus, indicating how effectively vRNPs recruit the host nuclear import factors. Supporting this observation, it was shown that NP adaptation to the importin-α isoforms of a particular species is crucial for productive IAV infections (86). While the bulk of the vRNP trafficking work has been carried out using various immortalized cell lines, the potential species related differences, and the essential role of vRNP trafficking in reassortment, emphasize the need for further methodology development to examine the details of IAV entry in primary cells and tissue explants.

REPLICATION OF THE vRNAs

Inside the nucleus, the heterotrimeric viral RNA-dependent RNA polymerase carries out the transcription and replication of the vRNAs [reviewed in Refs. (87, 88)]. The replication of the influenza genome involves two steps: transcription of complimentary RNA (cRNA), followed by transcription of new vRNA copies using the cRNAs as templates. The cRNAs are produced by an unprimed process that relies on the correct complementation of free rNTPs (generally GTP and ATP) with the 3′ end of the vRNA template (**Figure 3A**) (89, 90). The nucleotide complementation locks the vRNA template into the polymerase active site within the PB1 subunit and results in the formation of an A–G dinucleotide from which the cRNA is elongated (91). Upon exiting the polymerase, the cRNA associates with newly synthesized NP molecules and a single copy of the viral polymerase to assemble into a cRNP (90).

Currently, it is thought that the newly produced viral polymerases, which are incorporated into the cRNPs, generate multiple vRNA copies in a manner similar to cRNA transcription (**Figure 3B**). However, there is one distinction related to the difference in the positioning of the longer 3′ end of the positive-sense cRNA. Due to the increased length, the cRNA is positioned in the polymerase such that the rNTP annealing and dinucleotide formation is likely to occur at the nucleotides located 4 and 5 bases from the cRNA 3′ end (**Figure 3B**, pathway i) (90, 92–94). The dinucleotide primer then has to dissociate and reanneal to the nucleotides at the 3′ end prior to elongation (**Figure 3B**). Alternatively, the cRNA 3′ end could reposition within the polymerase due to rNTP binding, resulting in the generation of full-length vRNA transcripts directly (**Figure 3B**, pathway ii). The transient nature of the rNTP annealing and dinucleotide formation makes it technically challenging to exclude either possibility. The remaining task of assembling a vRNP is analogous to cRNP formation.

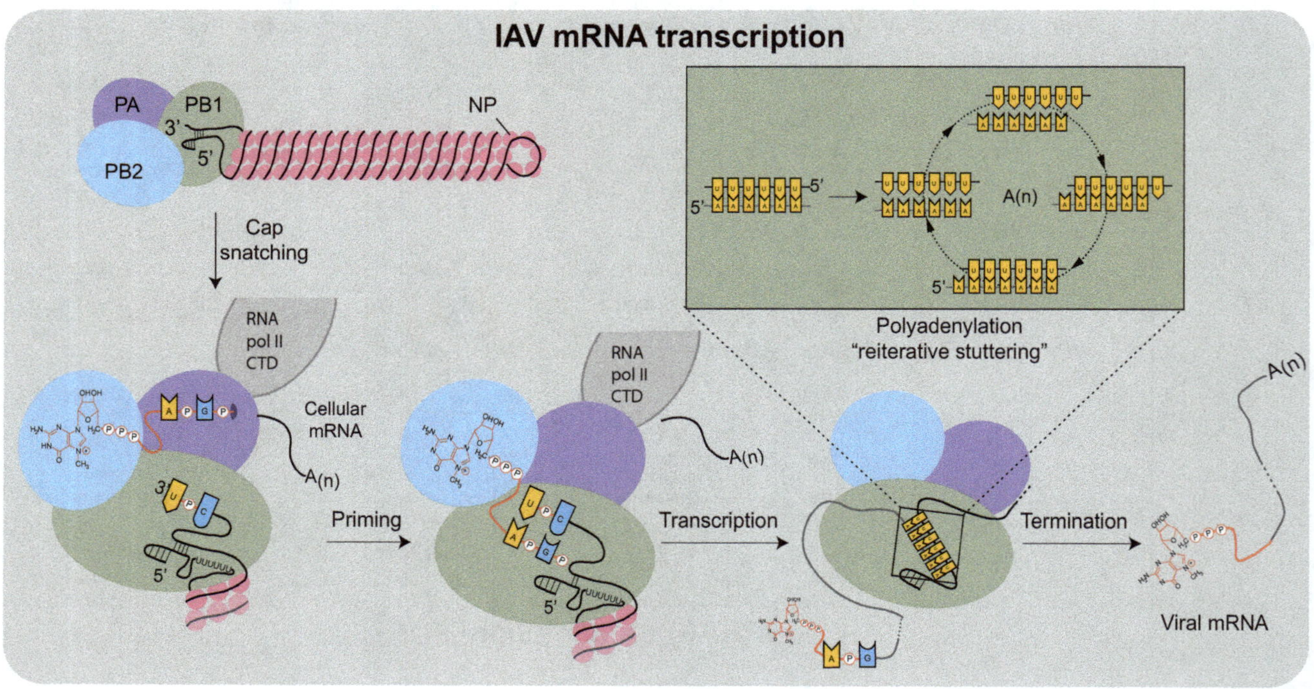

FIGURE 4 | Transcription of IAV mRNAs by the viral polymerase. Viral mRNA transcription occurs when the viral ribonucleoproteins reach the host cell nucleus and is assisted by the association of the viral polymerase (PA subunit) with the cellular RNA polymerase II C-terminal domain (RNA pol II CTD). Transcription initiates by a "cap-snatching" mechanism where the PB2 subunit binds to the 5′ cap of a host mRNA (red). Cap binding positions the region of the mRNA 10–13 nucleotides downstream for cleavage by the endonuclease domain in the PA subunit. Following cleavage, a conformational shift repositions the acquired mRNA capped primer to the PB1 subunit where the 3′ end base-pairs with a complimentary sequence at the vRNA 3′ end. Following the priming event, the viral polymerase extends the mRNA transcript. The transcription is terminated by a "reiterative stuttering" process (depicted in the box), which occurs when the polymerase encounters the 5–7 consecutive uracil bases at the vRNA 5′ end. The "reiterative stuttering" function likely involves multiple cycles of dissociation and reannealing, and effectively polyadenylates [A(n)] the viral mRNA by continuously repositioning the elongating 3′ end on the uracil-rich region of the vRNA template.

VIRAL mRNA TRANSCRIPTION

Viral mRNA transcription from the vRNA templates is primed, making it significantly more efficient than cRNA and vRNA transcription (95). The viral polymerase obtains the primers through a mechanism termed cap snatching (96), which is aided by the association with the cellular RNA polymerase II C-terminal domain (**Figure 4**) (97–99). For cap snatching, the viral polymerase uses the PB2 subunit to bind to 5′ caps of nascent host transcripts (100) and the PA subunit endonuclease domain to cleave 10–13 nucleotides downstream of the 5′ cap (101–103). The PB2 cap-binding domain then rotates to position the newly acquired capped primer into the PB1 catalytic center where it is extended using the vRNA as a template (95). Finally, each transcript is polyadenylated through a reiterative stuttering' process, which occurs when the polymerase encounters the short poly-U sequence at the vRNA 5′ end (**Figure 4** "box")(104, 105). This process likely involves multiple cycles of dissociation, repositioning, and reannealing of the mRNA to this template region of the vRNA to achieve polyadenylation.

During the course of infection, mRNA synthesis occurs before cRNA and vRNA transcription, and mRNA transcription is much more abundant because the use of primers significantly increases the initiation efficiency (106). The initial mRNAs are transcribed by the vRNP-associated polymerases and exported from the nucleus for translation by cytoplasmic ribosomes (93). However, the M and NS transcripts also possess donor and acceptor splice sites that match well with those in human transcripts (107). These sites recruit the cell spliceosome, which produces the spliced transcripts that encode for the M2 and NS2 proteins, respectively (108–112). The NS transcript has been reported to maintain a similar ratio of non-spliced and spliced transcripts throughout infection (113), whereas the ratio of the spliced M transcripts (encoding M2) have been shown to increase during infection (114). These observations imply that NS1 and NS2 are always equally expressed, while M2 expression is more biased toward the later stages of infection. However, it is likely that the splicing efficiency of the NS and M transcripts differs between IAV strains (115, 116).

ASSEMBLY AND TRAFFICKING OF vRNPs

IAV protein synthesis is entirely dependent on the translation machinery of the host cell. Following nuclear export [reviewed in Ref. (117)], the translation of the viral mRNAs is divided between cytosolic ribosomes (for PB1, PB2, PA, NP, NS1, NS2, and M1) and endoplasmic reticulum (ER)-associated ribosomes for the membrane proteins HA, NA, and M2 (**Figure 5**, steps i and ii).

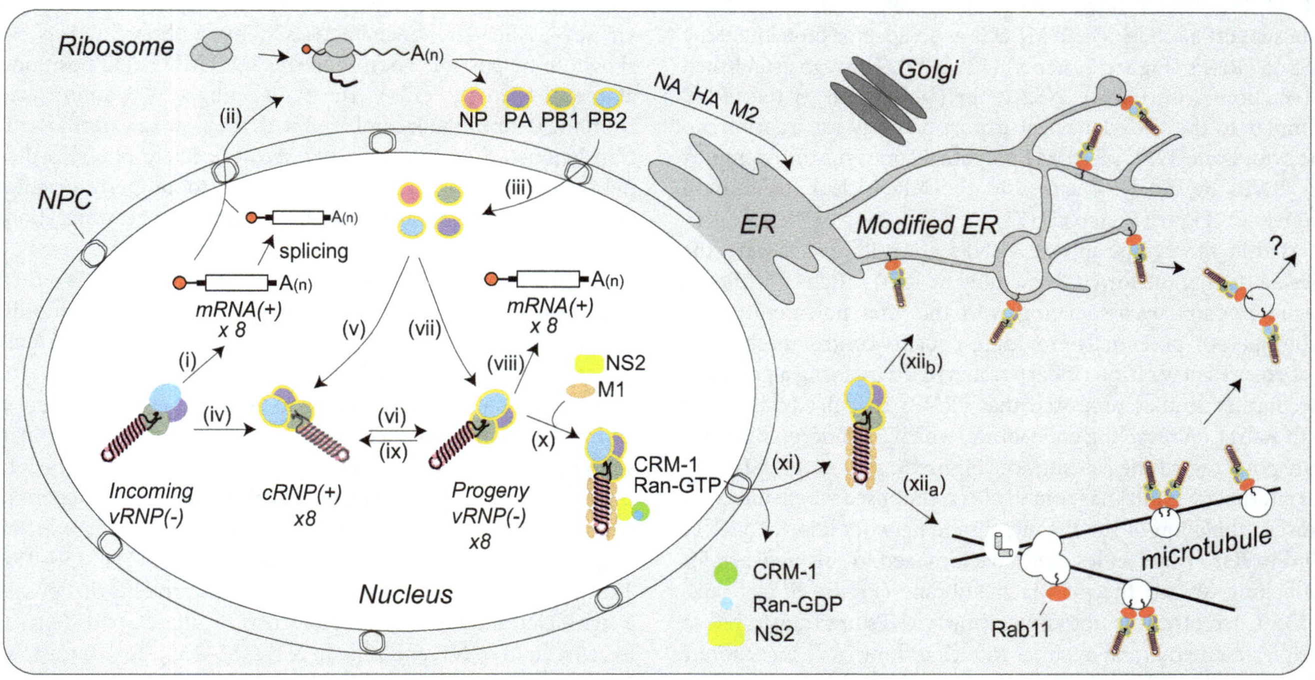

FIGURE 5 | Coordination of viral ribonucleoprotein (vRNP) assembly and trafficking to the plasma membrane. Upon entry into the host cell nucleus, (i) the vRNP-associated viral polymerase transcribes the viral mRNAs. (ii) The mRNAs are either directly, or after alternative splicing, exported for translation by cytosolic ribosomes. (iii) Newly synthesized viral polymerase subunits (PA, PB1, and PB2) and nucleoprotein (NP) are imported back into the nucleus. (iv) Due to the inefficient dinucleotide priming, the vRNP-associated viral polymerase also infrequently transcribes complimentary RNA (cRNA) copies that assemble into cRNPs *via* (v) binding of a newly synthesized viral polymerase (PA, PB1, and PB2) and NP. (vi) The polymerase transcribes viral RNA (vRNA) copies from the positive strand in the cRNPs and these assemble into vRNPs by (vii) association with a new viral polymerase (PA, PB1, and PB2) and NP. Once assembled, the new vRNPs can (viii) transcribe additional viral mRNAs, (ix) transcribe new cRNA copies, or (x) associate with the newly synthesized viral proteins M1 and NS2 to facilitate the recruitment of CRM1, which (xi) mediates the nuclear export of the vRNP. (xii_a) Once exported, the vRNPs then associate with Rab11 that assists in the trafficking of the vRNPs toward the cell surface. The vRNP trafficking either occurs by Rab11-containing vesicles associated with microtubules or (xii_b) through Rab11 located in the modified endoplasmic reticulum (ER) membranes. How the vRNPs reach the budding site at the plasma membrane is currently not known.

Nuclear localization sequences on the newly synthesized NP proteins and polymerase subunits (PB1, PB2, and PA) target these proteins into the nucleus by recruiting the importin-α-importin-β pathway that is utilized for vRNP nuclear import (**Figure 5**, step iii). The NP and PB2 proteins are imported individually, whereas the PB1 and PA proteins are imported as a heterodimer (81, 118). In the nucleus, these newly synthesized proteins assist in viral mRNA transcription and vRNA replication. NP monomers bind to 12 nucleotide stretches with a partial G bias in vRNAs, and presumably cRNAs, to assemble vRNPs and cRNPs through a process that may be regulated by the NP phosphorylation (**Figure 5**, steps v and vii) (119–121). The heterotrimeric polymerase assembles and binds to the newly formed cRNPs to transcribe vRNAs (**Figure 5**, step vi) that upon formation into vRNPs can generate additional viral mRNA (**Figure 5**, step viii), or cRNA transcripts (**Figure 5**, step ix) (90, 93).

The viral RNA-binding protein NS1 is synthesized early and also imported into the nucleus, where it can act as an inhibitor of interferon signaling [reviewed in Ref. (122)]. In addition, NS1 may contribute to viral mRNA export from the nucleus by linking the viral transcripts to the cellular nuclear export components TAP/NXF1, p15, Rae1, E1B–AP5, and the nucleoporin NUP98 (123). NS2 (alternatively known as the nuclear export protein) and M1 are imported into the nucleus as well. Multiple studies have implicated these two proteins in the nuclear export of vRNPs (70, 71, 124–127). While the mechanism remains unclear, current data support a model where M1 acts as an adaptor protein linking NS2 to vRNPs (**Figure 5**, step x) (128, 129). Through established interactions with CRM1, NS2 is then able to target the vRNP complex to the CRM1 nuclear export pathway for transport to the cytoplasm (127), where M1 potentially prevents the re-import of vRNPs by blocking access to the NP nuclear localization sequences (**Figure 5**, step xi) (71).

Within the cytoplasm the vRNPs are trafficked toward the plasma membrane for viral assembly by Rab11. Rab11 facilitates the interaction by associating with the viral polymerase PB2 subunit (130), potentially providing a quality control mechanism that ensures new virions incorporate vRNPs carrying a polymerase. Earlier studies proposed that vRNPs specifically associate with Rab11 on recycling endosomes, which use microtubules for transport toward the cell surface (**Figure 5**, step xii_a) (130–132). An alternative model has recently been proposed where infection causes tubulation of the ER membrane network and the vRNPs bind to Rab11 molecules that have localized to this network for trafficking toward the plasma membrane (**Figure 5**, step xii_b) (133). Currently, it is not known how vRNPs are transferred to the plasma membrane in either model, or how IAVs incorporate all eight of the different vRNPs in a "1 + 7" configuration. While several studies have indicated that specific vRNP associations likely contribute to the packaging of the eight vRNPs (35, 134, 135), the underlying mechanisms remain to be established.

ER TARGETING AND MATURATION OF THE IAV MEMBRANE PROTEINS

The IAV membrane proteins, which are ultimately destined for the viral envelope, are synthesized by ribosomes associated with the ER membrane. Similar to cellular secretory proteins, ribosome–nascent chain complexes containing NA, HA, or M2 are co-translationally directed to the ER by interactions of their hydrophobic targeting sequences with the signal recognition particle (SRP) (**Figure 6**, step ii) (136–139). The cleavable signal sequence on HA facilitates the interaction with SRP, whereas NA and M2 use their respective TMD as an ER targeting sequence. Once bound, SRP targets the ribosome–nascent chain complexes to the SRP receptor in the ER membrane (**Figure 6**, step iii), which transfers the ribosome to a Sec61 protein-conducting channel known as the translocon (140–142). Linked to the dependence on SRP, mutations that alter the targeting sequence hydrophobicity of cellular secretory proteins have been shown to decrease their ER targeting and subsequent synthesis (143, 144). Although this aspect has not been examined for the IAV membrane proteins, there is evidence that the hydrophobicity of their ER-targeting sequences change (138, 148), which suggests IAVs potentially use this mechanism to titrate NA and HA expression.

The translocon enables passage of the elongating NA, HA, and M2 polypeptides into the ER lumen and facilitates the membrane partitioning of their respective TMD segments through a lateral gate (145, 146). To activate the membrane integration, the TMD segments have to be of the appropriate length and hydrophobicity (146, 147). In human H1N1 and H3N2 viruses, these criteria are conserved in the TMDs of HA and M2, but not in the TMD of NA, as it has become progressively less hydrophobic in the H1N1 viruses (148). The uncharacteristic hydrophobicity loss was shown to be possible because of the NA TMD being positioned at the N-terminus (138). The positioning (~435 amino acids from the C-terminus), combined with the slow rate of ribosomal translation (~5 amino acids per second), likely provides these nontypical TMDs with significant time to properly orientate and facilitate membrane insertion during the co-translational translocation process.

During translocation, the N-terminus of HA and M2 is directly translocated into the ER lumen, whereas NA inverts, positioning the C-terminus in the ER lumen (137, 138). In addition, HA and NA receive multiple N-linked glycans. The glycans are transferred by the oligosaccharyltransferase to Asn–X–Ser/Thr sequences, and vary in number as well as positioning based on the strain, or subtype (149). One function of the glycans is to increase the folding efficiency of NA and HA by recruiting the lectin chaperones (calnexin and calreticulin) and the associated oxidoreductase ERp57, which aids in disulfide bond formation (136, 150–152). This is especially crucial for the HA and NA proteins that possess a significant number of intramolecular disulfide bonds (e.g., six in HAs, eight in N1, and nine in N2) (153–155). By contrast, M2 possesses two intermolecular disulfide bonds in its tetrameric conformation (156). Depending on the subtype, NA tetramers also possess 2 or more intermolecular disulfide bonds.

Oligomerization of HA involves the trimerization of independently folded monomers, whereas NA tetramerization has been proposed to result from the pairing of two co-translationally formed dimers, which assemble through a process involving the N-terminal TMD of NA (150, 157). In line with this model, it has been shown that the TMD is essential for proper NA folding, and that the decreasing hydrophobicity in the N1 TMDs functions to

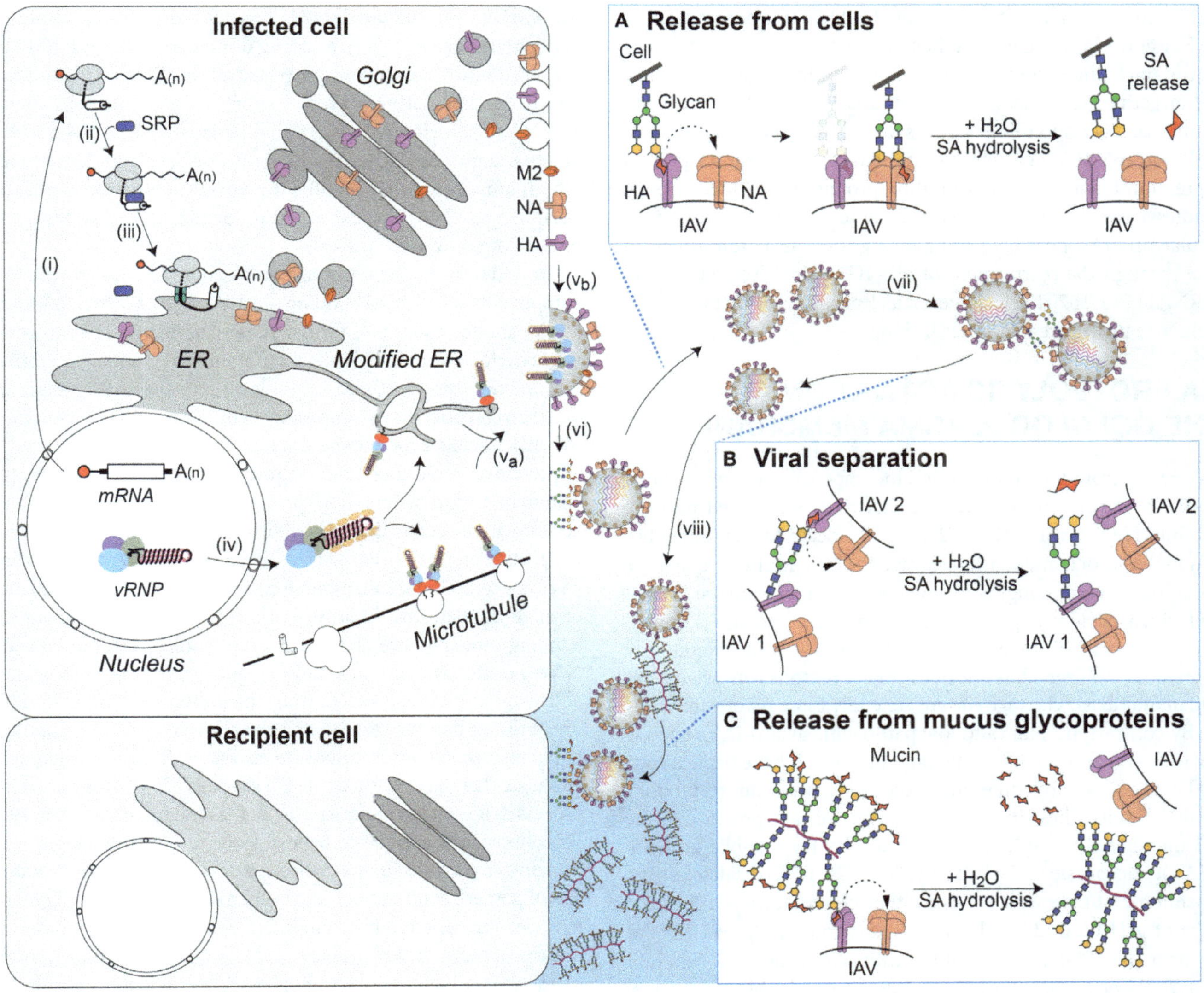

FIGURE 6 | NA contributions to viral release and intercellular movement. (i) Viral mRNAs encoding the membrane proteins NA, HA, and M2 are exported for translation by cytosolic ribosomes. (ii) Exposure of the N-terminal signal sequence (HA) or transmembrane domains (NA and M2) recruits the signal recognition particle (SRP), which (iii) targets the ribosome–nascent chain complex for synthesis at the endoplasmic reticulum (ER). Following synthesis, the proteins oligomerize and are trafficked through the *Golgi* to the plasma membrane. (iv) Late in replication, the viral ribonucleoproteins (vRNPs) are exported from the nucleus and (v_a) trafficked to the budding regions in the plasma membrane, where (v_b) HA and NA have co-localized, with M2 at the budding boundary. (vi) Following budding, progeny virus can remain associated with the infected cell's surface through HA binding to sialic acid (SA). (Box A) The envelope protein NA promotes release of the virus from the infected cell surface by hydrolyzing the glycosidic bond attaching the SAs. (vii) SAs present on the glycans of HA and NA can result in HA-mediated virus–virus association. (Box B) NA can separate the viruses by removing these SAs. (viii) In the respiratory tract, the epithelium is protected by mucus, rich in sialylated glycoproteins such as mucin, which can associate with HA and slow viral movement. (Box C) NA can cleave off the SAs from the glycoproteins within the mucus to facilitate movement of the virus to neighboring cells.

support the folding and oligomerization of the enzymatic head domain (158, 159). IAVs easily achieve the protein concentration-dependent requirement for oligomerization due to the abundance of HA and NA that is synthesized during an infection. However, these high synthesis levels at the ER can also be deleterious by activating the ER-stress response. Indeed, several studies have shown that IAV replication does activate the ER-stress induced unfolded protein response (160, 161), but this response is also mitigated by the inhibition of the eIF2α-kinase and stress granule formation through the functions of other viral proteins (162).

Despite everything that is known about the synthesis and assembly of the IAV membrane proteins, several aspects have yet to be addressed. These include obtaining atomic structures of full-length HA and NA in a membrane, something that should become easier to address with the advances in cryo-electron microscopy structure determination. Identifying if the NA protein removes SA residues directly from substrates within the *Golgi*, as this could decrease the effectivity of nonmembrane permeable NA inhibitors. It is also unclear how IAVs regulate the timing and expression levels of the viral proteins as viral mRNA transcription shows little temporal variation (163, 164). While it is likely that M2 is regulated in part by splicing (112, 114), this does not apply to HA and NA. Recent work has linked NA and HA regulation to the nucleotide composition of the 5′coding regions for their ER-targeting sequences, which dramatically differ from the profile of corresponding regions in human secretory protein mRNAs (165, 166). An obvious candidate for post-transcriptional regulation is the viral RNA-binding protein NS1. Indeed, many studies have shown that NS1 can increase translation of particular mRNAs, possibly by enhancing the translation initiation rate through the recruitment of eIF-4G to the 5′region of viral mRNAs (165, 167–171). However, a clear mechanistic picture for influenza protein regulation is lacking.

HA PROTEOLYTIC ACTIVATION AT THE *GOLGI* OR PLASMA MEMBRANE

HA traffics from the ER as a fusion incompetent precursor termed HA0. To gain its fusion function, HA must be cleaved into the subunits HA1 and HA2 (74, 172, 173). The cleavage occurs in either a monobasic, or a multibasic, cleavage site (55). Multibasic sites are commonly found in highly pathogenic avian IAVs and are cleaved by furin, a calcium-dependent serine endoprotease that is located within the *trans-Golgi* network (174). Furin is also ubiquitously expressed (175), which is one of the major reasons why avian IAVs with a multibasic cleavage site are generally more pathogenic.

By contrast, human (and low pathogenic avian) IAVs encode for HAs with a monobasic cleavage site, which have been shown to be processed by different proteases in human respiratory epithelial cells. These include the transmembrane protease serine S-1 member 2 (TMPRSS2), human airway trypsin-like protease (HAT), and possibly TMPRSS4 (176, 177). HAT localizes at the plasma membrane where it can either cleave newly synthesized HA or the HA found in cell-associated virions (178, 179). Similar to furin, TMPRSS2 resides in the *trans-Golgi* network, where it cleaves HA en route to the plasma membrane. The M2 ion channel is thought to prevent the premature activation of HA following cleavage by equilibrating the slightly acidic pH of the *Golgi* (180, 181). Distinct from furin, TMPRSS2 expression has been found to be more restricted to the upper and lower respiratory tract, whereas HAT was mainly shown to be expressed in the upper respiratory tract (182). These cell tropisms suggest that lower respiratory infections are likely mediated by TMPRSS2, and could be one of the primary reasons human IAVs are confined to the epithelial layer of the respiratory tract.

IAV ASSEMBLY AND BUDDING

Compared with the bulk lipid profile of the plasma membrane, IAV envelopes are enriched in cholesterol and sphingolipids (32), indicating that they bud from distinct apical plasma membrane regions often referred to as "rafts" (183). However, infectious IAVs must possess mechanisms to target the eight vRNPs, M1, HA, NA, and M2 to these sites in the membrane (184, 185). HA is believed to localize to these distinct regions based on fatty acid modifications of the C-terminal cysteine that occur in the *Golgi* (186–189), whereas NA enrichment has previously been attributed to a property in the C-terminus of the TMD (190). In contrast, M2 has been shown to accumulate at the boundaries of these budding domains (191), and the cytosolic protein M1 has been proposed to localize to the budding region by associating with the short cytoplasmic tails of HA and NA (192). However, it is equally plausible that NA and HA create membrane domains with a unique lipid profile that have a high affinity for M1. Finally, the vRNPs, delivered to the cell periphery by Rab11, are thought to localize to the budding site by binding to M1 (193, 194).

In addition to orchestrating the assembly of the correct viral components at the apical budding site, IAVs also have to remodel the membrane to induce bud formation, and ultimately scission of the viral envelope from the plasma membrane. To promote bud formation, the virus must first induce significant curvature in the membrane and then constrict the two opposing membranes of the viral envelope to help to facilitate membrane scission. Curvature can be induced by (i) protein or "molecular" crowding on one leaflet of a bilayer, (ii) association of curved or "bending" proteins with the bilayer, (iii) biased accumulation of cone shaped lipids in one leaflet of the bilayer, or (iv) the cytoskeleton (195). Based on cumulative data regarding budding, IAVs appear to induce membrane curvature through a combination of these mechanisms. Indicative of using molecular crowding and bending proteins, several studies have demonstrated that HA and NA expression is sufficient to induce budding, and that the efficiency and shape uniformity benefit from the presence of M1 (196–199). These results indicate that the abundance of HA and NA on one side of the membrane can contribute to curvature. It also is intriguing to speculate that the asymmetric (154) shape of NA plays a role in this process as it is often seen clustering in the viral membrane (16, 199). By contrast, M1 appears to be analogous to a membrane-bending protein as it recruited to the cytosolic side of the membrane budding site, oligomerizes upon reaching the membrane, and these oligomers have been modeled to form curved structures (200–202). Based on these properties, it is plausible that M1 significantly influences the membrane curvature at the budding site, potentially explaining its role in discerning whether IAVs form spheres or filaments (27, 203).

The ion channel M2 localizes to the budding site boundary and has also been shown to contribute to IAV scission by functioning as a membrane-bending protein (191, 204). The membrane-bending property of M2 is localized in an amphiphilic α-helix that can incorporate the amino acid side chains from its hydrophobic face into a leaflet of the bilayer. With this domain positioned in the cytosol, the intercalation results in negative membrane curvature, which has been proposed to facilitate viral bud neck formation and scission, presumably by decreasing the distance between the two opposing membranes of the viral envelope (204). While much of the framework concerning IAV budding has been established, it has been difficult to identify the details of the budding process, in part due to the mobility and heterogeneity of the plasma membrane. The lack of strong phenotypes from domains proposed to contribute to budding could also imply that IAVs have built redundancy into the budding process (205–207). The possibility of redundancy is certainly plausible, as IAVs contain the necessary components to allow for a combination of lipid recruitment, molecular crowding, and a membrane-bending protein.

IAV CELL RELEASE AND MOVEMENT

Once the newly assembled IAVs bud, their release is highly dependent on the sialidase activity of NA. NA is a homotetramer, and each subunit is comprised of a short N-terminal cytoplasmic tail (six amino acids), followed by a TMD, a length variable stalk, and a globular enzymatic head domain (208). The globular head domain forms a 6-bladed propeller structure, where each blade is comprised of four antiparallel β-sheets that are stabilized by disulfide bonds (155, 209, 210). The catalytic Tyr residue is found in a highly conserved active site that forms a deep pocket in the center of each monomer (211). All of the residues necessary for catalysis exist within each monomer (212), which has made it difficult to reconcile why NA evolved to function as a tetramer (208, 213, 214). Structures of the enzymatic head domain indicate that NA tetramers bind up to five calcium ions and calcium has been shown to contribute to NA activity (155, 208, 215). However, it remains unclear why influenza NA has evolved to position a calcium ion at the tetrameric interface.

NA facilitates viral release by catalyzing the hydrolysis of the glycosidic linkage that attaches SA to underlying sugar molecules (216–218). By removing local SA residues, NA prevents HA binding at the cell surface, which facilitates the release of the virus during budding (**Figure 6A** and step vi) (219, 220). NA has also been shown to promote the separation of IAVs by removing SA residues from the N-linked glycans located on the HA and NA molecules in the viral envelope (**Figure 6B** and step vii) (221). In contrast to HA, NAs from human IAVs show a general preference for α2,3-linked SA with variable abilities to cleave α2,6-linked SA residues (208, 222, 223). However, a thorough analysis of NA SA preference is lacking. More recent studies have found that some strains possess NAs that are inefficient enzymes, but still capable of SA binding, raising the question of whether a poor NA enzyme could contribute to, or replace, the HA receptor-binding function (224, 225).

The movement of IAVs from cell to cell in the respiratory epithelium is significantly different from that in immortalized cell lines grown in liquid culture due to the presence of different cell types and a mucus layer. The mucus layer provides a protective barrier for the epithelium and is rich in heavily glycosylated mucins that can interact with IAVs and limit cell binding (226, 227). Studies measuring viral movement through mucus and respiratory epithelial cells have shown that NA-mediated cleavage of SAs from mucins enhances IAV movement through the mucus layer and infectivity (**Figure 6C** and step viii) (226, 228, 229). Recent work showed that this function may also apply to transmission, as IAVs that possess low NA activity, and are inhibited by mucus, are deficient in aerosol and contact transmission (230).

PERSPECTIVES

IAVs are constantly exposed to negative and positive selection pressure, which shapes how the virus evolves. The functional requirements of each IAV protein, such as enzyme catalysis, substrate binding, oligomerization, and domains that perform essential interactions with host proteins all combine to create substantial negative selection pressure that often manifests in the form of sequence conservation. Negative pressure can also come from functions within the vRNA sequences. These include promoters and "packaging signals," but are also likely to involve aspects such as the formation of structural elements, or possibly mediating vRNP interactions that generate the 1 + 7 assembly in viral particles. In addition, the exposure of IAVs to the immune response and constantly changing environments such as host, temperature, pH, cell type, and antivirals result in positive selection pressure. Experimentally, addressing each type of selection has its caveats, but clearly a holistic picture of both IAV and host functions are required to begin predictions of evolutionary constraints on the virus.

Most studies on the influenza evolutionary process focus primarily on antigenic drift and antigenic shift. However, all the viral transcribed RNAs are subject to replication errors by the viral polymerase, which are estimated at 1 per 2,000–10,000 nucleotides (231–233). Consequently, both the viruses and the viral proteins are likely to exist as large heterogeneous populations during an infection. As many IAV proteins are homo-oligomers this can potentially generate heterogeneity within individual protein complexes that could have functional advantages. By applying single particle and single cell analysis, these types of aspects are beginning to be investigated (234). Another interesting approach is deep mutational scanning, which has been used to examine the site-specific amino acid tolerance of IAV proteins in general, and in the context of different selection pressure (235–238).

Currently, the best characterized protein in IAVs is HA, which has two primary functions, (i) to initiate binding to the host cell and (ii) to deliver the vRNPs to the host cell cytosol by fusing the viral and endosomal membranes. These functions are efficiently divided between the two domains of HA (HA1 and HA2), created by proteolysis. The receptor-binding site responsible for entry is located in the considerably larger HA1 subunit that is known to be immunodominant, explaining the high sequence variability in this region (239). By contrast, the smaller HA2 subunit, containing the fusion peptide that is necessary to deliver the viral genome to the host cell, shows considerably higher sequence conservation. This organization is logical from the viral perspective as the large HA1 subunit likely blocks antibody recognition of HA2. The viral downside is the need to escape antibodies that inhibit the receptor-binding pocket without losing specificity and the binding function.

Based on this knowledge, several exciting new strategies are being developed to elicit the production of antibodies that target the more conserved region of HA (240–242). The hope is that these strategies will generate broadly neutralizing antibodies that recognize multiple HA subtypes from IAVs and the distinct lineages in IBVs, providing longer lasting immunity and alleviating the threat of potential pandemics. A similar approach using NA would likely provide additional benefits. However, our knowledge of NA lags behind HA. Currently, it is still not known why NA has evolved to function as a tetramer, which is relevant because this property presumably restricts the potential antigenic drift (mutations) it can accommodate and still function.

A relatively overlooked feature in the replication process is the contributions of host RNA-binding proteins (RBPs). Human cells are predicted to encode over 1,500 RBPs, 700 of which are predicted to interact with mRNAs (243). As a RNA virus, it is highly likely that IAVs have evolved to utilize this enormous network of RBPs, which is supported by observations that some RBPs inhibit IAV replication, whereas others contribute (244–246). It should also be considered that changes in RBPs have been associated with various cancers, which could possibly influence the susceptibility to influenza infections (247, 248). With the growing interest in RNA biology, this aspect of IAV infections is likely to receive considerable attention in the future.

In terms of IAV antivirals, the recent progress in determining the structures and mechanisms of the viral polymerase should significantly aid in the current development of drugs aimed at inhibiting different aspects of IAV transcription (249). Through continued progress in defining the fundamental mechanisms that are necessary for IAV infections, replication and intercellular movement, it should become possible to minimize the annual burden caused by IAVs.

AUTHOR CONTRIBUTIONS

RD wrote the review with input from DD, RR, HÖ, and HW. DD, RR, HÖ, and HW put together the figures and wrote the figure legends.

REFERENCES

1. Hause BM, Collin EA, Liu R, Huang B, Sheng Z, Lu W, et al. Characterization of a novel influenza virus in cattle and swine: proposal for a new genus in the Orthomyxoviridae family. *MBio* (2014) 5:e31–14. doi:10.1128/mBio.00031-14
2. Palese P, Shaw ML. *Fields Virology*. Philadelphia: Lippincott Williams & Wilkins (2007).
3. Palese P, Schulman JL. Mapping of the influenza virus genome: identification of the hemagglutinin and the neuraminidase genes. *Proc Natl Acad Sci U S A* (1976) 73:2142–6. doi:10.1073/pnas.73.6.2142
4. McGeoch D, Fellner P, Newton C. Influenza virus genome consists of eight distinct RNA species. *Proc Natl Acad Sci U S A* (1976) 73:3045–9. doi:10.1073/pnas.73.9.3045
5. Houser K, Subbarao K. Influenza vaccines: challenges and solutions. *Cell Host Microbe* (2015) 17:295–300. doi:10.1016/j.chom.2015.02.012
6. Jagger BW, Wise HM, Kash JC, Walters KA, Wills NM, Xiao YL, et al. An overlapping protein-coding region in influenza A virus segment 3 modulates the host response. *Science* (2012) 337:199–204. doi:10.1126/science.1222213
7. Wise HM, Foeglein A, Sun J, Dalton RM, Patel S, Howard W, et al. A complicated message: identification of a novel PB1-related protein translated from influenza A virus segment 2 mRNA. *J Virol* (2009) 83:8021–31. doi:10.1128/JVI.00826-09
8. Yamayoshi S, Watanabe M, Goto H, Kawaoka Y. Identification of a novel viral protein expressed from the PB2 segment of influenza A virus. *J Virol* (2016) 90:444–56. doi:10.1128/JVI.02175-15
9. Zhang Y, Aevermann BD, Anderson TK, Burke DF, Dauphin G, Gu Z, et al. Influenza research database: an integrated bioinformatics resource for influenza virus research. *Nucleic Acids Res* (2017) 45:D466–74. doi:10.1093/nar/gkw857
10. Muramoto Y, Noda T, Kawakami E, Akkina R, Kawaoka Y. Identification of novel influenza A virus proteins translated from PA mRNA. *J Virol* (2013) 87:2455–62. doi:10.1128/JVI.02656-12
11. Chen W, Calvo PA, Malide D, Gibbs J, Schubert U, Bacik I, et al. A novel influenza A virus mitochondrial protein that induces cell death. *Nat Med* (2001) 7:1306–12. doi:10.1038/nm1201-1306
12. Webster RG, Bean WJ, Gorman OT, Chambers TM, Kawaoka Y. Evolution and ecology of influenza A viruses. *Microbiol Rev* (1992) 56:152–79.
13. Yoon SW, Webby RJ, Webster RG. Evolution and ecology of influenza A viruses. *Curr Top Microbiol Immunol* (2014) 385:359–75. doi:10.1007/82_2014_396
14. Hurt AC, Vijaykrishna D, Butler J, Baas C, Maurer-Stroh S, Silva-de-la-Fuente MC, et al. Detection of evolutionarily distinct avian influenza A viruses in Antarctica. *MBio* (2014) 5:e1098–1014. doi:10.1128/mBio.01098-14
15. Hurt AC, Su YC, Aban M, Peck H, Lau H, Baas C, et al. Evidence for the introduction, reassortment, and persistence of diverse influenza A viruses in Antarctica. *J Virol* (2016) 90:9674–82. doi:10.1128/JVI.01404-16
16. Harris A, Cardone G, Winkler DC, Heymann JB, Brecher M, White JM, et al. Influenza virus pleiomorphy characterized by cryoelectron tomography. *Proc Natl Acad Sci U S A* (2006) 103:19123–7. doi:10.1073/pnas.0607614103
17. Katz G, Benkarroum Y, Wei H, Rice WJ, Bucher D, Alimova A, et al. Morphology of influenza B/Lee/40 determined by cryo-electron microscopy. *PLoS One* (2014) 9:e88288. doi:10.1371/journal.pone.0088288
18. Gamblin SJ, Skehel JJ. Influenza hemagglutinin and neuraminidase membrane glycoproteins. *J Biol Chem* (2010) 285:28403–9. doi:10.1074/jbc.R110.129809
19. Arranz R, Coloma R, Chichon FJ, Conesa JJ, Carrascosa JL, Valpuesta JM, et al. The structure of native influenza virion ribonucleoproteins. *Science* (2012) 338:1634–7. doi:10.1126/science.1228172
20. Moeller A, Kirchdoerfer RN, Potter CS, Carragher B, Wilson IA. Organization of the influenza virus replication machinery. *Science* (2012) 338:1631–4. doi:10.1126/science.1227270
21. Pflug A, Guilligay D, Reich S, Cusack S. Structure of influenza A polymerase bound to the viral RNA promoter. *Nature* (2014) 516:355–60. doi:10.1038/nature14008
22. Fodor E, Seong BL, Brownlee GG. Photochemical cross-linking of influenza A polymerase to its virion RNA promoter defines a polymerase binding site at residues 9 to 12 of the promoter. *J Gen Virol* (1993) 74(Pt 7):1327–33. doi:10.1099/0022-1317-74-7-1327
23. Hsu MT, Parvin JD, Gupta S, Krystal M, Palese P. Genomic RNAs of influenza viruses are held in a circular conformation in virions and in infected cells by a terminal panhandle. *Proc Natl Acad Sci U S A* (1987) 84:8140–4. doi:10.1073/pnas.84.22.8140
24. Badham MD, Rossman JS. Filamentous influenza viruses. *Curr Clin Microbiol Rep* (2016) 3:155–61. doi:10.1007/s40588-016-0041-7
25. Kilbourne ED, Murphy JS. Genetic studies of influenza viruses. I. Viral morphology and growth capacity as exchangeable genetic traits. Rapid in ovo adaptation of early passage Asian strain isolates by combination with PR8. *J Exp Med* (1960) 111:387–406. doi:10.1084/jem.111.3.387
26. Seladi-Schulman J, Steel J, Lowen AC. Spherical influenza viruses have a fitness advantage in embryonated eggs, while filament-producing strains are selected in vivo. *J Virol* (2013) 87:13343–53. doi:10.1128/JVI.02004-13
27. Bourmakina SV, Garcia-Sastre A. Reverse genetics studies on the filamentous morphology of influenza A virus. *J Gen Virol* (2003) 84:517–27. doi:10.1099/vir.0.18803-0
28. Roberts PC, Lamb RA, Compans RW. The M1 and M2 proteins of influenza A virus are important determinants in filamentous particle formation. *Virology* (1998) 240:127–37. doi:10.1006/viro.1997.8916

29. Calder LJ, Wasilewski S, Berriman JA, Rosenthal PB. Structural organization of a filamentous influenza A virus. *Proc Natl Acad Sci U S A* (2010) 107:10685–90. doi:10.1073/pnas.1002123107
30. Hutchinson EC, Charles PD, Hester SS, Thomas B, Trudgian D, Martinez-Alonso M, et al. Conserved and host-specific features of influenza virion architecture. *Nat Commun* (2014) 5:4816. doi:10.1038/ncomms5816
31. Shaw ML, Stone KL, Colangelo CM, Gulcicek EE, Palese P. Cellular proteins in influenza virus particles. *PLoS Pathog* (2008) 4:e1000085. doi:10.1371/journal.ppat.1000085
32. Gerl MJ, Sampaio JL, Urban S, Kalvodova L, Verbavatz JM, Binnington B, et al. Quantitative analysis of the lipidomes of the influenza virus envelope and MDCK cell apical membrane. *J Cell Biol* (2012) 196:213–21. doi:10.1083/jcb.201108175
33. Ivanova PT, Myers DS, Milne SB, McClaren JL, Thomas PG, Brown HA. Lipid composition of viral envelope of three strains of influenza virus – not all viruses are created equal. *ACS Infect Dis* (2015) 1:399–452. doi:10.1021/acsinfecdis.5b00040
34. Noda T, Sagara H, Yen A, Takada A, Kida H, Cheng RH, et al. Architecture of ribonucleoprotein complexes in influenza A virus particles. *Nature* (2006) 439:490–2. doi:10.1038/nature04378
35. Moreira EA, Weber A, Bolte H, Kolesnikova L, Giese S, Lakdawala S, et al. A conserved influenza A virus nucleoprotein code controls specific viral genome packaging. *Nat Commun* (2016) 7:12861. doi:10.1038/ncomms12861
36. Nakatsu S, Murakami S, Shindo K, Horimoto T, Sagara H, Noda T, et al. Influenza C and D viruses package eight organized ribonucleoprotein complexes. *J Virol* (2018) 92(6):e02084-17. doi:10.1128/JVI.02084-17
37. Noda T, Murakami S, Nakatsu S, Imai H, Muramoto Y, Shindo K, et al. Importance of the 1+7 configuration of ribonucleoprotein complexes for influenza A virus genome packaging. *Nat Commun* (2018) 9:54. doi:10.1038/s41467-017-02517-w
38. Tong S, Li Y, Rivailler P, Conrardy C, Castillo DA, Chen LM, et al. A distinct lineage of influenza A virus from bats. *Proc Natl Acad Sci U S A* (2012) 109:4269–74. doi:10.1073/pnas.1116200109
39. Tong S, Zhu X, Li Y, Shi M, Zhang J, Bourgeois M, et al. New world bats harbor diverse influenza A viruses. *PLoS Pathog* (2013) 9:e1003657. doi:10.1371/journal.ppat.1003657
40. Zhu X, Yang H, Guo Z, Yu W, Carney PJ, Li Y, et al. Crystal structures of two subtype N10 neuraminidase-like proteins from bat influenza A viruses reveal a diverged putative active site. *Proc Natl Acad Sci U S A* (2012) 109:18903–8. doi:10.1073/pnas.1212579109
41. Zhu X, Yu W, McBride R, Li Y, Chen LM, Donis RO, et al. Hemagglutinin homologue from H17N10 bat influenza virus exhibits divergent receptor-binding and pH-dependent fusion activities. *Proc Natl Acad Sci U S A* (2013) 110:1458–63. doi:10.1073/pnas.1218509110
42. Maruyama J, Nao N, Miyamoto H, Maeda K, Ogawa H, Yoshida R, et al. Characterization of the glycoproteins of bat-derived influenza viruses. *Virology* (2016) 488:43–50. doi:10.1016/j.virol.2015.11.002
43. Morens DM, Taubenberger JK, Fauci AS. The persistent legacy of the 1918 influenza virus. *N Engl J Med* (2009) 361:225–9. doi:10.1056/NEJMp0904819
44. Rota PA, Wallis TR, Harmon MW, Rota JS, Kendal AP, Nerome K. Cocirculation of two distinct evolutionary lineages of influenza type B virus since 1983. *Virology* (1990) 175:59–68. doi:10.1016/0042-6822(90)90186-U
45. Bedford T, Suchard MA, Lemey P, Dudas G, Gregory V, Hay AJ, et al. Integrating influenza antigenic dynamics with molecular evolution. *Elife* (2014) 3:e01914. doi:10.7554/eLife.01914
46. Sobel Leonard A, McClain MT, Smith GJ, Wentworth DE, Halpin RA, Lin X, et al. The effective rate of influenza reassortment is limited during human infection. *PLoS Pathog* (2017) 13:e1006203. doi:10.1371/journal.ppat.1006203
47. Lowen AC. Constraints, drivers, and implications of influenza A virus reassortment. *Annu Rev Virol* (2017) 4:105–21. doi:10.1146/annurev-virology-101416-041726
48. Weis W, Brown JH, Cusack S, Paulson JC, Skehel JJ, Wiley DC. Structure of the influenza virus haemagglutinin complexed with its receptor, sialic acid. *Nature* (1988) 333:426–31. doi:10.1038/333426a0
49. Hamilton BS, Whittaker GR, Daniel S. Influenza virus-mediated membrane fusion: determinants of hemagglutinin fusogenic activity and experimental approaches for assessing virus fusion. *Viruses* (2012) 4:1144–68. doi:10.3390/v4071144
50. Sakai T, Nishimura SI, Naito T, Saito M. Influenza A virus hemagglutinin and neuraminidase act as novel motile machinery. *Sci Rep* (2017) 7:45043. doi:10.1038/srep45043
51. Rogers GN, Paulson JC. Receptor determinants of human and animal influenza virus isolates: differences in receptor specificity of the H3 hemagglutinin based on species of origin. *Virology* (1983) 127:361–73. doi:10.1016/0042-6822(83)90150-2
52. Nobusawa E, Aoyama T, Kato H, Suzuki Y, Tateno Y, Nakajima K. Comparison of complete amino acid sequences and receptor-binding properties among 13 serotypes of hemagglutinins of influenza A viruses. *Virology* (1991) 182:475–85. doi:10.1016/0042-6822(91)90588-3
53. Matrosovich M, Tuzikov A, Bovin N, Gambaryan A, Klimov A, Castrucci MR, et al. Early alterations of the receptor-binding properties of H1, H2, and H3 avian influenza virus hemagglutinins after their introduction into mammals. *J Virol* (2000) 74:8502–12. doi:10.1128/JVI.74.18.8502-8512.2000
54. Gambaryan AS, Tuzikov AB, Piskarev VE, Yamnikova SS, Lvov DK, Robertson JS, et al. Specification of receptor-binding phenotypes of influenza virus isolates from different hosts using synthetic sialylglycopolymers: non-egg-adapted human H1 and H3 influenza A and influenza B viruses share a common high binding affinity for 6'-sialyl(N-acetyllactosamine). *Virology* (1997) 232:345–50.
55. Bottcher-Friebertshauser E, Garten W, Matrosovich M, Klenk HD. The hemagglutinin: a determinant of pathogenicity. *Curr Top Microbiol Immunol* (2014) 385:3–34. doi:10.1007/82_2014_384
56. Tumpey TM, Maines TR, Van Hoeven N, Glaser L, Solorzano A, Pappas C, et al. A two-amino acid change in the hemagglutinin of the 1918 influenza virus abolishes transmission. *Science* (2007) 315:655–9. doi:10.1126/science.1136212
57. Imai M, Watanabe T, Hatta M, Das SC, Ozawa M, Shinya K, et al. Experimental adaptation of an influenza H5 HA confers respiratory droplet transmission to a reassortant H5 HA/H1N1 virus in ferrets. *Nature* (2012) 486:420–8. doi:10.1038/nature10831
58. Herfst S, Schrauwen EJ, Linster M, Chutinimitkul S, de Wit E, Munster VJ, et al. Airborne transmission of influenza A/H5N1 virus between ferrets. *Science* (2012) 336:1534–41. doi:10.1126/science.1213362
59. Linster M, van Boheemen S, de Graaf M, Schrauwen EJA, Lexmond P, Manz B, et al. Identification, characterization, and natural selection of mutations driving airborne transmission of A/H5N1 virus. *Cell* (2014) 157:329–39. doi:10.1016/j.cell.2014.02.040
60. Roy AM, Parker JS, Parrish CR, Whittaker GR. Early stages of influenza virus entry into Mv-1 lung cells: involvement of dynamin. *Virology* (2000) 267:17–28. doi:10.1006/viro.1999.0109
61. Rust MJ, Lakadamyali M, Zhang F, Zhuang X. Assembly of endocytic machinery around individual influenza viruses during viral entry. *Nat Struct Mol Biol* (2004) 11:567–73. doi:10.1038/nsmb769
62. Chen C, Zhuang X. Epsin 1 is a cargo-specific adaptor for the clathrin-mediated endocytosis of the influenza virus. *Proc Natl Acad Sci U S A* (2008) 105:11790–5. doi:10.1073/pnas.0803711105
63. Sieczkarski SB, Whittaker GR. Influenza virus can enter and infect cells in the absence of clathrin-mediated endocytosis. *J Virol* (2002) 76:10455–64. doi:10.1128/JVI.76.20.10455-10464.2002
64. de Vries E, Tscherne DM, Wienholts MJ, Cobos-Jimenez V, Scholte F, Garcia-Sastre A, et al. Dissection of the influenza A virus endocytic routes reveals macropinocytosis as an alternative entry pathway. *PLoS Pathog* (2011) 7:e1001329. doi:10.1371/journal.ppat.1001329
65. Lakadamyali M, Rust MJ, Babcock HP, Zhuang X. Visualizing infection of individual influenza viruses. *Proc Natl Acad Sci U S A* (2003) 100:9280–5. doi:10.1073/pnas.0832269100
66. Pinto LH, Lamb RA. The M2 proton channels of influenza A and B viruses. *J Biol Chem* (2006) 281:8997–9000. doi:10.1074/jbc.R500020200
67. White J, Helenius A, Gething MJ. Haemagglutinin of influenza virus expressed from a cloned gene promotes membrane fusion. *Nature* (1982) 300:658–9. doi:10.1038/300658a0
68. Yoshimura A, Ohnishi S. Uncoating of influenza virus in endosomes. *J Virol* (1984) 51:497–504.
69. Bullough PA, Hughson FM, Skehel JJ, Wiley DC. Structure of influenza haemagglutinin at the pH of membrane fusion. *Nature* (1994) 371:37–43. doi:10.1038/371037a0

70. Martin K, Helenius A. Nuclear transport of influenza virus ribonucleoproteins: the viral matrix protein (M1) promotes export and inhibits import. *Cell* (1991) 67:117–30. doi:10.1016/0092-8674(91)90576-K
71. Bui M, Whittaker G, Helenius A. Effect of M1 protein and low pH on nuclear transport of influenza virus ribonucleoproteins. *J Virol* (1996) 70:8391–401.
72. Harrison SC. Viral membrane fusion. *Virology* (2015) 479-480:498–507. doi:10.1016/j.virol.2015.03.043
73. White JM, Whittaker GR. Fusion of enveloped viruses in endosomes. *Traffic* (2016) 17:593–614. doi:10.1111/tra.12389
74. Klenk HD, Rott R, Orlich M, Blodorn J. Activation of influenza A viruses by trypsin treatment. *Virology* (1975) 68:426–39. doi:10.1016/0042-6822(75)90284-6
75. Lazarowitz SG, Choppin PW. Enhancement of the infectivity of influenza A and B viruses by proteolytic cleavage of the hemagglutinin polypeptide. *Virology* (1975) 68:440–54. doi:10.1016/0042-6822(75)90285-8
76. Eisfeld AJ, Neumann G, Kawaoka Y. At the centre: influenza A virus ribonucleoproteins. *Nat Rev Microbiol* (2015) 13:28–41. doi:10.1038/nrmicro3367
77. Martin K, Helenius A. Transport of incoming influenza virus nucleocapsids into the nucleus. *J Virol* (1991) 65:232–44.
78. Kemler I, Whittaker G, Helenius A. Nuclear import of microinjected influenza virus ribonucleoproteins. *Virology* (1994) 202:1028–33. doi:10.1006/viro.1994.1432
79. O'Neill RE, Jaskunas R, Blobel G, Palese P, Moroianu J. Nuclear import of influenza virus RNA can be mediated by viral nucleoprotein and transport factors required for protein import. *J Biol Chem* (1995) 270:22701–4. doi:10.1074/jbc.270.39.22701
80. Wang P, Palese P, O'Neill RE. The NPI-1/NPI-3 (karyopherin alpha) binding site on the influenza a virus nucleoprotein NP is a nonconventional nuclear localization signal. *J Virol* (1997) 71:1850–6.
81. Cros JF, Garcia-Sastre A, Palese P. An unconventional NLS is critical for the nuclear import of the influenza A virus nucleoprotein and ribonucleoprotein. *Traffic* (2005) 6:205–13. doi:10.1111/j.1600-0854.2005.00263.x
82. Wu WW, Weaver LL, Pante N. Ultrastructural analysis of the nuclear localization sequences on influenza A ribonucleoprotein complexes. *J Mol Biol* (2007) 374:910–6. doi:10.1016/j.jmb.2007.10.022
83. Chou YY, Heaton NS, Gao Q, Palese P, Singer RH, Lionnet T. Colocalization of different influenza viral RNA segments in the cytoplasm before viral budding as shown by single-molecule sensitivity FISH analysis. *PLoS Pathog* (2013) 9:e1003358. doi:10.1371/journal.ppat.1003358
84. Lakdawala SS, Wu Y, Wawrzusin P, Kabat J, Broadbent AJ, Lamirande EW, et al. Influenza a virus assembly intermediates fuse in the cytoplasm. *PLoS Pathog* (2014) 10:e1003971. doi:10.1371/journal.ppat.1003971
85. Dou D, Hernandez-Neuta I, Wang H, Ostbye H, Qian X, Thiele S, et al. Analysis of IAV replication and co-infection dynamics by a versatile RNA viral genome labeling method. *Cell Rep* (2017) 20:251–63. doi:10.1016/j.celrep.2017.06.021
86. Gabriel G, Klingel K, Otte A, Thiele S, Hudjetz B, Arman-Kalcek G, et al. Differential use of importin-alpha isoforms governs cell tropism and host adaptation of influenza virus. *Nat Commun* (2011) 2:156. doi:10.1038/ncomms1158
87. Fodor E. The RNA polymerase of influenza a virus: mechanisms of viral transcription and replication. *Acta Virol* (2013) 57:113–22. doi:10.4149/av_2013_02_113
88. Pflug A, Lukarska M, Resa-Infante P, Reich S, Cusack S. Structural insights into RNA synthesis by the influenza virus transcription-replication machine. *Virus Res* (2017) 234:103–17. doi:10.1016/j.virusres.2017.01.013
89. Newcomb LL, Kuo RL, Ye Q, Jiang Y, Tao YJ, Krug RM. Interaction of the influenza a virus nucleocapsid protein with the viral RNA polymerase potentiates unprimed viral RNA replication. *J Virol* (2009) 83:29–36. doi:10.1128/JVI.02293-07
90. York A, Hengrung N, Vreede FT, Huiskonen JT, Fodor E. Isolation and characterization of the positive-sense replicative intermediate of a negative-strand RNA virus. *Proc Natl Acad Sci U S A* (2013) 110:E4238–45. doi:10.1073/pnas.1315068110
91. Robb NC, Te Velthuis AJ, Wieneke R, Tampe R, Cordes T, Fodor E, et al. Single-molecule FRET reveals the pre-initiation and initiation conformations of influenza virus promoter RNA. *Nucleic Acids Res* (2016) 44:10304–15. doi:10.1093/nar/gkw884
92. Deng T, Vreede FT, Brownlee GG. Different de novo initiation strategies are used by influenza virus RNA polymerase on its cRNA and viral RNA promoters during viral RNA replication. *J Virol* (2006) 80:2337–48. doi:10.1128/JVI.80.5.2337-2348.2006
93. Jorba N, Coloma R, Ortin J. Genetic trans-complementation establishes a new model for influenza virus RNA transcription and replication. *PLoS Pathog* (2009) 5:e1000462. doi:10.1371/journal.ppat.1000462
94. Zhang S, Wang J, Wang Q, Toyoda T. Internal initiation of influenza virus replication of viral RNA and complementary RNA in vitro. *J Biol Chem* (2010) 285:41194–201. doi:10.1074/jbc.M110.130062
95. Reich S, Guilligay D, Pflug A, Malet H, Berger I, Crepin T, et al. Structural insight into cap-snatching and RNA synthesis by influenza polymerase. *Nature* (2014) 516:361–6. doi:10.1038/nature14009
96. Plotch SJ, Bouloy M, Ulmanen I, Krug RM. A unique cap(m7GpppXm)-dependent influenza virion endonuclease cleaves capped RNAs to generate the primers that initiate viral RNA transcription. *Cell* (1981) 23:847–58. doi:10.1016/0092-8674(81)90449-9
97. Engelhardt OG, Smith M, Fodor E. Association of the influenza A virus RNA-dependent RNA polymerase with cellular RNA polymerase II. *J Virol* (2005) 79:5812–8. doi:10.1128/JVI.79.9.5812-5818.2005
98. Martinez-Alonso M, Hengrung N, Fodor E. RNA-free and ribonucleoprotein-associated influenza virus polymerases directly bind the serine-5-phosphorylated carboxyl-terminal domain of host RNA polymerase II. *J Virol* (2016) 90:6014–21. doi:10.1128/JVI.00494-16
99. Lukarska M, Fournier G, Pflug A, Resa-Infante P, Reich S, Naffakh N, et al. Structural basis of an essential interaction between influenza polymerase and Pol II CTD. *Nature* (2017) 541:117–21. doi:10.1038/nature20594
100. Guilligay D, Tarendeau F, Resa-Infante P, Coloma R, Crepin T, Sehr P, et al. The structural basis for cap binding by influenza virus polymerase subunit PB2. *Nat Struct Mol Biol* (2008) 15:500–6. doi:10.1038/nsmb.1421
101. Dias A, Bouvier D, Crepin T, McCarthy AA, Hart DJ, Baudin F, et al. The cap-snatching endonuclease of influenza virus polymerase resides in the PA subunit. *Nature* (2009) 458:914–8. doi:10.1038/nature07745
102. Yuan P, Bartlam M, Lou Z, Chen S, Zhou J, He X, et al. Crystal structure of an avian influenza polymerase PA(N) reveals an endonuclease active site. *Nature* (2009) 458:909–13. doi:10.1038/nature07720
103. Rialdi A, Hultquist J, Jimenez-Morales D, Peralta Z, Campisi L, Fenouil R, et al. The RNA exosome syncs IAV-RNAPII transcription to promote viral ribogenesis and infectivity. *Cell* (2017) 169:679–692.e14. doi:10.1016/j.cell.2017.04.021
104. Robertson JS, Schubert M, Lazzarini RA. Polyadenylation sites for influenza virus mRNA. *J Virol* (1981) 38:157–63.
105. Poon LL, Pritlove DC, Fodor E, Brownlee GG. Direct evidence that the poly(A) tail of influenza A virus mRNA is synthesized by reiterative copying of a U track in the virion RNA template. *J Virol* (1999) 73:3473–6.
106. Reich S, Guilligay D, Cusack S. An in vitro fluorescence based study of initiation of RNA synthesis by influenza B polymerase. *Nucleic Acids Res* (2017) 45:3353–68. doi:10.1093/nar/gkx043
107. Dubois J, Terrier O, Rosa-Calatrava M. Influenza viruses and mRNA splicing: doing more with less. *MBio* (2014) 5:e70–14. doi:10.1128/mBio.00070-14
108. Lamb RA, Lai CJ. Sequence of interrupted and uninterrupted mRNAs and cloned DNA coding for the two overlapping nonstructural proteins of influenza virus. *Cell* (1980) 21:475–85. doi:10.1016/0092-8674(80)90484-5
109. Lamb RA, Choppin PW, Chanock RM, Lai CJ. Mapping of the two overlapping genes for polypeptides NS1 and NS2 on RNA segment 8 of influenza virus genome. *Proc Natl Acad Sci U S A* (1980) 77:1857–61. doi:10.1073/pnas.77.4.1857
110. Lamb RA, Lai CJ, Choppin PW. Sequences of mRNAs derived from genome RNA segment 7 of influenza virus: colinear and interrupted mRNAs code for overlapping proteins. *Proc Natl Acad Sci U S A* (1981) 78:4170–4. doi:10.1073/pnas.78.7.4170
111. Inglis SC, Brown CM. Spliced and unspliced RNAs encoded by virion RNA segment 7 of influenza virus. *Nucleic Acids Res* (1981) 9:2727–40. doi:10.1093/nar/9.12.2727
112. Mor A, White A, Zhang K, Thompson M, Esparza M, Munoz-Moreno R, et al. Influenza virus mRNA trafficking through host nuclear speckles. *Nat Microbiol* (2016) 1:16069. doi:10.1038/nmicrobiol.2016.69
113. Inglis SC, Brown CM. Differences in the control of virus mRNA splicing during permissive or abortive infection with influenza A (fowl plague) virus. *J Gen Virol* (1984) 65(Pt 1):153–64. doi:10.1099/0022-1317-65-1-153

114. Valcarcel J, Portela A, Ortin J. Regulated M1 mRNA splicing in influenza virus-infected cells. *J Gen Virol* (1991) 72(Pt 6):1301–8. doi:10.1099/0022-1317-72-6-1301
115. Robb NC, Fodor E. The accumulation of influenza A virus segment 7 spliced mRNAs is regulated by the NS1 protein. *J Gen Virol* (2012) 93:113–8. doi:10.1099/vir.0.035485-0
116. Backstrom Winquist E, Abdurahman S, Tranell A, Lindstrom S, Tingsborg S, Schwartz S. Inefficient splicing of segment 7 and 8 mRNAs is an inherent property of influenza virus A/Brevig Mission/1918/1 (H1N1) that causes elevated expression of NS1 protein. *Virology* (2012) 422:46–58. doi:10.1016/j.virol.2011.10.004
117. York A, Fodor E. Biogenesis, assembly, and export of viral messenger ribonucleoproteins in the influenza A virus infected cell. *RNA Biol* (2013) 10:1274–82. doi:10.4161/rna.25356
118. Huet S, Avilov SV, Ferbitz L, Daigle N, Cusack S, Ellenberg J. Nuclear import and assembly of influenza A virus RNA polymerase studied in live cells by fluorescence cross-correlation spectroscopy. *J Virol* (2010) 84:1254–64. doi:10.1128/JVI.01533-09
119. Lee N, Le Sage V, Nanni AV, Snyder DJ, Cooper VS, Lakdawala SS. Genome-wide analysis of influenza viral RNA and nucleoprotein association. *Nucleic Acids Res* (2017) 45:8968–77. doi:10.1093/nar/gkx584
120. Williams GD, Townsend D, Wylie KM, Kim PJ, Amarasinghe GK, Kutluay SB, et al. Nucleotide resolution mapping of influenza A virus nucleoprotein-RNA interactions reveals RNA features required for replication. *Nat Commun* (2018) 9:465. doi:10.1038/s41467-018-02886-w
121. Mondal A, Potts GK, Dawson AR, Coon JJ, Mehle A. Phosphorylation at the homotypic interface regulates nucleoprotein oligomerization and assembly of the influenza virus replication machinery. *PLoS Pathog* (2015) 11:e1004826. doi:10.1371/journal.ppat.1004826
122. Ayllon J, Garcia-Sastre A. The NS1 protein: a multitasking virulence factor. *Curr Top Microbiol Immunol* (2015) 386:73–107. doi:10.1007/82_2014_400
123. Satterly N, Tsai PL, van Deursen J, Nussenzveig DR, Wang Y, Faria PA, et al. Influenza virus targets the mRNA export machinery and the nuclear pore complex. *Proc Natl Acad Sci U S A* (2007) 104:1853–8. doi:10.1073/pnas.0610977104
124. O'Neill RE, Talon J, Palese P. The influenza virus NEP (NS2 protein) mediates the nuclear export of viral ribonucleoproteins. *EMBO J* (1998) 17:288–96. doi:10.1093/emboj/17.1.288
125. Cao S, Liu X, Yu M, Li J, Jia X, Bi Y, et al. A nuclear export signal in the matrix protein of influenza A virus is required for efficient virus replication. *J Virol* (2012) 86:4883–91. doi:10.1128/JVI.06586-11
126. Neumann G, Hughes MT, Kawaoka Y. Influenza A virus NS2 protein mediates vRNP nuclear export through NES-independent interaction with hCRM1. *EMBO J* (2000) 19:6751–8. doi:10.1093/emboj/19.24.6751
127. Huang S, Chen J, Chen Q, Wang H, Yao Y, Chen J, et al. A second CRM1-dependent nuclear export signal in the influenza A virus NS2 protein contributes to the nuclear export of viral ribonucleoproteins. *J Virol* (2013) 87:767–78. doi:10.1128/JVI.06519-11
128. Shimizu T, Takizawa N, Watanabe K, Nagata K, Kobayashi N. Crucial role of the influenza virus NS2 (NEP) C-terminal domain in M1 binding and nuclear export of vRNP. *FEBS Lett* (2011) 585:41–6. doi:10.1016/j.febslet.2010.11.017
129. Akarsu H, Burmeister WP, Petosa C, Petit I, Muller CW, Ruigrok RW, et al. Crystal structure of the M1 protein-binding domain of the influenza A virus nuclear export protein (NEP/NS2). *EMBO J* (2003) 22:4646–55. doi:10.1093/emboj/cdg449
130. Amorim MJ, Bruce EA, Read EK, Foeglein A, Mahen R, Stuart AD, et al. A Rab11- and microtubule-dependent mechanism for cytoplasmic transport of influenza A virus viral RNA. *J Virol* (2011) 85:4143–56. doi:10.1128/JVI.02606-10
131. Eisfeld AJ, Kawakami E, Watanabe T, Neumann G, Kawaoka Y. RAB11A is essential for transport of the influenza virus genome to the plasma membrane. *J Virol* (2011) 85:6117–26. doi:10.1128/JVI.00378-11
132. Momose F, Sekimoto T, Ohkura T, Jo S, Kawaguchi A, Nagata K, et al. Apical transport of influenza A virus ribonucleoprotein requires Rab11-positive recycling endosome. *PLoS One* (2011) 6:e21123. doi:10.1371/journal.pone.0021123
133. de Castro Martin IF, Fournier G, Sachse M, Pizarro-Cerda J, Risco C, Naffakh N. Influenza virus genome reaches the plasma membrane via a modified endoplasmic reticulum and Rab11-dependent vesicles. *Nat Commun* (2017) 8:1396. doi:10.1038/s41467-017-01557-6
134. Elton D, Simpson-Holley M, Archer K, Medcalf L, Hallam R, McCauley J, et al. Interaction of the influenza virus nucleoprotein with the cellular CRM1-mediated nuclear export pathway. *J Virol* (2001) 75:408–19. doi:10.1128/JVI.75.1.408-419.2001
135. Gavazzi C, Yver M, Isel C, Smyth RP, Rosa-Calatrava M, Lina B, et al. A functional sequence-specific interaction between influenza A virus genomic RNA segments. *Proc Natl Acad Sci U S A* (2013) 110:16604–9. doi:10.1073/pnas.1314419110
136. Daniels R, Kurowski B, Johnson AE, Hebert DN. N-linked glycans direct the cotranslational folding pathway of influenza hemagglutinin. *Mol Cell* (2003) 11:79–90. doi:10.1016/S1097-2765(02)00821-3
137. Bos TJ, Davis AR, Nayak DP. NH2-terminal hydrophobic region of influenza virus neuraminidase provides the signal function in translocation. *Proc Natl Acad Sci U S A* (1984) 81:2327–31. doi:10.1073/pnas.81.8.2327
138. Dou D, da Silva DV, Nordholm J, Wang H, Daniels R. Type II transmembrane domain hydrophobicity dictates the cotranslational dependence for inversion. *Mol Biol Cell* (2014) 25:3363–74. doi:10.1091/mbc.E14-04-0874
139. Hull JD, Gilmore R, Lamb RA. Integration of a small integral membrane protein, M2, of influenza virus into the endoplasmic reticulum: analysis of the internal signal-anchor domain of a protein with an ectoplasmic NH2 terminus. *J Cell Biol* (1988) 106:1489–98. doi:10.1083/jcb.106.5.1489
140. Gorlich D, Prehn S, Hartmann E, Kalies KU, Rapoport TA. A mammalian homolog of SEC61p and SECYp is associated with ribosomes and nascent polypeptides during translocation. *Cell* (1992) 71:489–503. doi:10.1016/0092-8674(92)90517-G
141. Deshaies RJ, Schekman R. A yeast mutant defective at an early stage in import of secretory protein precursors into the endoplasmic reticulum. *J Cell Biol* (1987) 105:633–45. doi:10.1083/jcb.105.2.633
142. Gilmore R, Walter P, Blobel G. Protein translocation across the endoplasmic reticulum. II. Isolation and characterization of the signal recognition particle receptor. *J Cell Biol* (1982) 95:470–7. doi:10.1083/jcb.95.2.470
143. Karamyshev AL, Patrick AE, Karamysheva ZN, Griesemer DS, Hudson H, Tjon-Kon-Sang S, et al. Inefficient SRP interaction with a nascent chain triggers a mRNA quality control pathway. *Cell* (2014) 156:146–57. doi:10.1016/j.cell.2013.12.017
144. Kang SW, Rane NS, Kim SJ, Garrison JL, Taunton J, Hegde RS. Substrate-specific translocational attenuation during ER stress defines a pre-emptive quality control pathway. *Cell* (2006) 127:999–1013. doi:10.1016/j.cell.2006.10.032
145. Bowie JU. Solving the membrane protein folding problem. *Nature* (2005) 438:581–9. doi:10.1038/nature04395
146. Van den Berg B, Clemons WM Jr, Collinson I, Modis Y, Hartmann E, Harrison SC, et al. X-ray structure of a protein-conducting channel. *Nature* (2004) 427:36–44. doi:10.1038/nature02218
147. Hessa T, Meindl-Beinker NM, Bernsel A, Kim H, Sato Y, Lerch-Bader M, et al. Molecular code for transmembrane-helix recognition by the Sec61 translocon. *Nature* (2007) 450:1026–30. doi:10.1038/nature06387
148. Nordholm J, da Silva DV, Damjanovic J, Dou D, Daniels R. Polar residues and their positional context dictate the transmembrane domain interactions of influenza a neuraminidases. *J Biol Chem* (2013) 288:10652–60. doi:10.1074/jbc.M112.440230
149. Mandon EC, Trueman SF, Gilmore R. Protein translocation across the rough endoplasmic reticulum. *Cold Spring Harb Perspect Biol* (2013) 5:a013342. doi:10.1101/cshperspect.a013342
150. Wang N, Glidden EJ, Murphy SR, Pearse BR, Hebert DN. The cotranslational maturation program for the type II membrane glycoprotein influenza neuraminidase. *J Biol Chem* (2008) 283:33826–37. doi:10.1074/jbc.M806897200
151. Daniels R, Svedine S, Hebert DN. N-linked carbohydrates act as lumenal maturation and quality control protein tags. *Cell Biochem Biophys* (2004) 41:113–38. doi:10.1385/CBB:41:1:113
152. Hebert DN, Zhang JX, Chen W, Foellmer B, Helenius A. The number and location of glycans on influenza hemagglutinin determine folding and association with calnexin and calreticulin. *J Cell Biol* (1997) 139:613–23. doi:10.1083/jcb.139.3.613

153. Wilson IA, Skehel JJ, Wiley DC. Structure of the haemagglutinin membrane glycoprotein of influenza virus at 3 A resolution. *Nature* (1981) 289:366–73. doi:10.1038/289366a0
154. Varghese JN, Laver WG, Colman PM. Structure of the influenza virus glycoprotein antigen neuraminidase at 2.9 A resolution. *Nature* (1983) 303:35–40. doi:10.1038/303035a0
155. Li Q, Qi J, Zhang W, Vavricka CJ, Shi Y, Wei J, et al. The 2009 pandemic H1N1 neuraminidase N1 lacks the 150-cavity in its active site. *Nat Struct Mol Biol* (2010) 17:1266–8. doi:10.1038/nsmb.1909
156. Holsinger LJ, Lamb RA. Influenza virus M2 integral membrane protein is a homotetramer stabilized by formation of disulfide bonds. *Virology* (1991) 183:32–43. doi:10.1016/0042-6822(91)90115-R
157. Saito T, Taylor G, Webster RG. Steps in maturation of influenza A virus neuraminidase. *J Virol* (1995) 69:5011–7.
158. da Silva DV, Nordholm J, Madjo U, Pfeiffer A, Daniels R. Assembly of subtype 1 influenza neuraminidase is driven by both the transmembrane and head domains. *J Biol Chem* (2013) 288:644–53. doi:10.1074/jbc.M112.424150
159. da Silva DV, Nordholm J, Dou D, Wang H, Rossman JS, Daniels R. The influenza virus neuraminidase protein transmembrane and head domains have coevolved. *J Virol* (2015) 89:1094–104. doi:10.1128/JVI.02005-14
160. Hassan IH, Zhang MS, Powers LS, Shao JQ, Baltrusaitis J, Rutkowski DT, et al. Influenza A viral replication is blocked by inhibition of the inositol-requiring enzyme 1 (IRE1) stress pathway. *J Biol Chem* (2012) 287:4679–89. doi:10.1074/jbc.M111.284695
161. Roberson EC, Tully JE, Guala AS, Reiss JN, Godburn KE, Pociask DA, et al. Influenza induces endoplasmic reticulum stress, caspase-12-dependent apoptosis, and c-Jun N-terminal kinase-mediated transforming growth factor-beta release in lung epithelial cells. *Am J Respir Cell Mol Biol* (2012) 46:573–81. doi:10.1165/rcmb.2010-0460OC
162. Khaperskyy DA, Emara MM, Johnston BP, Anderson P, Hatchette TF, McCormick C. Influenza a virus host shutoff disables antiviral stress-induced translation arrest. *PLoS Pathog* (2014) 10:e1004217. doi:10.1371/journal.ppat.1004217
163. Vester D, Lagoda A, Hoffmann D, Seitz C, Heldt S, Bettenbrock K, et al. Real-time RT-qPCR assay for the analysis of human influenza A virus transcription and replication dynamics. *J Virol Methods* (2010) 168:63–71. doi:10.1016/j.jviromet.2010.04.017
164. Kawakami E, Watanabe T, Fujii K, Goto H, Watanabe S, Noda T, et al. Strand-specific real-time RT-PCR for distinguishing influenza vRNA, cRNA, and mRNA. *J Virol Methods* (2011) 173:1–6. doi:10.1016/j.jviromet.2010.12.014
165. Nordholm J, Petitou J, Ostbye H, da Silva DV, Dou D, Wang H, et al. Translational regulation of viral secretory proteins by the 5' coding regions and a viral RNA-binding protein. *J Cell Biol* (2017) 216:2283–93. doi:10.1083/jcb.201702102
166. Palazzo AF, Springer M, Shibata Y, Lee CS, Dias AP, Rapoport TA. The signal sequence coding region promotes nuclear export of mRNA. *PLoS Biol* (2007) 5:e322. doi:10.1371/journal.pbio.0050322
167. Panthu B, Terrier O, Carron C, Traversier A, Corbin A, Balvay L, et al. The NS1 protein from influenza virus stimulates translation initiation by enhancing ribosome recruitment to mRNAs. *J Mol Biol* (2017) 429:3334–52. doi:10.1016/j.jmb.2017.04.007
168. Trapp S, Soubieux D, Lidove A, Esnault E, Lion A, Guillory V, et al. Major contribution of the RNA-binding domain of NS1 in the pathogenicity and replication potential of an avian H7N1 influenza virus in chickens. *Virol J* (2018) 15:55. doi:10.1186/s12985-018-0960-4
169. Aragon T, de la Luna S, Novoa I, Carrasco L, Ortin J, Nieto A. Eukaryotic translation initiation factor 4GI is a cellular target for NS1 protein, a translational activator of influenza virus. *Mol Cell Biol* (2000) 20:6259–68. doi:10.1128/MCB.20.17.6259-6268.2000
170. Enami K, Sato TA, Nakada S, Enami M. Influenza virus NS1 protein stimulates translation of the M1 protein. *J Virol* (1994) 68:1432–7.
171. de la Luna S, Fortes P, Beloso A, Ortin J. Influenza virus NS1 protein enhances the rate of translation initiation of viral mRNAs. *J Virol* (1995) 69:2427–33.
172. Huang RT, Rott R, Klenk HD. Influenza viruses cause hemolysis and fusion of cells. *Virology* (1981) 110:243–7. doi:10.1016/0042-6822(81)90030-1
173. Maeda T, Kawasaki K, Ohnishi S. Interaction of influenza virus hemagglutinin with target membrane lipids is a key step in virus-induced hemolysis and fusion at pH 5.2. *Proc Natl Acad Sci U S A* (1981) 78:4133–7. doi:10.1073/pnas.78.7.4133
174. Stieneke-Grober A, Vey M, Angliker H, Shaw E, Thomas G, Roberts C, et al. Influenza virus hemagglutinin with multibasic cleavage site is activated by furin, a subtilisin-like endoprotease. *EMBO J* (1992) 11:2407–14.
175. Schalken JA, Roebroek AJ, Oomen PP, Wagenaar SS, Debruyne FM, Bloemers HP, et al. fur gene expression as a discriminating marker for small cell and nonsmall cell lung carcinomas. *J Clin Invest* (1987) 80:1545–9. doi:10.1172/JCI113240
176. Bottcher E, Matrosovich T, Beyerle M, Klenk HD, Garten W, Matrosovich M. Proteolytic activation of influenza viruses by serine proteases TMPRSS2 and HAT from human airway epithelium. *J Virol* (2006) 80:9896–8. doi:10.1128/JVI.01118-06
177. Chaipan C, Kobasa D, Bertram S, Glowacka I, Steffen I, Tsegaye TS, et al. Proteolytic activation of the 1918 influenza virus hemagglutinin. *J Virol* (2009) 83:3200–11. doi:10.1128/JVI.02205-08
178. Zhirnov OP, Ikizler MR, Wright PF. Cleavage of influenza a virus hemagglutinin in human respiratory epithelium is cell associated and sensitive to exogenous antiproteases. *J Virol* (2002) 76:8682–9. doi:10.1128/JVI.76.17.8682-8689.2002
179. Bottcher-Friebertshauser E, Freuer C, Sielaff F, Schmidt S, Eickmann M, Uhlendorff J, et al. Cleavage of influenza virus hemagglutinin by airway proteases TMPRSS2 and HAT differs in subcellular localization and susceptibility to protease inhibitors. *J Virol* (2010) 84:5605–14. doi:10.1128/JVI.00140-10
180. Steinhauer DA, Wharton SA, Skehel JJ, Wiley DC, Hay AJ. Amantadine selection of a mutant influenza virus containing an acid-stable hemagglutinin glycoprotein: evidence for virus-specific regulation of the pH of glycoprotein transport vesicles. *Proc Natl Acad Sci U S A* (1991) 88:11525–9. doi:10.1073/pnas.88.24.11525
181. Takeuchi K, Lamb RA. Influenza virus M2 protein ion channel activity stabilizes the native form of fowl plague virus hemagglutinin during intracellular transport. *J Virol* (1994) 68:911–9.
182. Bertram S, Heurich A, Lavender H, Gierer S, Danisch S, Perin P, et al. Influenza and SARS-coronavirus activating proteases TMPRSS2 and HAT are expressed at multiple sites in human respiratory and gastrointestinal tracts. *PLoS One* (2012) 7:e35876. doi:10.1371/journal.pone.0035876
183. Lingwood D, Simons K. Lipid rafts as a membrane-organizing principle. *Science* (2010) 327:46–50. doi:10.1126/science.1174621
184. Rossman JS, Lamb RA. Influenza virus assembly and budding. *Virology* (2011) 411:229–36. doi:10.1016/j.virol.2010.12.003
185. Veit M, Thaa B. Association of influenza virus proteins with membrane rafts. *Adv Virol* (2011) 2011:370606. doi:10.1155/2011/370606
186. Zurcher T, Luo G, Palese P. Mutations at palmitylation sites of the influenza virus hemagglutinin affect virus formation. *J Virol* (1994) 68:5748–54.
187. Wagner R, Herwig A, Azzouz N, Klenk HD. Acylation-mediated membrane anchoring of avian influenza virus hemagglutinin is essential for fusion pore formation and virus infectivity. *J Virol* (2005) 79:6449–58. doi:10.1128/JVI.79.10.6449-6458.2005
188. Kordyukova LV, Serebryakova MV, Baratova LA, Veit M. S acylation of the hemagglutinin of influenza viruses: mass spectrometry reveals site-specific attachment of stearic acid to a transmembrane cysteine. *J Virol* (2008) 82:9288–92. doi:10.1128/JVI.00704-08
189. Takeda M, Leser GP, Russell CJ, Lamb RA. Influenza virus hemagglutinin concentrates in lipid raft microdomains for efficient viral fusion. *Proc Natl Acad Sci U S A* (2003) 100:14610–7. doi:10.1073/pnas.2235620100
190. Barman S, Adhikary L, Chakrabarti AK, Bernas C, Kawaoka Y, Nayak DP. Role of transmembrane domain and cytoplasmic tail amino acid sequences of influenza a virus neuraminidase in raft association and virus budding. *J Virol* (2004) 78:5258–69. doi:10.1128/JVI.78.10.5258-5269.2004
191. Rossman JS, Jing X, Leser GP, Lamb RA. Influenza virus M2 protein mediates ESCRT-independent membrane scission. *Cell* (2010) 142:902–13. doi:10.1016/j.cell.2010.08.029
192. Ali A, Avalos RT, Ponimaskin E, Nayak DP. Influenza virus assembly: effect of influenza virus glycoproteins on the membrane association of M1 protein. *J Virol* (2000) 74:8709–19. doi:10.1128/JVI.74.18.8709-8719.2000
193. Zhang J, Pekosz A, Lamb RA. Influenza virus assembly and lipid raft microdomains: a role for the cytoplasmic tails of the spike glycoproteins. *J Virol* (2000) 74:4634–44. doi:10.1128/JVI.74.10.4634-4644.2000

194. Noton SL, Medcalf E, Fisher D, Mullin AE, Elton D, Digard P. Identification of the domains of the influenza A virus M1 matrix protein required for NP binding, oligomerization and incorporation into virions. *J Gen Virol* (2007) 88:2280–90. doi:10.1099/vir.0.82809-0
195. Jarsch IK, Daste F, Gallop JL. Membrane curvature in cell biology: an integration of molecular mechanisms. *J Cell Biol* (2016) 214:375–87. doi:10.1083/jcb.201604003
196. Chen BJ, Leser GP, Morita E, Lamb RA. Influenza virus hemagglutinin and neuraminidase, but not the matrix protein, are required for assembly and budding of plasmid-derived virus-like particles. *J Virol* (2007) 81:7111–23. doi:10.1128/JVI.00361-07
197. Lai JC, Chan WW, Kien F, Nicholls JM, Peiris JS, Garcia JM. Formation of virus-like particles from human cell lines exclusively expressing influenza neuraminidase. *J Gen Virol* (2010) 91:2322–30. doi:10.1099/vir.0.019935-0
198. Yondola MA, Fernandes F, Belicha-Villanueva A, Uccelini M, Gao Q, Carter C, et al. Budding capability of the influenza virus neuraminidase can be modulated by tetherin. *J Virol* (2011) 85:2480–91. doi:10.1128/JVI.02188-10
199. Chlanda P, Schraidt O, Kummer S, Riches J, Oberwinkler H, Prinz S, et al. Structural analysis of the roles of influenza A virus membrane-associated proteins in assembly and morphology. *J Virol* (2015) 89:8957–66. doi:10.1128/JVI.00592-15
200. Harris A, Forouhar F, Qiu S, Sha B, Luo M. The crystal structure of the influenza matrix protein M1 at neutral pH: M1-M1 protein interfaces can rotate in the oligomeric structures of M1. *Virology* (2001) 289:34–44. doi:10.1006/viro.2001.1119
201. Shtykova EV, Dadinova LA, Fedorova NV, Golanikov AE, Bogacheva EN, Ksenofontov AL, et al. Influenza virus matrix protein M1 preserves its conformation with pH, changing multimerization state at the priming stage due to electrostatics. *Sci Rep* (2017) 7:16793. doi:10.1038/s41598-017-16986-y
202. Hilsch M, Goldenbogen B, Sieben C, Hofer CT, Rabe JP, Klipp E, et al. Influenza A matrix protein M1 multimerizes upon binding to lipid membranes. *Biophys J* (2014) 107:912–23. doi:10.1016/j.bpj.2014.06.042
203. Elleman CJ, Barclay WS. The M1 matrix protein controls the filamentous phenotype of influenza A virus. *Virology* (2004) 321:144–53. doi:10.1016/j.virol.2003.12.009
204. Rossman JS, Lamb RA. Viral membrane scission. *Annu Rev Cell Dev Biol* (2013) 29:551–69. doi:10.1146/annurev-cellbio-101011-155838
205. Jin H, Leser GP, Lamb RA. The influenza virus hemagglutinin cytoplasmic tail is not essential for virus assembly or infectivity. *EMBO J* (1994) 13:5504–15.
206. Garcia-Sastre A, Palese P. The cytoplasmic tail of the neuraminidase protein of influenza A virus does not play an important role in the packaging of this protein into viral envelopes. *Virus Res* (1995) 37:37–47. doi:10.1016/0168-1702(95)00017-K
207. Stewart SM, Pekosz A. Mutations in the membrane-proximal region of the influenza A virus M2 protein cytoplasmic tail have modest effects on virus replication. *J Virol* (2011) 85:12179–87. doi:10.1128/JVI.05970-11
208. Air GM. Influenza neuraminidase. *Influenza Other Respi Viruses* (2012) 6:245–56. doi:10.1111/j.1750-2659.2011.00304.x
209. Colman PM. Influenza virus neuraminidase: structure, antibodies, and inhibitors. *Protein Sci* (1994) 3:1687–96. doi:10.1002/pro.5560031007
210. Burmeister WP, Ruigrok RW, Cusack S. The 2.2 A resolution crystal structure of influenza B neuraminidase and its complex with sialic acid. *EMBO J* (1992) 11:49–56.
211. Kim JH, Resende R, Wennekes T, Chen HM, Bance N, Buchini S, et al. Mechanism-based covalent neuraminidase inhibitors with broad-spectrum influenza antiviral activity. *Science* (2013) 340:71–5. doi:10.1126/science.1232552
212. Colman PM, Varghese JN, Laver WG. Structure of the catalytic and antigenic sites in influenza virus neuraminidase. *Nature* (1983) 303:41–4. doi:10.1038/303041a0
213. Paterson RG, Lamb RA. Conversion of a class II integral membrane protein into a soluble and efficiently secreted protein: multiple intracellular and extracellular oligomeric and conformational forms. *J Cell Biol* (1990) 110:999–1011. doi:10.1083/jcb.110.4.999
214. Bucher DJ, Kilbourne ED. A 2 (N2) neuraminidase of the X-7 influenza virus recombinant: determination of molecular size and subunit composition of the active unit. *J Virol* (1972) 10:60–6.
215. Chong AK, Pegg MS, von Itzstein M. Influenza virus sialidase: effect of calcium on steady-state kinetic parameters. *Biochim Biophys Acta* (1991) 1077:65–71. doi:10.1016/0167-4838(91)90526-6
216. Burnet FM, Mc CJ, Anderson SG. Mucin as substrate of enzyme action by viruses of the mumps influenza group. *Nature* (1947) 160:404. doi:10.1038/160404b0
217. Burnet FM. Mucins and mucoids in relation to influenza virus action; the destruction of Francis inhibitor activity in a purified mucoid by virus action. *Aust J Exp Biol Med Sci* (1948) 26:389–402. doi:10.1038/icb.1948.40
218. Gottschalk A. Neuraminidase: the specific enzyme of influenza virus and Vibrio cholerae. *Biochim Biophys Acta* (1957) 23:645–6. doi:10.1016/0006-3002(57)90389-X
219. Webster RG, Laver WG. Preparation and properties of antibody directed specifically against the neuraminidase of influenza virus. *J Immunol* (1967) 99:49–55.
220. Palese P, Compans RW. Inhibition of influenza virus replication in tissue culture by 2-deoxy-2,3-dehydro-N-trifluoroacetylneuraminic acid (FANA): mechanism of action. *J Gen Virol* (1976) 33:159–63. doi:10.1099/0022-1317-33-1-159
221. Palese P, Tobita K, Ueda M, Compans RW. Characterization of temperature sensitive influenza virus mutants defective in neuraminidase. *Virology* (1974) 61:397–410. doi:10.1016/0042-6822(74)90276-1
222. Gulati U, Wu W, Gulati S, Kumari K, Waner JL, Air GM. Mismatched hemagglutinin and neuraminidase specificities in recent human H3N2 influenza viruses. *Virology* (2005) 339:12–20. doi:10.1016/j.virol.2005.05.009
223. Mochalova L, Kurova V, Shtyrya Y, Korchagina E, Gambaryan A, Belyanchikov I, et al. Oligosaccharide specificity of influenza H1N1 virus neuraminidases. *Arch Virol* (2007) 152:2047–57. doi:10.1007/s00705-007-1024-z
224. Lin YP, Gregory V, Collins P, Kloess J, Wharton S, Cattle N, et al. Neuraminidase receptor binding variants of human influenza A(H3N2) viruses resulting from substitution of aspartic acid 151 in the catalytic site: a role in virus attachment? *J Virol* (2010) 84:6769–81. doi:10.1128/JVI.00458-10
225. Zhu X, McBride R, Nycholat CM, Yu W, Paulson JC, Wilson IA. Influenza virus neuraminidases with reduced enzymatic activity that avidly bind sialic Acid receptors. *J Virol* (2012) 86:13371–83. doi:10.1128/JVI.01426-12
226. Cohen M, Zhang XQ, Senaati HP, Chen HW, Varki NM, Schooley RT, et al. Influenza A penetrates host mucus by cleaving sialic acids with neuraminidase. *Virol J* (2013) 10:321. doi:10.1186/1743-422X-10-321
227. Burnet FM. Mucoproteins in relation to virus action. *Physiol Rev* (1951) 31:131–50. doi:10.1152/physrev.1951.31.2.131
228. Yang X, Steukers L, Forier K, Xiong R, Braeckmans K, Van Reeth K, et al. A beneficiary role for neuraminidase in influenza virus penetration through the respiratory mucus. *PLoS One* (2014) 9:e110026. doi:10.1371/journal.pone.0110026
229. Matrosovich MN, Matrosovich TY, Gray T, Roberts NA, Klenk HD. Neuraminidase is important for the initiation of influenza virus infection in human airway epithelium. *J Virol* (2004) 78:12665–7. doi:10.1128/JVI.78.22.12665-12667.2004
230. Zanin M, Marathe B, Wong SS, Yoon SW, Collin E, Oshansky C, et al. Pandemic swine H1N1 influenza viruses with almost undetectable neuraminidase activity are not transmitted via aerosols in ferrets and are inhibited by human mucus but not swine mucus. *J Virol* (2015) 89:5935–48. doi:10.1128/JVI.02537-14
231. Cheung PP, Rogozin IB, Choy KT, Ng HY, Peiris JS, Yen HL. Comparative mutational analyses of influenza A viruses. *RNA* (2015) 21:36–47. doi:10.1261/rna.045369.114
232. Drake JW. Rates of spontaneous mutation among RNA viruses. *Proc Natl Acad Sci U S A* (1993) 90:4171–5. doi:10.1073/pnas.90.9.4171
233. Steinhauer DA, Holland JJ. Rapid evolution of RNA viruses. *Annu Rev Microbiol* (1987) 41:409–33. doi:10.1146/annurev.mi.41.100187.002205
234. Russell AB, Trapnell C, Bloom JD. Extreme heterogeneity of influenza virus infection in single cells. *Elife* (2018) 7:e32303. doi:10.7554/eLife.32303
235. Ashenberg O, Padmakumar J, Doud MB, Bloom JD. Deep mutational scanning identifies sites in influenza nucleoprotein that affect viral inhibition by MxA. *PLoS Pathog* (2017) 13:e1006288. doi:10.1371/journal.ppat.1006288
236. Thyagarajan B, Bloom JD. The inherent mutational tolerance and antigenic evolvability of influenza hemagglutinin. *Elife* (2014) 3:e03300. doi:10.7554/eLife.03300
237. Doud MB, Bloom JD. Accurate measurement of the effects of all amino-acid mutations on influenza hemagglutinin. *Viruses* (2016) 8:E155. doi:10.3390/v8060155

238. Doud MB, Lee JM, Bloom JD. How single mutations affect viral escape from broad and narrow antibodies to H1 influenza hemagglutinin. *Nat Commun* (2018) 9:1386. doi:10.1038/s41467-018-03665-3
239. Rathore U, Kesavardhana S, Mallajosyula VV, Varadarajan R. Immunogen design for HIV-1 and influenza. *Biochim Biophys Acta* (2014) 1844:1891–906. doi:10.1016/j.bbapap.2014.05.010
240. Krammer F, Garcia-Sastre A, Palese P. Is it possible to develop a "universal" influenza virus vaccine? Toward a universal influenza virus vaccine: potential target antigens and critical aspects for vaccine development. *Cold Spring Harb Perspect Biol* (2018) 10(7):a028845. doi:10.1101/cshperspect.a028845
241. Yassine HM, Boyington JC, McTamney PM, Wei CJ, Kanekiyo M, Kong WP, et al. Hemagglutinin-stem nanoparticles generate heterosubtypic influenza protection. *Nat Med* (2015) 21:1065–70. doi:10.1038/nm.3927
242. Kallewaard NL, Corti D, Collins PJ, Neu U, McAuliffe JM, Benjamin E, et al. Structure and function analysis of an antibody recognizing all influenza A subtypes. *Cell* (2016) 166:596–608. doi:10.1016/j.cell.2016.05.073
243. Gerstberger S, Hafner M, Tuschl T. A census of human RNA-binding proteins. *Nat Rev Genet* (2014) 15:829–45. doi:10.1038/nrg3813
244. Tsai PL, Chiou NT, Kuss S, Garcia-Sastre A, Lynch KW, Fontoura BM. Cellular RNA binding proteins NS1-BP and hnRNP K regulate influenza A virus RNA splicing. *PLoS Pathog* (2013) 9:e1003460. doi:10.1371/journal.ppat.1003460
245. Chen G, Liu CH, Zhou L, Krug RM. Cellular DDX21 RNA helicase inhibits influenza A virus replication but is counteracted by the viral NS1 protein. *Cell Host Microbe* (2014) 15:484–93. doi:10.1016/j.chom.2014.03.002
246. Younis S, Kamel W, Falkeborn T, Wang H, Yu D, Daniels R, et al. Multiple nuclear-replicating viruses require the stress-induced protein ZC3H11A for efficient growth. *Proc Natl Acad Sci U S A* (2018) 115(16):E3808–16. doi:10.1073/pnas.1722333115
247. Kechavarzi B, Janga SC. Dissecting the expression landscape of RNA-binding proteins in human cancers. *Genome Biol* (2014) 15:R14. doi:10.1186/gb-2014-15-1-r14
248. Pereira B, Billaud M, Almeida R. RNA-binding proteins in cancer: old players and new actors. *Trends Cancer* (2017) 3:506–28. doi:10.1016/j.trecan.2017.05.003
249. Yuan S, Wen L, Zhou J. Inhibitors of influenza A virus polymerase. *ACS Infect Dis* (2018) 4:218–23. doi:10.1021/acsinfecdis.7b00265

16

Respiratory Mononuclear Phagocytes in Human Influenza A Virus Infection: Their Role in Immune Protection and as Targets of the Virus

Sindhu Vangeti, Meng Yu and Anna Smed-Sörensen *

Division of Immunology and Allergy, Department of Medicine Solna, Karolinska Institutet, Karolinska University Hospital Solna, Stockholm, Sweden

***Correspondence:**
Anna Smed-Sörensen
anna.smed.sorensen@ki.se

Emerging viruses have become increasingly important with recurrent epidemics. Influenza A virus (IAV), a respiratory virus displaying continuous re-emergence, contributes significantly to global morbidity and mortality, especially in young children, immunocompromised, and elderly people. IAV infection is typically confined to the airways and the virus replicates in respiratory epithelial cells but can also infect resident immune cells. Clearance of infection requires virus-specific adaptive immune responses that depend on early and efficient innate immune responses against IAV. Mononuclear phagocytes (MNPs), comprising monocytes, dendritic cells, and macrophages, have common but also unique features. In addition to being professional antigen-presenting cells, MNPs mediate leukocyte recruitment, sense and phagocytose pathogens, regulate inflammation, and shape immune responses. The immune protection mediated by MNPs can be compromised during IAV infection when the cells are also targeted by the virus, leading to impaired cytokine responses and altered interactions with other immune cells. Furthermore, it is becoming increasingly clear that immune cells differ depending on their anatomical location and that it is important to study them where they are expected to exert their function. Defining tissue-resident MNP distribution, phenotype, and function during acute and convalescent human IAV infection can offer valuable insights into understanding how MNPs maintain the fine balance required to protect against infections that the cells are themselves susceptible to. In this review, we delineate the role of MNPs in the human respiratory tract during IAV infection both in mediating immune protection and as targets of the virus.

Keywords: emerging, virus, influenza, respiratory, monocyte, dendritic cell, macrophage

---

Abbreviations: AMϕ, alveolar macrophage; ARDS, acute respiratory distress syndrome; BAL, bronchoalveolar lavage; CM, classical monocyte; DC, dendritic cell; IAV, influenza A virus; IFN, interferon; IM, intermediate monocyte; IMϕ, interstitial macrophage; ISG, interferon-stimulated gene; LRT, lower respiratory tract; MDC, myeloid dendritic cell; MNP, mononuclear phagocyte; Mo-DC, monocyte-derived dendritic cell; Mϕ, macrophage; NCM, non-classical monocyte; PDC, plasmacytoid dendritic cell; RE, respiratory epithelium; tipDC, TNF/iNOS-producing dendritic cell; URT, upper respiratory tract.

INTRODUCTION

Emerging viruses including influenza viruses, contribute significantly to human morbidity and mortality. Influenza is one of the oldest diseases known to mankind, with historical reports of influenza outbreaks dating as far back as 1173 (1). Still, influenza viruses are considered emerging/re-emerging viruses due to their capacity to dramatically change and cause epidemics with high mortality rate (2–5).

There are two forms of influenza: seasonal and pandemic. Seasonal influenza epidemics are caused by influenza A and B viruses and seasonal strains undergo mutations referred to as antigenic drift. For influenza A viruses (IAVs) antigenic drift is typically more pronounced each season, while it is more gradual for influenza B (6–9). Seasonal influenza epidemics contribute heavily to global disease burden and to deaths associated with lower respiratory tract (LRT) infections. 3–5 million cases of severe illness and 290–650,000 deaths annually are estimated, especially in young children, immunocompromised, and elderly people (10–13). The clinical picture of IAV infection is broad, ranging from mild/no symptoms, to viral pneumonia, severe respiratory failure, or acute respiratory distress syndrome. IAV infection results in increased susceptibility to secondary bacterial infections, which also contribute to mortality (14–16). In addition, circulating IAV strains can, at unpredictable intervals, cause influenza pandemics when the virus undergoes more dramatic genetic changes known as antigenic shift. Four pandemics have occurred in the past century: the 1918 Spanish flu, the 1957 Asian flu, the 1968 Hong Kong flu, and the 2009 Swine flu. Influenza pandemics are usually characterized by higher mortality than seasonal epidemics, often in age groups that are not typically at risk for influenza infections (17–23).

The nature and severity of influenza disease are influenced by the properties of the virus, host genetics, pre-existing immunity, and the immune response generated to varying extents—their relative contributions remaining incompletely understood (24–30). Highly pathogenic strains, like the Spanish flu, induce massive immune responses, suggesting that too potent antiviral immune responses are pathogenic rather than protective and that immunopathology is central in influenza (19, 31–37). Still, robust immune responses against IAV are required to control and clear infection (38–40). Mononuclear phagocytes (MNPs)— monocytes, dendritic cells (DCs), and macrophages (Mϕ)—are important in IAV infection as they are capable of limiting virus release; sensing and phagocytosing pathogens; clearing virus and apoptotic cells; releasing cytokines to mediate inflammation; directing leukocyte traffic *via* chemokine release; processing and presenting viral antigens; and finally activating naïve T cells (41–49).

The distribution and function of immune cells, including MNPs, differ between anatomical compartments (50–53). However, the exact nature of MNP involvement in human IAV infection remains largely unclear. Sampling the human respiratory tract in patients during ongoing infection poses significant challenges of accessibility and risk of causing further injury to the mucosal barrier. Defining human respiratory MNP distribution, phenotype, and function during IAV infection can therefore offer valuable insights into understanding how the immune system maintains the fine balance required to protect against infections. In this review, we will summarize insights on the role of MNPs in the human respiratory tract during IAV infection both in mediating immune protection and as targets of the virus.

HUMAN RESPIRATORY MNPs

The human respiratory tract encompasses a large mucosal surface with the densest vasculature of all organ systems, that is constantly exposed to the external environment with every inhalation (54, 55). MNPs are positioned along the respiratory tree, in anticipation of exposure to foreign material and respiratory pathogens. MNPs are dually tasked with both promoting inflammation and maintaining tolerance, without disrupting the mucosal barrier that separates the air-filled alveolar spaces from sterile blood in the capillaries (56). A detailed understanding of the distribution and function of respiratory MNPs from the nasal cavities to the alveoli is essential, yet currently incomplete, largely due to the challenges of accessing these tissues in humans. However, recent studies have generated important insight in this area and Mϕs, monocytes, monocyte-derived DCs (mo-DCs), and bona fide DC subsets have been identified from healthy human respiratory tissues. **Figure 1** summarizes the current understanding of the phenotype and distribution of human MNP subsets in respiratory tissues at steady state, as reported (41, 51, 52, 57–62).

Alveolar macrophages (AMϕs) are the most abundant phagocytes of the human lungs, responsible for internalizing inhaled pathogens and antigens, and comprising 95% of cells sampled *via* bronchoalveolar lavage (BAL) (51, 58, 60, 77). Interstitial macrophages, a functionally distinct population of Mϕs residing in lung parenchymal tissue, are less accessible and thus less well studied (63, 78). Similar to monocytes in blood, respiratory monocytes have been characterized as classical monocytes (CMs: CD14+ CD16−), intermediate monocytes (IM: CD14+ CD16+), and non-classical monocytes (NCMs: CD14− CD16+) (51, 52, 58, 64–66). IMs are more frequent in the airways, as opposed to blood, where CMs are in abundance; while NCMs seem to be the rarest monocyte subset (51, 58–60). CMs are the first cells to migrate out of blood to infiltrate sites of inflammation, release chemokines to attract other leukocytes; and can differentiate into mo-DCs and Mϕs (67, 68). IMs represent a population of differentiating monocytes that have been reported to expand during inflammation and/or infection (79–82). NCMs have been attributed with patrolling functions, debris removal, promoting wound healing (64, 81), and to some extent, TLR3 mediated type I interferon (IFN) production (69). Mo-DCs are an interesting subset that transiently arises in tissues from (primarily classical) monocytes recruited to the site of inflammation (46). In comparison to monocytes, DCs are rare in blood, and rarer still in the airways. Subsets of CD11c-expressing myeloid DCs (MDCs); CD1c+ MDCs, CD141+ MDCs, and more recently, langerin+ MDCs (with variable CD1a expression), as well as CD123+ plasmacytoid DCs (PDCs) have been described in the human respiratory tract (51, 57–60, 70–72). MDCs are excellent

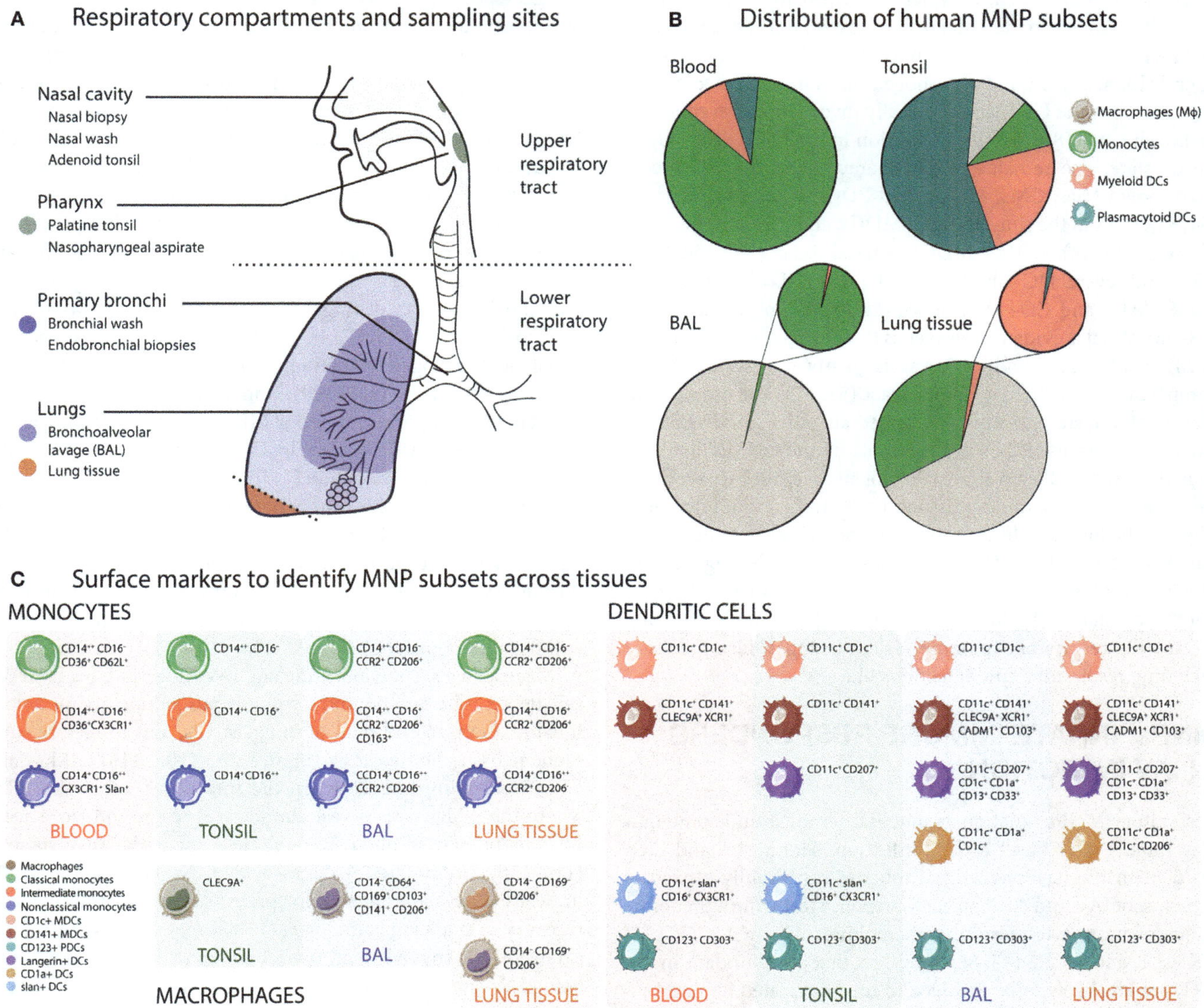

FIGURE 1 | Mononuclear phagocyte (MNP) phenotype and distribution vary across human respiratory compartments. **(A)** Respiratory compartments and sampling sites. In the human upper respiratory tract, the initial site of influenza A virus infection, immune cells including macrophage (Mϕ), monocyte, and dendritic cell (DC) subsets from the nasal cavity and sinuses can be collected with nasal biopsies or nasal wash sampling. Along with pharyngeal palatine tonsils (and tubal and lingual tonsils), the adenoids form the Waldeyer's ring, an anatomical structure comprising a ring of lymphoid tissue guarding the pharynx. In the lower respiratory tract, bronchoscopy allows sampling of discrete regions of the airways and lungs. Bronchial washes can be used to sample the cells lining the bronchi and bronchioles. Endobronchial biopsies can also be obtained from the mucosal tissue of the bronchial walls. Bronchoalveolar lavages (BALs) sample the most distal airways and alveolar sacs. Finally, lung resection samples allow sampling of lung parenchyma and tissue-resident immune cells. **(B)** Distribution of human MNP subsets. Pie charts illustrate broadly pooled data from 21 published studies on human MNP subset distribution in blood, tonsils, BAL, and lung tissue to demonstrate the differential distribution of MNPs across anatomical compartments reported from many research groups (51, 52, 57–61, 63–76). As different studies utilize different strategies to specifically define MNPs, the pie charts show groups of cells typically including several subsets of cells: Mϕs (beige), monocytes (green), myeloid DCs (MDCs) (coral), and plasmacytoid DCs (PDCs) (teal). **(C)** Surface markers to identify MNP subsets across human tissues. The various MNP subsets across tissues can be identified using flow cytometry from HLA-DR+ leukocytes that do not express lineage (T cells, B cells, NK cells, and granulocytes) markers. Apart from CD123+ PDCs, the MNP subsets express different levels of the myeloid marker CD11c. Mϕs have been studied in detail in both BAL and lung tissue, where CD169 expression distinguished alveolar from interstitial Mϕs. Monocyte subsets can be identified from most tissues based on relative expression of CD14 and CD16, as first defined in blood. The major MDC subsets are defined by expression of CD1c or CD141. The extended MDC subsets are now distinguished by expression of CD207 (langerin), CD1a, or slan (51, 52, 57–61, 63–76).

antigen-presenting cells, CD141+ MDCs specialize in cross presentation *via* MHC I; and PDCs excel at type I IFN-mediated antiviral protection.

In the human respiratory system, the upper respiratory tract (URT) is comprised of the nasal cavity, sinuses, and the pharynx (**Figure 1A**). The LRT including the trachea, bronchi, bronchioles, and alveoli, is typically divided into the proximal conducting zone and the distal respiratory zone (**Figure 1A**) (83). The LRT accounts for a larger cumulative surface area and consequently higher likelihood of pathogen–immune cell interactions. However, it is the URT that is initially involved in prevention of pathogen entry (83). MNP distribution in the URT, especially at steady state, also remains poorly characterized. Recent studies have shown Mϕs, CMs, MDCs, and PDCs in the nasal cavities (84, 85); CMs in the sinuses; CMs, MDCs, and PDCs in the nasopharynx (43, 44); CD1c+ MDCs in nasal tissue (86); and Mϕs, CMs, and several DC subsets (PDC, CD1c+, CD141+, CD207+, slan+, Axl+, and CD4+) have been described in human tonsils (73–76). What is evident, however, is that the relative distribution of MNP subsets at steady state varies greatly across the different compartments of the respiratory tract (51, 87). For example, in blood, monocytes greatly outnumber all other MNP subsets, whereas in tonsils, PDCs are the most abundant MNP subset. In BAL, AMϕs make up almost 95% of all cells, but IMs are more frequent than DCs. In lung tissues, both alveolar and interstitial Mϕs can be found at different frequencies. Monocytes and MDCs are also present at greater frequencies than PDCs (**Figure 1B**). The immunological map of the human respiratory tree is becoming more detailed (**Figure 1C**), enabling a better understanding of how the respiratory immune system changes during disease including respiratory viral infections like IAV.

MNPs: INNATE IMMUNE RESPONDERS IN IAV INFECTION

Respiratory MNPs function as mucosal sentinels and come into play rapidly after onset of IAV infection. Monocytes and DCs resident in the nasopharyngeal mucosa can rapidly sense the presence of IAV and elicit an early response featuring a predominance of monocyte-recruiting chemokines like CCL2, CCL17, CX3CL1, and MCP3 (45, 88, 89). Mϕs, that are abundant in the LRT, are less likely to be involved in uncomplicated human IAV infections, when the virus typically remains localized in the URT. However, when the virus spreads lower toward the lungs, not uncommon among pandemic IAV strains, Mϕs are likely central in the innate immune response.

The diverse functional capacity of monocytes translates into their involvement in several aspects of immunity to IAV, as depicted in **Figure 2**. Monocytes rapidly infiltrate the URT following IAV infection where increased nasal CM numbers and cytokine (MCP3, IFNα2, and CCL17) levels can predict disease severity (43–45). Similarly, in patients infected with the pandemic A/CA/07/09 (pH1N1) strain, high numbers of CD14+, TNF-producing monocytes were reported in blood, that positively correlated with disease severity in young, otherwise healthy adults (88, 90). In addition, exposure to IAV also drives differentiation of monocytes into mo-DCs *in vitro* (91). Studies on human IAV infections demonstrate causal association between CCR2-dependent lung monocyte and mo-DC recruitment and IAV-induced mortality in an NOS-2-dependent manner (91–95).

Mucosal tissue-resident DCs in peripheral tissues like the respiratory tract sense and take up antigens. They then migrate to draining lymph nodes to present processed antigen to T cells. Antigen-specific, clonally expanded T cells migrate back to the site of infection to control and clear infection (128–131) (**Figure 2**). This process is critical to restoration of homeostasis as well as for induction of potent adaptive immune responses. Murine models have elegantly demonstrated DC function during IAV infection (96–100, 132). What remains to be described is the exact role of human DC subsets. During pediatric IAV infection, MDCs and PDCs mobilize to the nasopharynx while DC numbers are reduced in blood (43, 44). The potential redistribution of DC subsets remains to be characterized in adults as well as over the course of infection. The different DC subsets each likely perform individualized tasks during IAV infection. CD1c+ MDCs are the most abundant MDCs in the airways (51, 58, 60), and are excellent at pathogen recognition (101, 133), inducing expansive T helper responses (107–109); and cytokine secretion (101). CD141+ MDCs possess superior MHC I cross-presenting abilities that can aid IAV clearance by CD8+ T cells (73, 107). TLR3 mediated cytokine production (TNF, IL-6, IL-12, and IFN-β) and importantly, type III IFN production by CD141+ MDCs, assist in enhanced innate MNP protection against IAV (57). PDCs mediate type I IFN-dependent antiviral protection that is beneficial during IAV infection. In addition to transcriptional activation of many IFN-stimulated genes (ISGs), PDCs also promote both T and B cell responses (75, 76, 102–104, 110–112).

Macrophages contribute during IAV infection by clearing cell debris, chemokine and cytokine production to modulate inflammation, recruitment of other MNPs, and to restore subsequent tissue homeostasis (**Figure 2A**) (105, 113). AMϕs are of particular importance when the infection reaches the LRT, where the AMϕs are in vast abundance. Severe influenza with LRT pathology is often accompanied by AMϕ involvement (114–118). Unhindered AMϕ-associated cytokinemia can result in devastating consequences for patients, ranging from delayed recovery to fatal lung pathology (116). Several factors control the extent of Mϕ involvement, two of the most likely contributors being IAV subtype/strain and Mϕ phenotype (90, 105, 113, 114, 118–120, 134) (**Figure 1C**). For example, Mϕ cytokine production differs across H5N1 and pandemic/seasonal H1N1 strains (119). The protective and pathologic roles of MNP subsets during IAV infection have also been summarized in **Figure 2B**.

Murine models of IAV infection have extensively characterized the role of MNPs in antiviral protection (92, 100, 132, 135–137). A potent immune response to human IAV infection is also likely dependent on synergy between the different MNP subsets and their functions (53, 138–141). However, MNP susceptibility to IAV infection can easily upset the balance, impacting both virus clearance and return to homeostasis.

MNPs AND RESPIRATORY EPITHELIUM (RE): MUCOSAL BARRIERS AND TARGETS OF IAV INFECTION

During IAV infection, the virus is largely confined to the airways, where the RE is primarily targeted (13, 106, 142–147). The RE and MNPs represent an interesting functional dichotomy—both are targets of the virus and also capable of

A

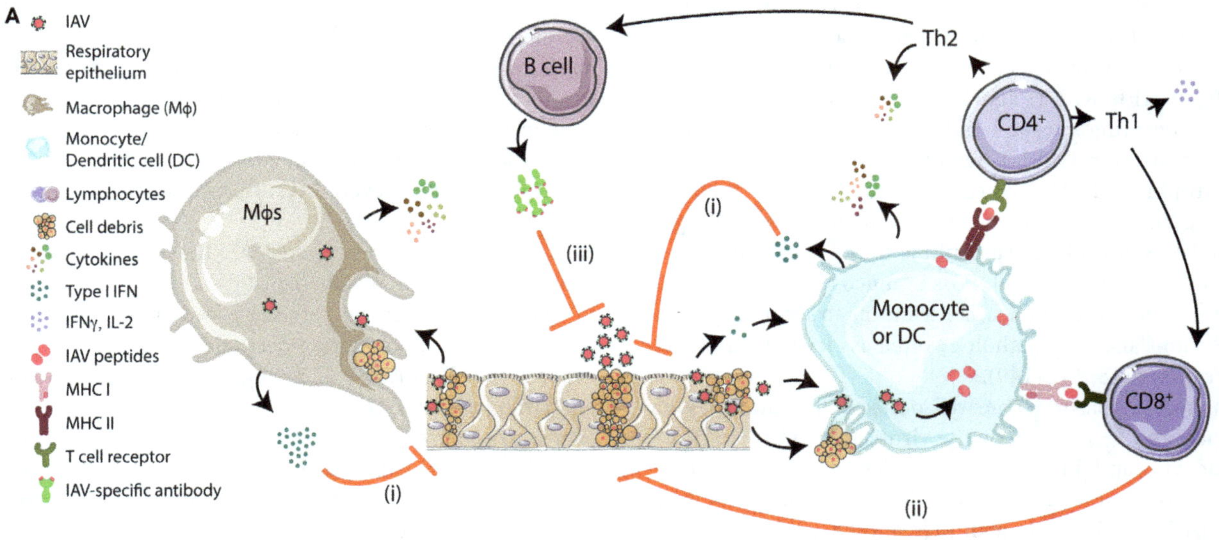

B

	Macrophages (Mϕ)	Monocytes	CD141+ MDCs	CD1c+ MDCs	PDCS
Normal function	phagocytose and clear cell debris, produce cytokines, restore homeostasis[117,118]	rapidly infiltrate site of inflamamtion, produce cytokines & chemokines, recruit other immune cells, differentiate into mo-DC[43-45]	cross present antigens i.e. necrotic cells via CLEC9A[83,108,154]	directly present antigens to naïve T cells, capable of Th1, Th2 & Th17 polarisation[108-110]	secrete type I IFN, mediate ISG signaling, Th1 & Th2 polarization, promote B cell responses[85,86,111-116]
Protective	+ clear debris from cytopathic effects of IAV[117,118]	+ recruit other innate cells to promote inflammation, differente into mo-DC[91]	+ contribute to CD8+ T effector response[83,108]	+ initiate CD4+ T cell responses[108-110]	+ promote antiviral state refractory to infection[85,86,111-116]
Pathologic	+ cause cytokine storm that leads to fatal lung pathology and death, especially during pandemic influenza[119-123]	+ sustained inflammatory state that causes irreversible damage to respiratory mucosal barrier integrity[43-45]	–	–	+ prolonged IFN signaling; can lead to systemic inflammation[150]
Susceptibility of MNP subset to infection	+ IAV replication can be productive or abortive, dependent on IAV strain and host factors; demonstrated in vitro[42,109,124,126,143,144]	+ IAV infection drives differentiation into mo-DCs; demonstrated in vitro[91]	– subvert IAV infection; attributed to RAB15-dependent antiviral pathway[154]	+ IAV infection results in cytopathic effects, impaired ability to cross-present antigens[143]	– refractory to infection; attributed to MxA and RAB15 pathways[115,116,154]
Effect of IAV infection on MNP function	augmented phagocytic capabilities, strong cytokine responses[37,124,152]	positive feedback loop maintains inflammation in pathologic manner[92,95] or efficient antigen uptake and presentation by mo-DCs[91,92]	upregulate CD141 and CLEC9A, may promote CD8 responses[154]	rapidly apoptose causing impaired function[143] or TNF/iNOS producing subset contributes to severe pathology[146]	rapidly apoptose, dysregulate IFN response (in pregnant women)[151] or sustain IFN response (contribute to cytokine storm)[25,150,151]

FIGURE 2 | Human mononuclear phagocytes (MNPs) play a multitude of roles to mediate immune protection during influenza A virus (IAV) infection. **(A)** MNP subsets have many overlapping functions. Macrophages (Mϕs) clear up cell debris and release cytokines. Monocytes and dendritic cells (DCs) can also release cytokines and present antigens to initiate adaptive responses. (i) Following IAV infection of respiratory epithelium, Mϕs, monocytes, and DCs respond to the virus and cell debris, launching potent cytokine responses (TNFα, IL-6, IL-12p40, and IL-10), including interferon (IFN)α. Induction of interferon-stimulated genes (ISGs) promotes an antiviral state in bystander cells, protecting them from infection. (ii) The antigens taken up by monocytes/DCs are processed and presented *via* MHC I and II to CD8+ and CD4+ T cells, respectively. Antigen-specific CD8+ T cells perform effector functions *via* cytotoxic granule- and FasL-mediated caspase-dependent apoptosis. (iii) CD4+ T cells mature into subsets with specific functions. Th1 cells primarily produce IFNγ, IL-2, and TNFβ; and aid CD8+ T cell proliferation. Th2 cells on the other hand, produce IL-4, IL-5, and IL-13 and assist B cells, especially during antibody class switching, promoting production of neutralizing antibodies. Induction of broadly neutralizing antibodies against all strains of influenza virus remains a challenge in the field of influenza immunology (45, 57, 75, 76, 96–106). **(B)** The table summarizes the individual functions of MNP subsets that can protect against IAV infection, but also contribute to pathology. Most MNP subsets are susceptible to IAV infection, as demonstrated by *in vitro* studies. As a consequence of IAV infection, MNP function can be directly affected, prompting them to respond in a protective or pathologic fashion (25, 37, 42–45, 73, 75, 76, 91, 102–105, 107–127).

immune functions to limit infection (25). The epithelial tight junctions constitute a mechanical barrier against the exterior and secrete antiviral molecules. The RE senses IAV *via* TLRs and RIG-I; with RIG-I signaling concentrated at the tight junctions, resulting in type I and type III interferon-mediated antiviral protection (106). Chemokines secreted from the RE aid neutrophil and MNP recruitment to the site of infection, enhancing innate protection. While potently responding to IAV, the RE is also highly susceptible to the cytopathic effects of IAV infection (**Figure 2A**). Loss of mucosal barrier integrity promotes bacterial adherence, contributing to secondary bacterial infections and lung pathology often associated with severe IAV infection (118, 147–149).

Mononuclear phagocytes are well located in the human respiratory mucosa to be targeted by the virus upon entry (135), and the endocytic and migratory properties of MNPs are likely favorable to viral infection and dissemination (120, 134). *In vitro* IAV infection of human Mϕs and DCs has been shown to result in productive infection with release of infectious particles (119–121) but has also been reported to result in abortive infection (42, 108, 121, 122), the contrast being discussed in great detail in Ref. (42). Which of these alternatives prevail in clinical cases, and what host factors determine their own fate, are questions that are yet to be answered. In addition, the negative implications of IAV infection, from an immunological perspective, they may be more pronounced for MNPs than for epithelial cells as MNPs are central in establishing a protective, specific immune response.

CONSEQUENCES OF IAV INFECTION OF MNPs

Mononuclear phagocyte susceptibility to IAV infection can impair their many functions. For example, MDCs are crucial for T cell activation but they are also readily susceptible to IAV infection, impairing their ability to present antigens *via* both the direct presentation and cross presentation pathways (46, 121, 150). Most seasonal and low-pathogenic IAV strains infect respiratory human Mϕs and DCs but replication is typically abortive and therefore skews in favor of host defense (120). However, highly pathogenic strains of IAV can overcome this barrier and productively infect Mϕs and DCs, which in turn can impact viral amplification, dissemination, as well as pathogenicity and immunogenicity (123). Primary human monocytes exposed to H5N1 or highly pathogenic avian influenza strains *in vitro* exhibit a reduced antiviral response, as a consequence of impaired NF-κB signaling (91, 114, 115). In a murine model of IAV infection, CCR2+ inflammatory monocytes accumulate in lungs (92, 94). Impaired virus clearance by MNPs triggers IFN-mediated recruitment of CCR2+ monocytes inflammatory in a positive-feedback loop, resulting in severe lung pathology (92) (**Figure 2B**).

Impaired MNP responses have also been observed in IAV patients. Peripheral blood monocytes and to some extent PDCs, exhibit attenuated IFN responses indicating dysregulation at a systemic level, in particular in infants and the elderly, two of the largest risk groups for severe influenza disease (151–153). Human PDCs that potently produce large amounts of type I IFN, in response even to low doses of IAV, can rapidly undergo apoptosis when exposed to high doses of the virus (25, 124). Possibly related to that, it has been reported that pregnant women, a risk group for influenza, have fewer PDCs in circulation that are also less efficient at IFN production, which could contribute to more severe IAV disease during pregnancy (125) (**Figure 2B**).

As undesirable as depressed MNP function is, excessive activation of MNPs can also be equally dangerous, by contributing to IAV-induced immune pathology leading to fatal respiratory distress. Human monocyte-derived pro-inflammatory Mϕs exposed to IAV *in vitro* exhibit augmented phagocytic capability and strong cytokine responses (119). While this can encourage adaptive responses, it also contributes to the cytokine storm that is a hallmark of severe influenza disease (37, 126). Prolonged IFN signaling can also destroy alveolar epithelium and contribute to development of secondary bacterial infections, the most common complication associated with influenza infections (93). TNF/iNOS-producing DCs, a subset of inflammatory DCs, accumulate in the LRT and promote CD8+ T cell responses in an IAV mouse model, but are also positively correlated with higher lethality (123). However, *in vitro*, human CD8+ T cells can rapidly induce monocyte differentiation into tip-DCs that in turn prime naïve CD4+ T cells and promote protective Th1 responses (154) (**Figure 2B**).

Not all respiratory MNP–IAV interactions have adverse implications. Virus-induced human *in vitro* mo-DCs express both CLEC9A and CD141, as do blood CD141+ MDCs. But uniquely, mo-DCs express CD141 on the cell surface and CLEC9A intracellularly (91). CD141+ DCs can efficiently prime and drive CD8+ T cell proliferation, while CLEC9A is linked to antigen uptake. CD141+ MDCs also subvert IAV infection by resisting virus entry in a RAB-15 dependent manner, instead relying on uptake of apoptotic virus-infected CD1c+ MDCs (and other cells) as a source of antigens (127) (**Figure 2B**). Virus-induced CD141+ DCs also exhibit type I IFN secretion and upregulate ISGs (tetherin, viperin, and IFITM3) and RIG-I/MDA5, suggesting an important protective role for them during infection; despite poor expression of co-stimulatory molecules (CD40, CD86, and HLA-DR), weaker pro-inflammatory cytokine expression, and impaired ability to activate naïve CD4+ T cells (46). Induction of CD141+ DCs could therefore be employed in vaccination/therapeutic strategies. To summarize, while IAV infection of MNP compromises some aspects of innate protection, biological redundancy due to the overlapping functions of MNP subsets can likely prevent loss of essential immune responses.

CONCLUDING REMARKS

Respiratory MNPs are important in the immune responses to IAV infection. At the same time, MNP susceptibility to IAV infection poses an interesting immunological challenge. Several key questions still remain to be further addressed to understand this dichotomy better. Does compromised MNP function result in altered innate immune responses? Do altered innate immune responses subsequently impair efficient induction of adaptive responses, ultimately contributing to increased host morbidity and mortality? If on the other hand, robust, unchecked innate responses lead to prolonged inflammation, causing irreparable damage to the host, is there a commonality in host responses across the various demographics affected by influenza? To answer these questions, and delineate the role of respiratory MNPs in human IAV infection, it will be critical to detail the function of the different MNP subsets—for example, functional assessment of sorted cells from the respiratory system and performing RNA sequencing or epigenetic analyses. Prospective studies of human IAV patients where detailed analyses of tissue samples can be correlated to clinical parameters are likely required to fully understand how MNPs contribute to disease severity.

AUTHOR CONTRIBUTIONS

SV and MY performed the literature review. SV designed the figures. SV, MY, and AS-S organized and wrote the manuscript. SV and AS-S edited the manuscript.

REFERENCES

1. Hirsch A. *Handbook of Geographical and Historical Pathology.* London: The New Sydenham Society (1883).
2. Potter CW. A history of influenza. *J App Microbiol.* (2001) 91:572–9. doi:10.1046/j.1365-2672.2001.01492.x
3. Dunn JJ, Miller MB. Emerging respiratory viruses other than influenza. *Clin Lab Med* (2014) 34(2):409–30. doi:10.1016/j.cll.2014.02.011
4. Hui DS, Zumla A. Emerging respiratory tract viral infections. *Curr Opin Pulm Med* (2015) 21(3):284–92. doi:10.1097/MCP.0000000000000153
5. Gao GF. From "A"IV to "Z"IKV: attacks from emerging and re-emerging pathogens. *Cell* (2018) 172(6):1157–9. doi:10.1016/j.cell.2018.02.025
6. Bedford T, Suchard MA, Lemey P, Dudas G, Gregory V, Hay AJ, et al. Integrating influenza antigenic dynamics with molecular evolution. *Elife* (2014) 3:e01914. doi:10.7554/eLife.01914
7. Drake JW. Rates of spontaneous mutation among RNA viruses. *Proc Natl Acad Sci U S A* (1993) 90:4171–5. doi:10.1073/pnas.90.9.4171
8. Drake JW, Holland JJ. Mutation rates among RNA viruses. *Proc Natl Acad Sci U S A* (1999) 96(24):13910–3. doi:10.1073/pnas.96.24.13910
9. Chen H, Deng Q, Ng SH, Lee RT, Maurer-Stroh S, Zhai W. Dynamic convergent evolution drives the passage adaptation across 48 years' history of H3N2 influenza evolution. *Mol Biol Evol* (2016) 33(12):3133–43. doi:10.1093/molbev/msw190
10. WHO. *The Top 10 Causes of Death – Fact Sheet No. 310 2014.* Geneva: WHO (2017). Available from: http://www.who.int/news-room/fact-sheets/detail/the-top-10-causes-of-death (Accessed: March 14, 2018).
11. Russell CA, Kasson PM, Donis RO, Riley S, Dunbar J, Rambaut A, et al. Improving pandemic influenza risk assessment. *Elife* (2014) 3:e03883. doi:10.7554/eLife.03883
12. Petrova VN, Russell CA. The evolution of seasonal influenza viruses. *Nat Rev Microbiol* (2018) 16(1):47–60. doi:10.1038/nrmicro.2017.118
13. Wootton S, Aguilera EA, Wanger A, Jewell A, Patel K, Murphy JR, et al. Detection of NH1N1 influenza virus in nonrespiratory sites among children. *Pediatr Infect Dis J* (2014) 33(1):95–6. doi:10.1097/INF.0b013e3182a09de7
14. Zhu L, Liu L, Zhang Y, Pu L, Liu J, Li X, et al. High level of neutrophil extracellular traps correlates with poor prognosis of severe influenza A infection. *J Infect Dis* (2018) 217(3):428–37. doi:10.1093/infdis/jix475
15. Wang K, Lai C, Li T, Wang C, Wang W, Ni B, et al. Basic fibroblast growth factor protects against influenza A virus-induced acute lung injury by recruiting neutrophils. *J Mol Cell Biol* (2017) 1–13. doi:10.1093/jmcb/mjx047
16. Buttignol M, Pires-Neto RC, Rossi ESRC, Albino MB, Dolhnikoff M, Mauad T. Airway and parenchyma immune cells in influenza A(H1N1) pdm09 viral and non-viral diffuse alveolar damage. *Respir Res* (2017) 18(1):147. doi:10.1186/s12931-017-0630-x
17. Iuliano AD, Roguski KM, Chang HH, Muscatello DJ, Palekar R, Tempia S, et al. Estimates of global seasonal influenza-associated respiratory mortality: a modelling study. *Lancet* (2018) 391(10127):1285–300. doi:10.1016/S0140-6736(17)33293-2
18. Summers JA, Stanley J, Baker MG, Wilson N. Risk factors for death from pandemic influenza in 1918-1919: a case-control study. *Influenza Other Respir Viruses* (2014) 8(3):329–38. doi:10.1111/irv.12228
19. Gagnon A, Miller MS, Hallman SA, Bourbeau R, Herring DA, Earn DJ, et al. Age-specific mortality during the 1918 influenza pandemic: unravelling the mystery of high young adult mortality. *PLoS One* (2013) 8(8):e69586. doi:10.1371/journal.pone.0069586
20. Ma J, Dushoff J, Earn DJ. Age-specific mortality risk from pandemic influenza. *J Theor Biol* (2011) 288:29–34. doi:10.1016/j.jtbi.2011.08.003
21. Viboud C, Simonsen L, Fuentes R, Flores J, Miller MA, Chowell G. Global mortality impact of the 1957-1959 influenza pandemic. *J Infect Dis* (2016) 213(5):738–45. doi:10.1093/infdis/jiv534
22. Taubenberger JK, Morens DM. The pathology of influenza virus infections. *Annu Rev Pathol* (2008) 3:499–522. doi:10.1146/annurev.pathmechdis.3.121806.154316
23. Taubenberger JK, Reid AH, Krafft AE, Bijwaard KE, Fanning TG. Initial genetic characterization of the 1918 "Spanish" influenza virus. *Science* (1997) 275:1793–6. doi:10.1126/science.275.5307.1793
24. Connors TJ, Ravindranath TM, Bickham KL, Gordon CL, Zhang F, Levin B, et al. Airway CD8(+) T cells are associated with lung injury during infant viral respiratory tract infection. *Am J Respir Cell Mol Biol* (2016) 54(6):822–30. doi:10.1165/rcmb.2015-0297OC
25. Gerlach RL, Camp JV, Chu YK, Jonsson CB. Early host responses of seasonal and pandemic influenza A viruses in primary well-differentiated human lung epithelial cells. *PLoS One* (2013) 8(11):e78912. doi:10.1371/journal.pone.0078912
26. Gerlach T, Hensen L, Matrosovich T, Bergmann J, Winkler M, Peteranderl C, et al. pH optimum of hemagglutinin-mediated membrane fusion determines sensitivity of influenza A viruses to the interferon-induced antiviral state and IFITMs. *J Virol* (2017) 91(11):1–16. doi:10.1128/JVI.00246-17
27. Kroetz DN, Allen RM, Schaller MA, Cavallaro C, Ito T, Kunkel SL. Type I interferon induced epigenetic regulation of macrophages suppresses innate and adaptive immunity in acute respiratory viral infection. *PLoS Pathog* (2015) 11(12):e1005338. doi:10.1371/journal.ppat.1005338
28. Travanty E, Zhou B, Zhang H, Di YP, Alcorn JF, Wentworth DE, et al. Differential susceptibilities of human lung primary cells to H1N1 influenza viruses. *J Virol* (2015) 89(23):11935–44. doi:10.1128/JVI.01792-15
29. Yang Y, Tang H. Aberrant coagulation causes a hyper-inflammatory response in severe influenza pneumonia. *Cell Mol Immunol* (2016) 13(4):432–42. doi:10.1038/cmi.2016.1
30. Peiris JS, Hui KP, Yen HL. Host response to influenza virus: protection versus immunopathology. *Curr Opin Immunol* (2010) 22(4):475–81. doi:10.1016/j.coi.2010.06.003
31. Kamal RP, Alymova IV, York IA. Evolution and virulence of influenza A virus protein PB1-F2. *Int J Mol Sci* (2018) 19(1):1–15. doi:10.3390/ijms19010096
32. Mok BW, Liu H, Chen P, Liu S, Lau SY, Huang X, et al. The role of nuclear NS1 protein in highly pathogenic H5N1 influenza viruses. *Microbes Infect* (2017) 19(12):587–96. doi:10.1016/j.micinf.2017.08.011
33. Shanks GD, Brundage JF. Pathogenic responses among young adults during the 1918 influenza pandemic. *Emerg Infect Dis* (2012) 18(2):201–7. doi:10.3201/eid1802.102042
34. Loo YM, Gale M Jr. Fatal immunity and the 1918 virus. *Nature* (2007) 445:267–8. doi:10.1038/445267a
35. Kobasa D, Jones SM, Shinya K, Kash JC, Copps J, Ebihara H, et al. Aberrant innate immune response in lethal infection of macaques with

the 1918 influenza virus. *Nature* (2007) 445(7125):319–23. doi:10.1038/nature05495
36. Bertoletti A, Sette A, Chisari FV, Penna A, Levrero M, De Carli M, et al. Natural variants of cytotoxic epitopes are T-cell receptor antagonists for antiviral cytotoxic T cells. *Nature* (1994) 369:407–10. doi:10.1038/369407a0
37. Berdal JE, Mollnes TE, Waehre T, Olstad OK, Halvorsen B, Ueland T, et al. Excessive innate immune response and mutant D222G/N in severe A (H1N1) pandemic influenza. *J Infect* (2011) 63(4):308–16. doi:10.1016/j.jinf.2011.07.004
38. Sridhar S, Begom S, Bermingham A, Hoschler K, Adamson W, Carman W, et al. Cellular immune correlates of protection against symptomatic pandemic influenza. *Nat Med* (2013) 19(10):1305–12. doi:10.1038/nm.3350
39. van de Sandt CE, Hillaire ML, Geelhoed-Mieras MM, Osterhaus AD, Fouchier RA, Rimmelzwaan GF. Human influenza A virus-specific CD8+ T-cell response is long-lived. *J Infect Dis* (2015) 212(1):81–5. doi:10.1093/infdis/jiv018
40. Reichman RC, Pons VG, Murphy BR, Caplan EA, Dolin R. Cell-mediated cytotoxicity following influenza infection and vaccination in humans. *J Med Virol* (1979) 4:1–14. doi:10.1002/jmv.1890040102
41. Baharom FRG, Blomberg A, Smed-Sörensen A. Human lung mononuclear phagocytes in health and disease. *Front Immunol* (2017) 8:499. doi:10.3389/fimmu.2017.00499
42. Short KR, Brooks AG, Reading PC, Londrigan SL. The fate of influenza A virus after infection of human macrophages and dendritic cells. *J Gen Virol* (2012) 93(Pt 11):2315–25. doi:10.1099/vir.0.045021-0
43. Gill MA, Long K, Kwon T, Muniz L, Mejias A, Connolly J, et al. Differential recruitment of dendritic cells and monocytes to respiratory mucosal sites in children with influenza virus or respiratory syncytial virus infection. *J Infect Dis* (2008) 198(11):1667–76. doi:10.1086/593018
44. Gill MA, Palucka KA, Barton T, Ghaffar F, Jafri H, Banchereau J, et al. Mobilization of plasmacytoid and myeloid dendritic cells to mucosal sites in children with respiratory syncytial virus and other viral respiratory infections. *J Infect Dis* (2005) 2005(191):1105–15. doi:10.1086/428589
45. Oshansky CM, Gartland AJ, Wong SS, Jeevan T, Wang D, Roddam PL, et al. Mucosal immune responses predict clinical outcomes during influenza infection independently of age and viral load. *Am J Respir Crit Care Med* (2014) 189(4):449–62. doi:10.1164/rccm.201309-1616OC
46. Cao W, Taylor AK, Biber RE, Davis WG, Kim JH, Reber AJ, et al. Rapid differentiation of monocytes into type I IFN-producing myeloid dendritic cells as an antiviral strategy against influenza virus infection. *J Immunol* (2012) 189(5):2257–65. doi:10.4049/jimmunol.1200168
47. Diao H, Cui G, Wei Y, Chen J, Zuo J, Cao H, et al. Severe H7N9 infection is associated with decreased antigen-presenting capacity of CD14+ cells. *PLoS One* (2014) 9(3):e92823. doi:10.1371/journal.pone.0092823
48. Lichtner M, Mastroianni CM, Rossi R, Russo G, Belvisi V, Marocco R, et al. Severe and persistent depletion of circulating plasmacytoid dendritic cells in patients with 2009 pandemic H1N1 infection. *PLoS One* (2011) 6(5):e19872. doi:10.1371/journal.pone.0019872
49. Soloff AC, Weirback HK, Ross TM, Barratt-Boyes SM. Plasmacytoid dendritic cell depletion leads to an enhanced mononuclear phagocyte response in lungs of mice with lethal influenza virus infection. *Comp Immunol Microbiol Infect Dis* (2012) 35(4):309–17. doi:10.1016/j.cimid.2012.01.012
50. Guilliams M, Lambrecht BN, Hammad H. Division of labor between lung dendritic cells and macrophages in the defense against pulmonary infections. *Mucosal Immunol* (2013) 6(3):464–73. doi:10.1038/mi.2013.14
51. Baharom F, Thomas S, Rankin G, Lepzien R, Pourazar J, Behndig AF, et al. Dendritic cells and monocytes with distinct inflammatory responses reside in lung mucosa of healthy humans. *J Immunol* (2016) 196(11):4498–509. doi:10.4049/jimmunol.1600071
52. Baharom F, Rankin G, Scholz S, Pourazar J, Ahlm C, Blomberg A, et al. Human lung dendritic cells: spatial distribution and phenotypic identification in endobronchial biopsies using immunohistochemistry and flow cytometry. *J Vis Exp* (2017) 119:e55222. doi:10.3791/55222
53. Pulendran B, Tang H, Denning TL. Division of labor, plasticity, and crosstalk between dendritic cell subsets. *Curr Opin Immunol* (2008) 20(1):61–7. doi:10.1016/j.coi.2007.10.009
54. Gehr P, Bachofen M, Weibel E. The normal human lung – ultrastructure and morphometric estimation of diffusion capacity. *Respir Physiol* (1978) 32:121–40. doi:10.1016/0034-5687(78)90104-4
55. Hamm H, Fabel H, Bartsch W. The surfactant system of the adult lung – physiology and clinical perspectives. *Clin Investig* (1992) 70:637–57. doi:10.1007/BF00180279
56. Wonderlich ER, Swan ZD, Bissel SJ, Hartman AL, Carney JP, O'Malley KJ, et al. Widespread virus replication in alveoli drives acute respiratory distress syndrome in aerosolized H5N1 influenza infection of macaques. *J Immunol* (2017) 198(4):1616–26. doi:10.4049/jimmunol.1601770
57. Granot T, Senda T, Carpenter DJ, Matsuoka N, Weiner J, Gordon CL, et al. Dendritic cells display subset and tissue-specific maturation dynamics over human life. *Immunity* (2017) 46(3):504–15. doi:10.1016/j.immuni.2017.02.019
58. Desch AN, Gibbings SL, Goyal R, Kolde R, Bednarek J, Bruno T, et al. Flow cytometric analysis of mononuclear phagocytes in nondiseased human lung and lung-draining lymph nodes. *Am J Respir Crit Care Med* (2016) 193(6):614–26. doi:10.1164/rccm.201507-1376OC
59. Patel VI, Booth JL, Duggan ES, Cate S, White VL, Hutchings D, et al. Transcriptional classification and functional characterization of human airway macrophage and dendritic cell subsets. *J Immunol* (2017) 198(3):1183–201. doi:10.4049/jimmunol.1600777
60. Yu YR, Hotten DF, Malakhau Y, Volker E, Ghio AJ, Noble PW, et al. Flow cytometric analysis of myeloid cells in human blood, bronchoalveolar lavage, and lung tissues. *Am J Respir Cell Mol Biol* (2016) 54(1):13–24. doi:10.1165/rcmb.2015-0146OC
61. Patel VI, Metcalf JP. Identification and characterization of human dendritic cell subsets in the steady state: a review of our current knowledge. *J Investig Med* (2016) 64(4):833–47. doi:10.1136/jim-2016-000072
62. Iwasaki A. Mucosal dendritic cells. *Annu Rev Immunol* (2007) 25:381–418. doi:10.1146/annurev.immunol.25.022106.141634
63. Fathi M, Johansson A, Lundborg M, Orre L, Skold CM, Camner P. Functional and morphological differences between human alveolar and interstitial macrophages. *Exp Mol Pathol* (2001) 70(2):77–82. doi:10.1006/exmp.2000.2344
64. Thomas GD, Hamers AAJ, Nakao C, Marcovecchio P, Taylor AM, McSkimming C, et al. Human blood monocyte subsets: a new gating strategy defined using cell surface markers identified by mass cytometry. *Arterioscler Thromb Vasc Biol* (2017) 37(8):1548–58. doi:10.1161/ATVBAHA.117.309145
65. Ziegler-Heitbrock L. Blood monocytes and their subsets: established features and open questions. *Front Immunol* (2015) 6:423. doi:10.3389/fimmu.2015.00423
66. Abeles RD, McPhail MJ, Sowter D, Antoniades CG, Vergis N, Vijay GK, et al. CD14, CD16 and HLA-DR reliably identifies human monocytes and their subsets in the context of pathologically reduced HLA-DR expression by CD14(hi)/CD16(neg) monocytes: expansion of CD14(hi)/CD16(pos) and contraction of CD14(lo)/CD16(pos) monocytes in acute liver failure. *Cytometry A* (2012) 81(10):823–34. doi:10.1002/cyto.a.22104
67. Serbina NV, Pamer EG. Monocyte emigration from bone marrow during bacterial infection requires signals mediated by chemokine receptor CCR2. *Nat Immunol* (2006) 7(3):311–7. doi:10.1038/ni1309
68. Patel AA, Zhang Y, Fullerton JN, Boelen L, Rongvaux A, Maini AA, et al. The fate and lifespan of human monocyte subsets in steady state and systemic inflammation. *J Exp Med* (2017) 214(7):1913–23. doi:10.1084/jem.20170355
69. Boyette LB, Macedo C, Hadi K, Elinoff BD, Walters JT, Ramaswami B, et al. Phenotype, function, and differentiation potential of human monocyte subsets. *PLoS One* (2017) 12(4):e0176460. doi:10.1371/journal.pone.0176460
70. Alcantara-Hernandez M, Leylek R, Wagar LE, Engleman EG, Keler T, Marinkovich MP, et al. High-dimensional phenotypic mapping of human dendritic cells reveals interindividual variation and tissue specialization. *Immunity* (2017) 47(6):1037–50.e6. doi:10.1016/j.immuni.2017.11.001
71. See P, Dutertre CA, Chen J, Gunther P, McGovern N, Irac SE, et al. Mapping the human DC lineage through the integration of high-dimensional techniques. *Science* (2017) 356(6342):1–13. doi:10.1126/science.aag3009
72. Villani AC, Satija R, Reynolds G, Sarkizova S, Shekhar K, Fletcher J, et al. Single-cell RNA-seq reveals new types of human blood dendritic cells, monocytes, and progenitors. *Science* (2017) 356(6335):1–12. doi:10.1126/science.aah4573
73. Jongbloed SL, Kassianos AJ, McDonald KJ, Clark GJ, Ju X, Angel CE, et al. Human CD141+ (BDCA-3)+ dendritic cells (DCs) represent a unique myeloid DC subset that cross-presents necrotic cell antigens. *J Exp Med* (2010) 207(6):1247–60. doi:10.1084/jem.20092140
74. De Monte AO, Olivieri CV, Vitale S, Bailleux S, Castillo L, Giordanengo V, et al. CD1c-related DCs that express CD207: Langerin, but are distinguishable

from Langerhans cells, are consistently present in human tonsils. *Front Immunol* (2016) 7:197. doi:10.3389/fimmu.2016.00197

75. Segura E, Durand M, Amigorena S. Similar antigen cross-presentation capacity and phagocytic functions in all freshly isolated human lymphoid organ-resident dendritic cells. *J Exp Med* (2013) 210(5):1035–47. doi:10.1084/jem.20121103
76. Segura E, Valladeau-Guilemond J, Donnadieu MH, Sastre-Garau X, Soumelis V, Amigorena S. Characterization of resident and migratory dendritic cells in human lymph nodes. *J Exp Med* (2012) 209(4):653–60. doi:10.1084/jem.20111457
77. Pinilla-Vera M, Xiong Z, Zhao Y, Zhao J, Donahoe MP, Barge S, et al. Full spectrum of LPS activation in alveolar macrophages of healthy volunteers by whole transcriptomic profiling. *PLoS One* (2016) 11(7):e0159329. doi:10.1371/journal.pone.0159329
78. Liegeois M, Legrand C, Desmet CJ, Marichal T, Bureau F. The interstitial macrophage: a long-neglected piece in the puzzle of lung immunity. *Cell Immunol* (2018). doi:10.1016/j.cellimm.2018.02.001
79. Duan M, Hibbs ML, Chen W. The contributions of lung macrophage and monocyte heterogeneity to influenza pathogenesis. *Immunol Cell Biol* (2017) 95(3):225–35. doi:10.1038/icb.2016.97
80. Shi C, Pamer EG. Monocyte recruitment during infection and inflammation. *Nat Rev Immunol* (2011) 11(11):762–74. doi:10.1038/nri3070
81. Lee J, Tam H, Adler L, Ilstad-Minnihan A, Macaubas C, Mellins ED. The MHC class II antigen presentation pathway in human monocytes differs by subset and is regulated by cytokines. *PLoS One* (2017) 12(8):e0183594. doi:10.1371/journal.pone.0183594
82. Kwissa M, Nakaya HI, Onlamoon N, Wrammert J, Villinger F, Perng GC, et al. Dengue virus infection induces expansion of a CD14(+)CD16(+) monocyte population that stimulates plasmablast differentiation. *Cell Host Microbe* (2014) 16(1):115–27. doi:10.1016/j.chom.2014.06.001
83. Standring S, Borley NR, Collins P, Crossman AR, Gatzoulis MA, Healy JC, et al. *Gray's Anatomy The Anatomical Basis of Clinical Practice*. 40th ed. Standring S, editor. London, United Kingdom: Elsevier (2008).
84. Jochems SP, Piddock K, Rylance J, Adler H, Carniel BF, Collins A, et al. Novel analysis of immune cells from nasal microbiopsy demonstrates reliable, reproducible data for immune populations, and superior cytokine detection compared to nasal wash. *PLoS One* (2017) 12(1):e0169805. doi:10.1371/journal.pone.0169805
85. Juliusson S, Bachert C, Klementsson H, Karlsson G, Pipkorn U. Macrophages on the nasal mucosal surface in provoked and naturally occurring allergic rhinitis. *Acta Otolaryngol* (2009) 111(5):946–53. doi:10.3109/00016489109138435
86. Lee H, Ruane D, Law K, Ho Y, Garg A, Rahman A, et al. Phenotype and function of nasal dendritic cells. *Mucosal Immunol* (2015) 8(5):1083–98. doi:10.1038/mi.2014.135
87. Kopf M, Schneider C, Nobs SP. The development and function of lung-resident macrophages and dendritic cells. *Nat Immunol* (2015) 16(1):36–44. doi:10.1038/ni.3052
88. Cole SL, Ho LP. Contribution of innate immune cells to pathogenesis of severe influenza virus infection. *Clin Sci (Lond)* (2017) 131(4):269–83. doi:10.1042/CS20160484
89. Sprenger H, Meyer RG, Kaufmann A, Bussfeld D, Rischkowsky E, Gemsa D. Selective induction of monocyte and not neutrophil-attracting chemokines after influenza A virus infection. *J Exp Med* (1996) 184:1191–6. doi:10.1084/jem.184.3.1191
90. Cole SL, Dunning J, Kok WL, Benam KH, Benlahrech A, Repapi E, et al. M1-like monocytes are a major immunological determinant of severity in previously healthy adults with life-threatening influenza. *JCI Insight* (2017) 2(7):e91868. doi:10.1172/jci.insight.91868
91. Hou W, Gibbs JS, Xiuju L, Brooke CB, Roy D, Modlin RL, et al. Viral infection triggers rapid differentiation of human blood monocytes into dendritic cells. *Blood* (2012) 119(13):3128–31. doi:10.1182/blood-2011-09-379479
92. Lin KL, Suzuki Y, Nakano H, Ramsburg E, Gunn MD. CCR2+ monocyte-derived dendritic cells and exudate macrophages produce influenza-induced pulmonary immune pathology and mortality. *J Immunol* (2008) 180(4):2562–72. doi:10.4049/jimmunol.180.4.2562
93. Lin SJ, Lee YC. Effect of influenza A infection on maturation and function of neonatal monocyte-derived dendritic cells. *Viral Immunol* (2014) 27(6):277–84. doi:10.1089/vim.2014.0007
94. Dawson TC, Beck MA, Kuziel WA, Henderson F, Maeda N. Contrasting effects of CCR5 and CCR2 deficiency in the pulmonary inflammatory response to influenza A virus. *Am J Pathol* (2000) 156(6):1951–9. doi:10.1016/S0002-9440(10)65068-7
95. Herold S, Steinmueller M, von Wulffen W, Cakarova L, Pinto R, Pleschka S, et al. Lung epithelial apoptosis in influenza virus pneumonia: the role of macrophage-expressed TNF-related apoptosis-inducing ligand. *J Exp Med* (2008) 205(13):3065–77. doi:10.1084/jem.20080201
96. McGill J, Van Rooijen N, Legge KL. Protective influenza-specific CD8 T cell responses require interactions with dendritic cells in the lungs. *J Exp Med* (2008) 205(7):1635–46. doi:10.1084/jem.20080314
97. Helft J, Manicassamy B, Guermonprez P, Hashimoto D, Silvin A, Agudo J, et al. Cross-presenting CD103+ dendritic cells are protected from influenza virus infection. *J Clin Invest* (2012) 122(11):4037–47. doi:10.1172/JCI60659
98. Lawrence CW, Braciale TJ. Activation, differentiation, and migration of naive virus-specific CD8+ T cells during pulmonary influenza virus infection. *J Immunol* (2004) 173(2):1209–18. doi:10.4049/jimmunol.173.2.1209
99. Lawrence CW, Ream RM, Braciale TJ. Frequency, specificity, and sites of expansion of CD8+ T cells during primary pulmonary influenza virus infection. *J Immunol* (2005) 174(9):5332–40. doi:10.4049/jimmunol.174.9.5332
100. Yu CI, Becker C, Wang Y, Marches F, Helft J, Leboeuf M, et al. Human CD1c+ dendritic cells drive the differentiation of CD103+ CD8+ mucosal effector T cells via the cytokine TGF-beta. *Immunity* (2013) 38(4):818–30. doi:10.1016/j.immuni.2013.03.004
101. Hemont C, Neel A, Heslan M, Braudeau C, Josien R. Human blood mDC subsets exhibit distinct TLR repertoire and responsiveness. *J Leukoc Biol* (2013) 93(4):599–609. doi:10.1189/jlb.0912452
102. Kool M, Geurtsvankessel C, Muskens F, Madeira FB, van Nimwegen M, Kuipers H, et al. Facilitated antigen uptake and timed exposure to TLR ligands dictate the antigen-presenting potential of plasmacytoid DCs. *J Leukoc Biol* (2011) 90(6):1177–90. doi:10.1189/jlb.0610342
103. Matsui T, Connolly JE, Michnevitz M, Chaussabel D, Yu CI, Glaser C, et al. CD2 distinguishes two subsets of human plasmacytoid dendritic cells with distinct phenotype and functions. *J Immunol* (2009) 182(11):6815–23. doi:10.4049/jimmunol.0802008
104. Haller K. Human MxA protein – an interferon-induced dynamin-like GTPase with broad antiviral activity. *J Interferon Cytokine Res* (2011) 31(1):79–87. doi:10.1089/jir.2010.0076
105. Sakabe S, Iwatsuki-Horimoto K, Takano R, Nidom CA, Le M, Nagamura-Inoue T, et al. Cytokine production by primary human macrophages infected with highly pathogenic H5N1 or pandemic H1N1 2009 influenza viruses. *J Gen Virol* (2011) 92(Pt 6):1428–34. doi:10.1099/vir.0.030346-0
106. Short KR, Kasper J, van der Aa S, Andeweg AC, Zaaraoui-Boutahar F, Goeijenbier M, et al. Influenza virus damages the alveolar barrier by disrupting epithelial cell tight junctions. *Eur Respir J* (2016) 47(3):954–66. doi:10.1183/13993003.01282-2015
107. Schlitzer A, McGovern N, Teo P, Zelante T, Atarashi K, Low D, et al. IRF4 transcription factor-dependent CD11b+ dendritic cells in human and mouse control mucosal IL-17 cytokine responses. *Immunity* (2013) 38(5):970–83. doi:10.1016/j.immuni.2013.04.011
108. Faith A, McDonald J, Peek E, Richards D, Caulfield J, Chevretton E, et al. Functional plasticity of human respiratory tract dendritic cells: GM-CSF enhances T(H)2 development. *J Allergy Clin Immunol* (2005) 116(5):1136–43. doi:10.1016/j.jaci.2005.08.002
109. Bogiatzi SI, Guillot-Delost M, Cappuccio A, Bichet JC, Chouchane-Mlik O, Donnadieu MH, et al. Multiple-checkpoint inhibition of thymic stromal lymphopoietin-induced TH2 response by TH17-related cytokines. *J Allergy Clin Immunol* (2012) 130(1):233–40.e5. doi:10.1016/j.jaci.2012.04.038
110. Di Pucchio T, Chatterjee B, Smed-Sorensen A, Clayton S, Palazzo A, Montes M, et al. Direct proteasome-independent cross-presentation of viral antigen by plasmacytoid dendritic cells on major histocompatibility complex class I. *Nat Immunol* (2008) 9(5):551–7. doi:10.1038/ni.1602
111. Fonteneau JF, Gilliet M, Larsson M, Dasilva I, Munz C, Liu YJ, et al. Activation of influenza virus-specific CD4+ and CD8+ T cells: a new role for plasmacytoid dendritic cells in adaptive immunity. *Blood* (2003) 101(9):3520–6. doi:10.1182/blood-2002-10-3063
112. Haller O, Gao S, von der Malsburg A, Daumke O, Kochs G. Dynamin-like MxA GTPase: structural insights into oligomerization and implications for

antiviral activity. *J Biol Chem* (2010) 285(37):28419–24. doi:10.1074/jbc.R110.145839

113. Wang J, Nikrad MP, Travanty EA, Zhou B, Phang T, Gao B, et al. Innate immune response of human alveolar macrophages during influenza A infection. *PLoS One* (2012) 7(3):e29879. doi:10.1371/journal.pone.0029879
114. Friesenhagen J, Boergeling Y, Hrincius E, Ludwig S, Roth J, Viemann D. Highly pathogenic avian influenza viruses inhibit effective immune responses of human blood-derived macrophages. *J Leukoc Biol* (2012) 92(1):11–20. doi:10.1189/jlb.0911479
115. Friesenhagen J, Viemann D, Börgeling Y, Schmolke M, Spiekermann C, Kirschnek S, et al. Highly pathogenic influenza viruses inhibit inflammatory response in monocytes via activation of Rar-related orphan receptor RORa. *J Innate Immun* (2013) 5:505–18. doi:10.1159/000346706
116. Kuiken T, van den Brand J, van Riel D, Pantin-Jackwood M, Swayne DE. Comparative pathology of select agent influenza a virus infections. *Vet Pathol* (2010) 47(5):893–914. doi:10.1177/0300985810378651
117. Guarner J, Falcon-Escobedo R. Comparison of the pathology caused by H1N1, H5N1, and H3N2 influenza viruses. *Arch Med Res* (2009) 40(8): 655–61. doi:10.1016/j.arcmed.2009.10.001
118. Nakajima N, Sato Y, Katano H, Hasegawa H, Kumasaka T, Hata S, et al. Histopathological and immunohistochemical findings of 20 autopsy cases with 2009 H1N1 virus infection. *Mod Pathol* (2012) 25(1):1–13. doi:10.1038/modpathol.2011.125
119. Hoeve MA, Nash AA, Jackson D, Randall RE, Dransfield I. Influenza virus A infection of human monocyte and macrophage subpopulations reveals increased susceptibility associated with cell differentiation. *PLoS One* (2012) 7(1):e29443. doi:10.1371/journal.pone.0029443
120. Yu WC, Chan RW, Wang J, Travanty EA, Nicholls JM, Peiris JS, et al. Viral replication and innate host responses in primary human alveolar epithelial cells and alveolar macrophages infected with influenza H5N1 and H1N1 viruses. *J Virol* (2011) 85(14):6844–55. doi:10.1128/JVI.02200-10
121. Smed-Sorensen A, Chalouni C, Chatterjee B, Cohn L, Blattmann P, Nakamura N, et al. Influenza A virus infection of human primary dendritic cells impairs their ability to cross-present antigen to CD8 T cells. *PLoS Pathog* (2012) 8(3):e1002572. doi:10.1371/journal.ppat.1002572
122. Baharom F, Thomas OS, Lepzien R, Mellman I, Chalouni C, Smed-Sorensen A. Visualization of early influenza A virus trafficking in human dendritic cells using STED microscopy. *PLoS One* (2017) 12(6):e0177920. doi:10.1371/journal.pone.0177920
123. Aldridge JRJ, Moseley CE, Boltz DA, Negovetich NJ, Reynolds C, Franks J, et al. TNF/iNOS-producing dendritic cells are the necessary evil of lethal influenza virus infection. *Proc Natl Acad Sci U S A* (2009) 106(13):5306–11. doi:10.1073/pnas.0900655106
124. Thomas JM, Pos Z, Reinboth J, Wang RY, Wang E, Frank GM, et al. Differential responses of plasmacytoid dendritic cells to influenza virus and distinct viral pathogens. *J Virol* (2014) 88(18):10758–66. doi:10.1128/JVI.01501-14
125. Vanders RL, Gibson PG, Murphy VE, Wark PA. Plasmacytoid dendritic cells and CD8 T cells from pregnant women show altered phenotype and function following H1N1/09 infection. *J Infect Dis* (2013) 208(7):1062–70. doi:10.1093/infdis/jit296
126. Wu W, Booth JL, Duggan ES, Wu S, Patel KB, Coggeshall KM, et al. Innate immune response to H3N2 and H1N1 influenza virus infection in a human lung organ culture model. *Virology* (2010) 396(2):178–88. doi:10.1016/j.virol.2009.10.016
127. Silvin A, Yu CI, Lahaye X, Imperatore F, Brault J-B, Cardinaud S, et al. Constitutive resistance to viral infection in human CD141+ dendritic cells. *Sci Immunol* (2017) 2(13):1–12. doi:10.1126/sciimmunol.aai8071
128. Banchereau J, Briere F, Caux C, Davoust J, Lebecque S, Liu YJ, et al. Immunobiology of dendritic cells. *Annu Rev Immunol* (2000) 18:767–811. doi:10.1146/annurev.immunol.18.1.767
129. Merad M, Sathe P, Helft J, Miller J, Mortha A. The dendritic cell lineage: ontogeny and function of dendritic cells and their subsets in the steady state and the inflamed setting. *Annu Rev Immunol* (2013) 31:563–604. doi:10.1146/annurev-immunol-020711-074950
130. Pulendran B. The varieties of immunological experience: of pathogens, stress, and dendritic cells. *Annu Rev Immunol* (2015) 33:563–606. doi:10.1146/annurev-immunol-020711-075049
131. Randolph GJ, Angeli V, Swartz MA. Dendritic-cell trafficking to lymph nodes through lymphatic vessels. *Nat Rev Immunol* (2005) 5(8):617–28. doi:10.1038/nri1670
132. Waithman J, Mintern JD. Dendritic cells and influenza A virus infection. *Virulence* (2012) 3(7):603–8. doi:10.4161/viru.21864
133. Clark GJ, Kupresanin F, Fromm PD, Ju X, Muusers L, Silveira PA, et al. New insights into the phenotype of human dendritic cell populations. *Clin Transl Immunol* (2016) 5(1):e61. doi:10.1038/cti.2015.40
134. Perrone LA, Plowden JK, Garcia-Sastre A, Katz JM, Tumpey TM. H5N1 and 1918 pandemic influenza virus infection results in early and excessive infiltration of macrophages and neutrophils in the lungs of mice. *PLoS Pathog* (2008) 4(8):e1000115. doi:10.1371/journal.ppat.1000115
135. Idoyaga J, Fiorese C, Zbytnuik L, Lubkin A, Miller J, Malissen B, et al. Specialized role of migratory dendritic cells in peripheral tolerance induction. *J Clin Invest* (2013) 123(2):844–54. doi:10.1172/JCI65260
136. GeurtsvanKessel CH, Bergen IM, Muskens F, Boon L, Hoogsteden HC, Osterhaus AD, et al. Both conventional and interferon killer dendritic cells have antigen-presenting capacity during influenza virus infection. *PLoS One* (2009) 4(9):e7187. doi:10.1371/journal.pone.0007187
137. Cella M. Plasmacytoid monocytes migrate to inflamed lymph nodes and produce large amounts of type I interferon. *Nat Med* (1999) 5(8):919–23. doi:10.1038/11360
138. Pulendran B, Maddur MS. Innate immune sensing and response to influenza. *Curr Top Microbiol Immunol* (2015) 386:23–71. doi:10.1007/82_2014_405
139. Chen X, Liu S, Goraya MU, Maarouf M, Huang S, Chen JL. Host immune response to influenza A virus infection. *Front Immunol* (2018) 9(320):1–13. doi:10.3389/fimmu.2018.00320
140. Ascough S, Paterson S, Chiu C. Induction and subversion of human protective immunity – contrasting influenza and respiratory syncytial virus. *Front Immunol* (2018) 9(323):1–23. doi:10.3389/fimmu.2018.00323
141. Miyauchi K. Helper T cell responses to respiratory viruses in the lung: development, virus suppression, and pathogenesis. *Viral Immunol* (2017) 30(6):421–30. doi:10.1089/vim.2017.0018
142. Gan H, Hao Q, Idell S, Tang H. Transcription factor Runx3 is induced by influenza A virus and double-strand RNA and mediates airway epithelial cell apoptosis. *Sci Rep* (2015) 5:17916. doi:10.1038/srep17916
143. Kim S, Kim MJ, Park DY, Chung HJ, Kim CH, Yoon JH, et al. Mitochondrial reactive oxygen species modulate innate immune response to influenza A virus in human nasal epithelium. *Antiviral Res* (2015) 119:78–83. doi:10.1016/j.antiviral.2015.04.011
144. McAuley JL, Corcilius L, Tan HX, Payne RJ, McGuckin MA, Brown LE. The cell surface mucin MUC1 limits the severity of influenza A virus infection. *Mucosal Immunol* (2017) 10(6):1581–93. doi:10.1038/mi.2017.16
145. Shin N, Pyo CW, Jung KI, Choi SY. Influenza A virus PB1-F2 is involved in regulation of cellular redox state in alveolar epithelial cells. *Biochem Biophys Res Commun* (2015) 459(4):699–705. doi:10.1016/j.bbrc.2015.03.010
146. Oughton M, Dascal A, Laporta D, Charest H, Afilalo M, Miller M. Evidence of viremia in 2 cases of severe pandemic influenza A H1N1/09. *Diagn Microbiol Infect Dis* (2011) 70(2):213–7. doi:10.1016/j.diagmicrobio.2010.12.013
147. Sobata R, Matsumoto C, Igarashi M, Uchida S, Momose S, Hino S, et al. No viremia of pandemic (H1N1) 2009 was demonstrated in blood donors who had donated blood during the probable incubation period. *Transfusion* (2011) 51(9):1949–56. doi:10.1111/j.1537-2995.2011.03109.x
148. Jamieson AM, Yu S, Annicelli CH, Medzhitov R. Influenza virus-induced glucocorticoids compromise innate host defense against a secondary bacterial infection. *Cell Host Microbe* (2010) 7(2):103–14. doi:10.1016/j.chom.2010.01.010
149. Nita-Lazar M, Banerjee A, Feng C, Amin MN, Frieman MB, Chen WH, et al. Desialylation of airway epithelial cells during influenza virus infection enhances pneumococcal adhesion via galectin binding. *Mol Immunol* (2015) 65(1):1–16. doi:10.1016/j.molimm.2014.12.010
150. Baharom F, Thomas S, Bieder A, Hellmer M, Volz J, Sandgren KJ, et al. Protection of human myeloid dendritic cell subsets against influenza A virus infection is differentially regulated upon TLR stimulation. *J Immunol* (2015) 194(9):4422–30. doi:10.4049/jimmunol.1402671
151. Levy O, Zarember KA, Roy RM, Cywes C, Godowski PJ, Wessels MR. Selective impairment of TLR-mediated innate immunity in human newborns: neonatal blood plasma reduces monocyte TNF-α induction by bacterial lipopeptides, lipopolysaccharide, and imiquimod, but preserves

the response to R-848. *J Immunol* (2004) 173(7):4627–34. doi:10.4049/jimmunol.173.7.4627

152. Marr N, Wang TI, Kam SH, Hu YS, Sharma AA, Lam A, et al. Attenuation of respiratory syncytial virus-induced and RIG-I-dependent type I IFN responses in human neonates and very young children. *J Immunol* (2014) 192(3):948–57. doi:10.4049/jimmunol.1302007
153. Molony RD, Nguyen JT, Kong Y, Montgomery RR, Shaw AC, Iwasaki A. Aging impairs both primary and secondary RIG-I signaling for interferon induction in human monocytes. *Sci Signal* (2017) 10(509):1–11. doi:10.1126/scisignalaan2392
154. Chong SZ, Wong KL, Lin G, Yang CM, Wong SC, Angeli V, et al. Human CD8(+) T cells drive Th1 responses through the differentiation of TNF/iNOS-producing dendritic cells. *Eur J Immunol* (2011) 41(6):1639–51. doi:10.1002/eji.201041022

17

Two is Better than One: Evidence for T-Cell Cross-Protection Between Dengue and Zika-Implications on Vaccine Design

Krishanthi S. Subramaniam [1], *Suzannah Lant* [1], *Lynsey Goodwin* [1], *Alba Grifoni* [2], *Daniela Weiskopf* [2] *and Lance Turtle* [1,3]*

[1] *NIHR Health Protection Research Unit in Emerging and Zoonotic Infections, Centre for Global Vaccine Research, Institute of Infection and Global Health, University of Liverpool, Liverpool, United Kingdom,* [2] *Division of Vaccine Discovery, La Jolla Institute for Immunology, La Jolla, CA, United States,* [3] *Tropical and Infectious Disease Unit, Liverpool University Hospitals, Liverpool, United Kingdom*

***Correspondence:**
Lance Turtle
lance.turtle@liverpool.ac.uk

Dengue virus (DENV, family *Flaviviridae*, genus *Flavivirus*) exists as four distinct serotypes. Generally, immunity after infection with one serotype is protective and lifelong, though exceptions have been described. However, secondary infection with a different serotype can result in more severe disease for a minority of patients. Host responses to the first DENV infection involve the development of both cross-reactive antibody and T cell responses, which, depending upon their precise balance, may mediate protection or enhance disease upon secondary infection with a different serotype. Abundant evidence now exists that responses elicited by DENV infection can cross-react with other members of the genus Flavivirus, particularly Zika virus (ZIKV). Cohort studies have shown that prior DENV immunity is associated with protection against Zika. Cross-reactive antibody responses may enhance infection with flaviviruses, which likely accounts for the cases of severe disease seen during secondary DENV infections. Data for T cell responses are contradictory, and even though cross-reactive T cell responses exist, their clinical significance is uncertain. Recent mouse experiments, however, show that cross-reactive T cells are capable of mediating protection against ZIKV. In this review, we summarize and discuss the evidence that T cell responses may, at least in part, explain the cross-protection seen against ZIKV from DENV infection, and that T cell antigens should therefore be included in putative Zika vaccines.

Keywords: dengue, Zika, T-cells, cross-reactivity, vaccine, epitope, animal models

INTRODUCTION

During the last two decades, the rate of infections with flaviviruses, particularly dengue virus (DENV) and Zika virus (ZIKV), has risen significantly (**Figure 1**). At present, half of the world's population is considered at risk for DENV and cases of ZIKV continue to be reported globally, including the first local cases in southern Europe (1, 2). DENV and ZIKV are spread via the bite of infected mosquitoes, *Aedes spp.*, whose expanding ecological niches beyond the tropical and sub-tropical regions pose a major public health threat (3). Infection with DENV can present with a spectrum of clinical manifestations ranging from an asymptomatic illness to an acute

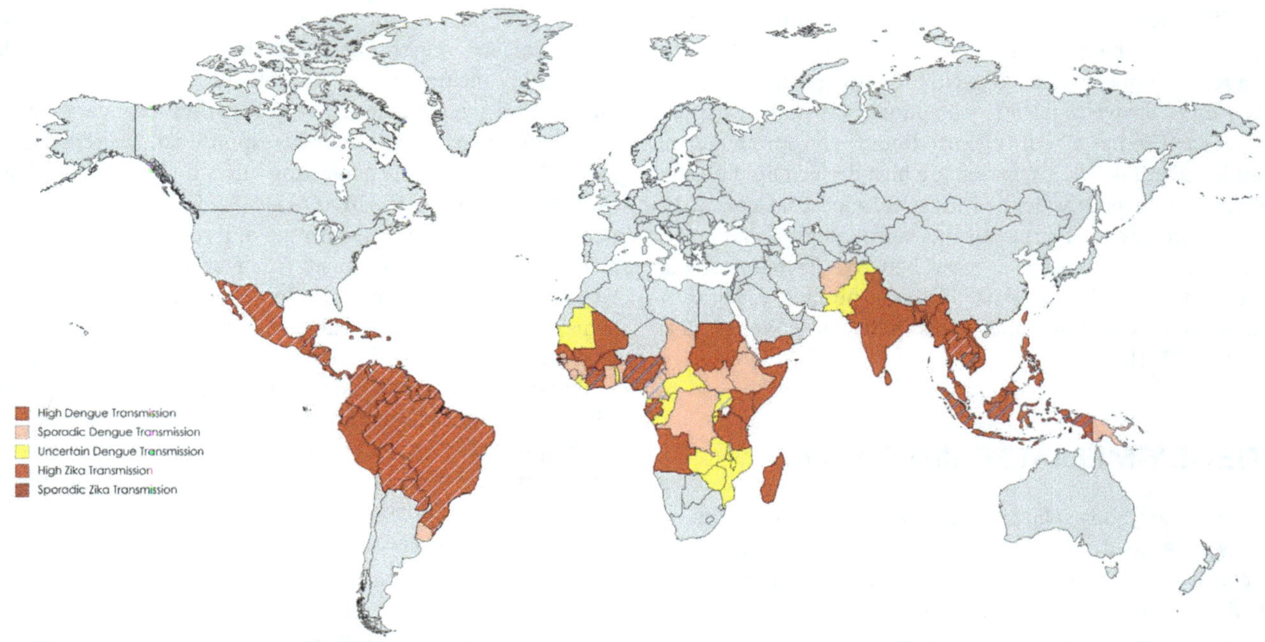

FIGURE 1 | Distribution of countries with Dengue and Zika transmission. Data compiled using the CDC yellow book and HealthMap©. Each color reflects a varying transmission rate from high dengue transmission (in red) to uncertain dengue transmission (in yellow). Countries with cross-hatched lines reflect those with high or sporadic Zika transmission.

fever/arthralgia/rash (dengue fever, DF) that usually is self-limiting, to more severe disease (dengue hemorrhagic fever/dengue shock syndrome, DHF/DSS) that is characterized by vascular leakage and/or hemorrhage (4). ZIKV causes a similar febrile illness that is often mild, with the exception of rare cases of neurological disease, such as Guillain-Barré syndrome (5). In pregnancy, ZIKV infection is associated with adverse fetal/neonatal outcomes such as congenital Zika syndrome (CZS) (6). Given that these viruses share similar geographic distributions and high sequence homology, immunological cross-reactivity between DENV and ZIKV is a well-recognized and unsurprising phenomenon. In this review, we will focus on the role of T cells during DENV and ZIKV infections in humans and in animal models, summarizing the major findings, discussing how cross-reactivity might impact immunity, and providing evidence why incorporating T cell epitopes into vaccine design is favorable.

VIROLOGY

There are four dengue viruses, DENV1-4, which are antigenically distinct (hence called serotypes) and possibly represent four distinct introductions into humans from the sylvatic cycle in non-human primates (7). On occasion several serotypes can circulate concomitantly within endemic areas, or as individual serotypes in sequence (8). A primary dengue infection generally results in lifelong immunity against the same serotype, although homotypic DENV re-infections have also been described (9). DENV infections can generate cross-reactive, poorly neutralizing antibodies that bind the other serotypes (10). Upon secondary infection with a heterologous DENV serotype, there is then a risk of severe disease, thought to be mediated via a mechanism called antibody-mediated enhancement (ADE) (11, 12). ADE arises when antibodies against one serotype can bind to, but not fully neutralize, another DENV serotype. These virus-antibody complexes can bind to the Fcγ receptors on the surface of mononuclear phagocytes enhancing viral entry and facilitating viral replication (13).

ZIKV has three genotypes, East African, West African and Asian (14). Recent Zika outbreaks have indicated a role for pre-existing immunity against DENV to modulate ZIKV infection (15). Data from a large pediatric cohort in Nicaragua found that prior DENV infection reduced the risk of symptomatic ZIKV infection by about one third (16) and in a Brazilian cohort high pre-existing antibody titers to DENV were associated with reduced risk of ZIKV infection and symptoms (17). Furthermore, protection against congenital Zika syndrome was shown to be associated with prior DENV immunity (18).

VIRAL STRUCTURE

The flavivirus virion is enveloped, and contains a single-stranded, positive-sense RNA that is ~11 kb size. The viral genome encodes three structural proteins [capsid, precursor membrane (prM) and envelope (E)] involved in virion assembly and seven non-structural (NS) proteins (NS1, NS2a, NS2b, NS3, NS4a, NS4b, and NS5) that function in the viral life cycle (19). The canonical role of NS proteins is in viral replication where with host factors they function in the assembly of the membrane-bound multi-protein replication complex (RC). NS proteins are also the target of most of the flavivirus CD8 T cell epitopes (20–22). A mature flavivirus particle has a well-organized outer glycoprotein shell with an icosahedral T = 3 symmetry, a host derived lipid bilayer membrane and a poorly defined inner nucelocapsid core (23). Flavivirus particles can assume various morphologies (immature, mosaic-like, and mature) that vary between flaviviruses and have important implications on antibody binding specifically regarding the availability and accessibility of epitopes (24) [reviewed in (25)].

ANTIBODY-MEDIATED IMMUNITY

Neutralizing antibody plays a crucial role in immunity to flaviviruses. Animal models show that robustly neutralizing monoclonal antibodies are sufficient for protection against many flaviviruses (24, 26, 27). However, antibody responses against flaviviruses can also be notoriously cross-reactive and the neutralization potential of these antibodies can vary considerably. The neutralizing antibody response is directed against the E protein, but responses against other proteins such as prM and NS1 also form a significant fraction of the response after both DENV and ZIKV infections (25, 28–30).

In recent years, much has been learned about anti-flavivirus antibody responses by cloning antibodies from infected or previously infected humans. These studies have demonstrated that, while many different classes of antibody are made, those which most potently neutralize frequently recognize quaternary epitopes on the viral surface and bind across multiple Envelope proteins (24, 31–33). The probable mechanism of neutralization by antibodies against quaternary epitopes is through interfering with viral fusion by locking the particle in a non-fusogenic form (24). Although some of these antibody classes can neutralize all four DENV serotypes and ZIKV (34, 35), they may not be durable in humans and their effectiveness may wane with time (36). In fact, a period of cross-protection exists even after a primary DENV infection, as observed by Sabin who found that subjects re-challenged with heterotypic DENV infection were protected if the re-challenge occurred 2–3 months after the original infection (37).

A major epitope recognized by the human antibody response is the viral fusion-loop of E domain II (25). Fusion loop antibodies are highly cross-reactive and strongly binding, but weakly neutralizing, not able to cross-neutralize other viruses, and can mediate ADE (38). During secondary flavivirus infections, the resulting antibody response can be predominantly focused upon the earlier infecting virus, a phenomenon known as "original antigenic sin (OAS);" and thus may be poorly neutralizing against the current infection (39). It may be challenging for new vaccines (such as those against ZIKV), when introduced in areas of intense flavivirus transmission, to protect if the balance of enhancing and neutralizing antibody is not optimal, or the development of new antibody responses is impaired (38). In addition, the development of congenital Zika syndrome has been linked to ADE (40) and could be due to the presence of cross-reactive fusion loop antibodies. Prior DENV immunity can protect against ZIKV, and, in the cases where inefficient antibody responses arise, possibly due to OAS, it might be that a cross-reactive CD8+ T cell response contributes to protection.

T CELL RESPONSES TO DENV IN HUMANS

Early work on cellular immunity to DENV demonstrated that T cell responses were readily detectable, and serotype cross-reactive responses of both CD4+ and CD8+ T cells were described (20–22, 41–46). The existence of serotype cross-reactivity at the level of individual T cell epitopes was found in both subjects given an experimental DENV vaccine (47, 48) and after natural exposure (49). In fact, a single DENV infection can elicit a cross-reactive T cell response against several serotypes (50), and the same T cell receptor (TCR) can recognize epitopes from multiple serotypes (51–53). Although variant epitopes may be recognized by the same TCR, the degree of overall serotype cross-reactivity is also likely to be influenced by the targeting of immunodominant responses, for example non-structural (NS) proteins are more highly conserved than structural proteins (**Table 1**). Responses biased toward sequences that are conserved between serotypes (possibly in NS proteins) give rise to higher potential for serotype cross-reactivity (55). The factors that determine whether responses are focused on conserved or variant epitopes are not known. However, interestingly, the pattern of conserved/serotype specific epitope recognition was remarkably similar in two different populations studied (**Figure 2**), implying

TABLE 1 | Percent homology across structural and non-structural proteins between Zika and DENV serotypes 1–4.

	ZIKA										
	Polyprotein%	**C%**	**prM%**	**E%**	**NS1%**	**NS2A%**	**NS2B%**	**NS3%**	**NS4A%**	**NS4B%**	**NS5%**
DENV1	55	50	43	57	54	46	35	66	43	51	67
DENV2	56	41	41	55	54	44	41	67	52	53	67
DENV3	57	50	42	58	55	46	38	67	39	52	67
DENV4	57	49	47	56	54	45	41	67	44	49	68

The results of this table was generated from data available in Grifoni et al. (54).

that the factors underlying the phenomenon are not constrained to specific populations (55). The immunodominant targets of the T-cell response can vary between CD4+ and CD8+ T cells (**Figure 3**), and also between DENV serotypes (22, 55), as well as with exposure to other flaviviruses. Interestingly, the stimulus for the most cross-reactive T cell responses of all appears to be the tetravalent live attenuated DENV vaccine TV003, which includes the NS protein from DENV serotypes 1, 3, and 4, where the vast majority of the response is directed against NS proteins (**Figure 4**) (56). CD8+ T cells from TV003 vaccines can also cross-recognize ZIKV peptides, suggesting that the tetravalent DENV vaccination can induce T cell cross-reactivity across DENV serotypes and the closely related ZIKV (54).

Demonstrating a clear role for DENV specific T cell responses in protection or disease has been more challenging. Initially, it was thought that the T cell response against DENV was pathological to the host. Some variant DENV epitopes may function as inefficient TCR agonists (58), and during acute disease CD8+ T cell responses can be more focused on variant epitopes from a previous infection (original antigenic sin) (51), possibly leading to less efficient responses. Moreover, many of these DENV specific T cells were found to be apoptotic (51). Some studies have demonstrated that *ex-vivo* T cell cytokine responses are greater with more severe disease, when tested shortly after disease onset (59, 60), suggesting a role for T cells in mediating excessive inflammation. In addition, degranulation of T cells [a surrogate marker for cytotoxicity (61)] was not greater in DHF (60, 62), implying that it is in fact the balance between cytokine production (pathological?) and killing (protective?) that may influence disease phenotype.

However, not all studies have shown a relationship between acute responses and disease phenotype, with some authors pointing out that the appearance of DENV specific T cells occurs after resolution of clinical outcomes in severe dengue (63). Furthermore, not all studies show a relationship between higher cytokine production and disease severity in DHF (64). In fact,

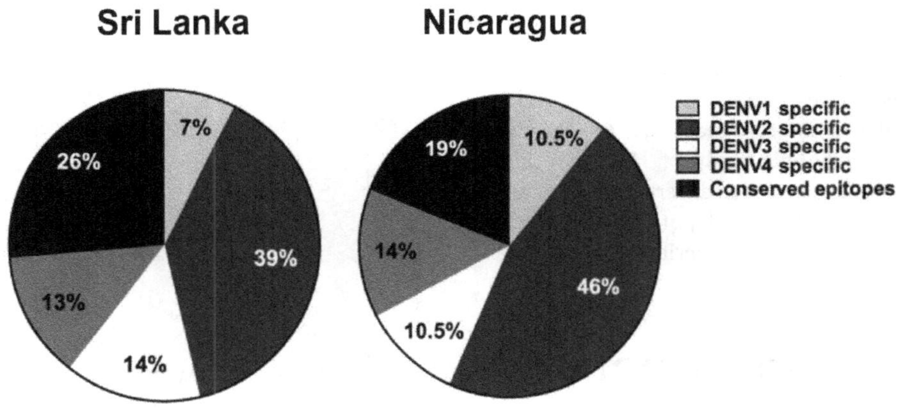

FIGURE 2 | Distribution of CD8+ T cell epitopes across the four DENV serotypes in two clinically characterized cohorts from Sri Lanka and Nicaragua. Adapted from results in Gordon et al. (16), Weiskopf et al. (55).

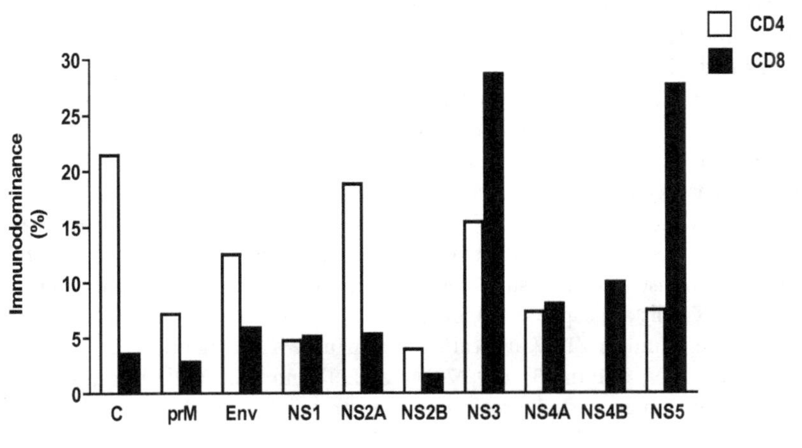

FIGURE 3 | Immunodominant protein pattern of DENV-specific CD4 and CD8 T cell response based on IEDB data. HLA class I and class II restricted epitopes for CD4 and CD8 DENV-specific T cell responses, respectively, have been derived querying IEDB database (www.IEDB.org) on 02-Aug-2019. Epitope list was filtered using Immunobrowser, selecting epitope lists tested in at least 10 donors. Protein immunodominance was calculated as percentage of epitopes per protein per HLA restriction.

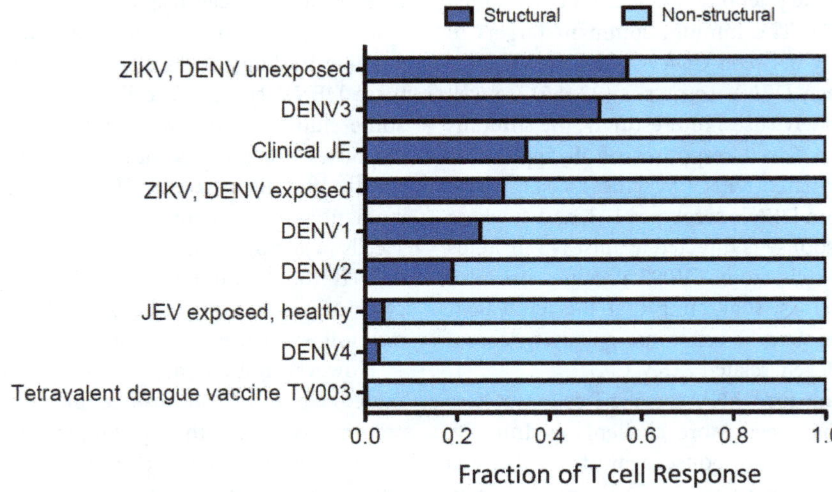

FIGURE 4 | Distribution of the T cell response to structural and non-structural components is influenced by prior clinical history. Data for this figure was compiled from the following studies: Turtle et al. (20), Weiskopf et al. (21, 56), Grifoni et al. (54), and Delgado et al. (57). T cell responses are from subjects with natural infections or vaccine recipients. Responses were identified by ELISPOT and intracellular cytokine staining (ICS) assays.

when sampled early in the disease course, or as in one prospective study before disease onset, T cell cytokine production correlated with lower viremia and less severe disease (65, 66), implying a protective role for T cells. One study of HLA association with disease severity of dengue showed certain alleles to be protective whilst others were detrimental, potentially explaining why studies of T cells and disease severity give discrepant results (21, 67, 68).

DENV/ZIKV T CELL CROSS-REACTIVITY

Given the potential for T cell responses to DENV to be protective, at least in some circumstances, it is therefore possible that T cells primed by DENV could recognize ZIKV and be protective. Grifoni et al. found that in DENV exposed individuals, the T cell response to ZIKV is earlier, larger and exhibits greater cytotoxic capacity (54). In the same study it was shown that in two large cohorts from Sri Lanka and Nicaragua (54), the imprint of previous DENV exposure is clearly detectable, and that the resulting T cell response to Asian ZIKV was biased toward the non-structural proteins (**Figure 4**). Similarly, evidence of pre-existing flavivirus immunity has been shown to result in enhanced T cell responses directed to NS3 of DENV and African ZIKV (69). Whether such responses are protective is unknown, but two studies have demonstrated that short-term T cell cultures of flavivirus specific T cells are capable of killing targets pulsed with peptides that are found in ZIKV, indicating that they likely have anti-viral function (**Figure 5**) (20, 70). With DENV infection appearing to confer partial protection against Zika illness (16, 18), cross-reactive T cell responses may be one such mechanism by which this protection is mediated. Additionally, transcriptomic profiles of ZIKV-specific CD8+ T cells in DENV naïve or pre-exposed patients showed no qualitative differences in ZIKV- specific CD8+ T cell responses

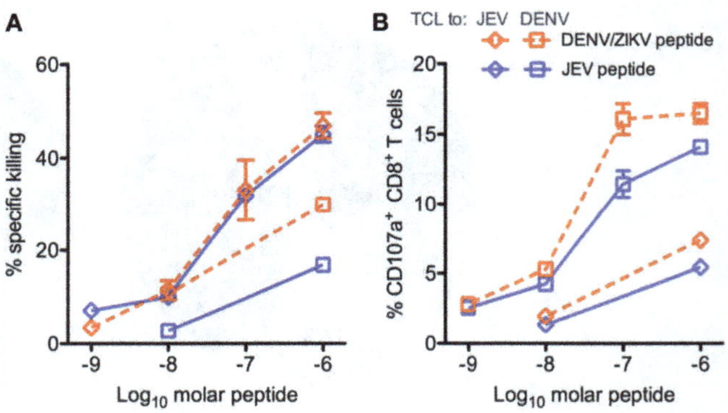

FIGURE 5 | Peptide-pulsed, CFSE-labeled, HLA-matched targets were incubated with CD8+ T cell line effector cells, and the percent specific killing was measured by flow cytometry in response to JEV and DENV/ZIKV peptides. Percent killing **(A)** and the percent of CD107+ CD8+ T cells **(B)** are shown. Diamonds indicate T cell lines expanded with JEV peptide, and squares indicate lines expanded with DENV/ZIKV peptide. Assays were performed in duplicate for each T cell line/peptide pair. Error bars represent standard error of the mean. This figure was adapted from Turtle et al. (20).

supporting the fact that cross-reactive T cell responses share the same protective phenotype observed after single flavivirus exposure (71). This phenomenon may also not be confined to ZIKV. There is some evidence that partial protection against Japanese Encephalitis (JE) appears to be conferred by prior DENV infection, with the number of JE cases lower than expected in areas with DENV outbreaks (72). Also it has been shown that the severity of JE is reduced by previous flavivirus infection (73). These effects may be mediated by T cell responses (20). The degree to which T cell responses are targeted to structural vs. non-structural flavivirus proteins may vary according to previous exposure. For example, in the case of ZIKV, being affected by prior DENV infection biases the response toward the non-structural proteins (**Figure 4**). Responses against non-structural proteins tend to be more cross-reactive, meaning that previous dengue infection has the potential to bias the T cell response to ZIKV toward more cross-reactive epitopes. In an environment where multiple flavivirus exposure occurs, such epitopes, are likely to receive a great number of re-stimulations and may rise to the top of a "hierarchy of immunodominance." Including such epitopes in vaccines, therefore, has merit in that such a vaccine may be made more effective if there is a degree of pre-existing immunity in the population, lowering the threshold for vaccine responses to be generated. Although further studies are required to unequivocally show that DENV-primed T cell responses can mediate protection against ZIKV in humans, mouse studies provide convincing evidence that T cells can mediate cross-protection.

T CELL RESPONSES IN MICE AND NON-HUMAN PRIMATES (NHP)

Mice are not natural hosts for flaviviruses as the murine type I IFN system provides a very effective defense, which thwarts viral dissemination and thus prevents them being useful models of severe disease phenotypes (74). As such, to establish a model of productive viral infection, which can be used to examine T cell function and test potential vaccine candidates, multiple strains of immunocompromised mice have been generated (74). These strains include mice deficient in either type I or type II or both IFN receptors, mice with STAT2 knocked-out, mice with mouse STAT2 replaced by human STAT2, and more nuanced models where type I IFN receptors are absent in specific cells or tissues (74). In combination with either mouse-adapted or human viral strains, this has established an infection model that closely, but not perfectly, mimics human disease. For DENV and ZIKV, strains that are commonly used either lack type I IFN receptor (IFNAR$^{-/-}$ and A129) or both type I and II receptors (AG129 mice) (74). Human Leucocyte Antigen (HLA)-transgenic mice have also been used to model CD8+ and/or CD4+ T cell responses in flavivirus infection. Work in HLA-transgenic mice show a broad epitope repertoire, whilst some HLA variants, such as HLA-B*0702, have been specifically studied due to a known association with high T cell response frequency and magnitude in humans, as well as decreased susceptibility to severe dengue disease (75, 76).

Control of primary DENV infection in mice requires CD8+ T cells to a greater extent than CD4+ cells. In IFNAR$^{-/-}$ mice, depletion of CD8+ cells was directly associated with increased viral burden in tissues that was not ameliorated by the transfer of serum or B cells (77). Protection in the study was mediated by increased cytotoxic activity in DENV-specific CD8+ T cells; activity which was further enhanced when mice received a peptide vaccination (77). However, challenge experiments in other mouse models (HEPG2-grafted SCID) find that DENV-specific CD8+ T cell responses were associated with reduced mortality, which suggests that T cells may contribute to disease severity in some instances, and prevent mortality in others (78).

Crossing IFNAR$^{-/-}$ mice with HLA transgenic mice showed that protective CD8+ T cell responses tended to be polyfunctional and principally targeted non-structural proteins such as NS3 and NS5, similar to that in humans (75). Responses targeted against NS proteins have also shown their protective potential in homotypic secondary DENV infections where wildtype mice primed with a non-lethal DENV2 strain ACS46 were challenged with a lethal encephalitic homotypic strain JHA1 (79). In this model, protective immunity was reduced when both CD4+ and CD8+ T cells were depleted. In most challenge models CD4+ T cells play an accessory and non-essential role in which they contribute to viral clearance when induced by immunization (80).

Models of heterologous DENV infection also demonstrate the importance of T cells during the anti-DENV response. Collectively these studies show that CD8+ responses can protect against heterologous DENV challenge in non-lethal (81) and lethal models (82). CD8+ T cell responses contribute to protection during heterotypic reinfection, whereas homotypic reinfection can be contained by neutralizing antibodies against the infecting serotype (81), as is believed to be the case in humans. Comparison of specific and cross-reactive T cell responses in IFNAR$^{-/-}$ mice reveal that, despite their relatively low magnitude and avidity, cross-reactive CD8+ T cells from prior DENV exposure reduce viral load and exhibit a polyfunctional response in a manner comparable to that of serotype-specific cells (46). However, in a model of secondary DENV infection resulting in severe disease, cross-reactive CD4+ and CD8+ T cells were found to be pathogenic in wildtype mice infected with a non-mouse adapted DENV strain (83). In summary, the contribution of T cells to disease and protection in dengue mouse models is still not fully understood. The variability in current data are likely shaped by factors such as differences in mouse immune function, infection methods, strain difference, and experimental end-points.

Similar to observations for DENV, experiments in mice in which T cell responses are lacking, or on the other hand are enhanced (e.g., through peptide immunization or adoptive cell transfer), demonstrate a protective role for CD8+ T cells against ZIKV (84, 85). CD8+ T cell responses in primary ZIKV infection appear to be essential for immunity. In LysMCre^{+} IFNAR$^{fl/fl}$ (type I IFN receptor absent only in myeloid cells) and IFNAR$^{-/-}$ mice, ZIKV-immune CD8+ T cells protect against infection through cytotoxic, polyfunctional cellular responses (46, 86). However, in some instances, the resulting cytotoxicity may damage the host, in a tissue specific manner. For example, in IFNAR$^{-/-}$ mice ZIKV infection of astrocytes results in a breakdown of the blood-brain barrier, allowing an influx of CD8+ T cells into the central nervous system (CNS) where they mediate apoptosis of ZIKV-infected neurons, but also results in severe neuropathology (87). Similarly, CD8+ cellular infiltration was also found in the CNS following ZIKV infection in C57/BL6 neonatal mice who developed hind limb collapse, cerebellar degeneration (88) and in the case of adult wildtype C57BL/6 mice, encephalitis (89). Whilst the CD8+ T cell response may be detrimental in the CNS, in IFNAR$^{-/-}$ pregnant mice cross-reactive DENV-specific CD8+ cells are protective against ZIKV infection of the fetus, including the fetal central nervous system, and are associated with increased fetal growth and viability (90). The CNS may represent a special case, where infection in the absence of CD8+ T cells results in severe viral pathology, and in the presence of CD8+ T cells in immunopathology, with little difference in survival in either case, as is seen in Japanese encephalitis (91).

Responses to sequential DENV-ZIKV infection (summarized in **Figure 6**) share similarities with secondary heterotypic DENV infection. Firstly, DENV-immune CD8+ T cell responses—either from prior exposure, peptide immunization or transfer of DENV-immune CD8+ T cells—can protect against ZIKV infection (90, 92, 93). This is an important result, which corroborates human studies that demonstrate prior DENV immunity can reduce the risk of Zika infection (16). Likewise, prior exposure to DENV provided IFNAR$^{-/-}$ mice protection against maternal and fetal ZIKV infection as compared with non-immune controls (90). As in heterotypic DENV, in mice as well as humans—the immunodominance pattern of the CD8+ T cell response to ZIKV infection was altered by prior DENV immunity and focused on conserved cross-reactive epitopes (93). ZIKV/DENV cross-reactive T cells performed comparably to ZIKV-specific T cells in viral load reduction in the serum and brain of knockout mice, which have key implications for ZIKV vaccine development.

Contrary to mice, non-human primates (NHP) are natural hosts for DENV and ZIKV. Several different primate models have been employed, including rhesus and cynomolgus macaques. In line with epidemiological observations in humans, experiments in NHP demonstrate that dengue immunity may curb Zika replication and potentially symptoms (94). Performing the order of viral challenge the other way around gave a similar result, where macaques with prior ZIKV immunity mounted strong humoral and cellular responses against DENV (95). Furthermore, this model found that a longer convalescence between ZIKV and DENV challenge was associated with higher and more durable antibody and T cell responses suggesting that ZIKV immune memory can contribute to protection against DENV (95).

DENGUE AND ZIKA VACCINES IN DEVELOPMENT

There are currently three dengue vaccines that have either been tested in, or are currently in, phase III trials. At the time of writing the only licensed dengue vaccine is Sanofi-Pasteur's Dengvaxia® (CYD-TDV), a live-attenuated, chimeric, tetravalent vaccine, in which the genes encoding prM and E of the four DENV serotypes have been inserted into YFV-17D (**Figure 7**) (96). The vaccine was developed to produce DENV neutralizing antibodies in human subjects, but protection against disease is incomplete despite high levels of seroconversion (97, 98), and one trial found no efficacy at all against DENV2 (99). During longer follow up of clinical trial participants, it was observed that young children in the vaccinated group had excess hospital admissions due to dengue compared with the placebo group (100). Dengvaxia is

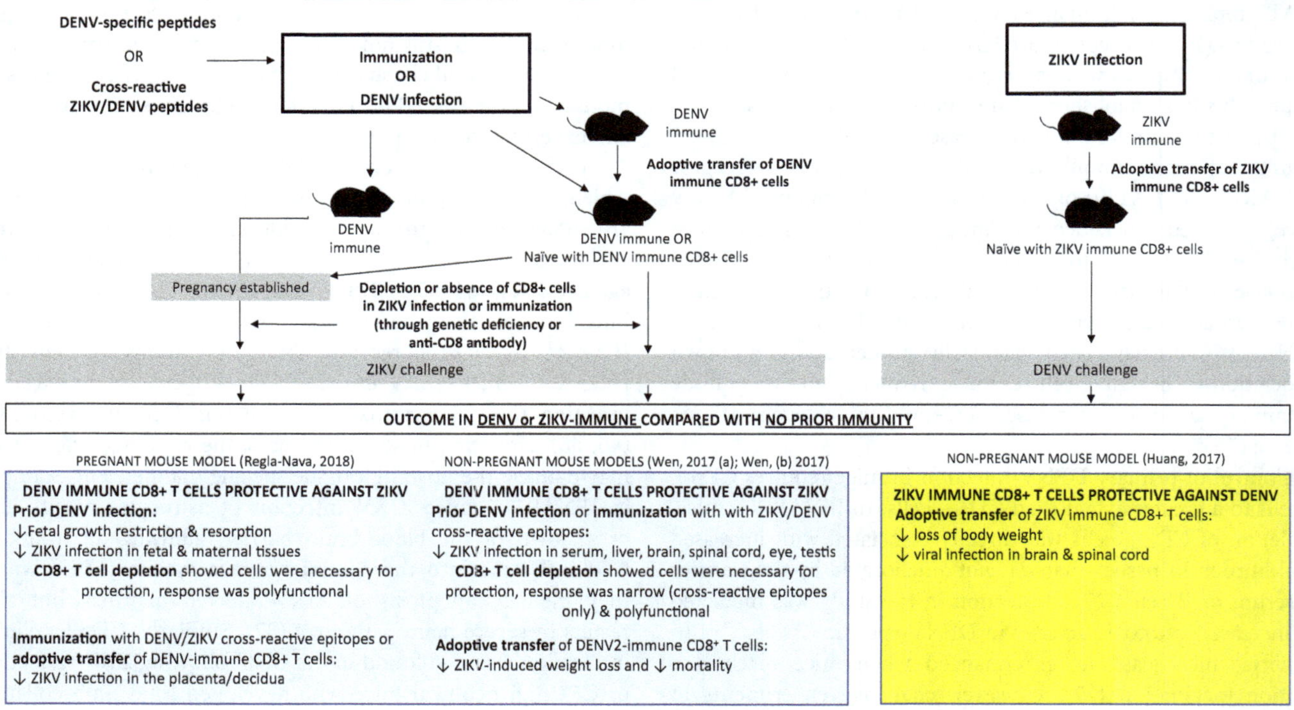

FIGURE 6 | The CD8+ T cell response and impact of prior flavivirus immunity in secondary flavivirus infection in mice. Summary of experiments (infections, immunizations, adoptive cell transfer, and depletions) demonstrating the protective effect of prior DENV immunity on ZIKV challenge and prior ZIKV immunity on DENV challenge in pregnant and non-pregnant mouse models.

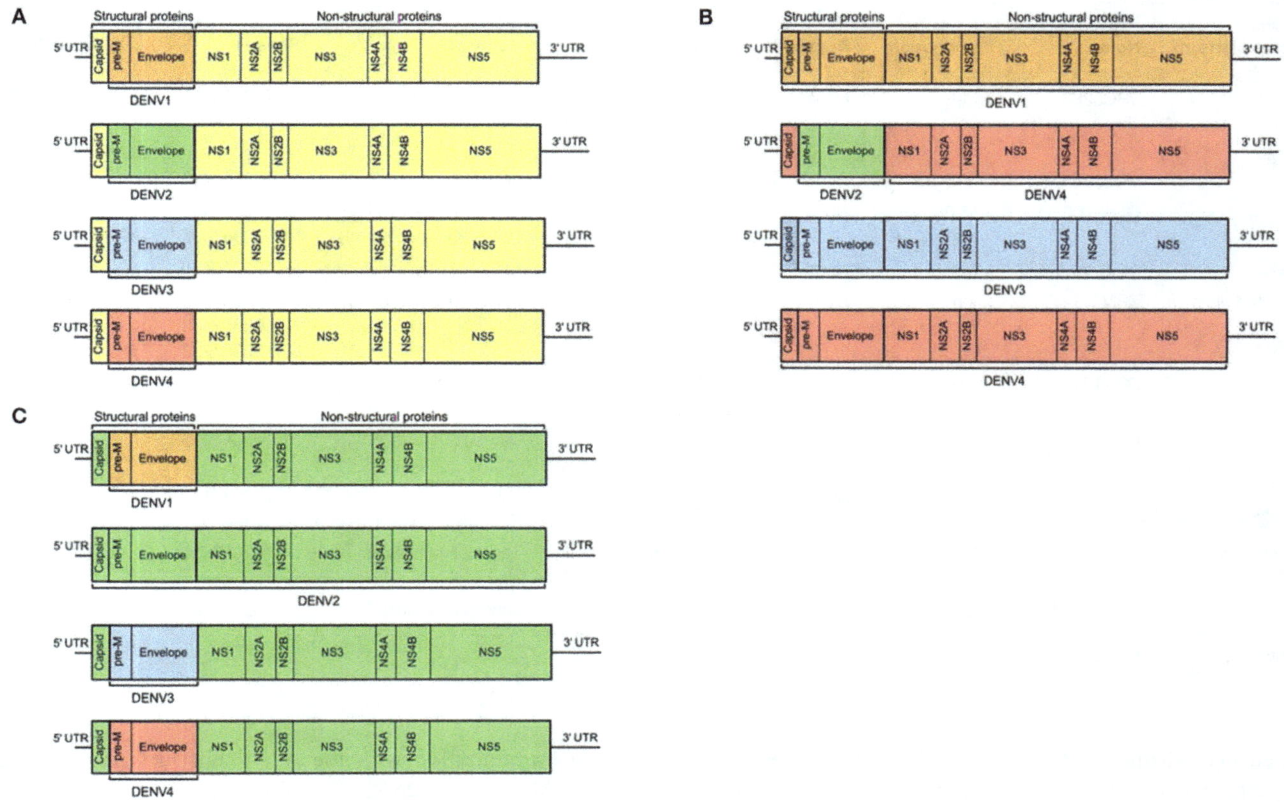

FIGURE 7 | Design schematic of three dengue vaccines. **(A)** represents Sanofi's licensed vaccine, Dengvaxia®, **(B)** represents the NIH live attenuated tetravalent dengue vaccine candidate (TV003), and **(C)** represents Takeda's tetravalent dengue vaccine (TDV). Each color represents regions from different flaviviruses: yellow, YFV; orange, DENV1; green, DENV2; blue, DENV3; and red, DENV4.

most effective in individuals who are DENV-seropositive at the time of immunization, while in seronegative subjects the vaccine is not protective and increases the risk of severe disease (101). One hypothesis for failure to protect DENV-naïve subjects may be that the T cell response generated was directed against the yellow fever NS proteins present within the vaccine, rather than DENV NS proteins (68, 102). These observations suggest the need to determine the optimal T cell antigens and incorporate them into new vaccines. The other two dengue vaccines in development are based on full length DENV. One [Takeda, tetravalent dengue vaccine (TAK-003)] uses an attenuated strain of DENV2, with the prM and E genes of the other serotypes inserted into it (103). Regardless of dengue serostatus, TAK-003 elicited strong humoral responses against all four DENV serotypes (104), and generated a polyfunctional CD8+ T cell response to the non-structural proteins of DENV2, which cross-reacted against DENV1, DENV3, and DENV4 (105). Preliminary findings of a phase III trial show TAK-003 to have ∼81% efficacy against symptomatic dengue (106), though protection against DENV3 was slightly lower. Therefore, a vaccine that induces better—and potentially more cross-reactive T cell responses also seems to have higher efficacy. However, these vaccines have not been compared directly and TAK-003 may still enhance disease in DENV naïve people, and could protect through a mechanism not involving CD8+ T cells. The other dengue vaccine in phase III trials is TV003, which is a tetravalent formulation of DENV1-3 with an additional chimeric DENV4 with the DENV2 prM and E genes inserted (**Figure 7**). Administration of TV003 induced a T cell response which predominantly targeted conserved epitopes of NS3 and NS5 (55) and was found to be immunogenic in subjects with prior flavivirus exposure (107). Field efficacy data are not yet available for TV003, but the vaccine protects against rash and viremia in a dengue human challenge model (108).

The majority of Zika vaccines are still in phase I/II trials (**Table 2**). These vaccines include DNA/mRNA, purified inactivated ZIKV, and recombinant virus-vectored vaccines; with most vaccine constructs containing the prM and E antigens as the main immunogen, as these proteins are targets for neutralizing antibodies (109). Three DNA-based vaccines (GLS-5700, VRC5283, and VRC5288) that have entered human testing show promising results, with one, VRC5283 advancing into phase II. VRC5283 and VRC5288 are both chimeric vaccines that utilize a JE virus (JEV) prM signal sequence followed by either the full-length E protein from wildtype ZIKV (VRC5283) or a modified E region in which the terminal 98 amino acids are exchanged with the analogous JEV sequence (VRC5288) (110). Both vaccines were shown to be immunogenic in mouse and NHP models (110) and a phase I trial found that vaccination with VRC5283

TABLE 2 | Current Zika vaccines in clinical trial.

Vaccine platform	Name	Immunogen	Adjuvant	Dose*	Sponsor	Phase I	Phase II
DNA	VRC5283	prM-E	None	4 mg IM (Phase I) and 4 mg vs. 8 mg IM (Phase II)	NIAID/VRC	NCT02996461	NTC03110770
	VRC5288	prM-E	None	4 mg IM	NIAID/VRC	NCT02840487	–
	GLS5700	prM-E	None	1,2 mg ID	GeneOne Life Science Inovio Pharmaceuticals	NCT02809443 NCT02887482	–
mRNA	mRNA-1325	prM-E	None	–	Moderna Therapeutics	NCT03010489	–
Inactivated Virus	ZPIV	virion	Alum	5 μg IM	NIAID/WRAIR/BIDMC	NCT02963909 NCT02952833 NCT02937233	–
	BBV121	virion	Alum	2.5 μg vs. 5 μg vs. 10 μg IM	Bharat Biotech	CTRI/2017/05/008539	–
	PIZV	virion	Alum	2 μg vs. 5 μg vs. 10 μg IM	Takeda	NCT03343626	–
	VLA1601	virion	Alum	2.5 μg vs. 5 μg vs. 10 μg IM	Valneva Emergent Biosolutions	NCT03425149	–
Viral Vectored	MV-ZIKV	prM-E	None	Low dose vs. High dose IM	Themis Biosciences	NCT02996890	–
	Ad26.ZIKV.001	M-E	None	–	Janssen Vaccines	NCT03356561	–

**IM, intramuscular; ID, intradermal.*

elicited neutralizing antibodies and cellular responses in all of the participants (111). A randomized placebo-controlled phase II study of VRC5283 is currently underway. A limitation of VRC5283 is whether the incorporation of a sequence from a different flavivirus (JEV prM) will provide protection against congenital Zika infection (111). To address this point, the vaccine was tested in a non-human primate pregnancy model. Vaccinated animals displayed fewer fetal losses and had reduced placental and fetal pathology; vaccine protection correlated with serum neutralizing antibody and antiviral T cell responses (112). However, these results may have to be considered cautiously as the model does not reflect early gestational exposure to ZIKV (112).

In addition to DNA-based vaccines, a ZIKV purified inactivated vaccine (ZPIV) based on the Puerto Rican strain PRVABC59 was found to be immunogenic at phase I with an acceptable safety profile (113). Vaccination with ZPIV elicited neutralizing antibody responses in the majority of tested individuals (113). One vaccine recipient from the trial produced cross-neutralizing antibodies to both ZIKV and DENV; responses which were linked to the individual's prior flavivirus exposure (114). These antibodies were shown to target the E domain I/III linker and could protect IFNAR$^{-/-}$ mice challenged either with ZIKV or DENV-2 (114). The durability of these protective responses were only evaluated up to 8 weeks post-vaccination (114) and longer follow up is still needed to fully demonstrate the longevity of these responses.

Enhanced immunogenicity associated with viral vectors (115) make these attractive candidates for Zika antigen delivery. Of the vaccines in clinical testing, two use viral vectors: one an attenuated measles strain (116) and the other a replication-incompetent human adenovirus serotype 26 (Ad26) (117). A single immunization with the Ad26 construct containing the Zika prM and E (Ad26.ZIKV.M-Env) antigens was able to elicit protective humoral and cellular responses in mice and NHP (117). Ad26.ZIKV.M-Env also protected IFNAR$^{-/-}$ dams and fetuses from ZIKV in a pregnancy model (118).

As discussed previously, all of vaccine constructs in clinical testing target structural proteins and may therefore not be optimal in their ability to induce cellular responses or boost pre-existing responses. Therefore, vaccines that include non-structural proteins should be considered, given that vaccination with non-structural proteins can induce cytotoxic T cell and polyfunctional helper T cell responses (119). Furthermore, given that non-structural proteins can elicit cross-reactive T cell responses, vaccines that incorporate these proteins may provide suitable priming for the development of memory responses during secondary flavivirus challenge (74, 94, 95, 109, 110, 115, 120–140).

CONCLUSION

There still remains a need to develop Zika vaccines, and also to better understand the cross-reactivity of flavivirus immune responses so that this can be harnessed for the emergent flaviviruses of the future. Dengue infection appears to be protective against ZIKV through mechanisms mediated by cross-reactive T cell responses against NS proteins. Given that in general, non-structural proteins elicit the most cross-reactive responses, and that these responses are likely to be protective against other viruses beyond dengue, there is a strong argument for including non-structural proteins to act as CD8 T cell antigens in novel flavivirus vaccines. As the majority of the population in flavivirus endemic areas are repeatedly exposed, vaccines incorporating non-structural antigens may be more efficient and may require fewer doses due to the constant boosting of an existing T cell response. Finally, the degree of cross-reactivity seen with human CD8+ T cell responses to flaviviruses raises the possibility of engineering a single component containing T cell antigens that could be used in multiple vaccines, or even in a multivalent vaccine, provided suitable B cell antigens can be found.

AUTHOR CONTRIBUTIONS

KS contributed to the conceptualization of the article, wrote the first draft, and reviewed the manuscript. SL and LG contributed to conceptualization of the article and wrote the first draft of sections of the article. AG contributed viral homology measures and also to conceptualization of the article. DW and LT contributed to conceptualization of the article, contributed to early drafts, and reviewed the article. All authors reviewed the final draft.

FUNDING

This article is an independent research funded by the National Institute for Health Research (NIHR, www.nihr.ac.uk) Health Protection Research Unit in Emerging and Zoonotic Infections (grant No. IS-HPU-1112-10117), Global Health Research Group on Brain Infections (No. 17/63/110) and National Institutes of Health contracts HHSN27220140045C and HHSN75N9301900065. LT is a Wellcome clinical career development fellow, supported by grant number 205228/Z/16/Z. SL, LT, and DW were supported by the European Union Zika Preparedness Latin American Network consortium (ZikaPLAN). ZikaPLAN has received funding from the European Union's Horizon 2020 research and innovation programme under grant agreement no 734584.

REFERENCES

1. Brady OJ, Gething PW, Bhatt S, Messina JP, Brownstein JS, Hoen AG, et al. Refining the global spatial limits of dengue virus transmission by evidence-based consensus. *PLoS Negl Trop Dis.* (2012) 6:e1760. doi: 10.1371/journal.pntd.0001760
2. Brady OJ, Hay SI. The first local cases of Zika virus in Europe. *Lancet.* (2019) 394:1991–2. doi: 10.1016/S0140-6736(19)32790-4
3. Reinhold JM, Lazzari CR, Lahondere C. Effects of the environmental temperature on aedes aegypti and aedes albopictus mosquitoes: a review. *Insects.* (2018) 9:E158. doi: 10.3390/insects9040158
4. Hasan S, Jamdar SF, Alalowi M, Al Ageel Al Beaiji SM. Dengue virus: a global human threat: review of literature. *J Int Soc Prev Community Dent.* (2016) 6:1–6. doi: 10.4103/2231-0762.175416
5. Reid S, Rimmer K, Thakur K. Zika virus and neurologic disease. *Neurol Clin.* (2018) 36:767–87. doi: 10.1016/j.ncl.2018.06.003
6. Lima GP, Rozenbaum D, Pimentel C, Frota ACC, Vivacqua D, Machado ES, et al. Factors associated with the development of Congenital Zika Syndrome: a case-control study. *BMC Infect Dis.* (2019) 19:277. doi: 10.1186/s12879-019-3908-4
7. Vasilakis N, Cardosa J, Hanley KA, Holmes EC, Weaver SC. Fever from the forest: prospects for the continued emergence of sylvatic dengue virus and its impact on public health. *Nat Rev Microbiol.* (2011) 9:532–41. doi: 10.1038/nrmicro2595
8. Chen R, Vasilakis N. Dengue–quo tu et quo vadis? *Viruses.* (2011) 3:1562–608. doi: 10.3390/v3091562
9. Waggoner JJ, Balmaseda A, Gresh L, Sahoo MK, Montoya M, Wang C, et al. Homotypic dengue virus reinfections in nicaraguan children. *J Infect Dis.* (2016) 214:986–93. doi: 10.1093/infdis/jiw099
10. Smith SA, de Alwis AR, Kose N, Harris E, Ibarra KD, Kahle KM, et al. The potent and broadly neutralizing human dengue virus-specific monoclonal antibody 1C19 reveals a unique cross-reactive epitope on the bc loop of domain II of the envelope protein. *MBio.* (2013) 4:e00873-13. doi: 10.1128/mBio.00873-13
11. Halstead SB. Dengue. *Lancet.* (2007) 370:1644–52. doi: 10.1016/S0140-6736(07)61687-0
12. Katzelnick LC, Gresh L, Halloran ME, Mercado JC, Kuan G, Gordon A, et al. Antibody-dependent enhancement of severe dengue disease in humans. *Science.* (2017) 358:929–32. doi: 10.1126/science.aan6836
13. Flipse J, Smit JM. The complexity of a dengue vaccine: a review of the human antibody response. *PLoS Negl Trop Dis.* (2015) 9:e0003749. doi: 10.1371/journal.pntd.0003749
14. Poland GA, Kennedy RB, Ovsyannikova IG, Palacios R, Ho PL, Kalil J. Development of vaccines against Zika virus. *Lancet Infect Dis.* (2018) 18:e211–9. doi: 10.1016/S1473-3099(18)30063-X
15. Gunawardana SA, Shaw RH. Cross-reactive dengue virus-derived monoclonal antibodies to Zika virus envelope protein: panacea or pandora's box? *BMC Infect Dis.* (2018) 18:641. doi: 10.1186/s12879-018-3572-0
16. Gordon A, Gresh L, Ojeda S, Katzelnick LC, Sanchez N, Mercado JC, et al. Prior dengue virus infection and risk of Zika: a pediatric cohort in Nicaragua. *PLoS Med.* (2019) 16:e1002726. doi: 10.1371/journal.pmed.1002726
17. Rodriguez-Barraquer I, Costa F, Nascimento EJM, Nery NJ, Castanha PMS, Sacramento GA, et al. Impact of preexisting dengue immunity on Zika virus emergence in a dengue endemic region. *Science.* (2019) 363:607–10. doi: 10.1126/science.aav6618
18. Pedroso C, Fischer C, Feldmann M, Sarno M, Luz E, Moreira-Soto A, et al. Cross-protection of dengue virus infection against congenital zika syndrome, Northeastern Brazil. *Emerg Infect Dis.* (2019) 25:1485–93. doi: 10.3201/eid2508.190113
19. Perera R, Kuhn RJ. Structural proteomics of dengue virus. *Curr Opin Microbiol.* (2008) 11:369–77. doi: 10.1016/j.mib.2008.06.004
20. Turtle L, Bali T, Buxton G, Chib S, Chan S, Soni M, et al. Human T cell responses to Japanese encephalitis virus in health and disease. *J Exp Med.* (2016) 213:1331–52. doi: 10.1084/jem.20151517
21. Weiskopf D, Angelo MA, de Azeredo EL, Sidney J, Greenbaum JA, Fernando AN, et al. Comprehensive analysis of dengue virus-specific responses supports an HLA-linked protective role for CD8+ T cells. *Proc Natl Acad Sci USA.* (2013) 110:e2046–53. doi: 10.1073/pnas.1305227110
22. Rivino L, Kumaran EA, Jovanovic V, Nadua K, Teo EW, Pang SW, et al. Differential targeting of viral components by CD4+ versus CD8+ T lymphocytes in dengue virus infection. *J Virol.* (2013) 87:2693–706. doi: 10.1128/JVI.02675-12
23. Kuhn RJ, Zhang W, Rossmann MG, Pletnev SV, Corver J, Lenches E, et al. Structure of dengue virus: implications for flavivirus organization, maturation, and fusion. *Cell.* (2002) 108:717–25. doi: 10.1016/s0092-8674(02)00660-8
24. Fibriansah G, Ibarra KD, Ng TS, Smith SA, Tan JL, Lim XN, et al. DENGUE VIRUS. Cryo-EM structure of an antibody that neutralizes dengue virus type 2 by locking E protein dimers. *Science.* (2015) 349:88–91. doi: 10.1126/science.aaa8651
25. Slon Campos JL, Mongkolsapaya J, Screaton GR. The immune response against flaviviruses. *Nat Immunol.* (2018) 19:1189–98. doi: 10.1038/s41590-018-0210-3

26. Oliphant T, Engle M, Nybakken GE, Doane C, Johnson S, Huang L, et al. Development of a humanized monoclonal antibody with therapeutic potential against West Nile virus. *Nat Med.* (2005) 11:522–30. doi: 10.1038/nm1240
27. Fernandez E, Dejnirattisai W, Cao B, Scheaffer SM, Supasa P, Wongwiwat W, et al. Human antibodies to the dengue virus E-dimer epitope have therapeutic activity against Zika virus infection. *Nat Immunol.* (2017) 18:1261–09. doi: 10.1038/ni.3849
28. Culshaw A, Mongkolsapaya J, Screaton G. The immunology of Zika Virus. *F1000Res.* (2018) 7:203. doi: 10.12688/f1000research.12271.1
29. Dejnirattisai W, Jumnainsong A, Onsirisakul N, Fitton P, Vasanawathana S, Limpitikul W, et al. Cross-reacting antibodies enhance dengue virus infection in humans. *Science.* (2010) 328:745–8. doi: 10.1126/science.1185181
30. Stettler K, Beltramello M, Espinosa DA, Graham V, Cassotta A, Bianchi S, et al. Specificity, cross-reactivity, and function of antibodies elicited by Zika virus infection. *Science.* (2016) 353:823–6. doi: 10.1126/science.aaf8505
31. Beltramello M, Williams KL, Simmons CP, Macagno A, Simonelli L, Quyen NT, et al. The human immune response to Dengue virus is dominated by highly cross-reactive antibodies endowed with neutralizing and enhancing activity. *Cell Host Microbe.* (2010) 8:271–83. doi: 10.1016/j.chom.2010.08.007
32. Smith SA, de Alwis AR, Kose N, Jadi RS, de Silva AM, Crowe JE, Jr. Isolation of dengue virus-specific memory B cells with live virus antigen from human subjects following natural infection reveals the presence of diverse novel functional groups of antibody clones. *J Virol.* (2014) 88:12233–41. doi: 10.1128/JVI.00247-14
33. Rouvinski A, Guardado-Calvo P, Barba-Spaeth G, Duquerroy S, Vaney MC, Kikuti CM, et al. Recognition determinants of broadly neutralizing human antibodies against dengue viruses. *Nature.* (2015) 520:109–13. doi: 10.1038/nature14130
34. Dejnirattisai W, Wongwiwat W, Supasa S, Zhang X, Dai X, Rouvinsky A, et al. Corrigendum: a new class of highly potent, broadly neutralizing antibodies isolated from viremic patients infected with dengue virus. *Nat Immunol.* (2015) 16:785. doi: 10.1038/ni0715-785a
35. Barba-Spaeth G, Dejnirattisai W, Rouvinski A, Vaney MC, Medits I, Sharma A, et al. Structural basis of potent Zika-dengue virus antibody cross-neutralization. *Nature.* (2016) 536:48–53. doi: 10.1038/nature18938
36. Collins MH, McGowan E, Jadi R, Young E, Lopez CA, Baric RS, et al. Lack of durable cross-neutralizing antibodies against zika virus from dengue virus infection. *Emerg Infect Dis.* (2017) 23:773–81. doi: 10.3201/eid2305.161630
37. Sabin AB. Research on dengue during world war II. *Am J Trop Med Hyg.* (1952) 1:30–50. doi: 10.4269/ajtmh.1952.1.30
38. Dejnirattisai W, Supasa P, Wongwiwat W, Rouvinski A, Barba-Spaeth G, Duangchinda T, et al. Dengue virus sero-cross-reactivity drives antibody-dependent enhancement of infection with zika virus. *Nat Immunol.* (2016) 17:1102–8. doi: 10.1038/ni.3515
39. Halstead SB, Rojanasuphot S, Sangkawibha N. Origin0061l antigenic sin in dengue. *Am J Trop Med Hyg.* (1983) 32:154–6. doi: 10.4269/ajtmh.1983.32.154
40. Robbiani DF, Olsen PC, Costa F, Wang Q, Oliveira TY, Nery N Jr. et al. Risk of Zika microcephaly correlates with features of maternal antibodies. *J Exp Med.* (2019) 216:2302–15. doi: 10.1084/jem.20191061
41. Kurane I, Innis BL, Nisalak A, Hoke C, Nimmannitya S, Meager A, et al. Human T cell responses to dengue virus antigens. Proliferative responses and interferon gamma production. *J Clin Invest.* (1989) 83:506–13. doi: 10.1172/JCI113911
42. Kurane I, Meager A, Ennis FA. Dengue virus-specific human T cell clones. Serotype crossreactive proliferation, interferon gamma production, and cytotoxic activity. *J Exp Med.* (1989) 170:763–75. doi: 10.1084/jem.170.3.763
43. Bukowski JF, Kurane I, Lai CJ, Bray M, Falgout B, Ennis FA. Dengue virus-specific cross-reactive CD8+ human cytotoxic T lymphocytes. *J Virol.* (1989) 63:5086–91. doi: 10.1128/JVI.63.12.5086-5091.1989
44. Shrestha B, Diamond MS. Role of CD8+ T cells in control of West Nile virus infection. *J Virol.* (2004) 78:8312–21. doi: 10.1128/JVI.78.15.8312-8321.2004
45. St John AL, Rathore APS. Adaptive immune responses to primary and secondary dengue virus infections. *Nat Rev Immunol.* (2019) 19:218–30. doi: 10.1038/s41577-019-0123-x
46. Elong Ngono A, Vizcarra EA, Tang WW, Sheets N, Joo Y, Kim K, et al. Mapping and role of the CD8(+) T cell response during primary zika virus infection in mice. *Cell Host Microbe.* (2017) 21:35–46. doi: 10.1016/j.chom.2016.12.010
47. Zivny J, Kurane I, Leporati AM, Ibe M, Takiguchi M, Zeng LL, et al. A single nine-amino acid peptide induces virus-specific, CD8+ human cytotoxic T lymphocyte clones of heterogeneous serotype specificities. *J Exp Med.* (1995) 182:853–63. doi: 10.1084/jem.182.3.853
48. Livingston PG, Kurane I, Dai LC, Okamoto Y, Lai CJ, Men R, et al. Dengue virus-specific, HLA-B35-restricted, human CD8+ cytotoxic T lymphocyte (CTL) clones. Recognition of NS3 amino acids 500 to 508 by CTL clones of two different serotype specificities. *J Immunol.* (1995) 154:1287–95.
49. Mathew A, Kurane I, Green S, Stephens HA, Vaughn DW, Kalayanarooj S, et al. Predominance of HLA-restricted cytotoxic T-lymphocyte responses to serotype-cross-reactive epitopes on nonstructural proteins following natural secondary dengue virus infection. *J Virol.* (1998) 72:3999–4004. doi: 10.1128/JVI.72.5.3999-4004.1998
50. Friberg H, Burns L, Woda M, Kalayanarooj S, Endy TP, Stephens HA, et al. Memory CD8+ T cells from naturally acquired primary dengue virus infection are highly cross-reactive. *Immunol Cell Biol.* (2011) 89:122–9. doi: 10.1038/icb.2010.61
51. Mongkolsapaya J, Dejnirattisai W, Xu XN, Vasanawathana S, Tangthawornchaikul N, Chairunsri A, et al. Original antigenic sin and apoptosis in the pathogenesis of dengue hemorrhagic fever. *Nat Med.* (2003) 9:921–7. doi: 10.1038/nm887
52. Dong T, Moran E, Vinh Chau N, Simmons C, Luhn K, Peng Y, et al. High pro-inflammatory cytokine secretion and loss of high avidity cross-reactive cytotoxic T-cells during the course of secondary dengue virus infection. *PLoS ONE.* (2007) 2:e1192. doi: 10.1371/journal.pone.0001192
53. Imrie A, Meeks J, Gurary A, Sukhbataar M, Kitsutani P, Effler P, et al. Differential functional avidity of dengue virus-specific T-cell clones for variant peptides representing heterologous and previously encountered serotypes. *J Virol.* (2007) 81:10081–91. doi: 10.1128/JVI.00330-07
54. Grifoni A, Pham J, Sidney J, O'Rourke PH, Paul S, Peters B, et al. Prior Dengue virus exposure shapes T cell immunity to Zika virus in humans. *J Virol.* (2017)91:e01469–17. doi: 10.1128/JVI.01469-17
55. Weiskopf D, Cerpas C, Angelo MA, Bangs DJ, Sidney J, Paul S, et al. Human CD8+ T-cell responses against the 4 dengue virus serotypes are associated with distinct patterns of protein targets. *J Infect Dis.* (2015) 212:1743–51. doi: 10.1093/infdis/jiv289
56. Weiskopf D, Angelo MA, Bangs DJ, Sidney J, Paul S, Peters B, et al. The human CD8+ T cell responses induced by a live attenuated tetravalent dengue vaccine are directed against highly conserved epitopes. *J Virol.* (2015) 89:120–8. doi: 10.1128/JVI.02129-14
57. Delgado FG, Torres KI, Castellanos JE, Romero-Sanchez C, Simon-Loriere E, Sakuntabhai A, et al. Improved immune responses against zika virus after sequential dengue and zika virus infection in humans. *Viruses.* (2018) 10:E480. doi: 10.3390/v10090480
58. Zivny J, DeFronzo M, Jarry W, Jameson J, Cruz J, Ennis FA, et al. Partial agonist effect influences the CTL response to a heterologous dengue virus serotype. *J Immunol.* (1999) 163:2754–60.
59. Appanna R, Huat TL, See LL, Tan PL, Vadivelu J, Devi S. Cross-reactive T-cell responses to the nonstructural regions of dengue viruses among dengue fever and dengue hemorrhagic fever patients in Malaysia. *Clin Vaccine Immunol.* (2007) 14:969–77. doi: 10.1128/CVI.00069-07
60. Duangchinda T, Dejnirattisai W, Vasanawathana S, Limpitikul W, Tangthawornchaikul N, Malasit P, et al. Immunodominant T-cell responses to dengue virus NS3 are associated with DHF. *Proc Natl Acad Sci USA.* (2010) 107:16922–7. doi: 10.1073/pnas.1010867107
61. Betts MR, Brenchley JM, Price DA, De Rosa SC, Douek DC, Roederer M, et al. Sensitive and viable identification of antigen-specific CD8+ T cells by a flow cytometric assay for degranulation. *J Immunol Methods.* (2003) 281:65–78. doi: 10.1016/S0022-1759(03)00265-5
62. Mongkolsapaya J, Duangchinda T, Dejnirattisai W, Vasanawathana S, Avirutnan P, Jairungsri A, et al. T cell responses in dengue hemorrhagic fever: are cross-reactive T cells suboptimal? *J Immunol.* (2006) 176:3821–9. doi: 10.4049/jimmunol.176.6.3821

63. Dung NT, Duyen HT, Thuy NT, Ngoc TV, Chau NV, Hien TT, et al. Timing of CD8+ T cell responses in relation to commencement of capillary leakage in children with dengue. *J Immunol.* (2010) 184:7281–7. doi: 10.4049/jimmunol.0903262
64. Simmons CP, Dong T, Chau NV, Dung NT, Chau TN, Thao le TT, et al. Early T-cell responses to dengue virus epitopes in vietnamese adults with secondary dengue virus infections. *J Virol.* (2005) 79:5665–75. doi: 10.1128/JVI.79.9.5665-5675.2005
65. Wijeratne DT, Fernando S, Gomes L, Jeewandara C, Ginneliya A, Samarasekara S, et al. Quantification of dengue virus specific T cell responses and correlation with viral load and clinical disease severity in acute dengue infection. *PLoS Negl Trop Dis.* (2018) 12:e0006540. doi: 10.1371/journal.pntd.0006540
66. Hatch S, Endy TP, Thomas S, Mathew A, Potts J, Pazoles P, et al. Intracellular cytokine production by dengue virus-specific T cells correlates with subclinical secondary infection. *J Infect Dis.* (2011) 203:1282–91. doi: 10.1093/infdis/jir012
67. Loke H, Bethell DB, Phuong CX, Dung M, Schneider J, White NJ, et al. Strong HLA class I–restricted T cell responses in dengue hemorrhagic fever: a double-edged sword? *J Infect Dis.* (2001) 184:1369–73. doi: 10.1086/324320
68. Screaton G, Mongkolsapaya J, Yacoub S, Roberts C. New insights into the immunopathology and control of dengue virus infection. *Nat Rev Immunol.* (2015) 15:745–59. doi: 10.1038/nri3916
69. Herrera BB, Tsai WY, Chang CA, Hamel DJ, Wang WK, Lu Y, et al. Sustained Specific and cross-reactive T cell responses to zika and dengue virus NS3 in West Africa. *J Virol.* (2018) 92:e01992–17. doi: 10.1128/JVI.01992-17
70. Lim MQ, Kumaran EAP, Tan HC, Lye DC, Leo YS, Ooi EE, et al. Cross-Reactivity and anti-viral function of dengue capsid and NS3-specific memory T cells toward zika virus. *Front Immunol.* (2018) 9:2225. doi: 10.3389/fimmu.2018.02225
71. Grifoni A, Costa-Ramos P, Pham J, Tian Y, Rosales SL, Seumois G, et al. Cutting edge: transcriptional profiling reveals multifunctional and cytotoxic antiviral responses of zika virus-specific CD8(+) T cells. *J Immunol.* (2018) 201:3487–91. doi: 10.4049/jimmunol.1801090
72. Grossman RA, Edelman R, Gould DJ. Study of Japanese encephalitis virus in Chiangmia Valley, Thailand. VI. Summary and conclusions. *Am J Epidemiol.* (1974) 100:69–76. doi: 10.1093/oxfordjournals.aje.a112010
73. Libraty DH, Nisalak A, Endy TP, Suntayakorn S, Vaughn DW, Innis BL. Clinical and immunological risk factors for severe disease in Japanese encephalitis. *Trans R Soc Trop Med Hyg.* (2002) 96:173–8. doi: 10.1016/S0035-9203(02)90294-4
74. Alves Dos Santos E, Fink K. Animal models for Dengue and Zika vaccine development. *Adv Exp Med Biol.* (2018) 1062:215–39. doi: 10.1007/978-981-10-8727-1_16
75. Weiskopf D, Yauch LE, Angelo MA, John DV, Greenbaum JA, Sidney J, et al. Insights into HLA-restricted T cell responses in a novel mouse model of dengue virus infection point toward new implications for vaccine design. *J Immunol.* (2011) 187:4268–79. doi: 10.4049/jimmunol.1101970
76. Weiskopf D, Angelo MA, Sidney J, Peters B, Shresta S, Sette A. Immunodominance changes as a function of the infecting dengue virus serotype and primary versus secondary infection. *J Virol.* (2014) 88:11383–94. doi: 10.1128/JVI.01108-14
77. Yauch LE, Zellweger RM, Kotturi MF, Qutubuddin A, Sidney J, Peters B, et al. A protective role for dengue virus-specific CD8+ T cells. *J Immunol.* (2009) 182:4865–73. doi: 10.4049/jimmunol.0801974
78. An J, Zhou DS, Zhang JL, Morida H, Wang JL, Yasui K. Dengue-specific CD8+ T cells have both protective and pathogenic roles in dengue virus infection. *Immunol Lett.* (2004) 95:167–74. doi: 10.1016/j.imlet.2004.07.006
79. Amorim JH, dos Santos Alves RP, Bizerra R, Araujo Pereira S, Ramos Pereira L, Nascimento Fabris DL, et al. Antibodies are not required to a protective immune response against dengue virus elicited in a mouse encephalitis model. *Virology.* (2016) 487:41–9. doi: 10.1016/j.virol.2015.10.006
80. Yauch LE, Prestwood TR, May MM, Morar MM, Zellweger RM, Peters B, et al. CD4+ T cells are not required for the induction of dengue virus-specific CD8+ T cell or antibody responses but contribute to protection after vaccination. *J Immunol.* (2010) 185:5405–16. doi: 10.4049/jimmunol.1001709
81. Zellweger RM, Tang WW, Eddy WE, King K, Sanchez MC, Shresta S. CD8+ T cells can mediate short-term protection against heterotypic dengue virus reinfection in mice. *J Virol.* (2015) 89:6494–505. doi: 10.1128/JVI.00036-15
82. Zompi S, Santich BH, Beatty PR, Harris E. Protection from secondary dengue virus infection in a mouse model reveals the role of serotype cross-reactive B and T cells. *J Immunol.* (2012) 188:404–16. doi: 10.4049/jimmunol.1102124
83. Talarico LB, Batalle JP, Byrne AB, Brahamian JM, Ferretti A, Garcia AG, et al. The role of heterotypic DENV-specific CD8(+)T lymphocytes in an immunocompetent mouse model of secondary dengue virus infection. *EBioMedicine.* (2017) 20:202–16. doi: 10.1016/j.ebiom.2017.04.033
84. Roth C, Delgado FG, Simon-Loriere E, Sakuntabhai A. Immune responses to dengue and zika viruses-guidance for T cell vaccine development. *Int J Environ Res Public Health.* (2018) 15:E385. doi: 10.3390/ijerph15020385
85. Huang H, Li S, Zhang Y, Han X, Jia B, Liu H, et al. CD8(+) T cell immune response in immunocompetent mice during zika virus infection. *J Virol.* (2017) 91:e00900–17. doi: 10.1128/JVI.00900-17
86. Hassert M, Brien JD, Pinto AK. Mouse models of heterologous flavivirus immunity: a role for cross-reactive T cells. *Front Immunol.* (2019) 10:1045. doi: 10.3389/fimmu.2019.01045
87. Jurado KA, Yockey LJ, Wong PW, Lee S, Huttner AJ, Iwasaki A. Antiviral CD8 T cells induce Zika-virus-associated paralysis in mice. *Nat Microbiol.* (2018) 3:141–7. doi: 10.1038/s41564-017-0060-z
88. Manangeeswaran M, Ireland DD, Verthelyi D. Zika (PRVABC59) infection is associated with T cell infiltration and neurodegeneration in CNS of immunocompetent neonatal C57Bl/6 mice. *PLoS Pathog.* (2016) 12:e1006004. doi: 10.1371/journal.ppat.1006004
89. Hayashida E, Ling ZL, Ashhurst TM, Viengkhou B, Jung SR, Songkhunawej P, et al. Zika virus encephalitis in immunocompetent mice is dominated by innate immune cells and does not require T or B cells. *J Neuroinflammation.* (2019) 16:177. doi: 10.1186/s12974-019-1566-5
90. Regla-Nava JA, Elong Ngono A, Viramontes KM, Huynh AT, Wang YT, Nguyen AT, et al. cross-reactive dengue virus-specific CD8(+) T cells protect against Zika virus during pregnancy. *Nat Commun.* (2018) 9:3042. doi: 10.1038/s41467-018-05458-0
91. Larena M, Regner M, Lee E, Lobigs M. Pivotal role of antibody and subsidiary contribution of CD8+ T cells to recovery from infection in a murine model of Japanese encephalitis. *J Virol.* (2011) 85:5446–55. doi: 10.1128/JVI.02611-10
92. Wen J, Elong Ngono A, Regla-Nava JA, Kim K, Gorman MJ, Diamond MS, et al. Dengue virus-reactive CD8(+) T cells mediate cross-protection against subsequent Zika virus challenge. *Nat Commun.* (2017) 8:1459. doi: 10.1038/s41467-017-01669-z
93. Wen J, Tang WW, Sheets N, Ellison J, Sette A, Kim K, et al. Identification of Zika virus epitopes reveals immunodominant and protective roles for dengue virus cross-reactive CD8(+) T cells. *Nat Microbiol.* (2017) 2:17036. doi: 10.1038/nmicrobiol.2017.36
94. Pantoja P, Perez-Guzman EX, Rodriguez IV, White LJ, Gonzalez O, Serrano C, et al. Zika virus pathogenesis in rhesus macaques is unaffected by pre-existing immunity to dengue virus. *Nat Commun.* (2017) 8:15674. doi: 10.1038/ncomms15674
95. Perez-Guzman EX, Pantoja P, Serrano-Collazo C, Hassert MA, Ortiz-Rosa A, Rodriguez IV, et al. Time elapsed between Zika and dengue virus infections affects antibody and T cell responses. *Nat Commun.* (2019) 10:4316. doi: 10.1038/s41467-019-12295-2
96. Prompetchara E, Ketloy C, Thomas SJ, Ruxrungtham K. Dengue vaccine: global development update. *Asian Pac J Allergy Immunol.* (2019). doi: 10.12932/AP-100518-0309. [Epub ahead of print].
97. Capeding MR, Tran NH, Hadinegoro SR, Ismail HI, Chotpitayasunondh T, Chua MN, et al. Clinical efficacy and safety of a novel tetravalent dengue vaccine in healthy children in Asia: a phase 3, randomised, observer-masked, placebo-controlled trial. *Lancet.* (2014) 384:1358–65. doi: 10.1016/S0140-6736(14)61060-6
98. Villar L, Dayan GH, Arredondo-Garcia JL, Rivera DM, Cunha R, Deseda C, et al. Efficacy of a tetravalent dengue vaccine in children in Latin America. *N Engl J Med.* (2015) 372:113–23. doi: 10.1056/NEJMoa1411037

99. Sabchareon A, Wallace D, Sirivichayakul C, Limkittikul K, Chanthavanich P, Suvannadabba S, et al. Protective efficacy of the recombinant, live-attenuated, CYD tetravalent dengue vaccine in Thai schoolchildren: a randomised, controlled phase 2b trial. *Lancet.* (2012) 380:1559–67. doi: 10.1016/S0140-6736(12)61428-7
100. Hadinegoro SR, Arredondo-Garcia JL, Capeding MR, Deseda C, Chotpitayasunondh T, Dietze R, et al. Efficacy and long-term safety of a dengue vaccine in regions of endemic disease. *N Engl J Med.* (2015) 373:1195–206. doi: 10.1056/NEJMoa1506223
101. Sridhar S, Luedtke A, Langevin E, Zhu M, Bonaparte M, Machabert T, et al. Effect of dengue serostatus on dengue vaccine safety and efficacy. *N Engl J Med.* (2018) 379:327–40. doi: 10.1056/NEJMoa1800820
102. Halstead SB. Which dengue vaccine approach is the most promising, and should we be concerned about enhanced disease after vaccination? there is only one true winner. *Cold Spring Harb Perspect Biol.* (2018) 10:a030700. doi: 10.1101/cshperspect.a030700
103. Osorio JE, Wallace D, Stinchcomb DT. A recombinant, chimeric tetravalent dengue vaccine candidate based on a dengue virus serotype 2 backbone. *Expert Rev Vaccines.* (2016) 15:497–508. doi: 10.1586/14760584.2016.1128328
104. Saez-Llorens X, Tricou V, Yu D, Rivera L, Jimeno J, Villarreal AC, et al. Immunogenicity and safety of one versus two doses of tetravalent dengue vaccine in healthy children aged 2-17 years in Asia and Latin America: 18-month interim data from a phase 2, randomised, placebo-controlled study. *Lancet Infect Dis.* (2018) 18:162–70. doi: 10.1016/S1473-3099(17)30632-1
105. Chu H, George SL, Stinchcomb DT, Osorio JE, Partidos CD. CD8+ T-cell responses in flavivirus-naive individuals following immunization with a live-attenuated tetravalent dengue vaccine candidate. *J Infect Dis.* (2015) 212:1618–28. doi: 10.1093/infdis/jiv258
106. Biswal S, Reynales H, Saez-Llorens X, Lopez P, Borja-Tabora C, Kosalaraksa P, et al. Efficacy of a tetravalent dengue vaccine in healthy children and adolescents. *N Engl J Med.* (2019) 381:2009–19. doi: 10.1056/NEJMoa1903869
107. Whitehead SS, Durbin AP, Pierce KK, Elwood D, McElvany BD, Fraser EA, et al. In a randomized trial, the live attenuated tetravalent dengue vaccine TV003 is well-tolerated and highly immunogenic in subjects with flavivirus exposure prior to vaccination. *PLoS Negl Trop Dis.* (2017) 11:e0005584. doi: 10.1371/journal.pntd.0005584
108. Kirkpatrick BD, Whitehead SS, Pierce KK, Tibery CM, Grier PL, Hynes NA, et al. The live attenuated dengue vaccine TV003 elicits complete protection against dengue in a human challenge model. *Sci Transl Med.* (2016) 8:330ra36. doi: 10.1126/scitranslmed.aaf1517
109. Lin HH, Yip BS, Huang LM, Wu SC. Zika virus structural biology and progress in vaccine development. *Biotechnol Adv.* (2018) 36:47–53. doi: 10.1016/j.biotechadv.2017.09.004
110. Dowd KA, Ko SY, Morabito KM, Yang ES, Pelc RS, DeMaso CR, et al. Rapid development of a DNA vaccine for Zika virus. *Science.* (2016) 354:237–40. doi: 10.1126/science.aai9137
111. Gaudinski MR, Houser KV, Morabito KM, Hu Z, Yamshchikov G, Rothwell RS, et al. Safety, tolerability, and immunogenicity of two Zika virus DNA vaccine candidates in healthy adults: randomised, open-label, phase 1 clinical trials. *Lancet.* (2018) 391:552–62. doi: 10.1016/S0140-6736(17)33105-7
112. Van Rompay KKA, Keesler RI, Ardeshir A, Watanabe J, Usachenko J, Singapuri A, et al. DNA vaccination before conception protects Zika virus-exposed pregnant macaques against prolonged viremia and improves fetal outcomes. *Sci Transl Med.* (2019) 11:eaay2736. doi: 10.1126/scitranslmed.aay2736
113. Modjarrad K, Lin L, George SL, Stephenson KE, Eckels KH, De La Barrera RA, et al. Preliminary aggregate safety and immunogenicity results from three trials of a purified inactivated Zika virus vaccine candidate: phase 1, randomised, double-blind, placebo-controlled clinical trials. *Lancet.* (2018) 391:563–71. doi: 10.1016/S0140-6736(17)33106-9
114. Dussupt V, Sankhala RS, Gromowski GD, Donofrio G, De La Barrera RA, Larocca RA, et al. Potent Zika and dengue cross-neutralizing antibodies induced by Zika vaccination in a dengue-experienced donor. *Nat Med.* (2020) 26:228–35. doi: 10.1038/s41591-019-0746-2
115. Garg H, Mehmetoglu-Gurbuz T, Joshi A. Recent advances in Zika virus vaccines. *Viruses.* (2018) 10:e631. doi: 10.3390/v10110631
116. Nurnberger C, Bodmer BS, Fiedler AH, Gabriel G, Muhlebach MD. A measles virus-based vaccine candidate mediates protection against zika virus in an allogeneic mouse pregnancy model. *J Virol.* (2019) 93:e01485-18. doi: 10.1128/JVI.01485-18
117. Cox F, van der Fits L, Abbink P, Larocca RA, van Huizen E, Saeland E, et al. Adenoviral vector type 26 encoding Zika virus (ZIKV) M-Env antigen induces humoral and cellular immune responses and protects mice and nonhuman primates against ZIKV challenge. *PLoS ONE.* (2018) 13:e0202820. doi: 10.1371/journal.pone.0202820
118. Larocca RA, Mendes EA, Abbink P, Peterson RL, Martinot AJ, Iampietro MJ, et al. Adenovirus vector-based vaccines confer maternal-fetal protection against Zika virus challenge in pregnant IFN-alphabetaR(-/-) mice. *Cell Host Microbe.* (2019) 26:591–600 e4. doi: 10.1016/j.chom.2019.10.001
119. Grubor-Bauk B, Wijesundara DK, Masavuli M, Abbink P, Peterson RL, Prow NA, et al. NS1 DNA vaccination protects against Zika infection through T cell-mediated immunity in immunocompetent mice. *Sci Adv.* (2019) 5:eaax2388. doi: 10.1126/sciadv.aax2388
120. Osorio JE, Brewoo JN, Silengo SJ, Arguello J, Moldovan IR, Tary-Lehmann M, et al. Efficacy of a tetravalent chimeric dengue vaccine (DENVax) in Cynomolgus macaques. *Am J Trop Med Hyg.* (2011) 84:978–87. doi: 10.4269/ajtmh.2011.10-0592
121. Sumathy K, Kulkarni B, Gondu RK, Ponnuru SK, Bonguram N, Eligeti R, et al. Protective efficacy of Zika vaccine in AG129 mouse model. *Sci Rep.* (2017) 7:46375. doi: 10.1038/srep46375
122. Shan C, Muruato AE, Nunes BTD, Luo H, Xie X, Medeiros DBA, et al. A live-attenuated Zika virus vaccine candidate induces sterilizing immunity in mouse models. *Nat Med.* (2017) 23:763–7. doi: 10.1038/nm.4322
123. Wang R, Liao X, Fan D, Wang L, Song J, Feng K, et al. Maternal immunization with a DNA vaccine candidate elicits specific passive protection against post-natal Zika virus infection in immunocompetent BALB/c mice. *Vaccine.* (2018) 36:3522–32. doi: 10.1016/j.vaccine.2018.04.051
124. Wang R, Gao N, Li Y, Fan D, Zhen Z, Feng K, et al. Cross-protection against four serotypes of dengue virus in mice conferred by a Zika DNA vaccine. *Front Cell Infect Microbiol.* (2019) 9:147. doi: 10.3389/fcimb.2019.00147
125. Griffin BD, Muthumani K, Warner BM, Majer A, Hagan M, Audet J, et al. DNA vaccination protects mice against Zika virus-induced damage to the testes. *Nat Commun.* (2017) 8:15743. doi: 10.1038/ncomms15743
126. Li A, Yu J, Lu M, Ma Y, Attia Z, Shan C, et al. A Zika virus vaccine expressing premembrane-envelope-NS1 polyprotein. *Nat Commun.* (2018) 9:3067. doi: 10.1038/s41467-018-05276-4
127. Brault AC, Domi A, McDonald EM, Talmi-Frank D, McCurley N, Basu R, et al. A Zika vaccine targeting NS1 protein protects immunocompetent adult mice in a lethal challenge model. *Sci Rep.* (2017) 7:14769. doi: 10.1038/s41598-017-15039-8
128. Sariol CA, White LJ. Utility, limitations, and future of non-human primates for dengue research and vaccine development. *Front Immunol.* (2014) 5:452. doi: 10.3389/fimmu.2014.00452
129. Ambuel Y, Young G, Brewoo JN, Paykel J, Weisgrau KL, Rakasz EG, et al. A rapid immunization strategy with a live-attenuated tetravalent dengue vaccine elicits protective neutralizing antibody responses in non-human primates. *Front Immunol.* (2014) 5:263. doi: 10.3389/fimmu.2014.00263
130. Sims S, Willberg C, Klenerman P. MHC-peptide tetramers for the analysis of antigen-specific T cells. *Expert Rev Vaccines.* (2010) 9:765–74. doi: 10.1586/erv.10.66
131. Kanthaswamy S, Ng J, Satkoski Trask J, George DA, Kou AJ, Hoffman LN, et al. The genetic composition of populations of cynomolgus macaques (Macaca fascicularis) used in biomedical research. *J Med Primatol.* (2013) 42:120–31. doi: 10.1111/jmp.12043
132. Osuna CE, Whitney JB. Nonhuman Primate Models of Zika Virus Infection, Immunity, and Therapeutic Development. *J Infect Dis.* (2017) 216:S928–34. doi: 10.1093/infdis/jix540
133. Dudley DM, Aliota MT, Mohr EL, Weiler AM, Lehrer-Brey G, Weisgrau KL, et al. A rhesus macaque model of Asian-lineage Zika virus infection. *Nat Commun.* (2016) 7:12204. doi: 10.1038/ncomms12204
134. Abbink P, Larocca RA, De La Barrera RA, Bricault CA, Moseley ET, Boyd M, et al. Protective efficacy of multiple vaccine platforms against Zika virus challenge in rhesus monkeys. *Science.* (2016) 353:1129–32. doi: 10.1126/science.aah6157

135. Muthumani K, Griffin BD, Agarwal S, Kudchodkar SB, Reuschel EL, Choi H, et al. *In vivo* protection against ZIKV infection and pathogenesis through passive antibody transfer and active immunisation with a prMEnv DNA vaccine. *NPJ Vaccines*. (2016) 1:16021. doi: 10.1038/npjvaccines.2016.21
136. Brewoo JN, Kinney RM, Powell TD, Arguello JJ, Silengo SJ, Partidos CD, et al. Immunogenicity and efficacy of chimeric dengue vaccine (DENVax) formulations in interferon-deficient AG129 mice. *Vaccine*. (2012) 30:1513–20. doi: 10.1016/j.vaccine.2011.11.072
137. Zust R, Dong H, Li XF, Chang DC, Zhang B, Balakrishnan T, et al. Rational design of a live attenuated dengue vaccine: 2'-o-methyltransferase mutants are highly attenuated and immunogenic in mice and macaques. *PLoS Pathog*. (2013) 9:e1003521. doi: 10.1371/journal.ppat.1003521
138. Zellweger RM, Shresta S. Mouse models to study dengue virus immunology and pathogenesis. *Front Immunol*. (2014) 5:151. doi: 10.3389/fimmu.2014.00151
139. Bente DA, Melkus MW, Garcia JV, Rico-Hesse R. Dengue fever in humanized NOD/SCID mice. *J Virol*. (2005) 79:13797–9. doi: 10.1128/JVI.79.21.13797-13799.2005
140. Becker R. Missing link: animal models to study whether Zika causes birth defects. *Nat Med*. (2016) 22:225–7. doi: 10.1038/nm0316-225

Permissions

All chapters in this book were first published by Frontiers; hereby published with permission under the Creative Commons Attribution License or equivalent. Every chapter published in this book has been scrutinized by our experts. Their significance has been extensively debated. The topics covered herein carry significant findings which will fuel the growth of the discipline. They may even be implemented as practical applications or may be referred to as a beginning point for another development.

The contributors of this book come from diverse backgrounds, making this book a truly international effort. This book will bring forth new frontiers with its revolutionizing research information and detailed analysis of the nascent developments around the world.

We would like to thank all the contributing authors for lending their expertise to make the book truly unique. They have played a crucial role in the development of this book. Without their invaluable contributions this book wouldn't have been possible. They have made vital efforts to compile up to date information on the varied aspects of this subject to make this book a valuable addition to the collection of many professionals and students.

This book was conceptualized with the vision of imparting up-to-date information and advanced data in this field. To ensure the same, a matchless editorial board was set up. Every individual on the board went through rigorous rounds of assessment to prove their worth. After which they invested a large part of their time researching and compiling the most relevant data for our readers.

The editorial board has been involved in producing this book since its inception. They have spent rigorous hours researching and exploring the diverse topics which have resulted in the successful publishing of this book. They have passed on their knowledge of decades through this book. To expedite this challenging task, the publisher supported the team at every step. A small team of assistant editors was also appointed to further simplify the editing procedure and attain best results for the readers.

Apart from the editorial board, the designing team has also invested a significant amount of their time in understanding the subject and creating the most relevant covers. They scrutinized every image to scout for the most suitable representation of the subject and create an appropriate cover for the book.

The publishing team has been an ardent support to the editorial, designing and production team. Their endless efforts to recruit the best for this project, has resulted in the accomplishment of this book. They are a veteran in the field of academics and their pool of knowledge is as vast as their experience in printing. Their expertise and guidance has proved useful at every step. Their uncompromising quality standards have made this book an exceptional effort. Their encouragement from time to time has been an inspiration for everyone.

The publisher and the editorial board hope that this book will prove to be a valuable piece of knowledge for researchers, students, practitioners and scholars across the globe.

List of Contributors

Sophia Davidson
Inflammation Division, The Walter and Eliza Hall Institute of Medical Research, Parkville, VIC, Australia

Tsz-Fung Yip, Aisha Sami Mohammed Selim and Suki Man-Yan Lee
HKU-Pasteur Research Pole, School of Public Health, The University of Hong Kong, Hong Kong

Ida Lian
School of Life Sciences and Chemical Technology, Ngee Ann Polytechnic, Singapore

Mathilde Laureti, Divya Narayanan, Julio Rodriguez-Andres, John K. Fazakerley and Lukasz Kedzierski
Department of Microbiology and Immunology, Peter Doherty Institute for Infection and Immunity, University of Melbourne, Melbourne, VIC, Australia
Faculty of Veterinary and Agricultural Sciences, University of Melbourne, Melbourne, VIC, Australia

Kim Blom, Angelica Cuapio, J. Tyler Sandberg, Renata Varnaite, Jakob Michaëlsson, Niklas K. Björkström, Johan K. Sandberg, Jonas Klingström and Hans-Gustaf Ljunggren
Department of Medicine Huddinge, Center for Infectious Medicine, Karolinska Institutet, Karolinska University Hospital, Stockholm, Sweden

Lars Lindquist
Department of Infectious Diseases, Karolinska University Hospital, Stockholm, Sweden
Unit of Infectious Diseases, Department of Medicine Huddinge, Karolinska Institutet, Karolinska University Hospital, Stockholm, Sweden

Sara Gredmark Russ
Department of Medicine Huddinge, Center for Infectious Medicine, Karolinska Institutet, Karolinska University Hospital, Stockholm, Sweden
Department of Infectious Diseases, Karolinska University Hospital, Stockholm, Sweden

Sophie A. Valkenburg, Maireid B. Bull and Athena P. Y. Li
HKU Pasteur Research Pole, The University of Hong Kong, Pokfulam, Hong Kong
WHO Collaborating Centre for Infectious Disease Epidemiology and Control, School of Public Health, The University of Hong Kong, Pokfulam, Hong Kong

Nancy H. L. Leung, Li-meng Yan, Leo L. M. Poon and Benjamin J. Cowling
WHO Collaborating Centre for Infectious Disease Epidemiology and Control, School of Public Health, The University of Hong Kong, Pokfulam, Hong Kong

Hui Yee Yong
Lee Kong Chian School of Medicine, Nanyang Technological University, Singapore, Singapore
NTU Institute of Structural Biology, Nanyang Technological University, Singapore
School of Biological Sciences, Nanyang Technological University, Singapore

Dahai Luo
Lee Kong Chian School of Medicine, Nanyang Technological University, Singapore, Singapore
NTU Institute of Structural Biology, Nanyang Technological University, Singapore

Kuldeep Dhama and Rajendra Singh
Division of Pathology, ICAR-Indian Veterinary Research Institute, Bareilly, India

Kumaragurubaran Karthik
Central University Laboratory, Tamil Nadu Veterinary and Animal Sciences University, Chennai, India

Rekha Khandia and Ashok Munjal
Department of Biochemistry and Genetics, Barkatullah University, Bhopal, India

Sandip Chakraborty
Department of Veterinary Microbiology, College of Veterinary Sciences and Animal Husbandry, Agartala, India

Shyma K. Latheef
Immunology Section, ICAR-Indian Veterinary Research Institute, Bareilly, India

Deepak Kumar
Division of Veterinary Biotechnology, ICAR-Indian Veterinary Research Institute, Bareilly, India

Muthannan Andavar Ramakrishnan
Division of Virology, ICAR-Indian Veterinary Research Institute, Nainital, Uttarakhand, India

Yashpal Singh Malik
Division of Biological Standardization, ICAR-Indian Veterinary Research Institute, Bareilly, India

Satya Veer Singh Malik
Division of Veterinary Public Health, ICAR-Indian Veterinary Research Institute, Bareilly, India

Raj Kumar Singh
ICAR-Indian Veterinary Research Institute, Bareilly, Uttar Pradesh, India

Wanpen Chaicumpa
Center of Research Excellence on Therapeutic Proteins and Antibody Engineering, Department of Parasitology, Faculty of Medicine SIriraj Hospital, Mahidol University, Bangkok, Thailand

Tomas Strandin and Antti Vaheri
Department of Virology, Medicum, Faculty of Medicine, University of Helsinki, Helsinki, Finland

Satu Mäkelä and Jukka Mustonen
Department of Internal Medicine, Faculty of Medicine and Life Sciences, Tampere University Hospital, University of Tampere, Tampere, Finland

Joseph Prescott, Darryl Falzarano, Emmie de Wit, Elaine Haddock, Heinz Feldmann and Vincent Jacobus Munster
Laboratory of Virology, Division of Intramural Research, Rocky Mountain Laboratories, National Institute of Allergy and Infectious Diseases, National Institutes of Health, Hamilton, MT, United States

Kath Hardcastle, Friederike Feldmann and Dana Scott
Rocky Mountain Veterinary Branch, Division of Intramural Research, Rocky Mountain Laboratories, National Institute of Allergy and Infectious Diseases, National Institutes of Health, Hamilton, MT, United States

William S. J. Horman
Department of Microbiology and Immunology, University of Melbourne at the Peter Doherty Institute for Infection and Immunity, Parkville, VIC, Australia
Australian Animal Health Laboratory, Health and Biosecurity, Commonwealth Scientific and Industrial Research Organisation (CSIRO), East Geelong, VIC, Australia

Thi H. O. Nguyen and Katherine Kedzierska
Department of Microbiology and Immunology, University of Melbourne at the Peter Doherty Institute for Infection and Immunity, Parkville, VIC, Australia

Andrew G. D. Bean and Daniel S. Layton
Australian Animal Health Laboratory, Health and Biosecurity, Commonwealth Scientific and Industrial Research Organisation (CSIRO), East Geelong, VIC, Australia

Thi Hiep Nguyen, Xiaoming Liu, Paul S. Foster and Ming Yang
Priority Research Centre for Healthy Lungs, The University of Newcastle, Callaghan, NSW, Australia
Faculty of Health and Medicine, School of Biomedical Sciences and Pharmacy, The University of Newcastle, Callaghan, NSW, Australia

Zhen Zhong Su
Department of Respiratory Medicine, The Second Hospital, Jilin University, ChangChun, China

Alan Chen-Yu Hsu
Priority Research Centre for Healthy Lungs, The University of Newcastle, Callaghan, NSW, Australia
Faculty of Health and Medicine, School of Medicine and Public Health, The University of Newcastle, Callaghan, NSW, Australia
Viruses, Infections/Immunity, Vaccines & Asthma, Hunter Medical Research Institute, Newcastle, NSW, Australia

Leo Yi Yang Lee, Leonard Izzard and Aeron C. Hurt
World Health Organisation Collaborating Centre for Reference and Research on Influenza at the Peter Doherty Institute, Melbourne, VIC, Australia

Veera Westenius, Sanna M. Mäkelä and Pamela Österlund
Expert Microbiology Unit, Department of Health Security, National Institute for Health and Welfare, Helsinki, Finland

Ilkka Julkunen
Institute of Biomedicine, University of Turku, Turku, Finland

Dan Dou, Rebecca Revol, Henrik Östbye, Hao Wang and Robert Daniels
Department of Biochemistry and Biophysics, Stockholm University, Stockholm, Sweden

Alba Grifoni and Daniela Weiskopf
Division of Vaccine Discovery, La Jolla Institute for Immunology, La Jolla, CA, United States

Sindhu Vangeti, Meng Yu and Anna Smed-Sörensen
Division of Immunology and Allergy, Department of Medicine Solna, Karolinska Institutet, Karolinska University Hospital Solna, Stockholm, Sweden

Krishanthi S. Subramaniam, Suzannah Lant and Lynsey Goodwin
NIHR Health Protection Research Unit in Emerging and Zoonotic Infections, Centre for Global Vaccine Research, Institute of Infection and Global Health, University of Liverpool, Liverpool, United Kingdom

Lance Turtle
NIHR Health Protection Research Unit in Emerging and Zoonotic Infections, Centre for Global Vaccine Research, Institute of Infection and Global Health, University of Liverpool, Liverpool, United Kingdom
Tropical and Infectious Disease Unit, Liverpool University Hospitals, Liverpool, United Kingdom

Index